NURSING
JURISPRUDENCE

NURSING JURISPRUDENCE

Mary (Maureen) Cushing, R.N., J.D.

Mooney, Mahoney & Cushing
Boston, Massachusetts

APPLETON & LANGE
Norwalk, Connecticut/San Mateo, California

0-8385-7039-9

Copyright © 1988 by Appleton & Lange *1-203-838- 4400*
A Publishing Division of Prentice Hall

88 89 90 91 92 / 10 9 8 7 6 5 4 3 2 1

Prentice-Hall of Australia, Pty. Ltd., Sydney
Prentice-Hall Canada, Inc.
Prentice-Hall Hispanoamericana, S.A., Mexico
Prentice-Hall of India Private Limited, New Delhi
Prentice-Hall International (UK) Limited, London
Prentice-Hall of Japan, Inc., Tokyo
Prentice-Hall of Southeast Asia (Pte.) Ltd., Singapore
Whitehall Books Ltd., Wellington, New Zealand
Editora Prentice-Hall do Brasil Ltda., Rio de Janeiro

Library of Congress Cataloging-in-Publication Data

Cushing, Maureen.
    Nursing jurisprudence.

    Includes bibliographies and index.
    1. Nurses—Malpractice—United States. 2. Nursing—
Law and legislation—United States. 3. Medical
jurisprudence—United States. I. Title. [DNLM:
1. Ethics, Nursing—United States. 2. Jurisprudence—
United States. 3. Nursing—United States.
WY 33 AA1 C93n]
KF2915.N83C87   1988   346.7303'3   87-27097
ISBN 0-8385-7039-9   347.30633

Production Editor: Karen W. Davis
Designer: Kathleen Peters Ceconi

PRINTED IN THE UNITED STATES OF AMERICA

*To my parents, John and Delia Cushing
who first taught me the value of high standards.*

CONTENTS

PREFACE

I began writing this book under the premise that nurses are more enlightened with respect to knowing the function of the courts and the significance of malpractice case law than they were a few years ago. This is due in part to the tremendous number of legal articles in professional journals, nursing law lectures, and changes in curriculum design dealing with legal principles impacting upon current nursing practice.

In the early planning stage of the book, I decided to cover the cases in sufficient depth to show how important even seemingly minor factual differences may have on the outcome. Some cases, such as the *Fraijo* case placed in Chapter 3: Nursing Judgment, are presented in considerable depth because of their factual complexity and legal analysis. In the planning of the book, I subscribed to the belief that nurses need to listen to the language of the courts and I made a deliberate attempt to use that language, frequently by including exact quotes. Language in a legal opinion gives insight into how the court and jury viewed the facts and evidence and helps in understanding the manner in which the court analyzed the case in light of the facts.

Apart from the unusual case which creates a new theory of liability or defense, nurses have less of a need to hear more cases than a need to understand from any one case the implications for their nursing care activities. I wanted to show the process rather than cite an exhaustive list of cases. Except in a very few cases it is not the outcome of a case which provides the lesson, but how the court looked at the events and arrived at its judgment.

The facts of a case are very important, and some of the fact patterns are helpful because they provide insight into how the courts and jury view what nursing does and how it does it. I have tried to show that the facts of a case are very important in deciding the outcome. For example, the fact that a patient vomited several times while in the postanesthesia room has a direct bearing on the extent of monitoring done by the nurses after his return to the regular hospital ward. I know a trial lawyer who says, "Forget the law and argue the facts." Of course, he does not mean that the substantive law has no place in legal decisions, but that frequently the case will turn on a subtle fact which distinguishes it from other cases. Pay attention to the facts of the cases, especially the negligence cases, as they tend to be more subtle. Also, some chapters, such as Chapter 7: Care and Treatment of the Mentally Ill, require slow and deliberate reading because of their complexity. This is no more or less deliberate reading than is necessary to process a complex nursing theory or a scientific theory.

In selecting the chapters and content for the book I naturally drew from my own nursing background, and its genesis is in some compelling aspect of my own nursing or legal experience. If I had not been a teacher of nursing I would not have included a chapter on educational law. Having served on admissions and promotions committees in nursing schools the case of *Russell v. Salve Regina College*, decided in 1986—which held that a young nursing student has the right to her "day in court" and to have a jury decide whether her dismissal was warranted—is of particular interest to me.

For exactly 20 years, I practiced nursing, always in an acute care hospital setting. I taught in a diploma nursing program using a conceptual framework approach, which gave me less of a difficult time than it gave my colleagues because law school had already taught me how to think conceptually. For 9 years after finishing law school I continued to practice nursing and tried to practice law "on the side." During this time hospitals and special interest groups asked me to lecture to nurses on legal subjects and this experience exposed me to the problems associated with other than my own area of nursing expertise. It also gave me the opportunity to listen to nurses across the country tell about their practice problems.

During this time I became active in law associations, particularly those that had committees working on health law issues. I volunteered for every committee dealing with any aspect of health care. Even though I knew I did not want to practice in the health law area the exposure to specific health law issues was helpful and forced me to read the literature and case law in areas I would not ordinarily read.

The first chapter, Anatomy of a Suit, was in fact the last chapter to be written. I could not have written it when I began the book because I did not yet have enough jury trial experience to have the "feel" of the cases. What I mean by the feel of the cases is the ability to understand some of the strategy behind them. In this first chapter, I give a general overview of the process of a civil suit so that the reader better understands how the process fits into the final disposition.

The second chapter in the book was actually the first one I wrote. I felt comfortable starting the task of writing the Standard of Care because it was an old friend. Establishing the standard is one of the first concepts a young lawyer becomes skilled in developing, and besides I had been talking about this concept to so many nurses for many years at nursing law lectures. In addition, the term standard of care is familiar in nursing parlance. I never thought much about nursing standards while I was practicing nursing. They were ever present in one stage or another. They were either being created, evaluated, or revised. Nursing standards are an integral part of every nurse's activity.

The materials in the Standard of Care chapter are important for three reasons. First, the chapter sets out the importance of proving the legal elements of "duty" and violation or "breach" of the duty in malpractice cases. Second, it tells how the court and/or jury makes a determination that what the nurse did or did not do failed to measure up to what should have been done. Third, the cases tell who may or may not serve as an expert nursing witness to establish the applicable standard.

Legal cases are not decided in a vacuum; the applicable test or way to measure the alleged nursing wrong must be laid out for the jury so that it can apply the yardstick in deciding whether the allegations have merit. When I did the first draft of this Standard of Care chapter, I had to resort largely on the case law as it applied to medical cases; however, when I updated the content in the fall of 1985, I found that the courts had begun to require that nurses establish the applicable nursing standard.

The idea to include the Chapter 3: Nursing Judgment is directly traced to the debates I had with a nursing instructor colleague in the early seventies. I took great pride, as all nurses do, in my ability to reach quick and well-reasoned decisions in clinical situations. However, I was troubled about the lack of formal content in nursing curriculums to teach this essential skill. This has changed but it was not always easy to identify learning activities specifically designed to teach this skill. I was sometimes at a loss to clearly articulate that nursing judgment was not simply a matter of differing opinions. How often I heard a student say to me, "But that's just your opinion." It was and it was not. I eventually came to use the legal phrase "reasoned analysis" and became quite comfortable with that response. As an attorney, the judgment concept surfaced again in the form of the legal defense of "error in judgment." I am destined never to get away from the judgment concept, but at least I have reconciled myself to it.

Chapter 4: Safety deals with the more common injuries, such as falls, and patient identification problems as well as some of the newer malpractice concepts. Patient abandonment and the failure to teach the patient critical information, for example, are relatively new nursing liability concepts. It is too soon to tell whether these few cases represent an emerging trend or are simply factually isolated cases. They bear watching from both a plaintiff and defense perspective.

Chapter 5: Medications was for me the most intimidating to write for a number of reasons. In reading every case I was mentally transported back to the medication cart or medication closet. I felt the same degree of alertness as I felt when preparing medications. For me, administering medications required a kind of discipline or control I was not consciously aware of in carrying out other nursing activities.

There is something unsettling in the fact that the potential for error is always at your elbow. Perhaps no other type of error is critiqued more than the medication error and, perhaps, most harshly by the nurse who committed the error. I subscribed to three personal rules when giving medications: don't give it until you know enough about it and the patient's situation to give it safely; go slowly and methodically; and never allow yourself to become distracted at any phase of the procedure. Some of the medication cases will intimidate you, just as they did me, but focus on where the breakdown occurred, not the result. The cases once read become a valuable lesson if they are read from that perspective.

Chapter 6: Communication and Documentation is included because both written and verbal communication are essential to an orderly process of managing patient care and treatment and as such become important in any legal proceeding where that care is questioned. In recent years there has been considerable emphasis in the nursing literature placed upon the importance of documentation in negligence cases. The objective of this chapter is to emphasize the duty to communicate and document essential patient findings in a timely, complete, and professional manner. Special problems, such as correcting records and the effect of altered records, present sometimes insurmountable problems for the defense and are included to show a balance between the need to correct or add to a record without risking an allegation by the opposing attorney that the change was a self-serving alteration. The content on incident reports is necessarily couched in legal parlance and cannot be read with any speed because the content by its nature is complex. Save this section for a time when you are in the mood to be challenged.

We are all products of our experience and my experience as a nurse and an attorney impacted significantly on the selection of particular chapters over others which might have been included. My reasons for including Chapter 7: Care and Treatment of the Mentally Ill date back to one of my first law committees which dealt with issues of the physically and mentally disabled. Because the committee was closely following and arguing about the legal issues in the *Rogers I* case, I took an interest in its development and subsequently its precedent-setting ruling. The Rogers cases (*Rogers I* and *Rogers II*), which ultimately reached the U.S. Supreme Court, spanned over a 10-year period and illustrate the creativity, effort, and cost in defining rights.

The care and treatment of the mentally ill was a neglected area of the law until some patients through their legal advocates forced society and care giver alike to look at how things could be made better. As with every sleeping legal issue it simply took off and issues emerged which had run beneath the surface for many years. As in many areas of the law the balancing of rights of both the care giver and the patient became important.

Although there was case law involving the mentally ill prior to *Rogers I*, much of it dealt with interpretation of civil commitment laws. However, sometimes a case comes along which goes in a different direction because the liability theme is novel or unique. The California *Tarasoff* case decided in 1976 which dealt with the liability of care givers for harm to a third person was such a case. That decision set off a long line of cases in its wake. It would appear, at least for now, that the case law dealing with the care and treatment of the mentally ill has stabilized and we will see a steady stream of cases rather than the dramatic cases associated with the U.S. Supreme Court decisions.

I have included Chapter 8: Abortion because it impacts upon nurses practicing in a wide variety of settings, and it illustrates more than any other area of the law the process of refining a law and testing it in the courts again and again. The reader will note that many of the state statutes were rewritten after being stricken by the U.S. Supreme Court and made their way back to that same court in the hope that they would either survive or fail with further Constitutional scrutiny. It is expected that the abortion laws will be tested in both state and federal high courts because abortion remains a controversial legal issue.

Although there were a significant number of legal cases that dealt with Medical Treatment Issues (Chapters 9 and 10), it was not until the 1976 Quinlan decision that the everyday problems confronting patients, families, and care givers went beyond the doors of hospitals and nursing homes. In my last year of nursing practice two Massachusetts cases were decided that had dramatic impact on nursing care. The first case *Saikewicz*, decided in November 1977, resulted in many hospitals in Massachusetts coding patients unless a directive from the patient requested a "no code." A test case (*Dinnerstein*) decided in June 1978 resolved that particular problem, and terminally ill patients who arrested were not automatically coded. After that case hospitals across the country, many for the first time, developed *do not resuscitate* policies.

Quinlan, Saikewicz, and the *Eichner* cases opened the floodgate of treatment decisions and court petitions. The body of case law is extensive in this area and there are many factual distinctions in these cases. The sheer number of cases although seemingly lacking in uniform decision-making models has provided a consensus. The extensive number of cases which reflects situations facing nurses in both acute-care and long-term facilities lent itself to placing the materials in two chapters. The first treatment decisions chapter identifies the decision-making models, whereas, the following chapter deals with specific treatment problems.

The cases in Chapter 11: Impact of the Law on Nursing Practice deal with issues surrounding employment problems, disciplinary proceedings before licensing boards, recognition of nurses' rights, and discrimination in education. The law as it relates to employment issues reflects a slight departure from the old legal rulings that an employer can "fire at will." In recent years the courts have started to pay closer attention to employment policies and under the right factual pattern the court has required good faith and fair dealing on the part of the employer. In the wake of federal legislation enacted to protect the rights of handicapped individuals, there have been cases involving both practicing nurses and nursing students.

The final chapter, Educational Law, is included because of my teaching experience. There is a growing body of law dealing with the due process rights of higher education school dismissals, as well as admission criteria. You will note that there are no specific cases dealing with nursing student negligence. This is because the principles of a malpractice suit are the same whether the alleged negligent act involves a student or a more experienced nurse.

Two points should be made to the reader: (1) I have used "she" for nurse and "he" for lawyer without meaning to imply that all nurses are female or all lawyers are male. (2) This book is not intended to provide legal counsel, and if you have a legal problem you should consult with your own legal counsel.

Writing was not a new experience for me, however writing a book was. It evoked a response similar to law school; having completed one semester it was too late to turn back. I knew I was in for serious business when I asked for "a really big dictionary" for a Christmas present. I found that there is happiness in finding just the right case to illustrate a legal concept. Because one of my nursing values was professionalism, with every section I asked myself was it written as a professional would write it? On that score I am happy with the outcome.

One day while I was laboring over a particularly difficult section I looked out of the window searching for the right phrase which sometimes lives in the oak tree at the end of the back walk. I live on a main street in a growing town which has a good amount of traffic and I saw a turtle the size of a large salad plate trying to cross the road. As the nearest lake is 2 miles away I could not believe my eyes and for some minutes I watched it darting its head in and out of its shell as drivers coming upon it suddenly veered to avoid hitting it. I finally ran out with a hastily marshalled rescue team, dishpan and shovel, and effected the rescue. After watching it swim off towards the middle of the lake my father said that no lawyer would stop in the middle of writing a book to rescue a turtle; only a nurse would. Since then whenever I'm writing I look for turtles.

ACKNOWLEDGMENTS

I am indebted to the thousands of nurses across the country who over the last 12 years never failed to confront me with the most intriguing and practical legal questions. Some of those questions stumped several competent Boston litigation attorneys (both defense and plaintiff) when I later posed the same questions to them. Truly, I learned much from these nurses. I was frequently overwhelmed by their noble demeanor and obviously high professional standards.

I am especially indebted to my editor Stu Horton, who always had enough faith for the both of us that this book would be written. It was particularly trying for him because it took place during my transition from nursing to law. He stands a breed apart. I am grateful to my production editor Karen Davis who was so supportive and understanding during the most difficult time for me, the "real" deadline.

I am particularly grateful to the following who reviewed chapters and made helpful suggestions even though all of them were overextended with their own demanding nursing endeavors: Joyce Passos, Marjorie Gordon, Tina DiMargio, Mary Beth Strauss, Eleanor Murphy, and Mary Baroli. I am grateful to my friend and nursing colleague, Carol Coakley Genereux, for her exceptional command of nursing knowledge and for always being available to answer my tedious nursing questions and to do "emergency" nursing research when the facts of a case created a technical labyrinth.

Lastly, I am forever indebted to my two legal mentors, Benjamin and Meyer H. Goldman, Esqs., who in addition to reading my chapters as if they were the final draft of a U.S. Supreme Court brief, taught me what it means to be a creative and competent advocate. They taught me by example that the practice of law requires a commitment to high standards and relentless dedication.

NURSING
JURISPRUDENCE

1

ANATOMY OF A SUIT

When I completed the initial draft of this book I felt that something was missing and discovered that it lacked a concise explanation of the dynamics involved in a nursing malpractice case, that is, those aspects which were common to all the cases included in the book. Thus, some preliminary explanations are in order.

Understanding what factors come into play before the nurse is notified that she is a party defendant or just an ordinary witness will help in understanding the cases. This chapter is an effort to give the nurse a sense of what happens before she knows she will be involved in a law suit and what goes on between that time and the first day of trial through the appeal. Not all cases are appealed, but it is important that the nurse understand that the losing party at the trial level, whether it be plaintiff or defendant may get a second chance because of a major error committed at the trial level. The threat of a second trial may result in a different outcome or force the parties to settle the case without a trial.

One concept which is difficult for the non-lawyer to fully

1

grasp is that the case law from state to state may be quite different. This is because states have different rules of evidence, statutes, and they may be bound by prior cases which established precedent for subsequent cases. In addition, the American courts rely heavily on a jury system of justice and the composition of each jury is unique to the case. To a lawyer there is uniformity in the legal process although to the nonlawyer it appears that there are few similarities in either the judicial process or outcome. That can be an intimidating perspective.

The most logical place to start dissecting a malpractice suit is to briefly explain the federal and state court system and the significance of each court's ruling or decision. The practical distinction between "ordinary" negligence and professional malpractice are best explained by citing a case dealing with the legal doctrine of the statute of limitations. The statute and its few exceptions are also important because they may serve as both a defense and an obstacle. It should also be reassuring to know that plaintiff's lawyers have both a professional and economic need to evaluate a malpractice case carefully. Most attorneys practicing medical malpractice litigation from a plaintiff's perspective do not take anywhere near the number of cases that come into their office. The lawyer must be able to prove liability and the injury suffered by the patient must justify bringing suit.

The pretrial discovery phase is simply the gathering of information. It may be both helpful and potentially harmful to the patient's or defendant's case and must be evaluated with care before the case reaches the trial stage. It is said that cases are won and lost in trial preparation. That is of course an oversimplification, but it was coined by lawyers to stress the importance of the work and effort necessary to influence the outcome of a trial. The trial itself is the most intimidating, but least mysterious, because it follows a predictable format. It has a beginning, a middle, and an end and each side has the opportunity to tell its side of the story.

The activities that precede a trial are vital. Because essentially all of the legal matters presented in this book deal with civil cases the focus of this chapter is on civil suits as opposed to criminal suits. A civil suit is docketed as *Smith v. Jones*. Smith is the plaintiff and Jones, the defendant. In a criminal case the parties are docketed as *State v. Jones*. A civil trial provides a forum to judicially examine issues that are in dispute between adversarial parties. A dispute may involve an allegation of malpractice involving the manner in which medical or nursing care was given, an allegation of wrongful job termination, or a legal determination that a specific activity is within the scope of nursing practice.[1] The trial must be held in a court that has authority to hear the particular case. There are statutes and rules governing the whole legal process from the filing of the petition (complaint) to the conclusion and any appeal process. All trials are open to the public as guaranteed by the U.S. Constitution.

In addition to civil trials a nurse may be involved in an administrative-type hearing. Examples of administrative hearings include those held by a civil service or licensing board, and unemployment eligibility hearings. Although different rules apply to the conduct of such hearings they are all begun by a formal petition, evidence is heard, and generally an appeal of the agency decision may be made in a higher court. Administrative agencies have been referred to as the "fourth branch of the government." The formal branches are the executive, judicial, and legislative branches.

A case may be brought in a state court, or in a federal court if the dispute is one that involves nonstate issues. Suit is brought in a federal court if there is a diversity of citizenship, that is, where one party is a citizen of one state and the party on the other side is a citizen of another state. Civil rights cases based on the U.S. Constitution or federal legislation are brought in a federal court as are negligence suits against a government agency, such as the Veterans Administration. There are also rules that govern whether a case will be tried before a jury or whether a judge will decide the case. Most malpractice cases are tried before a jury. If the plaintiff wants the case tried before a jury his attorney will request a jury trial in his complaint.

THE DIFFERENCE BETWEEN STATE COURTS AND FEDERAL COURTS

The majority of cases in this book took place in state courts which means they have the greatest significance for the states in which they were decided. That does not mean that another state cannot follow the holding as to matters or principles of law. Precedent, such as that set out in *Darling v. Charleston Hospital*,* may be followed by the state in which the case was decided, or it may be followed in jurisdictions of other states. Lawyers prefer to cite cases from their own jurisdiction, but use other state decisions if they support a particular position. This can be done as long as the lawyer's state has not ruled differently in a case. Practically speaking, if state A does not permit certain evidence and state B does, this can have a significant impact on the final result. Certainly, judges even in the same jurisdiction rule differently on matters of law. One judge may permit a particular expert witness to testify,

---

* The *Darling* case is discussed in depth in Chapter 2.

whereas another judge may rule that the expert is not qualified; thus, the judge's ruling may be the subject of a later appeal of the case.

One often hears the question, "But, what is the law in my state?" A case should be looked at for its significance, not because it was a Utah or a North Dakota decision. Many factors influence a jury's decision, such as the demeanor and appearance of the parties and the witnesses, the evidence that was allowed in, and subtle differences which cannot be measured or duplicated in a similar case. The "facts" of a particular case are the most important reason a lawyer decides to handle it. Facts may be similar in different cases, but they are rarely the same. Remember that a jury decides the facts. It is the duty of the respective lawyers to make sure that their set of facts and law gets introduced into evidence and evidence that is not favorable does not get admitted. This is the nature of the adversary system.

Some cases are tried in the federal court system as opposed to the state court system. All decisions can go to the U.S. Supreme Court, although relatively few are accepted for review. A federal suit is begun when U.S. constitutional rights are involved, where one of the parties resides in another state, or where issues of a federal nature are in dispute. A number of the cases dealing with the care and treatment of the mentally ill are federal court cases, as are many abortion decisions. A suit against the federal government, such as one involving a federal hospital, must be brought in the federal court that has jurisdiction to hear the case. The federal court system is similar to state system in that there is a trial level and two appeal levels that precede bringing the case before the U.S. Supreme Court.

Just as state courts may vary in applying principles of law, the federal "circuit" courts may also rule differently in a similar case. The court hearing a case can only rule on the evidence put in front of it. This includes interpreting federal laws, and in some instances state laws, and applying the law to the facts of the case. There are ten circuit or jurisdiction courts in the federal system. States and U.S. possessions (e.g., Virgin Islands) are grouped together to form circuits. A Second Circuit case, which includes New York and Vermont, may not be followed by the Ninth Circuit, which includes California and Alaska. The U.S. Supreme Court establishes the broad legal principles to be followed.

A federal circuit system is a way of dividing up the states and U.S. possessions. A case may be decided by the Second Circuit and states within that circuit grouping must follow its ruling. Circuits may issue conflicting rulings.

TIME LIMIT FOR BRINGING SUIT

Two critical threshold factors must be present before a malpractice suit is filed. One is that the suit must be brought within the prescribed time limit. This is known as the *statute of limitations* and is spelled out in state laws. The statute of limitations begins when an alleged wrong comes into existence and ends at the time period set out in the statute. Presently in New York the time period to bring a malpractice suit is $2\frac{1}{2}$ years[2] and in Massachusetts the time period for both malpractice and other personal injury suits is 3 years.[3] The time frame for filing malpractice suits in most states is between 1 and 3 years. Failure to file the suit within the prescribed time frame is a bar to the suit and the defendant will raise it as an affirmative defense in his answer to the plaintiff's complaint.

Case Law Exceptions: Time of Discovery and Interpretation of Malpractice

There are two important exceptions to the statute of limitations rule. The first is the law on "discovery" and the second is the case law that deals with the question whether the term "malpractice" includes nursing negligence.

Most states hold that the beginning of the time frame for filing a malpractice suit starts at the time of the wrong or when a reasonable person would have discovered the wrong. Tolling of a statute means the exact date a case will be recognized in law as beginning. For example, in Massachusetts, if a nurse put a hot pack on a patient which injured the patient on January 1, 1987, the patient must file a suit by December 31, 1990. A 1980 Massachusetts court in *Franklin v. Albert* set aside prior court decisions, thus joining the majority of state decisions, and held that the tolling of the statute did not begin until the plaintiff "learns, or reasonably should have learned, that he has been harmed as a result of the physician's conduct."[4] In that case the patient's chest x-ray films showed suspicious findings and the radiologist had recommended further evaluation tests. No follow-up was done and 4 years later the patient was diagnosed with Hodgkin's disease. The patient alleged that the findings of the early x-ray films were early signs of Hodgkin's disease. The court reasoned that a plaintiff should not be penalized, if through no fault of his own, he failed to discover the wrong.

While admittedly the discovery rule has more application to medical malpractice, it does have some significance for nursing. Malpractice concepts, such as failure to diagnose a medical condition, have implications for nurse practitioners—nurses authorized by law to perform some medical acts under protocols—but not for other nurses. A delay in establishing a nursing diagnosis may well cause harm to a patient, but the time frame in a nursing context is not the same as in a medical situation where the delay may preclude the best treatment option. However, a state that permits extension of the statute of limitations would do so when the nursing act involved a lost sponge after an operation.

Some states have held that the concept of malpractice is not applicable to the occupation of nursing. Thus, a suit involving alleged malpractice by a nurse would be brought under the heading of "ordinary negligence." This difference is important because in some states the time frame for bringing suit in a malpractice action differs from that involving a suit alleging ordinary negligence.[5] During the "malpractice crisis" of the mid-1970s a number of states enacted legislation that reduced the time frame for malpractice.

The state of Ohio applies a 1-year statute of limitations to "medical claims." In *Richardson v. Doe*, a 1964 Ohio case that involved nursing "negligence," the court stated: "There is no compelling reason for a nurse to be given the protection of a 1-year statute of limitations. A nurse, although obviously skilled and well trained, is not in the same category as a physician who is required to exercise his independent judgment on matters which may mean the difference between life and death."[6] Further, the court said, "If the General Assembly had wished to protect groups other than those traditionally associated with malpractice, it should have listed the ones to be covered." The suit alleged nursing negligence in the death of a mother from postpartum hemorrhage. It was filed beyond the 1-year medical malpractice period, but before the 2-year ordinary negligence statute had expired.

Ohio courts dealt with a subsequent line of cases all upholding the decision that the longer ordinary negligence statute of limitations applies to cases involving departures from good and accepted nursing care.[7] They narrowly interpreted the statutory language, "medical claim," to exclude nursing. In *Kambas v. St. Joseph's Mercy Hospital*, a case involving an anticoagulant injection, a Michigan court applied the 3-year negligence statute rather than the shorter 2-year statute for malpractice.[8] Some states apply the same length of time for both malpractice and negligence. Where there is a difference and where the statutory language fails to provide direction the court may decide that the malpractice statute only protects physicians, who are traditionally associated with malpractice actions.

It is common for defense attorneys, in responding to the plaintiff's complaint, to take the position that the suit must fail because it was not filed within the proper time frame. The defense will prevail where the statute is narrowly interpreted, as in the Ohio cases, to include only the common law definition of malpractice.

EVALUATION OF THE CASE

The second critical factor to be considered before bringing suit is the evaluation of the case. A patient who believes he has been harmed by the actions of a health care provider frequently consults an attorney to see if there are grounds for a suit. The attorney evaluates the case on its merits and feasibility for success. After interviewing the patient in depth and reviewing the hospital or office records the attorney sends the record to an expert in the field to evaluate the merits of the case. The expert gives the attorney a report indicating whether grounds for suit exist. If grounds exist the physician or nurse expert spells out the departure from good and accepted professional practice. This departure is construed by the plaintiff's attorney as negligence. In addition, the expert must indicate that the departure was the proximate cause of the harm suffered by the patient. The plaintiff must show a "probability" that the defendant's departure from good and accepted practice caused the harm in order to hold him liable for malpractice. In a recent Arizona case, *Thompson v. Sun City,* the court held that where a physician negligently transferred an injured man from an emergency room to another hospital without first doing necessary surgery the jury could find that the transfer "increased the risk of the harm" that the patient would suffer permanent damage, and this increased risk would permit a jury to find a probability that the doctor's negligence was the cause of the damage.[9]

The expert's opinion is the foundation of the plaintiff's case. Relatively few cases can prevail without an expert opinion. From the facts of the case and the expert's opinion the attorney formulates the theory of liability. At this point the plaintiff's attorney is ready to file the court petition and initiate the suit within the statutory time frame.

Malpractice cases are taken on a contingency basis which means that the attorney collects a fee only if the case is settled or a jury finds in favor of the plaintiff. Contrary to popular belief most plaintiff attorneys do not take a medical malpractice case unless the liability is strong. Further, no matter how good the liability (negligence issues), unless there is money available for the damages, suit will not be brought. In legal parlance this is known as "the deep pocket" concept. In a 1981 Missouri case the plaintiff's lawyer sued a hospital and several operating room nurses instead of the surgeon when he negligently took out the woman's small bowel.[10] The surgeon was not named in the suit because he was not insured. The jury awarded the woman over five million dollars. An appeal by the defendant resulted in a settlement for a smaller amount.

INITIATING THE SUIT

After the plaintiff's attorney has investigated the case and determined the merits, he brings the suit in court. A negligence suit, as with all other legal proceedings, is initiated by filing a petition or complaint in the court that has jurisdiction over the case. The purpose of the complaint is to advise the defendant of the type of action and the general basis for the suit. The complaint must be drafted with care. It is possible for a case to be ultimately dismissed because the complaint failed to state a cause of action recognizable in law.

The Complaint

The complaint contains a number of counts or separate claims. For example, in a wrongful death suit there will be one count for death, one for conscious pain and suffering, and one for loss of consortium for the surviving next of kin. If the suit is against more than one defendant the complaint contains counts for each defendant. If the suit involves nursing malpractice the complaint alleges that the defendant nurse was negligent in providing nursing care or in carrying out medical treatment orders.

The complaint must be filed with the court before the expiration of the statute of limitations. With permission of the court it may be amended to include other defendants even after the statute of limitations has expired. When it is filed it is assigned an identifying number known as a *docket number*. All subsequent correspondence and papers filed with the court use this docket number. The defendant is notified of the suit by a summons with a copy of the complaint which is served on him by a sheriff or a constable. When the defendant is served he must immediately inform his insurer. The defendant has a set time period to respond to the complaint and his response (answer) is filed with the court and a copy sent to the plaintiff.

A nurse may suspect that a suit will be brought because the patient may have threatened to bring suit or the nurse may reason that the event itself is likely to result in litigation. A patient may not want to sue a particular physician or nurse for a number of reasons. If the patient elects to sue a nurse he will name the nurse, individually, in his complaint or sue the hospital or health care facility for the negligence of the nurse-employee. Whether or not the nurse is named individually, if she has liability insurance her insurer will be called on to defend the nurse. Her insurer will pay part or all of any damage award. Of course, if the nurse is named in the suit her insurer defends her.

The Defendant's Answer

The defendant's written response to the suit is as important as the plaintiff's complaint. When the defendant files his answer with the court he must answer every allegation or count in the plaintiff's complaint. If the defendant fails to deny or otherwise address each allegation he may have admitted liability. The defendant admits some or part of the allegations contained in a specific count (1) because these allegations are true or (2) because they do not specifically address the issue of wrongdoing. For example, a hospital named as a defendant admits that it is licensed to provide psychiatric care and services. However, it denies that it is responsible for providing medical treatment as only a licensed physician may provide medical treatment. This denial would be essential where the alleged negligent acts were provided by a physician who is not employed by the hospital. A physician who has staff privileges is an independent contractor and the hospital is not liable for the physician's negligent medical care. However, note that a hospital may be liable for failing to check a physician's references when giving staff privileges or where the hospital fails to have a system in place to monitor the quality of medical practice according to its by-laws.[11] Such a failure would make the hospital liable as a corporation.

The defendant raises affirmative defenses. Examples of affirmative defenses include failure to file the suit within time limitations, failure to state a claim against the defendant on which relief can be granted, and allegation that the plaintiff was negligent and the injury was the result of that negligence. At some point the defendant may concede negligence, but does not concede that the negligence of the defendant caused injury or death to the patient. The plaintiff must prove both negligence and causation.

Generally the affirmative defenses section of the defendant's answer is stated in broad terms. These affirmative defenses are developed fully at the trial. For example, the nurse's attorney may argue that under the facts of the case the nurse was acting in a reasonable way or that the nurse used her best judgment. Where the case involved an emergency situation the defense may argue that because of the emergency situation the nurse was deprived of an adequate time frame in which to deliberate and consider fully her actions, that is, albeit the emergency circumstances the nurse's conduct was reasonable. Where the alleged negligence of the nurse overlapped with medical treatment the nurse may argue that she can not substitute her judgment for that of the physician, or that she did not have any part in the complex judgment that went into the decision-making regarding the patient's medical care. The nurse may state that she was simply carrying out the physician's medical orders.

In summary, the plaintiff's complaint tells the defendant the theories on which the plaintiff relies in trying the case, and the defendant's answers indicate the manner in which his case will be defended. Both the complaint and answer must be drafted with care.

SCREENING PANELS

In the mid-1970s many states enacted medical malpractice tribunals or screening panels.[12] The legislative objective of such statutes was to discourage the filing of frivolous and nonmeritorious medical malpractice suits. In Massachusetts the members of the tribunal consist of a judge, attorney, and medical or nursing expert. The expert must be from outside the jurisdiction where any of the defendants live or practice. The plaintiff has the burden of showing that the evidence, if believed by a jury, is sufficient to support a verdict in his favor. The screening panel does not require a "minitrial" and consideration is given to the fact that in-depth discovery has not been done before the tribunal convenes. Apart from the facts, the most important evidence presented at the tribunal is an opinion letter or testimony from an expert in the discipline of the defendant's area of practice.

The plaintiff's offer of proof to the tribunal panel ordinarily consists of the following: facts relevant to the case; an affidavit (sworn statement) from the plaintiff; essential portions of the medical records; the expert opinion letter, along with the qualifications of the expert; applicable case law; and treatises that support the allegations of the plaintiff. The plaintiff orally argues his preliminary case before the panel members and the defendant's attorney responds to the argument. The panel collectively votes on whether the suit should go forward because the allegations have merit or the tribunal finds in favor of the defendant, imposing an additional burden on the plaintiff.

The decision of the panel can be appealed. In Massachusetts, for example, if the panel renders a decision in favor of the defendant the plaintiff must post a bond of $6,000 for each defendant in order to proceed with the suit. The money goes to the defendant for the cost of defending the suit if the jury finds against the plaintiff. At this point the plaintiff has to decide whether to drop the suit, file the bond, or appeal the tribunal's decision instead of filing the bond. If the plaintiff elects to appeal the decision rather than file the bond the decision of the highest appeals court will prevail. If the high court finds for the defendant the plaintiff no longer has the option of filing the bond. An appeal of the tribunal decision against the plaintiff will be elected where the plaintiff's attorney believes that the evidence contained in the offer of proof was sufficient to permit a jury to find for the plaintiff.

PRETRIAL DISCOVERY

After the initial pleadings have been filed and the tribunal proceeding has been completed the parties begin the phase of *discovery*. The objectives of discovery are to obtain all the facts relevant to a case, to narrow the legal issues, and to develop testimony that will be presented at the trial. Just as there are rules and case law that govern the trial procedure, there are rules that govern the discovery process.

Interrogatories

Both the plaintiff and the defendant send each other a list of questions that must be answered under oath. These are filed with the court and are a part of the pleadings. For example, the defendant asks about the number, reason, location, and dates of all hospitalizations or medical care rendered within a certain time period. He asks about the specifics of the injury suffered by the plaintiff. He asks what treatment has been provided since the alleged injury and whether there are permanent injuries. Interrogatories are sent to all plaintiffs. The defendant may also wish to know the names and addresses of experts the plaintiff plans to use at the trial and the substance of any and all conversations the plaintiff had, including the location and dates, with the defendant.

The plaintiff asks the defendant about insurance coverage, professional education and expertise in the area of the alleged malpractice, details of his legal relationship with other physicians in any group medical practice, and specific details of treatment and discussions the defendant had with the plaintiff while the defendant was treating or caring for the plaintiff.

In state courts only a specific number of questions can be asked, but in federal courts the number is not limited. As with all pleadings the answers to interrogatories must be carefully drafted as they may be introduced as evidence at the trial.

Depositions

A *deposition* is the pretrial recorded testimony of a party and enables both the plaintiff and defendant attorney to directly examine and cross-examine the deponent, that is, the one being questioned. The *deponent* may be other than the plaintiff or defendant. For example, the defendant's attorney may wish to take the testimony of the plaintiff's medical or nursing expert witness. The process of taking a deposition is begun by serving a notice of intent to take a deposition on the deponent. Depositions are taken under oath and all attorneys involved in the suit are present. There is a stenographic record and the party being deposed signs the stenographic copy after reviewing it for accuracy.

A deposition has many potential uses. It frequently helps in the discovery of new evidence, including the names of new witnesses and important documents. It also serves as a basis for developing liability and defense arguments. It may serve as a substitution for the testimony of a witness who is not available at trial. It may be used to refresh a witness's memory at trial as an aid to recall. It is frequently used to impeach or discredit the witness at trial in the event his trial statements are in conflict with the testimony given at the deposition.

During the deposition exhibits are introduced into the record. Ordinarily the party being deposed is asked to bring certain documents to the deposition. Obtaining certain documents may be the chief reason for deposing an individual. The deposition may last an hour or it may take several days. All parties being deposed should be prepared for the deposition. Although no attorney may coach a witness in his testimony all parties being deposed or testifying at trial should be thoroughly prepared for the experience. The deponent should have in-depth knowledge of the facts, allegations, and defenses as they relate to his area of expertise.

The attorney for the plaintiff needs to know the right question to ask of a specialist at a deposition. For example, the plaintiff's attorney may ask the defendant obstetric doctor if one can hear fetal tones in an obese pregnant woman as well as in a nonobese pregnant woman. This question would be important where a defensive argument is that the woman's obesity caused the fetal heart tones to be somewhat unreliable. A plaintiff may want to ask the surgeon, anesthesiologist, and operating room nurse, to state who is responsible for selecting the position the patient was placed on the operating table. The defense attorney may ask the plaintiff's nurse expert if she ever used the type of physical restraint used by the defendant while caring for the injured patient and that allegedly caused the harm complained of.

In one recent case a nurse who filled out an incident report following an incident involving a patient recovering from surgery was served a notice that a plaintiff's attorney wanted to depose her.[13] The nurse was told to bring the incident report and any other written reports or taped recordings to the deposition. Neither the hospital at which the alleged injury occurred nor the nurse was a party to the suit. However, the nurse had legal counsel representing her at the deposition which lasted over 10 hours. The nurse did not bring the requested materials to the deposition, claiming privilege. Subsequently a motion asking a judge to rule on the request was filed and appropriate appeals taken. The plaintiff was ultimately allowed access to the incident report and other recorded statements. The court held that there was no privilege enjoyed by the hospital preventing access. The materials the plaintiff's attorney requested included the incident report completed at the time of the injury, a written report completed by the nurse shortly after the incident which was requested by in-house legal counsel, and a tape recorded report that was prepared for the hospital insurer at their request. This does not mean that these materials will be admitted into evidence at the trial.

Motions

During this pretrial phase both parties file motions with the court. A *motion* is a formal request by one of the parties asking the court to grant its request. Motions may include a request for a speedy trial because of the age of the plaintiff, production of documents, a court order compelling one of the parties to answer interrogatories or questions posed at a deposition, consolidation of the parties, and the continuance of the trial date. There are many reasons for a motion. The party requesting to be heard on a motion must notify the opposing party to give him an opportunity to be heard. The opposing attorney either agrees to the motion or opposes it and presents arguments before a motions judge. Commonly, motions are supported with a written narrative known as a *brief*. The brief contains legal arguments in support of or in opposition to its allowance. After the motion is argued before a motions session judge the court issues an order on the request.

THE TRIAL

After all the discovery has been completed the parties seek a trial date. Normally, this is years after the event and may be from 3 to 7 years after the plaintiff's complaint was filed. If the liability is clear-cut there may be settlement talks. For example, a ureter cut during an abdominal procedure may be regarded as good liability. If both the liability and the damages are fairly straightforward it is more likely that the case will be settled before the trial date. Of course, a settlement may be offered any time from the beginning of a suit until a jury has decided on an amount. It is possible to settle with one or more defendants and proceed to trial with those defendants who did not participate in the settlement agreement. If the insurer has made an offer to settle, the amount must be conveyed to the plaintiff by his attorney. If the plaintiff accepts the settlement figure a settlement agreement is signed by the parties to the settlement.

Immediately before the trial begins there are pretrial conferences. During these conferences the attorneys stipulate to certain facts, settle on procedural matters, or ask the judge to act as a facilitator in exploring a settlement. The attorneys also present the trial judge with trial motions such as voir dire and a list of jury instructions. *Voir dire* is a motion requesting the trial judge to ask certain questions of the prospective jurors. For example, the plaintiff's attorney will want to exclude anyone who has been treated by a defendant physician or has been hospitalized at the defendant hospital. The defendant's attorney may want to exclude a woman who had a stillborn if the case involves a fetal death.

The actual trial is open to the public. Virtually all medical or nursing malpractice cases are tried before a jury. Other cases, by statute or practice, are tried before a judge without a jury. Malpractice cases brought against the federal government are tried in a federal court, without a jury. In cases where there is a jury the jurors are the "triers of fact." That is, they are the individuals who decide questions of fact such as whether the nurse informed the patient that smoking in bed was not permitted in the defendant hospital, as she testified, or whether, as the plaintiff testified, no one informed him that he should not smoke after receiving narcotics. In a jury trial the role of the judge is to rule on issues of law, such as what evidence is admissible and other procedural matters. Where the judge is also the trier of fact, the determination of negligence and causation also rests with him.

Early in the trial the hospital and office medical records are introduced into evidence. The original records will have been subpoenaed and delivered to the court shortly before the trial begins. They will be certified by the keeper of the records—by the medical records librarian, in the instance of a hospital—as the true and complete copy of the hospital record. The records are used frequently throughout the trial by both sides. Blowups of specific parts of a record may be used to emphasize a point to the jury. There are, of course, rules applicable to how one side or the other may use such evidence. In addition to subpoenaing the medical records, the plaintiff's attorney subpoenas the defendant and other witnesses. The defense attorney subpoenas witnesses, other than the experts.

Some plaintiff attorneys ask their clients to observe a trial so that they will better understand the process and procedure of a trial. The courtroom is the domain of judges and attorneys, but few other individuals are acquainted with it and it can be an intimidating setting. Sitting through a trial can help acquaint the witness with the dynamics of a trial, as well as taking some of the mystery out of the process. It can also prepare the witness for his actual testimony. A nurse, whether or not she is a defendant in a malpractice case, can learn much about how a case is tried by sitting in on all or key parts of a trial. Key parts include the opening statements, expert testimony, closing arguments, and the jury instructions. It is important to observe how the applicable standard of care is established or rebutted during the direct and cross-examination of an expert witness.

Selecting the Jury

As the trier of fact the jury decides the factual issues and which testimony is the most believable when there is a dispute in testimonial evidence. The jury is selected just before the start of the actual trial. When the prospective jurors arrive they complete a form sheet indicating their address, occupation, age, level of education, and their marital status and spouse's occupation, if they are married. There may be other general questions. The judge asks the prospective jury members the questions submitted by the attorneys. A judge may refuse to ask the prospective jurors a submitted question if judicial discretion allows such refusal. The judge may ask, "Have you or any member of your family ever sued a physician or hospital for care and treatment rendered?" An affirmative answer does not necessarily mean that the prospective juror will be disqualified by the judge although it is likely. The judge may ask a prospective juror if he can arrive at a fair verdict even though he may have sued a health care provider in the past. If the prospective juror says that he is unable to reach a just verdict, then he will be excused. It is unlikely that a defense attorney will permit such a juror to be empaneled. Nurses, physicians, lawyers, and even judges may serve as jurors. Each attorney is permitted to strike a stipulated number of prospective jurors from the list without stating any reason. After the full jury is seated (empaneled) both attorneys prepare a master sheet containing the names of each juror and any relevant information from the juror form sheet that may be particularly important to be aware of during the trial. Although much has been written recently about the psychology of selecting a jury it remains an uncharted course. However, it is important that the attorneys develop a rapport with the jurors as their role is not insignificant in the outcome of the trial. The same must be said for the witnesses.

Opening Statements

The actual trial begins with the opening statements that are made by the respective attorneys. The plaintiff's opening provides a concise overview of the facts. The attorney begins by identifying both the plaintiff(s) and the defendant(s). The plaintiff's theory of liability is outlined and he tells the jury who will be called on to establish the prevailing standard of care and how the defendant(s) departed from the professional standard. The list of witnesses is recited, as well as the substance of their testimony. Exhibits may be used in both the opening statement and the closing argument by either attorney.

After the plaintiff's opening the defendant's counsel has an opportunity to speak to the jury. The defense attorney introduces his client. He admits that what has happened to the plaintiff is tragic, or unfortunate, but that no act or failure to act on the part of the defendant produced the tragic result. Just as the plaintiff's attorney indicated how his case would progress and the substance of each witness's testimony so the defense attorney tells the jury his defense theories and how he will show that his client is not liable. At this time the defense attorney may inform the jury that he will introduce a study that is helpful to his client's position. Both attorneys remind the jury that nothing they say in their opening or closing is to be considered as evidence, and that the testimony and exhibits are the evidence.

Trial Testimony

The purpose of evidence at a trial is to persuade the jury or judge that a particular series of events supports the position of the plaintiff or defendant. Evidence takes two forms: testimony and physical evidence. *Testimony* is oral evidence. A deposition, even though the deponent is not present at trial, is still oral evidence. *Physical evidence* includes documents, mock-ups (small-scale models), pictures, equipment, and other demonstrative evidence. There are, of course, legal rules of procedure and case law that govern the admission of both testimonial and physical evidence. It is common at the conclusion of the trial for the judge to explain to the jury the weight to be given to some testimony. For example, where the nurse at her deposition stated that she was not told of certain findings concerning the patient, the judge may instruct the jury that it may consider in evaluating the deposition testimony of the nurse that she was deposed 5 years after the event in question.

The plaintiff begins his case first. Ordinarily, the plaintiff is one of the first witnesses, if not the first to take the stand because his story is the basis of the case. Neither plaintiff or defense attorney may ask "leading" questions of his own witness. An example of a leading question is, "Did the defendant, Miss Jones, tell you that she gave you double the dose of adrenalin?" It is called a *leading question* because the question suggests the answer. Although some judges may be somewhat liberal in permitting leading questions it is generally not a good practice as the jury gets the impression that the testimony, whether it is the plaintiff's or the defendant's, is rehearsed or less credible. Testimony that is elicited from a particular attorney's witness is called "direct" testimony.

During testimony the attorney introduces exhibits such as the original hospital record, certified death certificates, and medical textbooks. These become evidence. Of course, opposing counsel may object to certain testimony and physical evidence, and the judge will have to issue a ruling. Such rulings may be given immediately or after a "side-bar" conference at the judge's bench. The arguments are not heard by the jury. Arguments are heard and if the objection was anticipated an attorney may give the judge a copy of a case supporting his position. The trial resumes with the judge telling the jury to disregard the question or some other instruction if the objection is upheld. At this time one of the attorneys may raise a formal objection to the judge's ruling and thus preserve the issue for appeal if the jury finds against his client.

During the testimony the jury is studying the manner in which the testimony is given, as well as the effect of the testimony on the plaintiff or defendant. Although coaching of witnesses is not permitted, both sides have gone over the areas of testimony in-depth during the pretrial preparation. A lawyer may tell his client how to testify, but he may not tell the witness what to testify to. The best advice is to tell the truth in a believable way.

After the plaintiff has been examined by his attorney the defendant's attorney cross-examines the witness. The general purpose of any cross-examination is to discredit the witness in the eyes of the jury. The main objective of the attorney doing the cross-examination is to lead the witness in the direction the attorney wants him to go. During cross-examination the defense attorney is permitted to ask leading questions as he is trying to weaken or discredit plaintiff's testimony. Where the plaintiff's attorney may ask, "Did you talk with anyone in the pre-operative holding unit?" the defendant's attorney may frame his question, "In fact, you had three injections to put you to sleep an hour before you went to the operating room, didn't you?" The cross-examining lawyer is permitted to cast doubt on the plaintiff's story during cross-examination. There is, of course, opportunity for the attorney of the testifying witness to try to repair any damage or impression left with the jury. This is called "re-direct" testimony. Neither side wants any loose ends left in the minds of the jury. The rules applicable to direct and cross-examination apply to all witnesses, not just the plaintiff and defendant.

Expert Testimony

Both sides present expert testimony to establish the standard of care. The experts testify that the defendant complied with or failed to comply with the "accepted and recognized standard of care." The first line of questioning after an expert has been sworn in is to establish his level of expertise. Sometimes, if the expert's credentials are extraordinary the defendant's attorney may stipulate that the expert is qualified to testify. This is done so that the least amount of attention is drawn to the expert's qualifications. Sometimes there is an objection to the qualifications of the expert. For example, the defendant's attorney may argue that a nurse is not competent to render an opinion on certain findings. The courts have begun to recognize that nursing is based on a core of scientific courses which gives nurses standing as experts to testify on matters concerning nursing care. In the last decade plaintiff's attorneys have begun using nurses instead of physicians as experts when the departure from care involved a nursing action. In addition to establishing the applicable standard of care, the expert must render a professional opinion that the departure from care caused the patient's injury.

If the plaintiff's expert has published articles or a book on the subject the defense will be familiar with the materials and will cross-examine the expert on any inconsistencies with his present testimony. The same applies to the defense expert and the defendant. In some instances a plaintiff who has been unable to obtain an expert to testify on his behalf can use the testimony of the defendant physician or nurse to establish the standard of care.

The prime reason for using an expert witness at the trial is to establish an expert opinion. Also, the expert when shown the clinical records during the trial can serve as a factual witness by describing the events of treatment and injury. The expert differs from other witnesses because he is permitted to state an opinion.

After the plaintiff has presented his case the defendant begins his defense. The trial procedure is essentially the same, the defendant tells his story to the jury and the plaintiff's attorney tries to discredit his testimony. The defendant nurse or physician is also an expert, but other expert witnesses are brought in to support his testimony.

Closing Arguments

After both sides have presented all their evidence they give their closing arguments or summation. The defense attorney presents his closing argument first. The plaintiff, in his closing statement, stresses the personal tragedy aspect of the case. The defense counsel therefore begins his statement by acknowledging that the harm to the plaintiff is tragic or unfortunate, but stresses that its occurrence can in no way be laid at the feet of the nurse, physician, or hospital. Both closing arguments summarize the testimony and try to focus the jury's attention on the salient points. Each side pays particular attention to refuting the opposing party's arguments. Each side concludes by requesting that the jury find in their favor.

Jury Instructions

After both attorneys have finished presenting their case and given the jury their closing arguments, the judge instructs or "charges" the jury. The instructions are simply the laws which the jury is to consider in their deliberations in the jury room. The instructions include applicable state laws, rules of law, and specific requests of the attorneys which they deem favorable to their case. For example, if the case involved a wrongful death the judge tells the jury exactly what is covered under the law.[14] Most states include reasonable funeral and burial expenses, compensation for loss of income, and loss of consortium in the death statute as items which a jury may consider in awarding money. An example of a rule of law which is given at the end of every trial is the "standard of proof" concept. For example, in a criminal case the burden is on the prosecution or state to prove the allegiance "beyond a reasonable doubt." In a civil (negligence) case the burden is based "on a preponderance of the evidence." The judge defines what a preponderance of the evidence is in accordance with the specific law of the state. Simply, it means a "tipping of the scales" to one side or the other.

It is not uncommon for a jury to request the judge to repeat parts of a charge. In a recent New York case, *Bender v. Nassau Hospital*, a civil suit had to be remanded or sent back to the trial court level because the jury did not understand the judge's charge.[15] The plaintiff had suffered neurological damage allegedly as a result of the physician's setting her fractured arm. During their deliberations the jury requested the court to re-read the charge a total of five times. The higher court said that the initial court had an obligation to do more than read abstract principles of law to the jury and that its failure to instruct the jury in a meaningful way was sufficient grounds for the case to be retried.

The jury instructions prepared by the attorneys are important because they mirror their liability (negligence) or defense arguments. In addition, they are drafted to overcome, if possible, the arguments of the opposing side. A judge need not give the requested instruction using the precise wording in which the attorney submitted it or he may refuse to give the requested instruction. It is not uncommon for one side or the other to base an appeal of the case on the judge's failure to give requested jury instructions. An appeal may also be based on an unrequested instruction.

In a 1979 California case, *Fraijo v. Hartland Hospital*, the plaintiff unsuccessfully based the appeal on a jury instruction that dealt with nursing judgment.[16] Also, in *Hicks v. U.S.*, a federal case involving a wrongful death, the plaintiff's attorney requested the following jury instruction which was upheld[17]:

> When a defendant's negligent action or inaction has effectively terminated a person's chance of survival, it does not lie in the defendant's mouth to raise conjectures as to the measure of the chances that he has put beyond the possibility of realization. If there was any substantial possibility of survival and the defendant has destroyed it, he is answerable.

After the jury has deliberated and reached a verdict it will be given to the court and the judge will enter a judgment accordingly. After the jury verdict it is common for posttrial motions to be filed. An attorney may file a motion to set aside the verdict as it is against the weight of the evidence or an attorney may request the judge to reduce the amount of money given by the jury. It is not uncommon where the jury has awarded a large sum to the plaintiff for the defendant's attorney to argue that the amount was excessive and was based upon "emotional" feelings on the part of the jury. Such arguments are common in quadriplegia cases and where newborns are severely impaired. A judge may tell the plaintiff that unless the plaintiff accepts a lesser amount the judge will order a new trial.

APPEAL

After the trial either side may appeal the decision. An appeal must be based on the formal court record which is recorded by a stenographer during the trial. Both sides submit written briefs and orally argue the merit of the appeal before an appeals court. The case may be appealed to the highest appeal court in the state. If the case was tried in the federal court it is appealed through the federal appeals system. Appeals involving a U.S. public health hospital and most products liability cases will be brought in a federal court. An example of a products liability case is when an infant is burned because the heating controls in an incubator malfunctioned. Most of the cases reported in this book and in the legal literature are cases where the trial level decision was appealed to a higher court. The appellate higher court generally issues a written opinion after it has decided the case.

The process of a trial is both intimidating and instructive. Any nurse who is involved in a suit, either as a defendant, expert witness, or "general" witness can take a great deal of fear out of the experience if she takes the trouble and time to sit in on a full or partial jury trial. Observing from "behind the bar," that is, out of the arena can provide an important lesson in the value of nursing policies and procedure, continuing professional education, and excellence in nursing care.[18] While it is true that a malpractice trial tests and scrutinizes what every nurse holds dear, it can also be an affirmation of the high tenets of nursing as a profession.

REFERENCES AND NOTES

1. Sermchief v. Gonzales, 660 S.W. 2nd 682 (MO, 1983). The state high court held that the Missouri nursing practice act permitted nurses to diagnose and treat delineated physical problems under established protocols.
2. McKinney's CPLR (Civil Practice Law and Rules), §214-a.
3. MGL (Massachusetts General Laws) c. 260, §2A.
4. Franklin v. Albert, 411 N.E. 2nd 458 (MA, 1980).
5. 8 American Law Reports 3rd 1136.
6. Richardson v. Doe, 129 N.E. 2nd 878 (OH, 1964). But see also Davis v. Eubanks, 167 N.E. 2nd 386 (OH, 1960) where, in the presence of a statute, the court held that a nonlicensed individual who was practicing nursing as a registered nurse was practicing a profession and could be guilty of malpractice.
7. See Bell v. Coen, 357 N.E. 2nd 392 (OH, 1975) for a childbirth death; Neilson v. Barberton Citizens Hospital, 446 N.E. 2nd 209 (OH, 1982) for loss of a surgical needle; Lombard v. Good Samaritan Medical Center, 433 N.E. 2nd 162 (OH, 1982), Cert. denied, 103 S. Ct. 127 (1982) for a suit against a hospital laboratory technician.
8. Kambas v. St. Joseph's Mercy Hospital, 205 N.W. 2nd 431 (MI, 1973). However, 2 years later the Michigan legislature changed the statute to include registered and licensed practical nurses within the 2-year malpractice law.
9. Thompson v. Sun City Community Hospital, 688 P. 2nd 605 (AZ, 1984).
10. Cushing, M. (June 1982). A matter of judgment. *American Journal of Nursing, 82*(6), 990.
11. Elam v. College Park Hospital, 183 *California Reporter, 156* (CA, 1982).
12. Massachusetts General Laws, Chap. 231, §60B (MA, 1975); Arizona Revised Statutes, Chap. 5.1, §12-567 (AZ, 1976); Florida Revised Statutes, §768.44 (3) (FL, 1979); Revised Statutes of Nebraska, §44-2840 (NB, 1976); Louisiana Revised Statutes Anno-

tated, § 40:1299.47 (LA, 1978); Pennsylvania Consolidated Statutes, §1301.402 (PA, 1975); Maryland Courts and Judicial Proceedings Code Annotated, §3-2A-02 (MD, 1976); New York (Judiciary) Law, §148-a (McKinney, 1975); West's Annotated Indiana Code §16-9.5-9-2 (IN, 1979).

13. Villers v. Puritan-Bennett Corporation, C.A. no. 84 0076-CV, Appeals Court (MA, Feb. 2, 1984).

14. Massachusetts General Laws, Chap. 229, §2 (MA, 1973); Florida Statutes Annotated, §768.21 (FL, 1972); New York (Estates, Powers and Trusts) Law, §5-4.3 (McKinney, 1966); West's Annotated California Code (Code of Civil Procedure) §377 (CA, 1961).

15. Bender v. Nassau Hospital, 471 NY 2nd 657 (NY, 1984).

16. Fraijo v. Hartland Hospital, 160 *California Reporter, 246* (CA, 1979).

17. Hicks v. U.S., 368 F. 2nd 626 (1966).

18. See Bluhm, Michael. (1987). *The doctor goes to court—Basic anatomy of personal injury litigation procedures* (3rd ed.). The 14-page booklet is available by writing to Michael Bluhm, M.D., 72345 Beverly Way, Rancho Mirage, California 92270. Cost of booklet is $2.00 plus self-addressed and stamped (22 cents postage) long business size envelope.

ESTABLISHING THE STANDARD OF CARE

A professional association has an inherent obligation to create standards. One of the identifying characteristics of any professional association is its right to direct and control the nature of its activities. The nursing literature refers to this as the nature of the association's autonomy. The predominant characteristic it enjoys is the right to develop professional standards of practice; indeed, this right must be viewed as a responsibility. The creation of professional standards reflects the growth of nursing as a profession. In the event that the nursing profession fails to create standards, other groups will assume this responsibility and the likelihood is that those standards will not reflect the direction of growth that nursing wishes to pursue. The standards of a recognized authority are important from a legal perspective because they may be used at a trial to establish the applicable standard of care.

What About Standards That May Conflict?

There are many groups and administrative agencies in the health care spectrum publishing standards which may overlap and, on occasion, conflict with another published standard. An intriguing legal question could arise where two equally recognized professional nursing organizations publish conflicting standards. The question then is which standard should be the one recognized by the court as imposing a specific legal duty. An argument that a specific standard that has been published by an acknowledged authority is the only applicable standard, may be rebutted by the defendant. That is, it could be argued that the standard of care that the plaintiff wants applied, should not apply to the factual situation. Second, the argument may be that the defendant complied with a different standard.

It is probable that the court would view the conflicting standards in much the same manner as testimony on the standard of care offered by the plaintiff's and defendant's expert witness. Where the sources of the standard are not published by organizations representing the same discipline, for example, the American Nurses' Association (ANA) and the American Hospital Association (AHA), the more persuasive argument is that the professional nursing organization standard should apply, so long as the standard is contemporaneous with current nursing theories and practice.

Malpractice suits involving other professions illustrate the necessity to establish a standard of care in nursing. In recent years suits have been brought against school committees and school boards alleging malpractice in the area of education. To date they have been unsuccessful because the courts have been unable to determine the standard of care that should apply. For example, the courts have held that a skill such as reading involves a host of experiences. These may include supportive measures in the home and the responsibility for the student learner to aid in the process of acquiring this skill.

How Does the Standard Apply to a Factual Situation?

The *standard of care* is legally defined as those acts performed or omitted that an ordinary prudent person would have done or not done. It is a measurement against which the defendant's conduct is compared. Two important points must be stressed here. First, the definition includes acts of omission as well as acts of commission. Thus, negligence may result from a failure to do a wound irrigation every 4 hours as ordered by the physician, or carrying out the procedure in such a manner that it violates the principles of aseptic technique. Another example is where the alleged negligent act resulted from the instillation of the incorrect type or amount of fluid to irrigate a T-tube in the hepatic duct, or the failure to release the T-tube clamp according to either the surgeon's ordered schedule or when the patient exhibits signs of intolerance to the clamping procedure. The failure to release the clamp when the patient exhibits the signs of intolerance (increased pain, drainage around the tube, temperature, nausea and vomiting) may occur because the nurse failed to make a nursing decision or failed to act on that decision. Second, in a malpractice suit the "ordinary prudent person" becomes the reasonable prudent nurse whose actions must conform to the actions of like professionals performing in the same or similar circumstances.

As a general rule, the courts do not establish the standard to be applied to a factual situation, yet the court in *Helling v. Carey* did just that in awarding damages to a young woman who was treated over a long period.[1] If the court had only recognized the standards as professed by the members of the medical profession, it would have had to deny recovery based on an argument of negligence.

> The plaintiff, a 22-year-old woman, was fitted with contact lenses for myopia in 1959. She returned to the same ophthalmologist in 1963 complaining of irritation from the lenses and was seen many times over the next 5 years by one or the other of two doctors in a joint practice. Because they believed that her problems were solely related to complications associated with her contact lenses, they did not do a tonometry test until October 1968. At that time it was discovered that her peripheral vision was lost and her central vision reduced markedly.
>
> During the trial, expert testimony presented by both parties established that the professional standards did not require routine pressure testing in patients under the age of 40 years. However, the standards did require testing if a patient's complaints and symptoms indicate that glaucoma should be expected. Although the incidence of glaucoma, a condition whose signs and symptoms are silent and irreversible, was 1 in 25,000 in persons under the age of 40, its presence could be detected by a simple and harmless test.

The issue before the court was whether compliance with the professional standards should protect the defendants from liability in a situation where a simple test could have prevented the devastating harm suffered by the young woman. The court, citing Justice Holmes's opinion in an earlier case stated, "What usually is done may be evidence of what ought to be done, but what ought to be done is fixed by a standard of reasonable prudence, whether it usually is complied with or not."[2] A concurring opinion by one of the justices agreed with the majority opinion, but submitted that the theory of recovery should have been that of strict liability, rather than negligence. A "strict liability" theory, that is a legal concept where liability is imposed without the necessity of proving the defendant was to blame. For example, most states hold that the owner of a dog who bites someone is strictly liable for any injury. Under that concept the courts hold that the innocent bystander bitten by the dog should not have to bear any harm because of the bite. The owner should pay any medical bills and money for any pain and suffering or scarring. The court in essence said that, if the professional members are derelict in fulfilling their responsibility to create and promote reasonable standards of care the courts will provide relief to one who has suffered damage, by imposing reasonable standards.

The lesson in this case for nurses is that the court will apply its own higher standard of care if the standard of care proposed by the nursing profession falls below an acceptable standard. Although the courts are reluctant to impose a higher standard of care it will do so.

What Are the Elements of a Negligence Suit?

The beginning law student learns that there are legal elements embodied in a negligence or malpractice suit. The elements are (1) duty to the patient; (2) a failure or breach of that duty; (3) causation, specifically that the breach was the proximate cause of an injury; (4) foreseeability; and (5) harm or damages resulting from the negligent act. All these elements must exist before a plaintiff's case will be decided by a judge or a jury. A failure on the part of the plaintiff to prove any one of the elements will prove fatal to the case.

The elements of duty and breach are the most burdensome for the plaintiff's attorney. Causation can also be burdensome, but to a lesser extent. The elements of foreseeability and damages are more straightforward. In legal parlance, duty and breach translate into "the applicable standard of care." The plaintiff's attorney is more apt to fail to adequately prove the existence of these two elements than any of the others because of their intricacies. There is a considerable body of law dealing with the proof of the applicable standard. Much of it holds that the failure on the part of the plaintiff to establish the standard is fatal to a finding of malpractice.[3] The fundamental legal question in a malpractice suit is, "What standard of conduct must be met by the defendant to satisfy the duty owed to the plaintiff?" The law defines duty as an obligation imposed by law. It requires one person to conform to a certain standard of conduct for the protection or benefit of another. In order for a duty to exist, it requires some type of legal relationship, such as that which exists between the nurse or physician and the patient. Once it has been established that a duty exists the jury determines from the facts whether the defendant's conduct measured up to the legal standard that is required by the relationship.

The circumstances surrounding a particular activity are important in judging the defendant's conduct. Thus, the standard of care required in an emergency situation may differ from that which would be required in a nonemergency situation. Emergency situations, such as unanticipated inadequate staffing or a lack of equipment, still require compliance with minimum standards in light of the circumstances. There is a minimum standard below which no nurse's performance should fall.

Is There a Practical Distinction Between Negligence and Malpractice?

The distinction between ordinary negligence and malpractice is important to bear in mind. *Negligence* may be defined as the failure to do something which a "reasonable" person would do, or doing something which a reasonable and prudent person would not do. *Malpractice* refers to any professional misconduct or unreasonable lack of skill in carrying out professional duties.[4] When an individual drives through a red light and injures a pedestrian walking with the "walk" light, the driver is negligent. It requires no expert testimony for a jury to conclude that the driver's action was something which a reasonable and prudent driver would not do. However, when the injury involves an act or failure to act on the part of a nurse the claim is based in professional malpractice. The elements apply to both ordinary negligence suits and malpractice suits.

Why the Need for Expert Testimony?

There is a rule of law that where questions of medical or professional judgment are involved expert opinion testimony is required to show that the defendant acted improperly. This is because the "trier of fact" (jury) or the judge can not determine from their own knowledge and life experiences what the standard is when the issues involve intricate professional issues. The common knowledge and experience concept is not as easy to apply as one might think. For example, some judicial decisions have held that a decision whether to raise a patient's bed rails is beyond the common knowledge of the jury. Conversely, other jurisdictions have adopted the position that questions regarding the necessity of bed rails do not involve matters to be decided by a physician or nurse, but rather involve routine custodial care of the patient, and are therefore within the common knowledge and experience of the jury.[5]

The importance of providing expert opinion testimony if the jury is unable to draw upon their own knowledge can be further illustrated. If an attorney has rested the plaintiff's malpractice case without offering evidence on the applicable standard of care the opposing party will immediately file a motion for a directed verdict (favorable) for the defendant. A directed verdict, if granted by the court, ends the case and jury deliberations are precluded. The only avenue left to the plaintiff's attorney is to appeal the judge's decision to a higher court.

There is an extensive body of case law dealing with the issue of establishing or failing to establish the applicable standard of care. There are relatively few malpractice cases for which a jury, without the aid of expert testimony, can determine whether or not the standard was met. If an attorney tries a case without offering expert opinion testimony it is because of one of the following reasons: (1) the attorney is unable to obtain an expert, (2) the facts of the case clearly come within an exception to the rule that an expert is necessary, (3) the deviation can be shown by introducing a hospital policy that establishes the standard, or (4) the attorney intends to rely solely on an admission of liability by the defendant during pretrial discovery. An example of an exception to the need for expert testimony is the doctrine of res ipsa loquitur. Res ipsa loquitur translates into "the thing speaks for itself." Another exception is the common knowledge doctrine. The common knowledge doctrine is the principle that the jury is able to determine the standard because the subject matter is the type that lay people would understand without the aid of professional testimony. For example, an electric lamp can be turned on by pressing an electric switch. It has been traditionally used in "lost sponge" cases or where the plaintiff awoke from anesthesia with an injury that could not be explained in a reasonable manner, for example, where an arm is broken and surgery was performed on the lower extremities or where a physician ligates or cuts a ureter during a hysterectomy.

How Is the Standard of Care Established?

During a trial both sides introduce into evidence what is known as "exhibits." Exhibits become part of the evidence that will be considered by the jury. The inclusion or exclusion of a key exhibit may be pivotal to the case. Many exhibits introduced during a trial are used to help establish the standard of care.

A written philosophy of nursing care, provided it is not worded in general terms, may be useful in establishing the applicable standard. Most facilities and agencies spend time in the development of a philosophy and some spell it out in specific terminology. A philosophy of nursing care may state that it is the responsibility of a professional nurse to do the essential discharge teaching. Frequently a policy or job description is more specific in identifying teaching responsibilities so that the physician and the nursing staff can work collaboratively in the teaching process.

For example, a nurse may be held liable if the patient alleges that the harm occurred because the nurse failed to implement a teaching plan and as a result, the patient did not know to limit the number of nitroglycerin pills during an angina attack and continued to take the pills instead of calling a physician. The institutional or agency philosophy or the job description would serve to establish that the nurses owed a duty to teach the patient about drug therapy. Expert testimony and the nursing literature would establish that certain content should have been included in the discharge teaching plan.

Some of the less commonly known resources that help to establish nursing standards include institutional directives. These should be drafted with care. Also, they should be communicated in a manner that assures that those employees charged with the responsibility of implementing them are aware of their existence and application. Also, it is believed by many legal authorities that, as the Professional Standards Review Organization (PSRO) standards are defined and gain more credibility and status, they will eventually become recognized as legal standards.[6] Some states have passed legislation protecting the records, reports, and proceedings of hospital staff review committees and PSROs from discovery and admissibility in evidence.

Once the standard of care is established, counsel for both parties elicit testimony to show that, in the instance of the defendant, the standard was met, or in the instance of the plaintiff, that the standard was not met. Each state has its own procedural rules affecting the introduction and use of evidence at a trial. In addition, prior case law decided by the respective state courts will determine whether and how evidence, such as a rubber catheter, is introduced and used as evidence. It is quite common for a case heard at the trial court level to be appealed to a higher court solely on the question of the admission, exclusion, or use of evidence admitted at the trial.

Recent court decisions have shown a willingness to allow into evidence a variety of sources of information to aid in establishing the applicable standard of care. It is expected that this trend will continue and the list of possibilities will become more extensive. While the majority of these sources are not conclusive in proving the standard of care, they assist the jury in the determination of which standard is applicable to the facts. They can generally be grouped into three broad classifications: (1) *legal requirements:* state laws and regulations, such as licensing requirements for health care providers and health facilities; federal enactments and regulations, such as the National Health Planning and Resource Development Act and the Rehabilitation Act of 1973; state and federal executive orders issued by a governor or the President; (2) *professional associations:* national and state associations, such as the state nurses' associations and hospital associations; published standards and position statements; and professional codes of conduct; (3)

publications of health care facilities and agencies: directives, procedures and protocols, formal institutional philosophies, job descriptions, and patient information pamphlets, and bylaws.

In addition, information or instruction sheets published by pharmaceutical and equipment companies, treatises, accrediting association standards, and expert witnesses serve to aid the "trier of fact" in the quest for the truth.

Summary

One of the most important functions of any professional association is to define its standards so that its members can be guided in their activities. Such standards are used in judicial proceedings as a measurement in determining compliance or lack of compliance in carrying out a professional activity. Judicial decisions, just as nursing decisions, are made after analyzing the facts and applying them to a given situation. In the law this is referred to as identifying the standard and then applying the facts to it.

The standard measures what the nurse owes to the patient. During a trial much evidence is heard regarding whether the nurse's actions measure up to the duty. The chief means to measure this is by expert opinion testimony. Other equally important means used are published standards and internal policies. Usually without expert testimony, the triers of fact are not able to determine what the nurse "ought" to have done under the circumstances.

PROFESSIONAL STANDARDS

Standards of nursing practice are a continually evolving entity. Each nursing care provider, whether an emergency room nurse or a school nurse involved in community nursing, should know the specific standards of practice impacting on her activities. Failure of the reasonably prudent nurse to be aware of the standard would be no defense in a malpractice or disciplinary proceeding. This is why nurses are urged to subscribe to professional journals and attend programs of professional organizations. The more specialized the area of nursing practice, the greater the duty of the nurse to be aware of the technological advancements affecting the area of specialization.

In 1973, the ANA formulated and published its standards for nursing practice.[7] In response to the question "why standards of practice?" the Congress for Nursing Practice stated that it is the responsibility of a professional association to provide a mechanism whereby the competency of its members can be judged. The standards mandate a structure to be followed in planning and implementing nursing care. It is, in fact, a process that has evolved over a period of time; this process is generic to the nursing profession and has come to be called "the nursing process." Its application is appropriate to any health care setting requiring nursing services. It has as much application to nursing in an emergency room where traditionally care is immediate and decisions made quickly, as it has to a complex nursing problem in a nursing home.

Both national and state nursing organizations create and publish position statements on issues important to nursing practice. While a position paper published by these organizations may go a long way in clarifying an issue or provide direction for the profession, it does not have the force or mantle of the law. It may be allowed into evidence to aid in establishing a standard; however, it is not conclusive on the issue of the applicable standard.

Standards that are published by a recognized authority serve to notify the health care provider that the actions described connote minimal acceptable behavior. In this sense, the standards provide a deterrent to less than acceptable standards. However, when a nurse's actions are shown to not comply with the standard they represent a difficult obstacle for the nurse's attorney to overcome.

Some states have specifically redefined the generic definition of professional nursing to include the components of the nursing process.[8] When one analyzes the early case law relevant to nursing negligence it is obvious that, although the concept of the nursing process had not been articulated, the steps of the process can be readily identified. Because of its significance to the practice of nursing, failure to apply the process to a nursing situation, may itself be negligence where a patient suffers damage. This would be true especially where a quasigovernmental regulatory body, such as the board of registration in nursing, has included the nursing process in the generic definition of nursing. A nurse may incur liability where it can be shown that the nursing action was not founded on the dynamics of the nursing process.

In a legal context the term "standard" means the general recognition and conformity to established practice.[9] Because of the significance given to the term, some legal authorities recommend that the term "guidelines" be used in lieu of the term "standards." The supposition is that a more general term such as guidelines would be less legally binding in a legal proceeding because the guidelines connote a recommended course of action rather than a mandated course of action. Thus, the actions spelled out in the guidelines do not preclude the implementation of other courses of activity, but merely serve to suggest a single course of action. However, other factors impact on the significance to be accorded the "guidelines" in a legal proceeding, such as the committee or organization that developed them, the general tenor of the guidelines, and their accessibility to those providers having need to refer to them. For example, if they are distributed to, or their existence is made known to, all the nursing staff at a staff development program, an argument can be made that the intent of the committee that drafted them was that they be universally adopted and followed. Thus, the attorney wishing to use the "guideline" document to establish the standard of care may argue that it is not the term/phrase, "guideline" which will determine whether it constitutes the yardstick for measuring the standard, but the actions set out in the guideline document itself. In other words, do nurses rely on this document to direct their actions? A standard or guideline published by a special interest group, such as the Association of Operation Room Nurses and the Critical Care Nurse Association, may be of particular value in establishing a standard in court because the specialized groups can be more specific in the wording of the standards.

Summary

Because nursing is a continually evolving profession which is responsive to expanding and changing societal needs it is imperative that nurses keep abreast of changes applicable to their practice setting. Apart from the professional element, a nurse who fails to keep up with advances appears as a less than credible witness in the course of a legal proceeding, whether as a defendant, general witness, or expert witness.

The courts recognize the standards published by the American Nurses Association and other recognized specialty groups. In the right factual situation, admission of a state's nursing practice act may be helpful to the plaintiff, as are any rules promulgated by the state agency authorized to create such rules.

NURSING PROCESS

The *nursing process* refers to the method of professional practice. When the ANA first published the *Standards of Nursing Practice* in 1973, it was apparent that the standards focused on practice. The standards represent a systematic approach to the practice of nursing. The standards, which are applicable to any nursing practice setting, include the steps or components of nursing intervention. Reference to the nursing process as an entity began to appear in the nursing literature in the 1960s; however, reference to this concept merely formalized nursing actions as they had evolved in the practice setting. The nursing process includes the following components: assessment or data collection, identification of a nursing problem or nursing diagnosis, formulation of a nursing care plan, selection of a plan of care, implementation or testing of the plan selected, and evaluation of the approach used, with revision if warranted.

The first standard in the nursing process is the *assessment component* which serves as the foundation. The ANA standards state that the collection of data is continuous and all health status data must be available for all members of the health care team. Assessment is accomplished by interview, examination, observation, and by reading records and reports. An emergency admission may require that the initial nursing interview be brief, and not be fully completed within the customary 24-hour admission period. However, notwithstanding the emergency, a jury may find negligence if the nature of the omitted questions were critical to the patient's well-being. The question, "Do you have any allergies?" is critical for a patient undergoing surgery where it is foreseeable that some type of antibiotic will be given in the postoperative period; whereas the question "What is your sleep pattern at night?" under the circumstances may be delayed until the crisis has passed. There would be an increased duty to review the laboratory reports of a diabetic who has daily fasting blood levels for glucose and postprandials done; whereas a failure to read the daily fasting bloods of a nonlabile diabetic who has been stabilized may not incur liability.

Consider the potential for liability where the nurse fails to take a nursing history when it is a policy in the health care facility. As a result of this failure, the chart of a patient, who wears both framed glasses and contact lenses, does not contain these data and the patient is sent to the operating room with contact lenses in place. It is foreseeable that the lenses may lacerate the cornea when the patient is under anesthesia. This same result could conceivably occur when some of the items in the nursing history form are left blank or are overlooked during a critical period.

The hospital itself may incur liability where the policy states that either a professional or nonprofessional person may complete the form. Whether the form is filled in by the patient, or partially completed by an orderly or aide, it is the ultimate responsibility of the professional nurse to assure that it is completed accurately. Most facilities require that the history be done by a professional nurse, because it requires interviewing skill and knowledge which is integral to the profession.

Failure to establish a nursing diagnosis, such as "potential for injury,"[10] whether arising from suicide threats or from the lack of sensation specific to a medical diagnosis, such as syringomelia, may well incur liability in a negligence suit. While many nurses, practicing in both an episodic and distributive setting, may not be knowledgeable in the accepted diagnostic nomenclature associated with the nursing diagnosis, all nurses are prepared, in both skill and knowledge, to identify the host of nursing problems encountered in daily practice. In a professional sense it is important that the nursing literature define the term "nursing diagnosis" in such a way that the concept can be universally and consistently applied to all nursing care situations. A nursing diagnosis is an essential element in the nursing process and is as unique to the nursing profession as the medical diagnosis is to the practice of medicine. Where a nurse makes an incorrect or incomplete nursing diagnosis, but the patient doesn't suffer any harm as a result of implementation of the care plan, no liability will exist absent the damage element essential to a negligence cause of action.

The Standard Applicable to Nurse Practitioners

When the alleged negligence involves a nurse practitioner the threshold question is whether the nurse was carrying out an activity that was (1) generic to nursing, (2) a medical activity permitted by law, (3) a medical activity not permitted under the law, or (4) a nursing function that overlaps with medicine. If the activity was generic to nursing, any nursing expert familiar with the applicable standard is permitted to testify. If the activity was the kind of medical activity that the law permits the nurse to carry out then the standard can be established by either a medical practitioner who has experience working with nurse practitioners or a nurse practitioner who has experience in the specific delegated medical activity.

If the activity involved an unpermitted medical act then the standard will be established by a medical expert. In addition, testimony will be introduced to show that the nurse practitioner acted outside the law, thus strengthening the case for the plaintiff and placing a greater burden on the defense. For example, a member of the board of nursing may be subpoenaed to testify that the statute or regulations do not permit such activity. Nursing functions that overlap with medicine may be generic to nursing or may be uniquely identified with an advanced level nursing practitioner. The rule would require the testimony of a practitioner who is familiar with both the theory and practice of the specific overlapping function.

Nurse practitioners who carry out functions that are traditionally recognized as "medical functions" should be familar with the judicial holdings in specific medical treatment cases.[11] Suits brought for medical misdiagnosis and incorrect or inadequate medical treatment comprise a substantial proportion of the case law in medical malpractice. Liability is found where there is a lack of skill in the assessment, or a failure to follow up on patient complaints or diagnostic findings. It can be anticipated that future cases involving nurse practitioners will raise the issue of delay or failure to refer the patient to a medical doctor.[12] Whether the patient is medically treated by a nurse, functioning in the expanded role, or by a medical doctor the issue remains: What should have been done that was not done?

The legal literature has adequately addressed the liability in medical diagnosis situations, but has not to any extent addressed the liability for nursing diagnosis. The few articles in law journals that have dealt with nursing diagnosis, view it in the context of a nurse making a medical diagnosis.[13]

Practically speaking, a patient who has been harmed by a nurse practitioner carrying out a delegated medical act will likely sue both the practitioner and the supervising physician. A persuasive argument can be made that a patient who receives medical care from a nurse practitioner is entitled to the standard of care required of physicians.[14]

There are only a few cases to date which have raised the issue as to whether a medical or a nursing standard should be applied when a nurse practitioner or a physician's assistant "makes a medical diagnosis" and prescribes a treatment plan. Generally, the authority of a physician's assistant to perform medical acts is found in a state's medical practice act. However, even if the authorization is not formalized by statute there is a presumption that a physician can delegate certain activities to nonmedical health care providers. Of course, in delegating any activity to a nonmedical person, the physician would be held to the standard of other medical doctors when delegating.

In *Fein v. Permanente Medical Group* suit was brought against Permanente, not against the nurse practitioner who examined the patient first or the second physician who examined him later in the day.[15] The plaintiff, a 34-year-old man, experienced intermittent and moderate chest pain while bicycle riding and jogging. He made an appointment that day with the Kaiser Health Foundation (Permanente), a health maintenance organization. His history was taken and he was examined by a nurse practitioner who gave him a prescription for valium. She told him he had muscle spasms and he returned home. The nurse had consulted with her physician supervisor before giving the patient the prescription. Later that same day he awoke with excruciating chest pains and was taken to the Kaiser emergency room and examined by a medical doctor. That physician ordered a chest x-ray films and gave him a narcotic prescription. He reaffirmed the diagnosis of muscle spasms.

The man returned to the emergency room the following day because of a now constant pain and an electrocardiogram (EKG) done by a second physician revealed that he was suffering an acute myocardial infarction. There was testimony that the residual cardiac damage would reduce his life expectancy by about one half (approximately 17 years). The trial court found for the plaintiff and that decision was upheld by the state supreme court.

One of the issues raised by the defense in its appeal of the jury's decision was the jury instruction regarding the standard of care which was owed by the nurse practitioner. At the end of the trial the judge gave the general jury instruction on the duty of care of a graduate nurse:

> It is the duty of one who undertakes to perform the service of a trained or graduate nurse to have the knowledge and skill ordinarily pos-

sessed, and to exercise the care and skill ordinarily used in like cases, by trained and skilled members of the nursing profession practicing their profession in the same or similar locality and under similar circumstances. Failure to fulfill either of these duties is negligence.

The following paragraph was added to the general jury instruction at the plaintiff's request:

> I instruct you that the standard of care required of a nurse practitioner *is that of a physician and surgeon duly licensed to practice medicine* [emphasis mine] in the state of California when the nurse practitioner is examining a patient or making a diagnosis.

The high court looked to the changes the legislature made in the nursing practice act in 1974 and in 1977, the latter being specifically related to "nurse practitioners." The 1977 addition identified the criteria necessary to practice as a nurse practitioner: "a 'nurse practitioner' must be both a registered nurse and also meet the standards for nurse practitioner established by the Board of Registered Nursing." One of the board's mandated criteria was certification. The nurse practitioner who examined the plaintiff met all the board's practice criteria.

The court looked at the 1974 legislative changes in the nursing practice act for guidance. The preamble section of the statute reads as follows (in part):

> . . . the Legislature recognizes that nursing is a dynamic field, the practice of which is continually evolving to include more sophisticated patient care activities. It is the intent of the Legislature . . . to provide clear legal authority for functions and procedures which have common acceptance and usage. It is the legislature intent also to recognize the existence of overlapping functions between physicians and registered nurses and to permit additional sharing of functions within organized health care systems which provide for collaboration between physicians and registered nurses.*

The state high court held that the jury instruction given at the trial misstated the standard of care applicable to the nurse practitioner and was inconsistent with recent legislation affecting nurses, specifically, nurse practitioners. The court took note of the fact that the law makers explicitly declared a legislative intent to recognize overlapping func-

---

* California's nursing practice act (Deerings Annotated California Business and Professional) Code §2725 is unusual in that it contains a preamble statement. Not all state laws permit the inclusion of a preamble section. Where it is used it aids the courts in interpreting the law because it frequently indicates legislative intent in enactment of the law.

tions between the two disciplines and their desire to permit sharing of functions by collaboration.

It also noted the following provision in the statute:

> Nursing also includes, "observation of signs and symptoms of illness, reactions to treatment, general behavior, or general physical condition, and . . . determination of whether such signs, symptoms, reactions, behavior or general appearance exhibit abnormal characteristics. . . ."

The court said in "light of these provisions the 'examination' or 'diagnosis' of a patient cannot in all circumstances be said—as a matter of law—to be a function reserved to physicians rather than registered nurses or nurse practitioners." Further, the court said that the plaintiff was certainly *entitled* [emphasis mine] to have the jury as triers of fact decide the following:

> (1) whether defendant medical center was negligent in permitting a nurse practitioner to see a patient who exhibited the symptoms of which plaintiff complained and (2) whether Nurse Welch met the standard of care of a reasonably prudent nurse practitioner in conducting the examination and prescribing treatment in conjunction with her supervising physician, the court should not have told the jury that the nurse's conduct in this case must—as a matter of law—be measured by the standard of care of a physician or surgeon.

The significance of the term, "matter of law" is that the court determines what the law is, rather than the jury, thus something which is a matter of law is *decided* by the court.

The court held that although the instruction relative to the nurse practitioner was erroneous it did not affect the jury's decision in finding Permanente liable because they could have found liability because of the second physician's failure to take an EKG when the patient returned to the emergency room in the middle of the night.

Under the facts of *Fein* either a physician who works with nurse practitioners or a nurse practitioner functioning in a similar setting would be qualified to establish the standard of care.[16]

In a more recent case a North Carolina court in *Paris v. Kreitz* held that a physician's assistant was not subject to the same standard of practice as physicians.[17] The patient, who was 70 years old, went to the hospital with family members when he awoke shortly after 11:00 P.M. with pain in his leg and foot. When the hospital emergency room nurse contacted the physician covering for the patient's family physician she was told that he was out of town and his physician's assistant was covering for him. The nurse recorded that the patient had been in pain for about ½ hour prior to admission and that his leg was pale and cold, and his toenails were blue. When the physician's assistant examined the patient a short time later he made the same observations, noting additional symptoms of decreased blood supply to the leg and foot. The nursing staff and the defendants testified that the physician's assistant talked with the physician via telephone, but the plaintiff testified that no call was made. The physician's assistant wrote, "peripheral vascular insufficiency" and "probably surgical appointment in morning" in the record. He prescribed a mild painkiller and discharged him. He told him to stay in bed and to call the physician's office in the morning.

He was seen by the physician in the morning who referred him to a vascular surgeon who operated later in the day. At this first operation the vascular surgeon removed thrombus material from the man's leg. Subsequently the patient had two more vascular procedures, but the leg had to be amputated 2 months after the original symptoms appeared. The plaintiff sued the hospital for the alleged negligence of the emergency room nurse, the covering physician, and his physician's assistant. The plaintiff alleged that when the physician's assistant wrote peripheral vascular insufficiency it was an incorrect diagnosis. The medical doctor diagnosed, "occlusion of the lower leg" when he examined him at 10:30 the next morning. The symptoms were the same, except the pain had gone further up the leg. The vascular surgeon confirmed the diagnosis.

The plaintiff also alleged that the emergency room nurse should have known that the man's circulatory impairment condition was an emergency and that he should have been seen by a medical doctor in the emergency room. The nurse testified that she did not have the emergency room physician examine the patient because she had called the defendant physician, and spoke with his physician's assistant who said he was coming to see the man. The court held that the evidence (medical record) did not support the plaintiff's allegation that the physician and the physician's assistant's diagnosis was "obvious negligence," thus, requiring the nurse to go over their heads and intervene on the patient's behalf. Further, the court held

"While the negligence of Kreitz and Averett (the physician's assistant and the physician) may be a question of fact, it is clear that the negligence was not so obvious as to require Nurse Garrett to disobey an instruction or refuse to administer a treatment. Nurse Garrett's observations of Mr. Paris agreed with those of Kreitz. Any disagreement or contrary recommendation she may have had as to the treatment prescribed would have necessarily been premised on a separate diagnosis, which she was not qualified to render."

In finding for all the defendants, the court in specifically addressing the liability of the physician's assistant said "Plaintiff's argument that physicians' assistants are subject to the same standards of care as the physicians for whom they work is without merit." Citing a standard jury instruction which provided, "a health care provider is subject to the standards of practice among members of the same health care profession with similar training and experience situated in the same or similar communities . . ." the court said it was clear that a physician's assistant was not subject to the same practice standard as a medical doctor.

There is one more point for nurse practitioners to take note of and that is that the rule that a medical expert witness has to be from the same medical specialty has been somewhat eroded.[18] For example, an anesthesiologist would be permitted to testify regarding emergency cardiac resuscitation done in an emergency room even though the anesthesiologist had never practiced in an emergency room. Judges are permitted discretion to determine whether the expert can aid the jury in ascertaining the applicable standard. In a recent California case an obstetric nurse practitioner was permitted to testify against an obstetrician.[19] This is because the services provided were the same as that which could be legally provided by an obstetric nurse practitioner.

When the Courts Look at the Nursing Process

The formulation of a nursing care plan requires the identification of goals expressed in measurable activity or patient outcomes and which are prioritized. The ANA standards of practice for operating room nursing state that one patient outcome is freedom "of adverse effects from lack of improper use of safety measures, such as, chemical, physical, and electrical hazards."[20] This means that the potential for liability is present when the circulating nurse fails to include in the patient's care plan measures to assure that the patient is properly grounded when a cautery device is to be used during the surgical procedure.

Liability with respect to the selection of a plan of care is not as easy to demonstrate as some of the other components of the nursing process. The selection of a plan clearly involves a judgment component which must, by its nature, include "reasonableness." In those situations where only one course of action is open the selection component poses no legal question when it is followed. However, where several alternative approaches are possible, a single selection may be a critical issue. The test of reasonableness in light of the circumstances remains the key factor. The greatest potential for liability occurs when the nurse continues, for an unreasonable length of time, to implement one specific nursing action which does not bring about the desired result, especially where alternative nursing approaches could have been tested.

The actual implementation of the nursing care plan emphasizes the necessity to carry out nursing actions in compliance with the standard of care in existence at the time. The last element of the nursing process requires that some nursing judgment be made to determine the effectiveness of the plan and where necessary, make adjustments when possible and necessary. Without this last step in the nursing process, the accountability precept which is an essential aspect of any professional group would be lacking.

Nursing judgment is as generic to nursing as medical judgment is to medicine. It may be possible for a nurse to argue successfully that the failure to comply with nursing home state regulations requiring the use of a specific restraining device when restraining residents was due to the fact that recent studies identified the recommended device as likely to cause injury. An affirmative defense could be pleaded where the nurse departed from the published standard because nursing judgment required deviation from the standard. In sum, nursing judgment required that a safer type of restraint be applied. Factually, the argument would be strengthened if the state regulations were outdated.

When one reviews the early case law in nursing malpractice the different components of the process can be readily abstracted from the facts and language of the case. This is possible even though the nursing process nomenclature had not yet been formulated. As the attorneys for both the plaintiff and the defense become aware of the nomenclature of the process and recognize its impact on nursing actions, the specifics of the nursing process will be more identifiable in the written opinion of the case.

A recent case decided by the Connecticut Supreme Court affirmed a lower court ruling and awarded a substantial award to a young woman who suffered permanent brain damage while a patient in the psychiatric unit of a general hospital.[21] The patient in *Pisel v. Stamford Hospital* had been hospitalized for 10 days prior to the incident in which her neck became lodged between the bed rail and bed frame resulting in hypoxia with resultant coma. Expert testimony was offered to determine whether the accident was a result of inadequate nursing assessment and judgment or whether the injury was one that the nursing staff could not have forseen.

The defendant nurses testified that the patient had been visually observed through a window in the door of her room at 10-minute intervals during the preceding 4 hours. The expert witness for the plaintiff's case offered testimony indicating that the standard of care was breached because the nurses did not do a physical assessment, in addition to the visual assessment of the patient. She testified that a visual assessment alone would be inadequate to determine patient needs. In the absence of a full and complete assessment, the nurses would be unable to implement appropriate nursing interventions. The expert witness for the defendants testified that the visual assessment was adequate, especially in view of the fact that there existed the likelihood that verbal and physical stimulation would tend to exacerbate agitation. She further testified that the patient's hospital record indicated that she had become agitated on previous occasions. The case is significant because it uses the language of the nursing process in finding the nurses liable. There was considerable expert testimony dealing with "assessment" needs and failures.

Summary

It is only recently that the courts have incorporated some of the language of the nursing process into their legal opinions. However, this is not particularly significant because it is not difficult to find the elements of the nursing process in the old nursing malpractice cases. What is important is that the courts now recognize that there is a systematic approach taken by nurses in managing patient case. Courts now hold nurses legally accountable for deviations from this process.

The legal opinions incorporate the language of nursing where nurses use this in testimony. However, a practical point should be made: attorneys want language a jury can grasp. They do not want language that clouds the issues for the jury. The attorney will ask the witness to translate the professional language into language that the jury may readily understand if there is any chance that professional language is beyond the jury's comprehension. This does not mean that the attorney will not be able to make his message clear to the jury.

Establishing the standard of care owed by a nurse practitioner is more complex. This is because there are no judicial decisions to rely on and the issue of which standard is applicable is a material one. The activities of nurse practitioners are tested, not only in negligence cases, but in other civil suits.[22] Nurse practitioners should study medical malpractice cases because many of their functions are closer to those of medicine than nursing.

A generic nurse is liable for failing to review the results of a critical laboratory test, whereas a nurse practitioner may incur liability for failing to use proper judgment in ordering the test. One specific area of liability that is being examined in the courts is the failure of a nurse practitioner to refer a patient to a physician. Conceptually, this is akin to a generic nurse's liability for failure to bring substandard medical care to the attention of hospital authorities.

DEFINING THE STANDARD OF CARE BY STATUTE

In the wake of the "malpractice crisis" that occurred in the mid-1970s, a number of states enacted legislation in response to an increase in the number and type of malpractice suits. The legislation dealt with a number of related issues and included measures such as statute of limitations reform, medical mediation panels, joint underwriting association laws, pretrial discovery procedures, and the requirement of filing a certificate of meritorious claim by the plaintiff's attorney before the suit could be instituted.

More recently, statues have been enacted impacting on the standard of care. A 1978 California statute outlines the standard of care and expert witness qualification in emergency situations.[23] The statute provides that where the cause of action involves emergency medical care rendered in an acute care hospital emergency room, testimony on the issue of the applicable standard of care is admissible only if it is given by a physician who has had substantial professional experience in an acute care hospital emergency room within the previous 5 years. In more recent legislation, a Virginia statute provides for a statewide standard unless trial testimony supports the application of a local standard, because it is more appropriate under the facts than the statewide standard.[24] The statute, in part, revives the concept of the "locality rule" (see Modification of the Locality Rule; below).

Florida has recently enacted legislation defining the acceptable standard of care applicable in malpractice cases. Nurses are included in the class of persons identified as health care providers. Three provisions in the statute are germane to the standard of care issue. First, the statute identifies two broad categories and classifications of similar health care providers. Second, it sets out the reason for identifying the various categories of health care provider as being a means of identifying who may testify as to the applicable standard of care. A third provision provides that any health care provider may testify as an expert if the court is satisfied that the provider "possess sufficient training, experience, and knowledge as to the acceptable standard of care."

This last provision in the statute would allow a physician to give testimony as to the acceptable standard of care in a nursing context, unless it could be shown that the nursing activity in question was unique to the nursing profession. Such a finding would preclude a physician from testifying as a qualified expert. For example, most physicians would qualify as an expert witness where the standard of care issue was the correct identification or selection of a site for an injection. However, the physician may not qualify if the technique of administration involves an aspect in which the physician lacks skill or experience, such as the Z-track method of injection, essential in administering an iron dextran drug.

The Florida Statute provides:

1. In any action for recovery of damages based on the death or personal injury of any person in which it is alleged that such death or injury resulted from the negligence of a health care provider. . . . ,

the claimant shall have the burden of proving by the greater weight of evidence that the alleged actions of the health care provider represented a breach of the accepted standard of care for that health care provider. The prevailing professional standard of care for a given health care provider shall be that level of care, skill, and treatment which, in light of all relevant surrounding circumstances, is recognized as acceptable and appropriate by reasonably prudent similar health care providers.[25]

2. a. If the health care provider whose negligence is claimed to have created the cause of action is not certified by the appropriate American board as being a specialist, is not trained and experienced in a medical specialty, or does not hold himself out as a specialist, a "similar health care provider" is one who:

1. Is licensed by the appropriate regulatory agency of this state;

2. Is trained and experienced in the same discipline or school of practice; and

3. Practices in the same or similar medical community.

b. If the health care provider whose negligence is claimed to have created the cause of action is certified by the appropriate American board as a specialist, is trained and experienced in a medical specialty, or holds himself out as a specialist, a "similar health care provider" is one who:

1. Is trained and experienced in the same specialty; and

2. Is certified by the appropriate American board in the same speciality.[26]

The statute recognizes different levels of expertise in the same discipline and where the provider is not certified or a specialist, the applicable standard is that existing in the particular community or one similar to it.

In a malpractice case against a podiatrist, an Illinois court in *Dolan v. Galluzzo* held that the expert witness must be licensed as a podiatrist and a physician or surgeon would be prevented from testifying for the purpose of proving the standard of care.[27] However, where the physician may also be licensed as a podiatrist, the trial court, at its discretion, may determine if the witness is qualified to testify as an expert. The case held that inequities would result if the skill and care of one school of discipline could be applied to another distinct discipline. The court stated that where the legislature provided for the regulation of practitioners of medicine, nursing, pharmacy, podiatry, and dental surgery it was a clear expression of their intent to create public policy in the recognition and regulation of various health professionals. Such legislative intent requires different training and regulations to be followed in the treatment and care each profession may offer. The court concluded that the "defendant has the right to have his competence judged by the standards of his own distinct profession and not by those of any other."

It is worth noting that in a dissenting opinion in this case one justice viewed the requirement of licensure to be a purely mechanical rule, saying that under the rule "a physician would be unable to testify to nursing standards of care even though nurses operated under his supervision or to testify to standards for midwives, and this because the physician was not licensed as a nurse or a midwife."[28]

One of the results of the malpractice crisis of 1973 was that some states enacted legislation spelling out the standard of care for some areas. They also listed the qualifications of witnesses who were deemed to offer expert opinion testimony. Other states continue to rely on case law to determine the qualifications of experts.

EXPERT WITNESS

The expert witness is the most important factor in establishing the standard of care in a malpractice case. To qualify as an expert witness two elements must be present: "(1) possession of knowledge so distinctly [sic] related to some science, profession, or business which is beyond the understanding of laymen; and (2) the witness must have sufficient skill, knowledge or experience in a particular field whereby his opinion will probably aid the trier in search for the truth."[29] However, it is a general rule of law that the expert witness is not required to be the best witness on the subject.[30]

Ordinarily, an attorney seeks a witness who has the best qualifications from a theoretical and experiential perspective. It is common for both sides to challenge the expertise of the opponent's witness. A witness may be challenged because she lacks expertise or because she is too much of an expert to testify against the more general nurse. It is the job of the expert witness to explain to the court and jury the standard of care that should have been given. It is important that it be conveyed in language that is understandable to the jury. The witness is counseled by the attorney to "teach" the jury what it needs to know about the subject. After eliciting the qualifications of the expert, the attorney will say, "Nurse Smith, will you teach all of us about observing signs of increasing intracranial pressure." If the opposing attorney believes the nurse is including too much physiology or pathology an objection will be made on the basis that the nurse is testifying beyond her area of expertise. Both sides enter into discussions with the judge, out of the jury's hearing, and after hearing the arguments presented by the attorneys the judge either permits the nurse to continue or precludes further testimony that is of the same nature.

Although nurses were used as expert witnesses in cases decided before the 1980s it was not until the 1980s that a distinct body of law began to emerge. Attorneys and the courts looked to medicine when expert nursing opinion was needed. This was because of society's high regard for physicians. Also, nursing did not begin as a discipline that had to draw on a scientific body of knowledge.

A Pennsylvania case, *Baur v. Mesta Machine Company*, decided in 1962, articulates the well-recognized standard of care applicable to a registered nurse, "that which a reasonably prudent registered nurse would have exercised in the circumstances."[31] This case illustrates that where the facts all point to substandard care it it easy to apply the principle. The testimony of a physician established the deviation from nursing standards.

In this case an employee went to the plant dispensary complaining of severe chest pains and vomiting. He was perspiring and unable to breathe. In spite of the fact that a hospital was within 5 minutes of the plant the man was not sent there and no physician was called. The nurse did not do any vital signs and only instructed him to lie down on the cot. His condition deteriorated over the next 2 hours. Another employee finally took him in a cab to a hospital and during the ride the man became unconscious. He was dead on arrival of a coronary occlusion.

The court held that the nurse was negligent in diagnosing his condition as a virus, solely based upon the man's history of a recent viral infection. The court also said that the failure on the part of the nurse to recognize that the employee's condition was worsening was gross incompetence.

Although not truly tested in nursing malpractice cases until recently, the rule is that the scope of the witness's knowledge and experience governs the question of qualification as an expert witness.

The question of overlapping knowledge and experience between the different disciplines or between different levels of the same discipline pose interesting questions. In a malpractice suit against a hospital and two orthopedic surgeons who had applied a cast to a fractured ankle, the court allowed a podiatrist to testify as an expert for the plaintiff in *Alexander v. Mt. Carmel Medical Center*.[32] The court held that the application and removal of casts were not the exclusive domain of orthopedic surgeons. Further, the function is one in which the various fields of medicine overlap. The plaintiff testified he had been taught the principles of cast application. He further testified that his testimony concerned the *minimum* standards of care common to cast application.

An important point should be made here, one well known to litigators, but somewhat of a mystery to nonattorneys. That is, that the case just discussed establishes a point of law applicable to both medical and nursing malpractice suits. In short, the parties involved may be different, but the legal point or issue, as it is applied to the facts, is what an attorney argues before a judge to persuade the court to rule in his favor. A point of law that may emerge from a case involving legal malpractice may have important lessons for nurses in their daily practice. A lawyer must look to the "lessons" far more frequently than the people involved. If no case law exists specifically bearing on the alleged point of nursing malpractice under discussion, the attorney must apply a point of law from a nonnursing context to the nursing situation. The issue in the case just cited is overlapping functions. You will see in the section Nurse Permitted to Testify Against Physician, below, how a nurse may be allowed to testify against a physician if her knowledge overlaps with medical knowledge.

In selecting an expert the attorney seeks an expert similar in position and experience to the defendant. Obtaining such an expert is not always possible. By selecting a similar expert the attorney has reasonable expectation that the testimony of the expert will be allowed or at least will survive a challenge.

A nurse practitioner unskilled in assessing pulmonary sounds would be unsuitable to testify as an expert where the issue was the alleged failure of an adult nurse practitioner to detect abnormal chest sounds. Conversely, a nurse experienced in assessing pulmonary sounds in an intensive care unit would be competent to give testimony in a case in which the sole issue requiring expert testimony dealt with the abnormal findings common to both an intensive care and a thoracic nursing unit.

Nurse Qualified to Set the Standard

When a witness is to testify as an expert a foundation must first be laid as to the qualifications of the witness. This is done by eliciting from the witness his educational and experiential background and current knowledge of the subject matter. Of course, the witness's knowledge must be that which was known at the time the injury occurred, not knowledge in existence at the time of trial which may be many years later.[33] An opposing attorney who objects to the lack of qualifications will object to the testimony being given and may take an exception to it, thus saving the issue for appeal in the event the jury finds against him. Likewise, an attorney whose witness was not permitted to testify, as in the following case, will challenge the exclusion.

A Kansas appeals court overruled the jury verdict for the defendant and sent the case back for retrial because the trial judge would not admit into evidence the testimony of a nursing college professor.[34] He sought to testify about the cause and treatment of decubitis ulcers. The trial court ruled that only a physician would qualify as an expert in matters of cause and treatment. The higher court stated:

> A nurse who has had wide experience with bedsores is in fact an expert
> as to decubitus ulcers since their prevention, treatment, and cure are

largely nursing duties. Thus, if a proper foundation is laid as to the nurse's experience with decubitus ulcers, she or he can qualify as an expert as to causation and as to such parts of treatment and cure that are performed by such nurses.

In a similar case a North Carolina court in *Maloney v. Wake Hospital Systems* ordered a new trial because the plaintiff's expert nurse was not permitted to testify as to the properties and effect of intravenous potassium chloride.[35] The plaintiff testified that she saw the nurse inject undiluted potassium chloride into her IV tube and as a result she had to have skin grafts which were only partially successful.

She offered the testimony of a physician who testified that if the undiluted solution was injected it would have caused immediate death, however, if the needle was outside the vein the injuries were consistent with exposure to the high concentration of the drug. The plaintiff also offered the testimony of a nurse who was then a fifth year pharmacy student and who had worked as both a staff nurse and an IV therapy nurse for many years.

During the trial the nurse was permitted to testify, but not in the presence of the jury, that she was familiar with parenteral fluids and their effects. She testified that, "It is the duty of all nurses to be familiar with IV fluids because they are the people who administer them. It is not the pharmacists or the physicians." The appeals court held, "The role of the nurse is critical to providing a high standard of health care in modern medicine. Her expertise is different from, but no less exalted than that of the physician."

In another North Carolina case, *Page v. Wilson Memorial Hospital*, decided shortly afterward, the appeals court held that a nurse who was licensed in three states (North Carolina, Kansas, and Missouri) and who had taught nursing in these states was qualified to testify against a nurse and an aide that placing a confused elderly patient on a bedpan in a chair and leaving her unattended for short periods was a violation of the nursing standard.[36] The defendants had unsuccessfully argued that her testimony was not representative of nursing care in the North Carolina community or any similar community.

No Expert Testimony Needed to Establish Standard

In cases where the lack of skill or care of the nurse is so grossly apparent or the treatment is such a common occurrence as to be within the comprehension of laymen, expert testimony will not be necessary.[37] A jury would be able to determine without the necessity for expert nurse testimony that the instruments used during surgery must be sterile before they are handed to the surgeon. Thus, in *Suburban Hospital Association v. Hadary*, expert testimony was not necessary where the act complained of was using an unsterilized needle for the withdrawal of tissue for a liver biopsy.[38] However, the specific methodology used to achieve asepsis would require expert testimony if that issue were material to a suit.

An Indiana plaintiff was successful in his appeal that the judge erroneously instructed the jury that they might consider only the evidence presented by expert witnesses.[39] The higher court held that no expert testimony was needed where the case was premised on a common negligence theory. Thus, it would be measured by the "reasonable man" standard and not by a "reasonable professional" standard as required in the majority of professional malpractice suits.

> The facts in *Emig v. Physicians' Physical Therapy Service* were that an 83-year-old woman who was recovering from hip surgery fell from a wheelchair because she was unrestrained and unattended by the attendant. She had been taken from the hospital to a facility that provided physical therapy. She fractured her hip and her estate brought suit in malpractice. The court held that just because an order was written by a physician it did not automatically become the type of medical decision that could only be analyzed by medical opinion testimony. The decision not to restrain the woman was not a medical decision, but rather a routine, ministerial decision which could be analyzed by a jury using their common knowledge and experience.

No Standard Established Because No Nurse Opinion Provided

There are times when plaintiff's attorney needs to provide the jury with expert opinion testimony, but is unable to do so because the attorney is unable to get an expert. This may be due to a number of reasons, chief of which is that no one will testify against the defendant. This does not necessarily mean that the plaintiff does not have a "good suit." However, the reason may be that the case is not strong and the potential witness does not want to be placed in a situation where his reputation will be compromised. That is not to say that the reputation of an expert is compromised just because the jury votes in favor of the opposing party. In a litigation trial one side must lose.

The failure to offer expert nurse testimony can be fatal to a case in that the judge will not submit it to the jury because of insufficient evidence. Plaintiff attorneys are frequently heard to say, "We've met our burden of proof by getting it into the hands of the jury; now it's up to them."

A North Carolina case *Vassey v. Burch* held that an *affidavit* (sworn statement) of the plaintiff's medical expert did not establish a deviation from nursing standards.[40] The legal issues in the case were the applicable standard of nursing care, and failure on the part of the nurse to use her "best judgment." In this case there was a key factor missing to aid the jury in their deliberations. A case that was meritorious did not even get to the jury.

The case involved a young child who was taken to his physician's office complaining of abdominal pain and nausea. The defendant physician gave him penicillin and sent him home with his parents with a prescription. Later in the day they went to the defendant hospital because the child complained of intense abdominal pain and vomiting. The mother told the emergency room nurse that the child probably had appendicitis, but the nurse said he did not. The nurse telephoned the physician, but told him the condition was not appendicitis. There was no objective evaluation of the child's condition as no physical examination or blood tests were ordered or done. After being advised of the child's symptoms the physician prescribed two injections over the telephone. The child went home and the next day his condition worsened so his parents took him to the surgeon's office. He was sent to the hospital where he was operated on immediately. He had peritonitis and a ruptured appendix.

An affidavit submitted by the plaintiff showed that the physician left the ultimate decision to the nurse. He said to keep the patient 30 minutes and send him home if he seemed better. The court said that there was no evidence that the nurse did not exercise her "best judgment" in concluding the child's condition was not appendicitis. The mere fact that the child's mother suggested appendicitis does not indicate that the nurse negligently exercised her professional knowledge in concluding otherwise. There was, however, dissenting opinion which held that the physician's testimony was sufficient to establish a deviation on the nurse's part.

Physician Not Permitted to Give Expert Nurse Opinion

Although there are decisions holding that the case failed because the plaintiff relied on a physician to establish the applicable nursing standard there are few reported decisions holding that a physician may not establish the nursing standard. However, in *Young v. Board of Hospital Directors, Lee County*, a Florida trial court held that a psychiatrist who was not familiar with the day-to-day practices of psychiatric nurses, such as monitoring and the method of checking the patient and monitoring hospital egress sites, could not testify as to a deviation from nursing standards.[41] In this case, a mentally ill person who eloped from a hospital and was hit by an automobile alleged that the nurses were negligent in permitting him to escape.

Nurse Permitted to Testify Against Physician

Within strict guidelines and at the discretion of the trial judge a nurse may be permitted to testify as an expert against a defendant physician. However, the nurse's opinion testimony must deal with knowledge that overlaps with medical knowledge. In addition, the depth of the nurse's knowledge must be equal or similar to that of a physician expert.

In one of the earliest cases to decide the extent of the nurse expert's knowledge, the Georgia Supreme Court in *Avet v. McCormick* held that the trial judge erred when he allowed the defendant's motion for a directed verdict at the close of the plaintiff's case because there was no expert testimony heard by the jury.[42] The plaintiff's expert, a registered nurse who had experience in withdrawing blood and inserting IVs in more than 2000 patients, was not permitted to testify. Suit was brought because the plaintiff developed a severe infection of the radial nerve after her physician withdrew her blood with an unsterilized needle. The case was sent back for retrial.

A subsequent Louisiana case, although not involving a physician, demonstrates the extent to which courts scrutinize the depth of knowledge of a nurse expert.[43] Suit was brought in *Belmon v. St. Francis Cabrini Hospital* against a hospital for the negligence of a laboratory technician and the hospital's nursing staff. The court permitted a nurse experienced in giving heparin and caring for heparinized patients to testify as to a patient's tendency to bleed. She was permitted to testify that the duty of the nurse increases as a patient's partial thromboplastin time (PTT) value increases. The higher court held that the lower court had improperly ruled that the nurse's testimony went beyond her expertise.

Finding the Expert Nurse

In the past there has been a general reluctance among physicians and nurses to give testimony against a colleague. This has been referred to as "the conspiracy of silence." However, if the case has merit the plaintiff's attorney can usually get a witness with the skill to further evaluate the case and testify at the trial. Most attorneys select an expert by utilizing some type of referral service. A number of nursing associations have established a list of expert nurses willing to evaluate cases and serve as experts at trials.

The Maryland Nurses Association was one of the first to establish such a service. The Maryland service, which was established in 1979, was modeled after similar services offered by the Arizona and New York Nurses Associations. The nurses associations of both California and Washington have developed guidelines for nurses who wish to serve as expert witnesses.[44]

Some legal organizations that provide continuing education for trial attorneys maintain a list of experts who are willing to testify and consult with them. The list includes disciplines other than nursing and medicine. In addition, a number of litigation publications which report trial verdicts include the names of the experts who testified for both the plaintiff and the defendant. Nurses who speak at professional education programs are considered a valuable resource.

The nursing associations that have established such a service provide educational activities for the nurses to enable them to provide their services. These activities include an explanation of their role as consult or witness, and some of the dynamics of pretrial and trial activity, such as depositions and direct and cross-examination testimony. It is, of course, the responsibility of the attorney who secures the services of an expert to prepare the expert for a deposition or trial.

After the expert has agreed to testify on behalf of the plaintiff or defendant the witness is asked to review relevant records that are made available. The expert writes a professional opinion indicating the merits of the case. The opinion may include citations from recent professional literature in support of the expert's opinion. Many states have enacted legislation creating some type of pretrial hearing on the merits of the suit and the written opinion of the nurse expert will be presented to the tribunal if it is favorable to the plaintiff's position.

There is another factor to be aware of with respect to witness services. There is a well-organized educational concept that scientific theory and principles change over a period of time. Therefore, an expert who has not practiced or updated scientific theories for over 5 years will be challenged. While there is no case law directly on this point it is discretionary with the trial judge whether the expert may testify. This is so whether the opposing counsel challenges the qualifications or not. However, if it may be persuasively argued that the testimony involves opinion which is essentially unchanged the expert will probably be allowed to testify. Persuasive arguments may be made by the attorney whose witness is being challenged that the expert should be qualified.

In the absence of unusual circumstances it is difficult to qualify a nursing expert who has not had clinical experience during the last 5 years if the key issue involves clinical decision-making. Contrast testimony in which it is established that the nurse has irrigated more than 500 T-tubes after hepatic surgery with the testimony of a nurse who has only done it on a few occasions. There is an inherent willingness to attach more credibility to the nurse who has the greater experience. The plaintiff's case is helped immeasurably when the nurse expert testifies that the facts involve a minimum standard below which no nurse's performance should fall.

Summary

Proof of a bad result or a mishap is not evidence of a lack of skill or negligence in the care rendered.[45] In the first instance, a patient's back pain may persist in spite of a technically correct laminectomy and in the second instance, a patient, through no fault of the hospital or its employees, may fall from a hospital bed.

Both defense and plaintiff attorneys turn to experts to evaluate the merits of their case. The plaintiff needs to determine if a suit exists and whether it is "winable." The defense needs to know the weaknesses of plaintiff's case and the defenses available. Once the case is evaluated the attorneys face the task of securing an expert to testify at the trial. The majority of cases require expert opinion testimony.

Until recently the courts readily accepted physicians as competent to establish a nursing standard and offer an opinion as to the deviation from accepted nursing practice standards. Recent case law has closely examined the expertise of the expert, especially as it relates to nursing malpractice. The body of case law that has evolved is some evidence of the strides nursing has made in articulating what is the particular domain of the nursing profession.

MODIFICATION OF THE LOCALITY RULE

The prevailing rule of law until recent years was the *locality* or *community rule* which stated that the degree of due care exercised by other physicians in the same or similar communities was the yardstick to be used in determining whether a physician had met the standard of care. The rule came into existence in 1880 when a general practitioner practicing in a town of 2500 treated a wound which required a high degree of surgical skill. The court in *Small v. Howard* said that it would be unfair to hold the physician to city standards as he lacked the opportunity to keep abreast of advancements in the profession and could not be expected to have the most modern facilities at hand when treating his patients.[46] In essence, the physician needs to comply with local custom as followed by other physicians in the same or similar community.

In a state that continues to strictly adhere to the locality rule the standard of care required of a nurse caring for a postoperative patient in a rural hospital would differ from that required in an urban facility. The narrow locality rule failed to recognize the concept that minimal professional standards should prevail and not an arbitrary measurement such as the local custom. The change in the locality rule applies to all health care professionals and not just general practitioners or specialists.

The first major departure from the locality rule occurred in 1967 when in a suit against a dental surgeon, a hospital, and the referring physician, who also participated in the operation, the court stated, "No longer is it proper to limit the definition of standard of care which a medical doctor or dentist must meet solely to the practices and customs of a particular locality, a similar location or a geographical area.[47]

The case, *Pederson v. Dumouchel*, involved a child who had suffered a broken jaw in an automobile accident and was seen in the emergency room by the "on call" physician who referred him to a dental surgeon. The hospital bylaws required the presence of a surgeon in the operating room when a dentist does surgery. The surgeon was not competent in the administration of general anesthesia and had left the responsibility and control of the anesthesia to the nurse anesthetist employed by the hospital. The child arrested during the procedure, did not recover from anesthesia for almost a month, and suffered permanent brain damage. The case held that no extraordinary or emergency conditions existed to justify the absence of a physician who was competent to administer the anesthesia. Such negligence could not be excused on grounds that other hospitals in the same locality practiced the same kind of negligence.

While a few states still follow the locality rule, the majority of court decisions have significantly modified it by extending the geographic area and taking into consideration such other factors as accessibility to other medical facilities that have more modern equipment, techniques, and experience. In short, the locality may be a factor for the jury to consider when deciding the applicable standard but it is not the only factor the jury considers. The local custom factor may be a jury consideration, but it does not constitute an absolute limit on the skill required. Vestiges of the locality rule still exist and allow the defendant to introduce into evidence the medical resources available to the physician. This conclusion was stated in a case that would allow the locality to be taken into account as one of the circumstances, but not as an absolute limit on the skill required.[48] The court in *Viita v. Dolan* stated:

> We are unwilling to hold that the physician is to be judged only by the qualification that others in the same village or similar villages possess. Frequent meetings of the medical society, articles in the medical journals, books by acknowledged authorities and extensive experience in hospital work put the country doctor on more equal terms with his city brother.

The recognition of a higher standard of care required of a specialist occurred in a landmark case involving a mother who, while attempting to get out of bed 11 hours after giving birth, fell and injured her legs. There was evidence in *Brune v. Belinkoff* that the condition resulted from an excessive amount of the spinal anesthetic, pontocaine, given by the anesthesiologist. At that time good anesthetic practice required the administration of 5 mg or less. The anesthesiologist argued that 8 mg was the local custom in a vaginal delivery. He further argued that the dosage discrepancy was due to a difference in obstetric technique. The custom in the rural setting was to apply pressure to the uterus during delivery, necessitating a higher level of anesthesia. The issue before the court was whether the specialist was to be judged by the standard as practiced in the rural setting.

The plaintiff argued successfully that the locality rule was invalidated because the hospital was located 50 miles from a world medical center, which was accessible and served as an excellent resource to provide information on the latest advancements in the field of anesthesiologic techniques and procedures. The court said the fact that specialists have access to advancements in their field tends to promote a certain degree of standardization within the profession.[49]

Thus, where the health care provider is a specialist, the standard by which his competence is judged becomes identical to that of another specialist practicing the same speciality. Where a cause of action is brought against a psychiatric nurse mental health clinical specialist the standard would be determined by another like specialist and not a generic psychiatric nurse or a coronary care nurse. The advent of mandatory continuing education for nurses and physicians will serve as a structured means to give evidence that they keep abreast of changes within the health care profession and in particular, the advancements relative to their area of practice.

Summary

The locality rule evolved in the 19th century in order to protect rural physicians. It was thought at the time that the country physician should not have to know as much as the city physician because he lacked access to the latest in theories of medical science and could not readily consult with colleagues who had superior skills and knowledge. At that time professional publications and avenues of continuing professional education were nonexistent. Most jurisdictions have abandoned or significantly weakened the rule.

Many courts argued that the rule fostered substandard care instead of encouraging doctors to elevate the quality of medical care. The courts also took note of the fact that other professions were not shielded by a similar rule.[50] Other courts have held that the basic concepts of medicine do not vary from state to state. One recent decision involving inadequate postoperative care held, "A pulse rate of 140 per minute provides a danger signal in Pascagoula, Mississippi, the same as it does in Cleveland, Ohio."[51]

Physicians as well as nurses have access to the latest theories in patient care management, and consultations are a common occurrence. As it stands in most jurisdictions, a plaintiff can have an expert from any state give expert opinion testimony. The expert must give testimony that reflects what should have been done in the particular case. This testimony will not reflect what the expert would have done, but what should have been done because it was the prevailing standard of care.

CUSTOM AND USAGE

The preamble section of the California Nurse Practice Act is unique, in that it sets out legislative intent in passing the statute. The preamble states, "It is the intent of the Legislature in amending the Act to provide clear legal authority for functions and procedures which have common acceptance and usage."[52]

The provision recognizes the custom and usage concept which has attached itself to the medical and nursing profession. *Custom* is legally defined as "a course of action; a practice which by its continued and unvarying habit has become compulsory and has acquired the force of a law."[53] *Usage* is defined as "following a uniform course of conduct which is reasonable and not contrary to law." The legal distinction between the two terms is in application. Thus, "custom" has acquired a mantle of legal respectability, whereas, "usage" is acceptable because it neither violates any law nor is inappropriate under the circumstances. However, practically the phrase is invariably stated, "custom and usage," especially as it relates to laws. The term "custom and usage" has significant impact on a determination of the standard of practice and frequent reference is made to the concept in discussion of the locality rule and its modification. The custom and usage concept stands as an important factor in determining the applicable standard of care. The burden of proving the existence of the concept is on the party attempting to make use of it in establishing the applicable standard.[54] While showing that a defendant followed a community custom may be a factor in a finding of no liability, its impact has been modified with the advent of specialization. It is clear from the recent decisions that the fact a defendant followed a practice or custom in the community does not negate a practice which is in and of itself negligent. In a Louisiana case the court rejected the customary practice defense argument.[55] The court in *Favalora v. Aetna Casualty Co.* found that the community standards were below a minimum acceptable level when an elderly woman was left unattended in the x-ray department. A review of her medical record would have revealed that she was at risk for falling and fainting and that measures should have been taken to prevent injury.

PUBLICATIONS AND TREATISES

In recent years it has become easier to have professional publications introduced into evidence during a trial to show the existence of a certain standard of care. The publications include nursing and health care texts and learned treatises. In addition, medical texts or other publications may be used to cross-examine (during examination of a witness by opposing counsel) an expert witness so long as the expert recognizes the publication as authorative, or in the alternative, a trial court judge takes judicial notice of the publication as authorative.[56]

In the precedent-setting *Darling* case an important legal issue was whether an expert witness could be required to answer questions asked by opposing counsel concerning recognized treatises in his area of professional practice where the expert did not purport to base his opinions on the views of these authorities.[57] The *Darling* court concluded that such cross-examination was permissible to insure that expert testimony will be a more accurate and effective tool in the attainment of justice. Prior to *Darling*, the Illinois courts held that an expert witness could only be questioned by opposing counsel about those texts on which the expert specifically based an opinion. Not all courts follow the *Darling* rule.

Professional publications may be introduced into evidence for the purpose of proving a fact in issue, such as, the standard of care requires that some type of restraining device should be placed on hospitalized infants so that they will not fall from their hospital crib. Professional publications may also be admitted for the sole purpose of discrediting the testimony of an expert witness. Either party may give testimony indicating the reasons why it is not always good practice, under certain circumstances, to follow the procedure indicated in the professional literature.

> A recent California case, *Lowry v. Henry Mayo Newhall Memorial Hospital*, illustrates that expert opinion testimony as well as judicial recognition (court's acceptance of the treatise into evidence) may be necessary to establish the applicable standard.[58] The family of a deceased patient sued the physician and hospital alleging that the physician deviated from the American Heart Association standards and guidelines for advanced life support. The family said that the physician who was in charge of the resuscitation effort for the patient's cardiac arrest departed from accepted procedure when he administered atropine rather than epinephrine. The plaintiff did not present any expert testimony that the use of the epinephrine rather than atropine would have dramatically increased the patient's survival chances. The defendant physician testified that she gave the atropine because it was one of the drugs which may be used initially to start the heart in the presence of no cardiac activity. In addition, the state had a statute providing immunity to designated numbers of a hospital emergency team if the resuscitation effort was carried out in "good faith."

ACCREDITATION STANDARDS AND REGULATIONS

Hospital licensing regulations, accreditation standards, and bylaws are admissible as evidence of the standard of care against which the conduct of a defendant hospital can be measured.[59] However, where state regulations governing hospitals, national hospital accreditation standards, or hospital bylaws are admitted into evidence, they do not *conclusively* establish a standard of care. Nonetheless, they are relevant to assist the jury in deciding what is feasible and what the hospital should have known regarding their responsibility for the care of the patient.[60]

> The landmark decision in the mid-1960s *Darling* case involved a number of factual and legal issues which continue to have significance for nurses. In

addition to allowing state regulations, hospital bylaws, and national hospital accreditation standards into evidence to show that the hospital should assume responsibility for quality patient care, the case determined the effect to be given to evidence concerning the custom or community standard of care and diligence. The court held that "Custom is relevant in determining the standard of care because it illustrates what is feasible, it suggests a body of knowledge of which the defendant should be aware, and it warns of the possibility of far-reaching consequences if a higher standard is required."[61]

The suit was brought on behalf of an 18-year-old college student who broke his leg while playing football. He was brought to the emergency room where his leg was placed in a cast by the physician on duty. Shortly after the cast application the patient's toes became swollen and dark in color with subsequent lack of feeling and were cold to the touch. Darling continued to be in considerable pain and during the next 3 days, his cast was "notched," modified, and bivalved at which time the Stryker saw cut both sides of his leg. At the trial, testimony was given indicating that blood and other seepage came from the cast and there was a terrible stench. He was transferred to another hospital 2 weeks after the injury, but in spite of efforts to save the leg it had to be amputated 8 inches below the knee.

The case held that the hospital, as an institution, was liable for its own (corporate) negligence in failing to enforce its own rules. The corporate bylaws required a consultation in such cases as Darling's and regulations and accreditation standards required the review of physician's work and these measures were not done. Under the doctrine of respondeat superior, which holds the employer responsible for the negligent acts of its employees, the court found that the nurses failed to do the standard tests to determine the color, sensation, and motion of the injured leg as frequently as the patient's condition warranted. Expert testimony indicated that the circulation to the injured leg should have been monitored more frequently. The plaintiff was successful in arguing that it was the "duty of the hospital nursing staff to see that these procedures were followed, and that either the nurses were derelict in failing to report developments in the case to the hospital administrator, he was derelict in bringing them to the attention of the medical staff, or the staff was negligent in failing to take action."

Competent and skilled nurses would have assessed the patient's findings and established a nursing diagnosis, that is, that there was impairment of circulation to the limb, which, if allowed to continue would result in a loss of the leg. An essential component of the nursing process requires that some nursing action be implemented in response to the patient's findings.

The *Darling* case set a precedent when it imposed an additional duty on nurses. The new theory of liability was accepted by the court. Darling was successful in his argument that the nurses had a duty to convey their findings to the attending physician, and if he failed to act, they should have reported their findings to the hospital authorities in order that the necessary intervention could be carried out. Nurses will be held liable where they fail to take reasonable measures to assure that patients receive adequate care, even when it requires a judgment with respect to the quality of medical care. The hospital must have the mechanism to assure and promote good care and its employees should comply with that mechanism in order to carry out their duty to report less than acceptable care and treatment.

Accreditation standards, such as those established by the Joint Commission on Accreditation of Hospitals (JCAH), represent a national standard and those hospitals accredited by the JCAH are held to comply with the standards set forth in its Accreditation Manual to maintain their accreditation status. The Manual covers many areas of a hospital's operation and in recent years it has included specific requirements for direct patient services, such as nursing, nuclear medicine and emergency care. It also includes standards for indirect services, such as building and grounds safety and medical record services. While it is essential that nurses working in a health care facility accredited by the JCAH be aware of the implications of the JCAH standards affecting nursing services, they should also have a working knowledge of the standards impacting on other departments and recognize their relationship to the nursing department. The format of the Manual sets out the standard and includes an interpretative statement indicating measures to be taken to comply with the provision.

The section on emergency services sets out in Standard I: "A well-defined plan for emergency care, based on community need and on the capability of the hospital, shall be implemented by every hospital."

The interpretation of the standard, specifically addressing patient transfers, states:

> No patient shall be arbitrarily transferred to another hospital if the hospital where he is initially seen has the means for providing adequate care. The patient shall not be transferred until the receiving hospital or facility has consented to accept the patient, and the patient is considered sufficiently stabilized for transport. Responsibility for the patient during transfer shall be established.[62]

Failure to comply with the JCAH standards does not violate any law or regulation and it has no enforceability under the law unless a law or regulation specifically requires compliance with the JCAH Standards. However, the JCAH can cite the facility for failing to implement the standards and can withdraw the accredited status. Loss of an accredited status will make the facility ineligible for governmental funding which is vital for the operation of every health care facility.

The health care industry is highly regulated, as are many other sectors of our society. Because of this fact, an initial point of reference in any determination of the standard of care should be the relevant federal and state statutes and governing regulations. Regulations are the mechanism whereby the more specific aspects of a legislative mandate are spelled out and are essential to the implementation of the law. The regulations are created by the quasigovernmental agency mandated under the provisions of the legislative act to write rules and regulations. They are necessary to carry out the intent of the legislature when they passed the statute.

For example, the Department of Health and Human Services is a federal agency which develops rules and regulations. On a state level, an example is the board of nursing. An important function of any nursing board is to write regulations that are necessary to implement the state's nursing practice act. The regulations are not law, but "have the force of the law."

It is the responsibility of the administrative agency to promulgate regulations. Promulgation is the process whereby the regulations are made known to the sectors of the health care industry who are required to comply with them. Final promulgation occurs after public hearings are held. Negligence aside, failure to comply with a regulation may result in receiving a citation from the regulatory agency and may put the license granted by the state in jeopardy.

Not all evidence is given the same weight or value. Some evidence by its very nature is more valuable because it proves more than other kinds of evidence. Such evidence may serve to absolutely preclude the opposing party from defending against it. For example, the law may regard noncompliance with a statute as: (1) negligence per se; (2) prima facie evidence; or (3) merely some evidence of negligence. The latter is the most frequently seen type of evidence (proof) presented during a trial. If it is negligence "per se," some jurisdictions will not allow the opposing party to introduce *any* evidence to rebut (argue against) the statute.[63] In the Leahy case below, the issue was whether the nursing practice statute was a "per se" law. Conversely, if the statute constituted prima facie (on its face) evidence, then the opposing attorney could offer his own evidence to rebut the statute. When evidence is classified as "merely some evidence of negligence" it simply means that the court or jury may believe it or not as it sees fit. It has no greater value than other "mere" evidence.

Those states that hold that negligence per se precludes opposing arguments must also find that the statute was enacted for the "safety" of a "specific class of persons." The following nursing malpractice case illustrates this principle. In *Leahy by Heft v. Kenosha Memorial Hospital*, a child who sustained severe brain injuries and his family sued three physicians and a hospital for the negligence of its nurses in caring for him in the nursery.[64] A jury found in favor of the plaintiffs, but a higher court overturned that verdict and sent the case back for a retrial because the jury instructions read to the jury included the nursing practice act.

The plaintiff's attorney who requested that the court read his prepared instruction to the jury wanted to have the court declare (by reading the instruction) the nursing statute a "safety" statute, thus establishing per se negligence. Having the statute declared negligence per se precluded the hospital from submitting any evidence showing it was not negligent. In short, the judge's declaration would mean that the negligence would have been an established fact. The strategy behind this request was to take the issue of negligence out of the hands of the jury who were the "triers of fact." Thus, they could not deliberate on the negligence issue because the court had already established negligence. However, the jury would decide on the facts whether the nurses violated the statute, that is, breached their duty.

The plaintiff was an infant who sustained brain injuries allegedly because of the negligent staffing of the nursery. It was the plaintiff's position that the hospital violated its duty because it permitted licensed practical nurses and technicians to cover the nursery without the presence of a nurse or a physician. The physicians and the hospital sought to show that the infant's condition was caused by events which occurred prior to his birth at the hospital.

The definitions section of the nursing practice act read:

Practice of professional nursing. The practice of professional nursing within the terms of this chapter means the performance for compensation of any act in the observation or care of the ill, injured or infirm, or for the maintenance of health or prevention of illness of others, which act requires substantial nursing skill, knowledge or training, or application of nursing principles based on biological, physical and social sciences, such as the observation and recording of symptoms and reactions, the execution of procedures and techniques in the treatment of the sick under the general or special supervision or direction of a physician, podiatrist, or dentist and the execution of general nursing procedures and techniques. Except as provided . . . , *the practice of professional nursing includes the supervision of a patient and the supervision and direction of licensed practical nurses and less skilled assistants* [emphasis added].[65]

Practice of practical nursing. The practice of practical nursing under this chapter means the performance for compensation of any simple acts in the care of convalescent, subacutely or chronically ill, injured or infirm persons, or of any act or procedure in the care of the more acutely ill, injured, or infirm *under the specific direction of a nurse, physician, podiatrist, or dentist* [emphasis added]. A simple act is one which does not require any substantial nursing skill, knowledge or training, or the application of nursing principles based on biological, physical, or social sciences, or the understanding of cause and effect in such acts and is one which is of a nature of those approved by the board for the curriculum of schools for licensed practical nurses.[66]

By incorporating the nursing practice statute the plaintiff's attorney sought to show that by "illegally" placing practical nurses and technicians in the nursery without the specific direction of a registered nurse or physician, the hospital was in violation of the statute. However, the higher court found that the statute was only a regulatory statute (intended only to regulate nurses). In order to constitute negligence per se it would have to be shown that it was a "safety" statute. Thus, if the statute were a safety statute, the negligence per se instruction would have been proper. However, if it were a regulatory statute, the instruction would have been improper, incorrectly influencing the jury in their deliberations.

A safety statute is defined as a legislative enactment designed to protect a specified class of persons from a particular type of harm. Further, a negligence per se statute must demonstrate that the "harm" was the type the statute was designed to prevent and the person injured was within the class the legislature sought to protect. In interpreting the legislative intent in enacting the statute the court held that the purpose of the statute was to regulate the nursing profession by creating a board of nursing and provide a licensing mechanism. Nothing in the statute showed a legislative intent to grant a citizen (the plaintiff) a right to sue for a violation of the nursing practice act. The right belonged to the state.

In sum, unless the statute is a safety law, not a regulatory law, violation of it will not absolutely, and without any other evidence, establish the element of negligence.

Summary

During a trial, evidence such as state and federal laws, as well as their regulations may be admitted into evidence to help the jury establish the applicable standard. Mandatory accreditation standards may also be admitted. An accreditation standard is considered mandatory where the government requires accreditation by a private group, such as JCAH, in order to be eligible for federal reimbursement of money. The Medicaid program requires such accreditation. In a suit the failure to comply with the standards is evidence of negligence.

It was not until 1965 that a case decided that JCAH standards were admissible. JCAH standards are not admissible against a hospital unless the hospital is bound to comply with them. Where a hospital is mandated to comply with them or where the hospital voluntarily has sought JCAH accreditation and received it, the court will recognize violation of the standards as negligence. Violations of state laws and regulations have long been admitted as evidence of negligence.

MANUFACTURER'S INSTRUCTIONS AND WARNINGS

While ordinarily the proof of the proper standards to be applied to a given set of facts would be established by expert testimony, recent courts have held that explicit instructions furnished by the manufacturer in a drug pamphlet or a standard drug resource such as the *Physicians' Desk Reference*, constitute proof of the proper standards. The law applies the same rule where instructions in the use and maintenance of equipment, such as cystoscope and total body scanners, are written by the manufacturer. Drug package inserts are an example of instructions written by a manufacturer and set out the information necessary for the prescribing and proper technique in the administration of these drugs. These include a warning on the hazardous nature of the drug. Where not contraindicated, the manufacturer's warnings or instructions are sufficient evidence and expert testimony is not required.

An Illinois court held it was a question for the jury where the evidence showed that the physician deviated from the manufacturer's instructions and the nurses did not monitor the patient.[67] In *Ohligschlager v. Proctor Community Hospital* a patient was admitted for treatment of severe gastroenteritis and the physician ordered the intravenous administration of a drug which was introduced into the intravenous tubing by the nursing staff. The patient had perivascular extravasation requiring a skin graft. At the trial the plaintiff's counsel introduced evidence that the drug company cautioned that no greater than a certain concentration should be given or there would be an increased risk of a localized thrombophlebitis. The manufacturer also cautioned that the patient should be observed and care should be exercised to prevent extravasation. The court held that

> Where a drug manufacturer recommends to the medical profession conditions under which its drug should be prescribed, states the disorders it is designed to relieve and precautionary measures which should be observed, and warns of dangers which are inherent in its use, a physician's deviation from such recommendations is prima facie evidence of negligence.

The liability of the nursing staff was shown when the nursing supervisor testified that it was the duty of the nurses to make periodic visits to the patient to insure that the intravenous was infusing properly. She stated that both infiltration and extravasation, as complications, were included in the hospital's staff orientation plan and that nurses had been warned of the dangers that are incident to the administration of certain types of intravenous fluids. She testified that, "if a patient complained of pain at the injection site the intravenous feeding should be discontinued immediately and that pain and swelling are symptoms of extravasation."

The drug manufacturer's accompanying literature has implication for the nurse as well as for the treating physician. Where the directions indicate a specific type of medication diluent or minimum amount of diluent the nurse is required to comply specifically with the directions. It is virtually impossible for the nurse to introduce into evidence different standards to apply in mixing the drug. The directions constitute prima facie evidence of the standard to be followed. Where the role of the nurse practitioner includes the prescribing or dosage modification of medications, the package inserts serve to notify the practitioner of the standards to be followed. Package inserts will have as much significance for nurse practitioners as their practice expands, as they do for the physician.

A physician may order a dosage of medication that exceeds the manufacturer's recommended dose, but this is generally done in situations in which the physician determines that an unusual dose is required to treat the patient's condition. It is not an uncommon practice for a physician to order a higher dose of antibiotic than that set out in the package insert when treating a virulent organism. For example, the treatment of a patient with a diagnosis of a septic hip following a failed total hip replacement, may require aggressive and unusual drug management. In order to overcome an allegation that the physician failed to comply with a standard established by the drug manufacturer, the physician would have to show that the prescribed treatment of the organism was compatible with acceptable, albeit, unusual medical practice. The physician's decision to treat the patient with higher doses would have to be supported by scientific studies or case reports in the medical literature justifying deviation from the usual course of treatment. Such treatment decisions are generic to the science of medicine and the court will not substitute itself for decisions within the province of medical judgment.

Where there is medically acceptable deviation from the usual treatment, the physician is required to monitor the patient with greater care to compensate for any increase in risk to the patient as a result of the unusual therapy. Determining whether and to what extent a physician could transfer this duty of care to a nurse would be a factual consideration. If the drug literature identified the drug as nephrotoxic, the duty of care would require the physician to order periodic laboratory tests to monitor the effect of the drug and diagnose any harmful adverse effects at as early a stage as reasonable. A strong argument can be made that the nurses caring for the patient would be liable for failing to monitor the patient's urinary output, via the routine monitoring activities, such as accurate intake and output measurement and specific gravity tests. Many drug manufacturers indicate the most serious complications by citing them in a black box warning section of the package insert which is designed to call the attention of the person reading the insert to particular information. A reasonable standard of care would require that the nurses caring for the patient knew or should have known the serious side effects of the drug, whether prescribed within a normal range or not.

Summary

The implication for nurses with respect to a manufacturer's instructions and warnings is that they must be familiar with the literature that accompanies drugs and equipment. Failure to operate a machine as recommended by the manufacturer may transfer the liability from the company to the nurse. The plaintiff's attorney will subpoena the instruction booklet or leaflet that was in effect at the time a drug was given or a machine was used in patient care.

There is some flexibility when deviating from a recommended dose of medication, but this applies only to the prescribing physician. If the physician can justify the reason for the deviation, such testimony will serve as rebuttal to the plaintiff's position. There is not a similar allowance afforded in the use of equipment.

SUMMARY

The legal elements which must be proven in a malpractice case, as in any other personal injury case, are duty, breach, causation, foreseeability, and damages or harm. All of the elements of a negligence suit must coexist before the plaintiff has met his burden of proof. The first two elements, duty and breach of that duty, are embodied in the standard of care concept. Simply put, these are the resources which will be used by both the plaintiff and the defense to establish the applicable standard to measure whether the plaintiff's duty was not met or whether the defendant nurse performed in a reasonably prudent manner.

A vast amount of case law deals with the legal issue of what constitutes duty and breach. Among the most fascinating issues are those determining when a nurse may serve as an expert—ascertaining who else may serve as a nursing expert and under what criteria a nurse may give expert testimony about the applicable "medical" standard. What is meant by physical evidence and what rules govern whether the court will allow such evidence are important factors in determining the outcome of a case. This chapter shows how the formal professional standards, such as professional association position papers and resolves, aid the jury in deciding on the standards and the criteria for applying them.

REFERENCES AND NOTES

1. Helling v. Carey, 519 P. 2nd 981 (WA, 1974). See also Albritton v. Bossier City Hospital Commission, 271 S. 2nd 353 (LA, 1972).

2. Texas & Pacific Railway v. Behymer, 23 S. Ct. 622 (1903).

3. Walski v. Tiesenga, 381 N.E. 2nd 279 (IL, 1978).

4. Black, H. (1979). *Black's law dictionary* (5th ed.). St. Paul, MN: West Publishing.

5. Polonsky v. Union Hospital, 418 N.E. 2nd 620 (MA, 1981), where a jury found against the hospital for the negligence of the nurse, but without the aid of expert opinion as to the standard.

6. Edelman, J. (June 1975). Negligence law and the required standard of care. *Hospital Medical Staff, 4*(6), 29.

7. American Nurses' Association (1973). *Standards of nursing practice.* Kansas City, MO.

8. 244 Code of Massachusetts Regulations 3.02. Massachusetts General Laws, Chap. 112, §80B (Acts of 1975), effective April 1979.

9. Black, H. (1979). *Black's law dictionary* (5th ed.). St. Paul, MN: West Publishing.

10. Gebbie, K., & Lavin, M. (1975). *Proceedings of the First National Conference on Classification of Nursing Diagnosis.* St. Louis: C. V. Mosby. Gordon M. (Sept. 1979). The concept of nursing diagnosis. *Nursing Clinics of North America, 14*(3), 487.

11. Goedecke v. Price, 506 P. 2nd 1105 (AZ, 1973); Walden v. Jones, 439 S.W. 2nd 571 (KY, 1969).

12. Lustig v. The Birthplace, WA, Kings County Superior Court, no. 83-2-07528-9, Sept. 19, 1983, 27 *The Association of Trial Lawyers of America Law Reporter,* 87 (March 1984), where liability was incurred by a nurse midwife for failing to refer a woman to a physician.

13. Burg, C. et al. (1968). Diagnosis by nurses. *Denver Law Journal, 45,* 469. See, however, Bruce, J., & Snyder, M. (1982) The right and responsibility to diagnose. *American Journal of Nursing, 82*(4), 645. For a discussion of the nurse practitioner in both an expanded role and as medical care extender and state-by-state analysis, see Weintraub, D. (Summer 1984). A new role for nurses: The nurse practitioner, *Medical Trial Technique Quarterly, 31*(1).

14. Devlin, M. (1983). Nurse practitioners and physician's assistants: Standard of care. *Journal of the American Medical Association 249*(5), 652.

15. Fein v. Permanente Medical Group, 175 *California Reporter 117* (CA, 1981); in Fein v. Permanente, 695 P.II 665 (1985) California Compensation Act was held constitutional.

16. For an interesting discussion of Fein, see Kelly, M., & Garrick, T. (Dec. 1984). Nursing negligence in collaborative practice: Legal liability in California. *Law, Medicine and Health Care, 12*(6), 260. Also see a rebuttal: Hershey, N. (Apr. 1985). Nurses in expanded roles vs. the responsibility to patients. *Law, Medicine and Health Care, 13*(2), 1.

17. Paris v. Kreitz, 331 S.E. 2nd 234 (NC, 1985). Also, note: at p. 245, addressing the issue of qualification of a physician to testify against the emergency room nurse the court said, "Physicians are clearly acceptable experts with regard to the standard of care for nurses." See also Thompson v. U.S., 368 F. Supp. 466 (1973), where the court held that a practical nurse who negligently permitted a patient out of bed, knowing of his weakness, was negligent. Under Louisiana law nurses and doctors are held to different degrees of care.

18. Samii v. Baystate Medical Center, 395 N.E. 2nd 455 (MA, 1979).

19. Marco, C. (Sept. 1983). Can nurse practitioner testify against physician? *Legal Aspects of Medical Practice, 11*(9), 2.

20. American Nurses' Association and Association of Operating Room Nurses (1973).*Standard of nursing practice: Operating room.* Kansas City, MO, Standard III, p. 7.

21. Pisel v. Stamford Hospital, 430 A. 2nd 1 (CT, 1980).

22. See Sermchief v. Gonzales, 660 S.W. 2nd 683 (MO, 1983). Interpreting the state nursing practice act, the court held that the activities performed by nurse practitioners at a clinic were not medical acts.

23. Anon. (Dec. 1979). Professional liability—a status report. *Hospital Medical Staff Advocate, 3*(4), 2.

24. Ibid.

25. Florida Statutes Annotated, §768.45(1) (FL, 1985).

26. Florida Statutes Annotated, §768.45(2)(a) (FL, 1985).
27. Dolan v. Galluzzo, 396 N.E. 2nd 13 (IL, 1979). But see cases cited in refs. 17 and 18.
28. Ibid, Dolan, p. 17.
29. Davis v. Schneider, 395 N.E. 2nd 283 (IN, 1979).
30. 2 Wigmore on Evidence §569 (3rd) (1940).
31. Baur v. Mesta Machine Company, 176 A. 2nd 684 (PA, 1962).
32. Alexander v. Mt. Carmel Medical Center, 383 N.E. 2nd 564 (OH, 1978).
33. See Johnson v. Hermann Hospital, 659 S.W. 2nd 124 (TX, 1983), where a nurse was permitted to testify concerning the proper standards of care for patients by nurses in surgical intensive care units (SICU). A 17-year-old girl who had undergone oral surgery was found cyanotic 2 hours after arriving in the postanesthesia room, suffering permanent brain damage. At the time of the incident the nurse was a licensed vocational nurse. She graduated from a bacclaureate nursing program a year later. However, she was permitted to serve as an expert because she had extensive experience over a 5-year period prior to the hospital incident in the care of patients with an endotracheal tube and in the proper method of suctioning such tubes.
34. Anon. (March 1982). Nursing practice act issues update. *Kansas Nurse 57*(3), 2.
35. Maloney v. Wake Hospital Systems, 262 S.E. 2nd 680 (NC, 1980).
36. Page v. Wilson Memorial Hospital, 272 S.E. 2nd 8 (NC, 1981).
37. Crawford v. Anagnostopoulos, 387 N.E. 2nd 1064 (IL, 1979).
38. Suburban Hospital Association v. Hadary, 322 A. 2nd 258 (MD, 1974).
39. Emig v. Physicians' Physical Therapy Service, 432 N.E. 2nd 52 (IN, 1982).
40. Vassey v. Burch, 262 S.E. 2nd 865 (NC, 1980).
41. Young v. Board of Hospital Directors, Lee County, FL, Jan. 26, 1984, no. 82-429.
42. Avet v. McCormick, 271 S.E. 2nd 833 (GA, 1980).
43. Belmon v. St. Frances Cabrini Hospital, 427 S. 2nd 541 (LA, 1983).
44. Northrop, C., & Mech, A. (March 1981). The nurse as expert witness. *Nursing Law and Ethics, 2*(3), 1. See also Anon. (Sept. 1983). MNA establishes nurse witness service. *Massachusetts Nurse, 52*(9), 1.
45. Scardina v. Colletti, 211 N.E. 2nd 762 (IL, 1965).
46. Small v. Howard, 128 Mass. 131 (MA, 1880).
47. Pederson v. Dumouchel, 431 P. 2nd 976 (WA, 1967).
48. Viita v. Dolan, 155 N.W. 1077 (MN, 1916).
49. Brune v. Belinkoff, 235 N.E. 2nd 793 (MA, 1968). See also Macon-Bibb County Hospital Authority v. Ross, 335 S.E. 2nd 633 (GA, 1985), where a Georgia hospital was liable for its nurse's negligence when a woman received intravenous dopamine that infiltrated causing burns and scarring. The intravenous was inserted into her wrist although the manufacturer recommended the use of a large vein. It further recommended that if a smaller vein was initially used, for example, in an emergency, the IV should be switched to a more suitable site as soon as possible. The hospital unsuccessfully argued that the nurse expert was not qualified to testify because she was not familiar with the standard in similar hospitals in similar communities. However, the court said that the locality rule did not apply because the legal issue concerned the judgment of professionals, rather than the adequacy of the facilities of a small hospital. The nurse also testified that an infusion pump should have been used rather than a drip chamber. See also Shepherd v. Delta Medical Center, 502 S. 2nd 1188 (MS, 1987), where a world reknowned anesthesiologist was not permitted to testify because the trial judge ruled that he did not have sufficient knowledge of the local standard of care. Immediately after the ruling the attorney asked to be permitted to seek another expert and begin the trial again. The judge denied this request, but a higher court, noting that the locality rule had been abolished since the judge's ruling, held that the expert's testimony should have been admitted even under the law at the time of the trial.
50. Morrison v. MacNamara, 407 A. 2nd 555 (DC, 1979).

51. Hall v. Hilbun, 464 S.E. 2nd 856 (MS, 1985).
52. Deerings Annotated California (Business and Professional) Code, §2725 (1974).
53. Black, H. (1979). *Black's law dictionary* (5th ed.). St. Paul, MN: West Publishing.
54. Western State Bank of South Bend v. First Union Bank & Trust Co. of Winamac, 360 N.E. 2nd 254 (IN, 1979).
55. Favalora v. Aetna Casualty Co., 144 So. 2nd 544, (LA, 1962).
56. Jones v. Bloom, 200 N.W. 2nd 196 (MI, 1972).
57. Darling v. Charleston Community Memorial Hospital, 211 N.E. 2nd 253 (IL, 1965); see also Lawson v. G. D. Searle & Co., 356 N.E. 2nd 799 (IL, 1976).
58. Lowry v. Henry Mayo Newhall Memorial Hospital, 229 *California Reporter 620* (CA, 1986).
59. Ibid., Darling, p. 259.
60. Ibid., Darling, p. 257.
61. Ibid., Darling, p. 257. See also Morris, J. (1942). Custom and negligence. *Columbia Law Review, 42,* 1147; 2 Wigmore on Evidence §§459 and 461 (3rd) (1940).
62. Joint Commission on Accreditation of Hospitals (1981). Emergency services. *Accreditation manual for hospitals,* Chicago: JCAH, pp. 23–24.
63. Prosser, W. (1971). *Law of torts* (4th ed.). St. Paul, MN: West Publishing, pp. 190–204; Anon. (1979). Pharmacy, *Hospital law manual* (p. 4). Germantown, MD: Aspen Systems Corp.
64. Leahy by Heft v. Kenosha Memorial Hospital, 348 N.W. 2nd 607 (WI, 1984).
65. Wisconsin Statutes Annotated §441.11(1), (1977).
66. Wisconsin Statutes Annotated §441.11(2), (1977).
67. Ohligschlager v. Proctor Community Hospital, 303 N.E. 2nd 392 (IL, 1972).

NURSING JUDGMENT

Judgment is the ability to make a decision and act on it. For example, when a careful, prudent person sees a one-way sign in the other direction at the entrance to a street, he will not want to drive down the street. Therefore, he stops the automobile and does not drive down the street. The person who proceeds down the street has acted carelessly and not as a "reasonable prudent person." In a negligence suit brought by an individual who was injured by such a motorist, the motorist's defense will be that he made a "mistake" or that the accident occurred because of "inadvertence."

In professional malpractice cases, one of the defense theories available is the "error in judgment" argument. While a defense attorney may argue that there has been an "honest" error in judgment, he never argues that there has been a "poor" judgment error. By arguing that there was an error in judgment the attorney is trying to convey to the jury that the physician or nurse made a mistake or miscalculation, but that no liability should be attached to it.

This chapter deals with cases in which professional judgment was assailed. The error in judgment argument raises a viable defense. However, common sense tells us that it cannot apply to every mistake or careless nursing action that results in injury. On one side of the coin is the error in judgment argument; on the other side is the plaintiff's argument that the action or inaction that caused the injury was based in negligence. Thus, the error in judgment defense argument says that the patient was injured, but not because the nurse was negligent.

Where the plaintiff's nurse expert testifies that the nurse's action was not based on essential knowledge, experience, or skill, that testimony is evidence that the patient care decision was not reasonable under the circumstances. If the root of the failure to make a clinical judgment or decision is based on a lack of assessment skill, or for having done no assessment at all, that constitutes pure negligence.

Until fairly recently the error in judgment defense was not applied in suits against nurses. The defense was first raised in medical malpractice suits. Both nursing and medical clinical decisions must be based on good patient assessments. It is most helpful to begin by examining the early medical cases from which the defense theory evolved and proceed to its application to nursing actions. It is important that the reader understand that there is not a "law for nurses" and a separate body of law for physicians. A lawyer works from legal principles and applies them to a given set of facts. The body of law that deals with errors in judgment evolved from medical malpractice cases and to understand the concept the reader must be able to see how the principles apply to a nursing context.

One of the earliest medical judgment cases was the New York case *Pike v. Honsinger*, decided in 1898, where liability was found for failure to make a careful examination.[1] An earlier New York case had found liability for failure to use an "approved method" in treating a patient's illness.[2] The concept of error of judgment is a theory raised by the defense. The plaintiff attempts to overcome it by attacking the facts surrounding the examination or assessment phase and the method or manner in which nursing care or medical treatment was given. However, in the area of health care, the law has long recognized that patients may suffer harm or that complications may arise in the absence of negligence on the part of the nurse or doctor. Both case law and statutes refer to such harm as an unfortunate outcome. In negligence cases that involve a specific medical therapy choice, the physician will be given considerable latitude in the selection of treatment. In *Potock v. Turek*, the court said

> physicians and other professionals practice the arts and must be allowed a wide range in the exercise of judgment and discretion. They cannot insure results and cannot be held liable under the law for honest errors of judgment made while pursuing methods, courses, procedures, and practices recognized as acceptable by their professions.[3]

As in all malpractice cases the standard of care must be established and where the choice of therapy falls below the standard of care of a reasonable physician, the defense theory of error in judgment will not prevail. Conversely, an error in judgment made in accordance with recognized standards, although it is later shown to be incorrect, is not actionable.[4]

To date, few cases have found a nurse liable for failing to establish a "nursing diagnosis."[5] The fact that the courts have not made reference specifically to the concept of nursing diagnosis should not lull nurses into thinking that liability will not ensue for harm that results from the failure of the nurse to do a proper assessment or employ judgment in analyzing data to identify a nursing problem. *Judgment* was previously defined as the ability to make a decision, or form an opinion objectively and wisely,[6] especially in matters affecting action. The ability to make a decision and act upon it is the basis of all learned professions.

In nursing there is a two-tiered test for evaluating nursing competency. This involves possession of scientific theory and skills, and an ability to transfer the scientific theory to a patient situation or work environment. This two-tiered scrutiny of nursing competency begins during the formal educational process and continues throughout the nurse's professional life. The law expresses this process in terms of a duty—specifically that the nurse owes a legally defined duty to the patient. This is a duty to **possess** the required knowledge and skill such as is possessed by the average member of the profession, and a duty to **exercise** ordinary and reasonable care in the application of such professional knowledge and skill. The nurse need not possess extraordinary learning and skill or exercise the highest possible degree of care; she must merely exercise average skill equal to that of like practitioners. An argument that the harm to the patient was the result of a "mere error in judgment" or an "honest mistake" will not prevail where the plaintiff is able to show that the real cause of the harm was due to a lack of knowledge and skill, or the failure to act on that knowledge and skill in a prudent manner.

It is not uncommon for the plaintiff's attorney to object to the phrase, "mere error in judgment" when it is raised as a defense by the defendant's attorney. The argument is made that the word, "mere" tends to minimize the error in judgment in the minds of the jury. As in all negligence cases, the facts surrounding the clinical decision will determine the outcome of the error in judgment defense. In short, there is no legal rule that an error in judgment precludes liability on the part of the nurse. A mistake does not excuse negligence or ignorance.

In order for a nurse to make a reasonable judgment it follows that sufficient and relevant data are known and the nurse possesses sufficient decision-making skills to arrive at a judgment. Poor assessments, whether based on faulty skills or lack of completeness, almost surely lead the way to liability. Complete assessments form the basis for good decision making. If the harm that has been suffered by the plaintiff can be traced to an inadequate assessment or a failure to skillfully diagnose the nursing problem, then the error in judgment defense strategy will not be successful.

The fact that two professionals of the same discipline may not concur in the method of treatment is not sufficient to create liability when the patient fails to respond to the prescribed treatment or care, or responds adversely. For instance, one physician may recommend surgery for repair of a torn ligament whereas another may recommend application of a cast. So long as both forms of treatment are acceptable and recognized methods of treatment, the argument that the one selected that proved unsuccessful was the result of poor judgment will not stand. One nurse may treat a decubitus ulcer by employing Op-Site care while another may use saline or Betadine soaks or karaya powder.[7] Both approaches are recognized nursing treatments. Liability may also attach when it is shown that the selected methodology was not carried out in a skillful manner. One medicolegal writer cites a case in which the family of a deceased patient settled out of court after the mortician called the family to view the decedent's decubitus ulcerations which were so severe that bone was visible.[8]

A nurse is professionally and legally bound to carry out the lawful, that is, medically acceptable physician's order. A fairly significant proportion of clinical judgments made by nurses involve discretion. *Discretion* is the power or right to decide or act according to one's own judgment.[9] The term "discretion" is in contrast to a compulsory or mandatory requirement. There are many examples of situations where a nurse in carrying out a physician's order uses discretionary authority, but perhaps the most common one is deciding whether to use the minimum or maximum dose of a medication when the physician has written it in a "range of dose" form. Custom, so long as it is compatible with practice standards, may allow a certain practice in one clinical facility and not another. Further, the extent of discretionary practices may vary according to the practice setting or facility. In summary, the error-of-judgment strategy may be a viable defense, but it does not have broad application. Its inclusion in jury instructions has been successfully challenged in some cases where it has been inappropriately used. A nurse will not be liable for the exercise of good judgment.

In a recent North Carolina case, *Currie v. U. S.* the next of kin brought suit against a Veteran's Administration hospital for the negligence of its psychotherapists after a client suffering from posttraumatic stress disorder killed a co-worker after he was fired from his job.[10] The family of the dead man who was killed by a random shot alleged that the hospital had a duty to seek the client's involuntary commitment and the failure of the psychotherapist to do so in the presence of threats against both the IBM medical research facility where he worked and the psychotherapists themselves constituted actionable negligence. Applying a "psychotherapist judgment" rule (the standard to be applied to the facts of the case) the court said "liability should not be imposed on therapists for simple errors in judgment . . . instead, under a psychotherapist judgment rule, the court must examine the good faith, independence and thoroughness of a psychotherapist's decision not to commit a patient in determining whether psychotherapist is liable to third parties for the failure to commit a mental patient."

Citing earlier law the court said that "policy considerations favor giving psychotherapists, just as directors of a corporation, significant discretion to use their best judgment. . . ." In deciding whether a defendant acted in "good faith" entails an examination of the following factors: (1) the competence and training of the reviewing psychotherapists; (2) whether the relevant documents and evidence (of the patient's case) were adequately, promptly, and independently reviewed; (3) the psychotherapist's efforts to check his judgment against the opinions and advice of the other psychotherapists; (4) whether the evaluation was made in light of the proper legal standards (state laws) for commitment; and (5) other evidence indicating the physician's good or bad faith.

Factually, the court found the therapist competent and learned that he had the client's case reviewed twice by seven board-certified psychiatrists. In addition, the client had made serious and direct threats against some of the therapists themselves. The court said that the therapist's decision not to commit in the presence of serious personal risk to themselves was strong evidence of the utmost good faith. In summary, the court said that the proper test in measuring whether the therapist's judgment constituted negligence was the "good faith" test and under the facts of the case the defendants could not be found to have acted in "bad faith."

HONEST ERROR IN JUDGMENT RULE

A number of courts in this country have adopted a rule of law that allows the judge when giving instructions to the jury at the end of the trial to include an instruction that they may find the physician or nurse committed an "honest error in judgment." The instruction given generally includes words to the effect that medicine is not an exact science and some latitude should be given to the physician in the exercise of discretion in treatment decisions. Further, the instruction states that medicine is an art and not a science, and therefore a physician is not responsible for an honest error in judgment. The rule itself, and specifically the inclusion of the qualifier, "honest," has been subject to much analysis and attorneys for the plaintiff frequently try to exclude or limit its application. They argue that the rule will serve to excuse, in the minds of the jury, all harm, regardless of the extent of negligence proven by the plaintiff. Further, if a person suffers harm, whether by an "honest" error in judgment or otherwise, that individual should receive redress. Their main objection to an honest error in judgment instruction is that honesty speaks to a person's character and reputation. In most malpractice suits the health care provider's character and reputation are not germane to the negligence issue. In a negligence suit when the defendant raises the error-in-judgment defense, the issue is, and must always be, whether the defendant's action constituted negligence because it failed to measure up to the standard of accepted practice.

Some courts have overturned decisions because the standard of "best" judgment was used. One court held, "A standard (charge) which only requires the physician to use his best judgment is no standard at all."[11] Challenges to such instructions are based on the fact that the professional's "best" judgment may not measure up to accepted practice standards. Another court ruled that the jury instruction that a *presumption* that a physician possessed sufficient learning and skill and that he properly applied that degree of learning and skill was prejudicial to the plaintiff's case.[12] Such an assumption places too great a burden on the plaintiff. The *Pike v. Honsinger* case held that a medical malpractice theory was based on three component duties that a physician owed to his patient. They were identified as: (1) a duty to possess the requisite knowledge and skill such as is possessed by the average member of the medical profession, (2) a duty to exercise ordinary and reasonable care in the application of such professional knowledge and skill, and (3) the duty to use his best judgment in the application of his knowledge and skill.[13]

Best Judgment

A number of cases have addressed the best judgment argument. In one suit in which the plaintiff alleged that the physician was negligent in diagnosing and treating his poliomyelitis, the court ruled against the plaintiff.

> The plaintiff in *Cunningham v. State of New York* alleged that he had residual disabilities that were attributed to the failure to diagnose polio in a timely manner. The court held that New York malpractice law required that a physician use his "best judgment." "This does not mean he can be held liable for a mere error in judgment; it only means that he is liable if he does not do what he thinks is best to do after he has made a careful examination."[14]

In error in judgment cases the courts have had to respond to the "hindsight" argument.

In *Riggs v. Christie,* a case in which the physician did not diagnose peritonitis after an appendectomy, the court held, "In the usual case where matters of professional judgment are involved, a tribunal of fact, whether court or jury, unassisted by expert testimony or evidence from the profession concerned, should not retrospectively substitute its judgment for that of the person whose judgment had been sought and given." The jury was instructed that a

> physician possesses and will use the reasonable degree of learning skill and experience which is ordinarily possessed by others of his profession . . . and that he will in cases of doubt use his best judgment as to the treatment to be given in order to produce a good result. He does not warrant a cure.[15]

Adopting the rule in a later case, a court held a physician liable for failing to diagnose osteomyelitis and treat the condition properly.[16] As in any malpractice case, the facts (in this case these included a prolonged period of time during which the patient was being treated by the negligent physician) are important in finding for or against the defendant.

In *Delaney v. Rosenthal,* the negligent physician treated the patient's finger over a period of 16 visits. When the patient went to another physician his condition was immediately diagnosed by x-ray examination and the insertion of drains in the finger brought about immediate relief of his intense pain and swelling. The immediate good results obtained by the second physician were significant in finding that the first physician did not use his best judgment.

Juries have been reluctant to find against the defendant in matters of judgment unless the facts clearly mandate such a finding.

In *Cooper v. U.S.,* in which the patient was being treated over a long period the physicians were found to be negligent for failing to diagnose brucellosis.[17] The patient was hospitalized for a period of 15 months in a Veterans Administration hospital and during that time the physicians failed to order bacteriology tests although brucellosis was not uncommon in the region and the man's history as a meat packer was known. Relying on previous holdings the court held that: "A physician is entitled to an error of judgment or an honest mistake. However, the failure to make the brucellosis diagnosis in 1964 is more than an error judgment and does constitute negligence."

In a frequently cited case, *DeFalco v. Long Island College Hospital,* the plaintiff brought suit against an eye surgeon and a hospital for negligence of one of its nurse employees. The judgment issue arose in a medical context, but was not applicable in the nursing context.[18] The plaintiff was unsuccessful against both the hospital and the physician. The patient, who was operated on for the removal of a cataract, developed a postoperative infection which subsequently caused corneal scarring. He had to have the eye enucleated after several years of unsuccessful treatment for the infection. He lost his case against the eye surgeon when the court held, "A mere error of judgment, absent negligence, or a bad result would not impose legal liability on the doctor or hospital. From time immemorial, the disciplines of medicine have been recorded as an inchoate melange of science and art. The practice of clinical medicine involves the experimental study, diagnosis and treatment of disease. By undertaking to perform a medical service, a surgeon does not, nor does the law require him to guarantee a good result."

Although this case did not raise the error in judgment issue in a nursing context it illustrates the strict legal requirement that the plaintiff has the burden of proving a connection between the act and the resultant harm. A witness testifying on behalf of the plaintiff stated that she saw a nurse pick up an eye patch which had fallen to the floor and apply it directly to the patient's eye. The organisms cultured from the patient's eye were identified as *Enterobacter* and *Staphylococcus albus*. In spite of this graphic testimony the plaintiff lost his suit against the hospital because he failed to show that the fallen patch had picked up the organisms from the floor. The fatal flaw in the plaintiff's case was that he failed to prove a causal connection between the act and the harm caused. In commenting on the nurse's action the court stated

> It would be a matter of common knowledge that such an act was unsanitary, and obviously not in accord with good nursing practice. The act of placing a presumably soiled eye patch over a patient's eye, by its very nature bespeaks improper treatment and malpractice. Nevertheless, such an obviously unsanitary procedure lacked the requisite expert testimony to prove that the presumably unsterile eye patch carried the *Enterobacter* and *Staphylococcus albus* organisms from the floor to the plaintiff's eye and caused the infection.

Addressing the error in judgment issue in the context of the assessment process, a 1976 case found no cause for liability against physicians who treated a patient in an emergency room.[19] The decedent in *Ulma v. Yonkers General Hospital* went to the hospital emergency room complaining of abdominal pain and hyperventilation. He was examined by an intern who diagnosed his condition as gastroenteritis and prescribed Compazine. The patient, however, remained in the emergency room because he said he felt too ill to go home. His primary physician was contacted and went to the hospital where he thoroughly examined him and confirmed the original diagnosis. The physician elicited a careful history, reviewed previous tests, listened to the patient's heart, examined a vomitus specimen, palpated his abdomen and tested for a possible aortic aneurysm. The discharged patient collapsed next to his car in the parking lot and died. An autopsy revealed that the man had occlusive coronary arteriosclerosis and the medical examiner said his findings were consistent with "electrical death of the heart." The court found that the hospital intern and primary physician exercised due care in the diagnosis and treatment of the decedent and that his death was due to a tragic eventuality beyond the control of medicine today. Citing prior decisions, the court said, "Doctors are not liable for mistakes in professional judgment, provided that they do what they think best after careful examination."

Jury Instructions on the Issue of Judgment

At the conclusion of a trial the judge gives instructions to the jury in order to aid them in their deliberations. The instructions relate to the law to be applied in the case. Attorneys for both parties submit requests to the judge as to the wording of specific jury instructions. It is not uncommon for an appeal of a case to be based on a jury instruction. The objection may be because one lawyer was not allowed to have requested instructions submitted to the jury or because instructions were given that were objected to by a lawyer. It is a strict proposition of law that a party is entitled to have an instruction given that supports a theory on which the case is based or defended. Instructions given to a jury can be confusing and technical, especially when the case deals with complex legal issues, and much has been written in legal journals with respect to the inability of juries to follow and comprehend complex instructions. Instructions should not be confusing or misleading.

In a recent case the jury verdict was upheld on appeal in favor of the defendant hospital for the alleged negligence of its nurses.

> The plaintiff in *Whitaker v. St. Joseph's Hospital* appealed the case based on the instructions given to the jury.[20] The suit was brought when a woman fell or jumped from the window of her hospital room. The plaintiff's attorneys argued that the following instruction was ambiguous, confusing and misleading: "If any of the nurses employed by St. Joseph's Hospital, in rendering care and treatment to the plaintiff, Dorothy Whitaker, exercised that degree of care and skill which would be exercised by similar nurses in same or similar communities, under same or similar circumstances; and if, while exercising that degree of care and skill, made a mistake or error of diagnosis or a mistake or error in judgment, this would not constitute negligence on the part of such nurses while practicing their nursing profession." The plaintiff's attorneys argued that such an instruction, in effect, said that "if these nurses made a mistake—no matter how gross the error— it would not constitute negligence." The higher court held that such an interpretation of the instruction was totally unjustified.

The courts have not always applied a *professional* standard of care in suits against nurses. They were more apt to apply a simple negligence standard than a professional standard. One of the earliest professional standard cases was a California case decided in 1955.[21]

> In that case, *Cooper v. National Motor Bearing Co.*, a nurse was liable for failing to refer an employee, who suffered an injury to his forehead and which ultimately evolved into a cancerous lesion, to a physician. The nurse

failed to initially probe the wound and continued to care for the injury for several months in spite of the fact that it failed to heal.

The nurse was held liable for failing to comply with nursing standards. The defendant nurse unsuccessfully argued that the instructions given to the jury applied a medical standard because the charge referred to a "diagnosis." The instruction stated: "A patient is entitled to an ordinary careful physical examination, such as the circumstances, the condition of the patient and the nurse's opportunities for examination will permit. If there is a reasonable opportunity for examination, and the nature of the injury or ailment can be discovered by the exercise of ordinary care and treatment, then the nurse is answerable for failure to make such discovery." A second instruction was phrased, "The same degree of responsibility and the same duty of care is imposed upon a nurse in the making of a diagnosis as is imposed upon her in the prescribing and administering of treatment." A court of review held that the instructions were correct because the jury properly understood the instruction to mean that a "nurse's diagnosis of a condition must meet the standard of learning, skill, and care, to which such nurses practicing in that community are held."

A 1977 case decided in a California court is interesting both factually and because of the wording of the jury instruction which were objected to by the plaintiff. The suit was brought against the two treating physicians and the hospital for the nurse's alleged negligence. The trial court found in favor of the defendant hospital and the challenge by the plaintiff was unsuccessful on appeal.

The decedent, in *Fraijo v. Hartland Hospital*, a 39-year-old woman with a history of chronic asthma, was treated twice in the hospital emergency room in June 1973.[22] She suffered a third acute asthmatic attack in late June and was treated in the emergency room for 2 hours prior to being admitted to the hospital. During that time she received standard treatment which included dextrose and water for dehydration, aminophylline and Bronkosol to dilate her lungs, and intermittent positive-pressure breathing (IPPB) treatment. She was also given Vistaril for anxiety. Two physicians who treated her in the emergency room later stated that they diagnosed her respiratory distress as moderate and did not consider her to be in mortal danger.

She was admitted at 10 P.M. and one of the orders was for 75 mg Demerol with 25 mg Phenergan every 4 hours, PRN for pain. Drug literature pertaining to the use of Demerol was allowed into evidence. It said that in patients having an acute asthmatic attack Demerol should be used with extreme caution, as even normal doses may produce apnea. Shortly after being sent to the unit the patient was given a steroid drug because of an increase in her pulse and respirations. The physician asked the nurse to inform him of the response to the drug. Just before 11 P.M. the patient had a dramatic change in her condition which was manifested by an increase in her vital signs, dyspnea, and increased anxiety. The nurse did not call the physician as she testified she was too busy caring for the woman. At 11:05 P.M. the patient complained of chest pain. At that time the nurse in charge testified that she called the physician and inquired whether the Vistaril given in the emergency room had any effect on the patient. She testified that she was informed that it had limited effect. The nurse did not at that time tell the physician of the dramatic change in the patient's condition. The charge nurse directed the medication nurse to administer the Demerol which she did. The medication nurse, who was a licensed practical nurse (LPN), testified that she knew that Demerol had a depressing effect on respiration. She said that she gave it to relieve the chest pain and before she gave it she spoke with one of the physicians who told her to go ahead and give it. However, the physician denied speaking with either the charge nurse of the LPN about the patient's condition and denied that he assured the medication nurse that it was all right to give the Demerol. Both physicians testified that given the severity of an asthmatic attack, the administration of Demerol would have been contraindicated. A short time after the Demerol was given the patient became cyanotic, had a seizure, and went into respiratory arrest. Resuscitation was unsuccessful and she was pronounced dead at 12:15 A.M. Her physician refused to sign the death cerficiate, stating he did not know why the patient died. No autopsy was done and when the coroner's office investigated a specific cause could not be identified.

An expert witness for the plaintiff testified that the decedent's medical care was substandard and that the administration of Demerol was the final incident of substandard practice. This was disputed by experts testifying on behalf of the defendants. One of these experts found no fault on the part of the nurses in failing to notify the physician of the patient change as frequently nurses wait a short period to see if stabilization will ensue. Further, the witness declined to characterize the exercise of *discretion* by the nurse in giving the Demerol as substandard practice. Both experts for the defense testified that the intramuscular injection could not have caused the arrest within 5 minutes of its administration and that other causative factors, such as pulmonary embolism, myocardial infarction, or spontaneous pneumothorax may have led to the patient's death.

The plaintiff, after losing at the trial level, based his appeal on two different instructions given to the jury. There was no objection to the standard instruction on "Duty of a Nurse." The objections were based on the argument that two instructions ordinarily applicable to physicians and surgeons were tailored to include a nurse. One entitled, "Medical Perfection Not Required" stated:

> A physician or nurse is not negligent simply because their efforts prove unsuccessful. It is possible for a physician or nurse to err in judgment, or to be unsuccessful in their treatment without being negligent. However, if a physician or nurse does not possess that degree of learning and skill ordinarily possessed by physicians and nurses of good standing practicing in the same or a similar locality and under similar circumstances, or if they fail to exercise the care ordinarily exercised by reputable members of their professions in the same or a similar locality and under similar circumstances, it is no defense to a charge of negligence that they did the best they could and their efforts simply proved unsuccessful.

The other, entitled, "Alternative Methods of Diagnosis or Treatment," read as follows:

> Where there is more than one recognized method of diagnosis or treatment, and no one of them is used exclusively and uniformly by all practitioners of good standing, a physician or nurse is not negligent if, in exercising their best judgment, they select one of the approved methods, which later turns out to be a wrong selection or one not favored by certain other practitioners.[23]

In the appeal the plaintiff's attorney argued that the instructions relative to a nurse's error in judgment and the nurse's selection of one of several alternative treatment options was an extension of a nurse's professionalism into the realm of *independent* judgment and was therefore improper. In essence, the plaintiff objected to the physician delegating a *discretionary* exercise of judgment to the nurses. Ruling in favor of the defendants, the court said that when the physician wrote the "as needed" PRN order the physician was relying on the nursing staff to observe the patient and make an independent judgment to give the medication or not give it. Further, the court said that if the standard of medical practice "permits" the physician to confer on nurses in some medical situations, the exercise of "independent" judgment, then the nurses, when acting in those situations must be accorded some latitude in decision making. The jury instructions, objected to by the plaintiff, articulated that latitude. To hold nurses to a standard that did not recognize any flexibility in nursing judgments would impose on nursing a standard of care that exceeds that applicable to the medical profession. An error of judgment instruction tells the jury that an error in medical or nursing judgment is not considered in a vacuum, but must be weighed in terms of the professional standard of care.

In summary, *Fraijo* holds that sometimes, even in the absence of negligence, a patient may respond adversely to the nursing management of his problem. Adverse response alone is not proof of negligence. In the presence of negligence, doing "one's best" will not thwart a negligence allegation.

Another lesson of the *Fraijo* case is that if the law (both case law and statutory law) permits a nurse to make an "independent" clinical decision the standard is whether other nurses may have done the same under the circumstances. A nurse is not bound to do exactly what another nurse would do, only to select one approach among several that exists at the time and is reasonable. There must be some latitude in decision making.

Although much of case law refers to these types of judgments as "independent" judgments, they would more correctly be referred to as "discretionary judgments," which are defined as judgments that are authorized or delegated. Just as medical judgments are inherent in the practice of medicine, so nursing judgment is inherent in nursing practice. A number of state nurse practice acts incorporate the judgment component in their statutory definition of nursing practice.[24] Apart from the legal implication of a judgment itself, a physician may incur liability for the act of delegating. Traditionally, a physician has not been permitted to delegate the authority to make a medical judgment. Note that in this last case the court spoke in terms of medical practice standards permitting a physician to delegate discretionary judgment when carrying out a specific medical treatment order. A physician may be liable for delegating a medical activity, whether a judgment or other medical skill, if such delegation does not conform to accepted medical practice. It is not inconceivable that a nurse may be held liable for carrying out the delegated medical act if the nurse knew or should have known it was not within customary practice. The law has not addressed the issue of the delegatory limits of medical practice.

PHYSICIAN'S ORDERS

Much of the early case law dealing with liability of nurses for carrying out physician's orders involved injection cases. The liability was for the lack of nursing skill in the administration technique. Because the physician has a right to expect that a nurse is competent to carry out that particular nursing skill the courts have been fairly consistent in not holding the physician liable when the harm resulted from improper administration technique. Much of existing law holds the physician solely liable for writing an incorrect medical order. However, where a nurse implements a *patently* incorrect order both disciplines may be held liable. Nurses will be held liable if they blindly implement a physician's order. The courts increasingly have begun to recognize that the scientific knowledge base on which nursing relies increases the duty nurses owe to the health care consumer. Liability for professional acts carried out in a negligent manner has increased since nurses' "handmaiden to the physician" image has been shed. It is to be expected that, as nurses testify about nursing skill and knowledge, some of nursing's professional terminology and tenets will appear in legal opinions. Attorneys have begun to utilize nurses, rather than physicians, as expert witnesses when testimony is needed to establish nursing skill and knowledge.

A nurse transcribing a medical order always checks it for clinical accuracy. This means that the order, if it is a medication order, is within the dose range and time sequence ordinarily given in a similar patient situation. Any question is quickly referred to the ordering physician for confirmation. The nurse also checks that the order is completely written and appropriate for the patient's condition. For example, a physician, after reviewing the chest films of an intensive care unit (ICU) patient, may order Lasix for a patient already on Digoxin. Frequently, the orders are written before the morning laboratory slips are reported to the unit. If, after reviewing the laboratory slips the potassium levels are low the

ICU nurse knows that it would be potentially harmful to give both these potassium-depleting drugs and the order is not carried out until the ordering physician is informed of the new findings. The physician may then order potassium supplements. A similar problem can arise in an ICU setting where more than one physician does the ordering. Frequently it is the nurse who notes a discrepancy in the orders left by different physicians. Such orders should be reviewed with great care.

It is not only new orders that have to reviewed carefully. Older or existing orders need to be reviewed to determine their timeliness. Because nurses provide a continuum of care as opposed to the daily visit by the physician on the general unit, they are in a unique position to observe the patient for changes in status. Subtle changes observed by the nursing staff may elude the physician. Most physicians recognize the built-in liability protection when nurses collaborate with them about patient needs.

A judgment based on the above factors is not to be confused with a medical diagnosis made by a physician. Both nurses and physicians can interpret arrhythmias in an ICU. The nurse treats it in accordance with established protocols, whereas the physician independently prescribes the treatment in accordance with good and established medical practice. However, the nurse could not make a "differential" medical diagnosis because that is the domain of medicine. A differential diagnosis is made when the physician arrives at a firm diagnosis after distinguishing between two similar clinical entities. Neither statutory law or case law sanctions the making of a medical diagnosis by one not licensed or authorized by a licensing board to do so.

However, the precedent-setting *Darling* case did find the nurses liable for failing to communicate to their superiors the fact that the medical treatment of the young man's leg fracture was not within the boundaries of acceptable practice.[25] The facts in that case were unusual and the failure to properly treat the patient's leg fracture according to acceptable medical practice resulted in eventual amputation. In essence, the nursing negligence surrounding that particular omission consisted in the nurses' lack of prudence in not communicating critical observations to the appropriate sources. (See Chapter 2 for a fuller treatment of the *Darling* case.)

Courts are aware of the obligation of health care providers to use reasonable judgment skills when a conflict arises between care givers. Review of the case law which raised the issue of medical or nursing judgment seems to point out that the courts will not permit either discipline to make "absolute" judgments, that is, judgments without any restraints. If the courts permitted a nurse or a physician to make completely unrestricted decisions there would be no legal accountability for one's actions.

See *Tarasoff v. Regents of University of California* where psychotherapists and others were liable when a patient shot and killed a young woman. See Chapter 7 for an in-depth discussion of the Tarasoff case. Although the court, in a footnote, recognized the issue of conflicting opinions it did not issue any ruling on the conflict issue because the plaintiff's petition failed to set forth sufficient facts to support the allegation.[26] The plaintiff alleged that one of the therapists recommended that the patient be involuntarily committed because he believed that his threats towards the woman showed him to be dangerous. However, his decision was countermanded and the therapist later unsuccessfully argued that he was obliged to obey the decision of his superior and therefore he should not be held liable for any dereliction arising from his obedience to the orders of his superior. The plaintiff contended that the therapist's duty to members of the public who were put at risk by the superior's veto should take precedence over the therapist's duty to obey the superior.

Case Law

A physician's direct order may raise the issue of control over a nurse's action. This brings into operation the "borrowed servant" doctrine. The issue of control over the nurse's actions is critical when a physician "borrows" the nurse to specifically carry out a particular act. Where the employer of the nurse is successful in arguing that the nurse was under the control of the physician and not the employing facility the employer may escape liability for the nurse's negligent act. Ordinarily the respondeat superior doctrine applies. In essence, the respondeat superior doctrine says, "Let the master answer." The employer is legally responsible for the nurse/employee's negligence. The principle behind this rule is the nurse's work is "under the control" of the employer.

> Such was the legal ruling in *Minogue v. Rutland Hospital* when a nurse was directed by the obstetrician in the delivery room to apply pressure to the upper abdomen.[27] While pressure was being exerted the woman complained of being hurt and yelled, "Don't break a rib." The next day an x-ray film of the woman's ribs revealed a new fracture and she later brought suit. The principal issue in the case was whether the "borrowed servant" defense would shield the hospital from liability for the nurse's act. The court held that liability could not attach to the hospital because the physician was controlling the nurse's actions. The case also addressed the issue of physician's orders. Citing *Byrd v. Marion General Hospital*, the court held that "nurses," in the discharge of their duties, must obey and diligently execute the orders of the physician or surgeon in charge of the patient, unless, of course, such an order is so obviously negligent as to lead any reasonable person to anticipate that substantial injury would result to the patient from the execution of such order on performance of such directions."[28]

A Louisiana case decided in 1966, *Powell v. Fidelity Casualty Co.*, held that two licensed practical nurses (LPNs) were not negligent in the death of a woman who was in her 35th week of pregnancy.[29] The physician, who was also a defendant, settled before the trial. The physician who first saw the patient in her 27th week decided to give her blood transfusions after finding a low hemoglobin. The blood was given in the emergency room at a general hospital. He ordered 1000 cc, started the infusions, and regulated the flow rate. He did not give the nurses verbal or written orders concerning the rate of infusion or other instructions. The nurses maintained the flow rate as initially regulated by the physician. He visited the patient when the first unit was nearly infused and commented that it was flowing nicely. When the second unit was infused the nurses continued to observe the woman while a relative went to get the car. Fifteen minutes after the infusion, the relative escorted the pregnant woman to the car at which time she complained of dizziness, which the relative did not report to the nurses. A short time later the woman was readmitted for pulmonary edema and in spite of an emergency cesarean section, both the infant and mother died. The plaintiff's expert testified that extensive tests should have been done before giving that amount of blood to a woman in an advanced pregnant state because all pregnant women at that stage have considerably more fluid in their system. All experts agreed that pulmonary edema was a problem when that amount of blood is given, even if given at a slow rate. With respect to the nurses, there was no evidence that they were ever taught to precisely regulate the flow rate. In addition, the plaintiff failed to demonstrate that the nurse had a duty, in the absence of physician's orders, to monitor the woman for a longer period than 15 minutes. Testimony that a reaction could have occurred as late as 24 hours after the transfusions also aided the defense.

The case illustrates that in order to be successful the plaintiff would have had to show that the nurses should have judged that the infusion was too rapid, taken steps to slow the infusion, and monitored the patient for a longer period in order to detect complications. Even if the plaintiff had succeeded in establishing negligence on the part of the nurses, the attorney would have had to show a causal relationship between the negligence and the death.

In *Variety Children's Hospital v. Osle*, liability was found against a surgeon, as well as the hospital's operating room nurses for blindly following the surgeon's directive.[30] The scrub nurse asked the surgeon if he wanted the specimens from each breast separated and labeled before they were sent to the pathology laboratory. The surgeon said that it would be all right to send the specimens in a single container as they were not malignant. Although the pathologist did not approve of this break in procedure, he failed to identify which specimen came from which breast. One specimen was larger than the other, but the pathologist failed to distinguish between the specimens when he dissected them. The surgeon removed both breasts although only one of the specimens was malignant. The hospital unsuccessfully argued that the nurses acted as the borrowed servant of the surgeon and the hospital should not be liable for their negligence. There was conflicting testimony as to whether the hospital employees violated the standard of care and whether the nurses were acting under the direct orders of the surgeon. The court held that the negligence of the surgeon and that of the hospital were so intertwined as to constitute a single cause for the plaintiff's injury.

The nursing profession has persuasively argued that, as a professional group, it should be held accountable for individual and collective actions. As the profession advances, the risk of liability increases. Nurses will be held liable, even in the presence of a medical directive, if it can be shown that reason should have dictated a different action. It is, of course, important to remember that the law will not find a nurse liable for events that could not have been reasonably forseen before the event. Apart from their competency in decision making, nurses are in a unique position to make judgments by virtue of the fact that they can observe a patient's condition over continuous and extended periods of time. It is not uncommon for a nurse to disagree with a physician's directive. In those instances, the nurse should make known the reasons for the disagreement and attempt to work out a solution with the physician. There are, of course, times when a nurse should refuse outright to carry out a physician's medical directive. Nurses, by virtue of their specialized knowledge and skill, are expected to question the clinical accuracy of any medical order. Hospitals should have policies explaining the procedure to be followed when there is a disagreement between the physician and the nurses.

Liability for blindly following a physician's order is best illustrated by the famous *Norton v. Argonaut Insurance Company* case.[31] The facts and the legal principles involved are complex. This nursing negligence case demonstrates better than any other the battle lines of defendants when medical and nursing liability intertwine.

The suit was brought by the parents of an infant who was born with a congenital heart defect and who died as a result of a nurse administering 3 cc of Lanoxin via an intramuscular injection. Both the negligent pediatric cardiologist and the nurse were found liable for the wrongful death of the infant.

The infant, who was admitted for tests prior to cardiac surgery, was digitalized during a prior hospital admission. At that time the physician wrote the following order: "Elixir Pediatric Lanoxin 2.5 cc (0.125) q6h × 3, then once daily." The mother, who stayed with the infant most of the day, asked permission to administer the child's daily maintenance dose. After showing the mother how to administer the elixir the physician wrote in the order sheet that the mother would be giving the daily dose. The infant was discharged only to be readmitted 13 days later when her condition became worse. The cardiologist indicated on the order sheet that the mother was giving the infant some of her medications. He also ordered some medications to be given by the staff. Lanoxin was not one of these medications. On the day in question (the fifth day of the second hospitalization period) the defendant cardiologist decided to increase the dose from 2.5 to 3 cc and he went to the nurse's station and wrote on the doctor's sheet: "Give 3.0 cc Lanoxin today for 1 dose only." The mother gave the Lanoxin.

A nursing supervisor, who had gone to the unit to help the skeleton staff, transcribed the order. Never having worked in pediatrics, the nurse was unaware that Lanoxin came in an elixir form. Each cubic centimeter of elixir contained 0.05 mg, whereas each cubic centimeter of the injectable form contained 0.25 mg, or five times more than the elixir. The supervisor obtained two ampules of the drug from the medicine closet, but because she had some apprehension about such a divided dose, she consulted, at different times, with two physicians who were on the unit about the correctness of the dose. She testified that she showed them the ampules and indicated that the order was for 3 cc. Both physicians disputed her testimony. One physician testified that he thought she was referring to the oral form when she asked about a 3-cc dose and that she did not show him the ampules. The other physician testified that the impression she gave was that she intended to give only 1 cc of the injectable form. The supervisor then drew up 3 cc in a syringe and injected 1.5 cc in each buttock. The error became known when the mother requested a hot water bottle for the infant's buttocks. The supervisor then contacted the cardiologist for an order and the error came to light. In spite of emergency measures the infant died 1 hour and 15 minutes after the injection.

The defendant cardiologist readily admitted error in failing to note in the orders that either the mother had given the dose or that it would be administered by her. However, he said that it was accepted medical and nursing practice that when the route of administration is not indicated in the order, it means that it is to be administered by the oral route. He conceded that while it may be argued that he was negligent by not indicating that the mother gave or would be giving the dose, the proximate cause of the infant's death was the administration of a dose, patently lethal, by the nurse. He argued that he could not have "forseen" that a nurse who lacked the competency to administer a drug would do so. Arguing that if the nurse had given the drug in the elixir form, as all competent nurses familiar with pediatric medicines doses would have done, the results would have been the possible administration of 6 cc of Lanoxin elixir. He presented testimony that 3 cc of the injectable form was a lethal dose, whereas an overdose in the elixir form would not have been lethal. Experts for the plaintiff and the defendant cardiologist disagreed as to the effects of a double dose of 3 cc of the elixir within a 1-hour period. The cardiologist attempted to show that the nurse's action was so unforeseeable and unpredictable as to relieve him of liability for his negligence in the method of prescribing. The cardiologist's failure to specify a route was in the court's view calculated to produce confusion and uncertainty which may have forseeably resulted in the drug being administered in either form. The cardiologist unsuccessfully argued that the nurse's action was an "independent and intervening" cause of harm.

The hospital's insurer maintained that the cardiologist, alone, was the proximate cause of the infant's death, that his failure to designate the administration route was responsible for the administration of the injectable Lanoxin instead of the elixir Lanoxin, and that the nurse who administered the medication simply gave what the physician ordered. However, the court said that a nurse who is unfamiliar with the fact that the drug in question is prepared in oral form for administration to infants is not properly and adequately trained for duty in a pediatric ward. While not holding a nurse to the same degree of knowledge of drugs as is possessed by members of the medical profession, the court said, common sense dictates that no nurse should attempt to administer a drug in the circumstances described in this case. Additionally, the nurse violated a rule generally recognized in the nursing community, that of contacting the prescribing physician when in doubt. Such a rule, said the court, is most reasonable and prudent.

One further point regarding the *Norton* case should be made. It is not a universally accepted nursing practice that omission of the route of administration from the order automatically means the medication is to be given via the oral route. However, if such a policy is to be adopted it should be formalized and communicated to all parties who will be effected by such a policy.

One avenue that nurses frequently utilize in clarifying medication orders is the hospital pharmacist. The pharmacist, although not authorized to prescribe medications, may provide helpful information. The prudent pharmacist shares appropriate knowledge with the nurses when a question arises, but is careful not to overlap with the physician's prescribing role. Physicians too frequently seek out and rely on the expertise of the pharmacist when prescribing medications. The pharmacist can be extremely helpful in providing information, but the rule is that the prescribing physician is the person to be consulted when a question surrounding the order arises. Conferring with the pharmacist is prudent when trying to resolve questions about a particular order.

An incident reported by a nurse demonstrates the types of non-medical judgments that confront nurses quite frequently.[32]

A directive by an intern, new to the speciality service, conflicted with a patient care judgment made by a nurse who was more familiar with the patient and routine. The intern had ordered that a patient with cranial trauma be sent to the X-ray department, but the nurse refused to move the patient until his low intercranial pressure readings became more stable. Ten minutes later the patient's vital signs dropped to critically low levels and the resuscitation team kept him alive by initiating essential life-support systems. It would have been impossible to respond to the crisis if the patient was in the X-ray department or on-route.

Anecdotes such as this highlight the collaborative role essential to health care. It illustrates a "judgment call" which was in the best interest of the patient. The law requires that such judgment calls must be reasonable under the facts and reflect professional knowledge and skill. Disagreements such as this should not create battlegrounds, but rather, provide an opportunity to assess what seems best under the circumstances. At times a fine line may exist between interfering with the physician's right and duty to practice medicine, and intevening to prevent foreseeable or potential harm to the patient. There is of course, no sure way to identify which situation may turn out to be harmful and which may constitute inappropriate interference. It is reassuring that such conflicts arise infrequently.

A recent case at the trial level held that three operating room nurses should have intervened to protect the patient and their failure to do so made them liable.[33]

A young woman who was 3 months pregnant underwent surgery to remove a dead fetus. The surgeon perforated the uterus and mistakenly pulled out the small bowel through the perforated organ. The scrub nurse, who was receiving the substance in a basin, thought it might be the umbilical cord. However, her suspicions were sufficiently aroused to make motions with her head and eyes alerting the circulating nurse and the nurse anesthetist. The nurse anesthetist suggested that the substance might be the small bowel. By the time the procedure was completed the woman had suffered extensive damage to the small bowel and despite emergency surgery more than 19 feet of bowel was nonsalvageable. As a result of the surgery the woman would have to remain on hyperalimentation feedings for the remainder of her life and would be unable to bear more children, both important findings which influenced the high multimillion dollar damage award.

The question of nursing negligence centered on whether the nurses erred in not demanding that the surgeon stop the procedure before the irreparable damage occurred. Although the nurses testified that events occurred over a 90-second time span, evidence presented on behalf of the plaintiff indicated that the time span was closer to 10 minutes. Nurses who testified for the defense said that they often "defer to a doctor's judgment even if they feel something is wrong." The case illustrates that operating room nursing is recognized as an appropriate setting for nurses to practice a specialized type of nursing. Such practice is not confined to the technical aspects, and draws upon the nurse's knowledge and skills and ability to act in a reasonable manner in applying such knowledge and skills. In short, the nurses were faulted for not intervening in a situation in which application of reason would require some type of action. The plaintiff's attorney submitted nursing ethics standards to help establish that the nurses had a duty to intervene earlier. Expert testimony established that the woman could have retained near-normal small bowel function if 2 feet of bowel had remained intact.

Frequently nurses ponder whether to intervene and if so, what form the intervention should take. The reluctance to intervene is most frequently observed for medical situations, that is, those in which the nurse's judgment may conflict with that of the physician. When events occur such as in the preceding case involving surgical trauma to the bowel, nurses should be advised to seek the counsel of administrative superiors whose role it is to problem solve or set in motion a process leading to confronting the conflict. Judgment conflicts are apt to occur in any health care setting. The conflicts would be substantially reduced in number if there existed a true collaborative mindset toward health care. Hospitals and other facilities must identify and operationalize a support system so that nurses will know where to turn when faced with these types of dilemmas. Professional ethics require that nurses take reasonable measures to protect the patient.

Nurses will not be held liable for a breach of a duty owed by the physician where their own actions conformed to accepted nursing practice. The following case, *Taylor v. Baptist Medical Center*, illustrates the duty owed by nurses when the patient's physician did not directly assess her status.[34]

A woman who was 23 weeks pregnant underwent an emergency appendectomy and 3 weeks later went into labor. She called the physician at 3 A.M. and was instructed to go to the hospital. The labor room nurses kept the physician appraised of her progress via telephone. The woman was attended by two nurses throughout labor and delivery. The woman delivered at 11:30 A.M. and the physician arrived 10 minutes later. The infant was either stillborn or died minutes after delivery. It weighed 1 pound 8 ounces, had fused eyelids, transparent skin, and no subcutaneous tissue. The woman's claim against the hospital was based on the theory that the nurses were negligent in failing to obtain another physician in the primary physician's absence. Addressing the issue of whether the hospital nurses were negligent, the court held that they could reasonably conclude that no other physician would be needed when the physician told them he would be "right on over." Also, by having the two qualified nurses with considerable childbirth experience in the labor and delivery room the hospital was not liable for failing to supply the patient with competent medical attendants in the delivery phase.

Because judgment is inherent in nursing practice, the issue of judgment may arise in other than a negligence context. In *Murphy v. Rowland*, a 1980 decision by a state board of nurses to suspend a nurse's license was upheld.[35] The suspension was for "unprofessional or dishonorable conduct likely to injure the public." The court found that the decision by the Texas Board of Nurse Examiners was supported by substantial evidence.

A woman who was 8 months pregnant awoke in great pain and went to the lay midwife who had agreed to deliver the infant. When she was examined, the midwife concluded that the woman's problems were not within her expertise and sent the woman to a hospital. After being examined by two nurses at the hospital, who consulted with a physician via telephone, the patient was sent to a second hospital. The nurse at the second hospital examined her in the parking lot and told the family to take her to a hospital that had more extensive services. The nurse did not contact a physician because she said that she knew what the physician would tell her to do. Evidence at the nurse's suspension hearing indicated that the hospital had limitations in its ability to provide emergency surgery to pregnant women. The family refused the nurse's offer to obtain a police escort. Ambulance service was not feasible. The woman and her family went to their home and the woman died shortly afterward of a ruptured uterus.

The nurse at the second hospital testified that she believed that the pains were related to the woman's pregnant condition and that her conduct in sending the woman to the third hospital was appropriate because that hospital was better equipped to handle emergency surgery. The board determined that the nurse's action was unprofessional and as such was the type of conduct that the nursing rules and regulations were designed to prevent. The board determined that the nurse's lack of judgment in failing to consult with the on-call emergency room physician, as well as the failure to initiate appropriate nursing intervention to stabilize the woman's condition were sufficient to establish that such conduct was unprofessional and likely to injure the public.

One of the questions that falls within the realm of nursing judgment is, "At what point should a nurse judge that a patient requires closer monitoring in the absence of a physician's order?" Another question is, "When should a nurse call the physician when there is a change in the patient's condition?" Nurses clearly do not need a physician's order to institute or increase monitoring. By virtue of the fact that nurses are more closely proximate to the patient, at least in a hospital setting, they have a professional and a legal duty to monitor and assess changes that may indicate complications. It is the practice of nurses to increase patient monitoring, even when there is only a suspicion that all may not be right with the patient.[36] The reasons for increased monitoring may be different. For example, when a patient event occurs, increased monitoring is the norm. When a patient is found out of bed shortly after having a femoral angiogram, the appropriate nursing response would be to immediately place him on frequent vital signs until the immediate threat of hemorrhage has passed. Monitoring the vital signs, along with other assessment actions, reflects the nurse's scientific knowledge. When the nurse harbors a suspicion that a patient may be undergoing an event, the purpose of monitoring is to determine whether the subtle changes or findings represent a situation that requires medical or nursing intervention.

The rule to apply in notifying the physician is that when a patient's condition becomes unstable and there is reason to suspect that the welfare of the patient may be in jeopardy, the physician should be informed. This allows the physician to institute appropriate medical intervention. In nursing practice, as in law, the facts of a situation determine whether the situation is one in which the physician should be notified immediately or whether it is appropriate for the nurse to monitor the patient for a reasonable period before contacting the physician. There is considerable case law in which nurses were found liable for failure or delay in informing the physician of critical changes in the patient's condition. In contract law there is a legal maxim that holds that "time is of the essence." Reasonableness, rather than any precise time limit, is the measure for knowing when to communicate a change in a patient's condition. In determining what is a reasonable delay in reporting a change or event, time is a critical factor. All the facts surrounding the situation are important in determining when and whether patient findings should be reported to the physician. When a judgment is made that the circumstances require monitoring only, it is important that the monitoring measures be done with sufficient frequency and skill to determine further nursing action.

Where a physician gives explicit orders nurses are not authorized to change or modify the orders in the absence of custom. When custom allows some latitude in modifying orders, it is important that such modification, including the reason, be communicated to the physician. In some instances, the information should be communicated to the physician soon after the event and, at other times, it is appropriate to have a reasonable lapse of time between the event and conveyance of the information. Custom, hospital policy and practice, as well as nursing standards, dictate acceptable nursing action. Under appropriate circumstances, it may be sufficient to communicate the information via daily nursing notes. By way of example, it would be inappropriate in the absence of policy to omit a prescribed antipsychotic drug when the patient is having an acute episode, without informing the primary physician.

A California case, *Cline v. Lund*, illustates the liability of a nurse for failing to timely implement explicit orders and use good judgment in communicating patient findings.[37] Some findings by their nature require immediate reporting rather than waiting until all assessment data are obtained.

A 29-year-old woman had an uneventful abdominal hysterectomy. Postoperatively her vital signs were monitored every 4 hours. Her blood pressure, although without normal limits, was slightly elevated. She was visited by the anesthesiologist at noon the day following surgery. At 1 P.M. her family physician visited her and noted that she was elevated in bed, sipping water with her eyes open and blinking, but that she did not respond to conversation. He attributed this to her postoperative emotional state. At 2:30 P.M. the woman was dangled by a nurse who charted that she tolerated it well although the nurse later testified that she did not think it had been well tolerated. The woman had projectile vomiting at 3:30 P.M. and she remained unresponsive to verbal stimuli thereafter.

At 9 P.M. her blood pressure was $142/90$ and the nursing notes reflected that the patient was not responsive to verbal stimuli and probably not to physical stimuli. The nurse requested that a supervisor check the patient and shortly after 9 P.M. the surgeon was called. He checked the patient at 10:15 P.M. and although her blood pressure was rising the surgeon suspected that the woman was hemorrhaging. At 10:50 P.M. he ordered a complete blood count stat, vital signs every 30 minutes throughout the night, and a "keep-open" intravenous to provide access to a vein if necessary. The physician returned to his home, which was 5 to 10 minutes away, pending completion of the laboratory work. Although the nurse knew that the laboratory was not staffed around the clock she failed to notify the technician and he left the hospital at 11 P.M. Witnesses testified that the blood work could have been done within 20 minutes of receiving the stat order, but because of the delay in notifying the technician, who had to return to the hospital, the report was not completed until almost an hour and a half after the order. The nurse took the first blood pressure 55 minutes after the order and it was $160/90$. At that time (11:45 P.M.), the woman had rigid extremities. The nurse notified the supervisor but did not notify the surgeon until one-half hour later (12:15 A.M.) when the laboratory work was completed. The laboratory work indicated internal bleeding. The surgeon ordered the woman transferred to the ICU, but the nurse delayed the transfer because the patient's blood pressure had risen to $230/130$ and she feared that she would have a cerebral hemorrhage. The nurse testified that she also feared that the patient would regurgitate and aspirate the vomitus. At 12:40 A.M. the patient became apneic and suffered an arrest 2 minutes later. She was transferred to the unit at 1:05 A.M. and died at 4:45 A.M.

The court found nursing negligence in several critical areas: (1) failure to timely implement the stat orders that would have revealed the marked pressure elevation and the hemorrhage earlier; (2) failure to notify the surgeon of the critical findings at 11:45 P.M.; and (3) delay in the transfer of the patient to the ICU. In addition, the court found that the intake and output chart was inaccurately kept and thus, could not be relied on by the physician. The court said that although no single nursing laxity pointed to direct causation, the jury could find that a series of negligent nursing acts was sufficient to establish causal connection. The nurses were found liable and the physician was not.[37]

In summary, liability for physician's orders can result from a failure to carry them out in a reasonable manner, as well as a failure to obtain orders when the patient situation warrants it. The nurse has a duty to assess the clinical accuracy of any physician order. No nurse may blindly institute a physician's order. If that were the standard, then far more incidents and errors would be associated with transcriptions. Even in those situations where a person other than a nurse transcribes medical orders, good and accepted nursing practice requires that the order be reviewed by a professional nurse to determine its clinical accuracy.

ERRORS OF JUDGMENT BASED ON FAULTY ASSESSMENT

The nursing process, first referred to in a nursing context more than a decade ago, is important in arriving at clinical judgments. The process, which is not unique to nursing, has been adopted by the profession because it facilitates order in decision making and promotes consistency in practice standards. The initial step in the process is assessment. In a medical context the courts have found liability for failing to diagnose or for a misdiagnosis. Although the theory of liability more often cites a failure to order appropriate diagnostic tests, follow-up on patient complaints, or failure to call in consultant(s), it translates into inadequate assessment. Legal opinions infrequently make reference to specific nursing concepts, such as physical assessment or nursing diagnosis. However, it is not difficult to abstract from the case law the liability for inadequate or incomplete nursing assessment. Presumably, liability for failure to make a nursing diagnosis will be recognized as increasingly more states include the concept in their nurse practice act, thus giving it legal standing. However, even though the legal opinion in a nursing negligence case does not specifically cite the term nursing diagnosis, the case law clearly holds nurses liable for failing to establish and act on a defined patient problem. On a practical level attorneys will shy away from using the term nursing diagnosis because they try to use terminology which lay people can readily grasp. However, the concept will be an integral part of the testimony.

The potential for liability for both nurses and physicians for inadequate patient assessment is considerable. In the following case, *Pigno v. Bunim,* suit was brought on behalf of an infant who was not given an exchange transfusion for blood incompatability.[38] The court held that liability may be found for the physician's negligence, but the suit against the hospital for the nurses negligence was dismissed before the jury decided the case. However, there were two dissenting opinions which would have the jury decide the issue of the nurses' negligence for failing to monitor the infant to determine when the aborted exchange transfusion should have been resumed. There are a number of lessons in the case:

> The infant (second child) of an Rh negative mother had the transfusion stopped after receiving only 120 cc because of cyanosis. The problem was that transfusions were not resumed until 4 days later. In the interim the infant had developed jaundice and by the 20th day showed signs of kernicterus which indicated that the bilirubin had invaded the brain. At the trial

the defendant pediatrician testified that the bilirubin tests were important and good medical practice required that they be ordered.

The physician testified that he ordered constant monitoring of the infant and left an order that the bilirubin tests be done every 8 hours. However, there were many problems with the infant's medical record because it was deficient in several aspects: (1) there was no written order for the 8-hour bilirubin tests and the order sheet was missing, (2) there were no laboratory reports, (3) there was no documentation in either the physician's or nurses' progress notes indicating how long the infant remained cyanotic, and (4) there was no documentation by either the nurses or physician of any test results or their impact on a proposed course of treatment.

Liability was imposed on the physician for being remiss in failing to check that his orders were being carried out, both the tests and the monitoring. In view of cases following *Darling* it would not have been unwarranted for the court to find that the physician's failure to eventually do the exchange transfusion placed a duty on the nursing staff to report such a failure. The opinion did not indicate whether the nursing monitoring should be confined to jaundice observations or laboratory results or both. Some courts impose liability because the function of patient monitoring is relatively simple.

This is especially true when the results are as devastating as in *Pigno v. Bunim*. The case is important, not because the suit against the nurses was dismissed, but because of the two dissenting opinions that would have sent the issue of nursing negligence to the jury. Thus, the lesson in some cases is not the actual decision, but rather the issues raised and the language of the court.

Independent Judgment

The courts have held that the concept of "independent" judgment imposes a duty on the nurse to modify a physician's order when new information about a patient situation would make implementation of the physician's order unsafe. Presumably, the courts have adopted the term "independent judgment" to make an exception to the rule that a nurse must implement a medical order unless it is patently incorrect. In reality, however, the potential need to modify an order is inherent in every clinical decision a nurse makes. Such deliberation is the rule, not the exception. For instance, nurses frequently "hold" a patient's medication or a prescribed treatment because of an adverse finding or other new information.

The issue of independent judgment was raised on *Osborn v. Public Hospital District No. 2*, in which the court held that the issue of reasonable prudence on the part of the nurses should have been submitted to the jury.[39]

In this case an 84-year-old man was admitted with a diagnosis of pneumonia, acute bronchitis, and bowel dysfunction. He was examined by his physician who ordered routine workup and Demerol every 3 to 4 hours. The physician did not leave any orders restricting the patient's mobility, but trial testimony of the nursing director showed that, in the absence of specific orders, a patient would be allowed bathroom privileges. She further testified that general hospital policy required elevation of the bed rails of elderly patients at night. The rails were lowered around 5 A.M. for morning care.

The record showed that the man received Demerol every 3 hours beginning 2 hours after admission at noon the day before the fall. A nurse testified that the patient was reasonably rational and alert when she gave him Demerol at 2:45 A.M. and an antibiotic at 4 A.M. The patient either fell out of bed or fell after getting out of the bed to go to the bathroom. The fall occurred shortly after 5 A.M. A nurse testified that the man was not confused when found after his fall although he vascillated in judging whether he was hurt or not. In fact, he had fractured his hip.

At the trial the court held that the nurse's actions were in accordance with the implied orders of the physician. However, on appeal the higher court held that the duty of care owed by the employees of the hospital was independent of the care which may be chargeable to the attending physician. The court stated, "Under these circumstances it would appear unreasonable to say that the staff who had opportunity to observe the mental condition of this weak and ill 84-year-old man the following morning, could blindly follow the implied direction of the doctor for the patient to have bathroom privileges, to be relieved of any responsibility of this patient's physical safety in the administering of his care."

The court stated that the nursing staff were responsible for administering to the physical safety of the patient as dictated by their reasonable observation of his state of mind and physical condition at a given time and that such observation was independent of the implied directive from the physician as of the day before. As the court stated, "The jury, from this record, could have concluded that reasonable prudence for Mr. Osborn's safety would have required the bed rails to have remained raised and assistance given Mr. Osborn in the exercise of his bathroom needs."

In summary, the court said that nurses do not "blindly" carry out medical treatment care. A physician's order, whether implied, as in this case, or expressly written is to be carried out in light of current patient findings. What the opinion did not say is that the nurse must notify the physician that there is a need to modify the order.

Although nurses may take exception to the use of the phrase, "independent judgment," it may be useful in other kinds of litigation against nurses. In some instances it may be advantageous to affirmatively argue the defense of "independent" judgment. For example, using the language of the court at a hearing before a nursing board where the alleged wrong was a failure to carry out a physician's order, may be more persuasive than simply arguing that nursing custom permitted the nurse to modify an order. "Nursing custom" means that an activity is an accepted practice because it is generally done in a certain manner. Thus, the nurse can rely on and quote "legal language" in arguing her case.

Failure to Take a History

When the nurse fails to take the patient's history and as a result the patient is harmed, liability will be found. In the following case, liability was found against the nurse, a radiologist, and an X-ray technician. Testimony established that each deviated from their respective responsibility.

> In this case, *Favalora v. Aetna Casualty*, the patient was admitted for diagnostic studies because of a recent history of fainting.[40] The policy in the hospital required the nurse to complete the requisition slip which required a statement indicating why the test was being done. Although the nurse knew why the patient was admitted, she did not include the history of fainting on the slip. During the diagnostic tests the woman fell, fracturing her femur, and a preexisting vascular condition was aggravated, necessitating vena cava ligation because of emboli.
>
> The court said that the nurse was liable for her failure to obtain a clinical history which would have given notice that the woman was subject to falling. In addition, the plaintiff's expert testified that a failure to note any patient data on the requisition slip was evidence of negligence. If that had been done, the radiologist would have been alerted to the problem.
>
> The radiologist raised the defense of "best judgment," but the court said that "the failure of the radiologist to take and rely on a history is not an error of judgment or diagnosis occasioned by a disparity of innate skill and ability against which the law offers the physician protection, but rather constituted failure of the physician to exercise reasonable care and diligence *along* (emphasis added) with his best judgment in his application to the patient of the degree of skill of which he is possessed." The court also said that the physician should have either reviewed the record or conducted some type of patient examination, eliciting information from the patient. There was no duty incumbent on the patient that would absolve the defendants, for example, the patient was not compelled to give them her history when she arrived for the x-ray films.
>
> The technician was found negligent because he left the room. Expert testimony established that the hospital orientation plan for technicians included patient safety measures. The court noted that three methods existed that would have prevented the injury: (1) securing her to the x-ray table by a strap or other device, (2) support by an attendant who remained constantly at her side, (3) a level of alertness by those in attendance which would have enabled them to come to the woman's aid, even if the fainting occurred without advance warning.

The plaintiff's attorney argued that all the defendants failed to take note of such factors as her age, the 12-hour fast prior to the examination, and the length of time estimated for completion of the test.

Lack of Assessment and Causation

Assessment of the patient includes both past and present history. A course of action based on inadequate or no information is a perilous course, and one that will certainly increase the risk of a lawsuit. The following case which alleged patient abandonment is an example of a situation in which there was a total lack of assessment in a situation requiring at the very least, a minimum assessment.

In this case, *Maslonka v. Hermann,* the trial court held that, while demonstrating negligence, the plaintiff failed to causally connect the lack of due care to the woman's death.[41] The case also shows what the plaintiff has to prove to meet the causation test. No autopsy was done to pinpoint the exact cause of death and the range of possibilities included pulmonary emboli, amniotic fluid embolism, a ruptured uterus, and intravascular coagulation.

When the case was appealed the court held that sufficient evidence had been presented, thus permitting a jury to find that the woman was neglected (abandoned) and this neglect was the proximate cause of her death.

> The decedent, a 33-year-old woman who had had three uneventful previous vaginal deliveries, was admitted at 5:30 A.M. At that time her blood pressure was $130/90$ and immediately after her delivery at 6:45 A.M. it was $180/100$. Her physician had administered Methergine after the delivery. A known side effect of the drug is elevated blood pressure. No vital signs were taken after 6:45 A.M. She was transferred to a semiprivate room at 7:30 A.M. At that time the nurse's notes reflected that she was bleeding moderately and passing clots. At 8:30 A.M. the nurse's notes indicated that the woman was pale and restless, with labored respirations and that her blood pressure could not be obtained. The woman was pronounced dead at 9:30 A.M.

Another patient in the room testified that the patient's efforts to get assistance and then her own efforts proved to no avail. During this period the decedent was delerious and had very heavy bleeding, sufficient to cover both her clothing and the bed sheets. The nurses failed to respond to either patients' calls for assistance, and no physician examined the woman until her condition had deteriorated substantially. The husband testified that the physician told him that no autopsy was necessary because he knew more or less that the cause of death was a pulmonary embolism. In fact, his orders indicated bleeding problems because he ordered a "type and cross-match." Both medical and nursing witnesses testifying on behalf of the plaintiff concluded that the decedent was poorly attended.

The plaintiff's nurse expert testified that both the nursing notes and pretrial discovery were evidence of poor care. She cited the lack of nursing notes which suggested poor communication among the nursing staff with regard to the woman's care and condition; an absence of vital signs indicating poor monitoring; and further, that a "nursing diagnosis" could have led the nurses to conclude that hemorrhage was possible.[42] The witness concluded her analysis by saying that one of the nurses caring for the patient had "not exercised all of the skills and knowledge that she should have gained as part of her basic professional training in behalf of the decedent. . . . The nurse's progress notes depict her neglect of the decedent."

The law requires that the plaintiff show that the negligent acts were "more *probable* than not" the cause of the decedent's death. Mere possibility is insufficient, because it is too speculative. The court held that the evidence could reasonably lead a jury to conclude that the abandonment and neglect were a proximate cause of the woman's bleeding to death.

SUMMARY

Nursing judgment, like medical judgment, requires the acquisition of the necessary knowledge and skills and the ability to use them in a reasonable manner. The nursing process is the means whereby the nurse arrives at clinical judgments. Any breakdown in any phase of the process may result in poor judgment. Simply stated, the two main requisites for nursing judgment are to *possess* knowledge and to *act* upon it.

As previously stated, a *judgment* is defined as the ability to make a decision and act on it. A critical question in exercising a judgment is what served as a basis for the particular judgment. A patient's record should reflect the exercise of a judgment. The law does not require perfection in matters of judgment, but it does not permit a defendant to escape liability for substandard judgments.

A defense of error in judgment is not an uncommon pleading. The error in judgment cases began early in the century and were confined to medical suits. However, as nursing shed its "handmaiden" image and showed that it is based in a defined body of scientific knowledge, the courts have imposed liability for failures in the decision-making process. When the defense of error in judgment is used, the plaintiff tries to overcome it by attacking either the patient assessment phase or the selection of the specific treatment or plan of nursing care.

Much of the error in judgment case law came about because of problems with the instructions given to juries. Once the error in judgment defense was acknowledged by the court variations of the theme appeared. Jury verdicts were set aside because of the use of such terms as "mere error in judgment," "best judgment," "honest error in judgment," and "good faith judgment."[43] The test in the error in judgment cases is always whether reasonable care in accordance with recognized and accepted nursing standards was given. Thus, an error in judgment argument has no meaning if the minimum standard was not met.

The courts recognize that there may be more than one accepted method in managing a patient problem and a nurse will not be found liable for electing one accepted method over another. The test is: Were both methods recognized?

The majority of error in judgment cases result from a failure to assess the patient in a skillful manner. Physicians' orders may also pose special judgment problems for the nurse. On one hand there is the rule that a nurse must carry out a physician's order, but there is liability if the nurse should have known that it was a clinically inaccurate order. The test then is whether a reasonable nurse should have known the order was not clinically accurate. It is inappropriate for any nurse to substitute her judgment in matters of medical treatment, for that of the physician. That does not mean that the nurse should remain passive in the presence of questionable medical practice. Professional ethics and the law mandate some type of intervention.

In determining whether a nurse has the authority to make a particular judgment pertaining to the modification of a medical treatment order, consideration should be given to whether the area under consideration is one usually left by a physician to the discretion of the nursing staff.

One last point, in the form of a caveat, should be made before concluding this chapter. It is inevitable that the error in judgment concept will be applied to nurses who make a medical diagnosis in conjunction with the advanced nurse practitioner role. It is not that the law applies a higher standard with respect to nurses practicing in that role, rather that the law requires specialists to conform to a standard different to that of generalists when functioning in the advanced role. The law requires evidence of competency; this means that the nurse practitioner has average skills and knowledge in her area of expertise.

REFERENCES AND NOTES

1. Pike v. Honsinger, 49 N.E. 760 (NY, 1898). The earliest case found by the author is Leighton v. Sargent, 27 New Hampshire 460 (NH, 1853) where a patient sued for negligence in managing an ankle fracture. That court said, "Every man is liable to error . . . the party must go further, and prove by other evidence that the defendant assumed that character, and undertook to act as a physician, without the education, knowledge, and skill which entitled him to act in that capacity; that is, he must show that he had not reasonable and ordinary skill; or he is bound to prove, in the same way, that having such knowledge and skill, he neglected to apply them with such care and diligence as in his judgment, properly exercised, the case must have appeared to require; in other words, that he neglected the proper treatment from inattention and carelessness." A 1986 New Hampshire decision, Morrill v. Tilney, 128 NH 773 (NH, 1986) reaffirmed that "a professional is not liable 'for errors of judgment' . . . (but) shall consider only whether the person . . . has acted with the due care having in mind the standards and recommended practices and procedures of his profession. . . ." See also, Gelsomino v. Gorov, 502 N.E. 2nd 264 (IL, 1986) where clients brought a professional malpractice action against former attorneys for negligence in the investigation,

preparation, and presentation of their lawsuit against their insurance carrier. The court said, "Generally an attorney cannot be held liable for every mistake in the practice of law . . . but merely characterizing an act or omission as a matter of judgment does not end the inquiry." Case held that an attorney is not liable for tactical trial decisions based on professional judgment, but bound to exercise a reasonable degree of skill and care in professional dealings.

2. DuBois v. Decker, 29 N.E. 313 (NY, 1891).
3. Potock v. Turek, 227 S. 2nd 724 (FL, 1969).
4. Brannigan, V. (July 9, 1981). Letters to the editor, Surgical mishaps. *New England Journal of Medicine, 305*(2), 109. Response to article reporting cases of surgical misadventure.
5. Maslonka v. Hermann, 414 A. 2nd 1350 (NJ, 1980), p. 1353, where the plaintiff's nurse expert testified that the nurses departed from acceptable nursing practice by failing to establish a nursing diagnosis; that decision for defendants overruled in 428 A. 2nd 504 (Supreme Court, 1981).
6. Stein, J. (Ed.) (1979). *Random House dictionary of the English language.* New York: Random House.
7. Ahmed, M. (Jan. 1982). Op-Site for decubitus care. *American Journal of Nursing, 82*(1), 61.
8. Averbach, A. (1970). Handling accident cases (Vol. 2A). Rochester, NY: Lawyers Cooperative Publishing (p. 199, footnote 12).
9. Stein, J. (Ed.) (1979). *Random House dictionary of the English language.* New York: Random House.
10. Currie v. U.S., 644 F. Supp. 1074 (NC, 1986).
11. Downs v. American Employer Insurance Co., 423 F. 2nd 1160 (1970). See also, Levermann v. Cartell, 393 S.W. 2nd 931 (TX, 1965) where a jury instruction that the defendant was not responsible for "an honest mistake in judgment" was improper.
12. Peacock v. Piper, 504 P. 2nd 1124 (WA, 1973).
13. Pike v. Honsinger, 155 NY 209 (NY, 1898).
14. Cunningham v. State of NY, 197 NYS 2nd 542 (NY, 1960); affirmed at Cunningham v. State of NY, 181 N.E. 2nd 852 (NY, 1962).
15. Riggs v. Christie, 342 MA 402 (MA, 1961).
16. Delaney v. Rosenthal, 347 MA 143 (MA, 1964).
17. Cooper v. U.S., 313 F. Supp. 1207 (1970).
18. DeFalco v. Long Island College Hospital, 393 NYS 2nd 859 (NY, 1977).
19. Ulma v. Yonkers General Hospital, 384 NYS 2nd 201 (NY, 1976).
20. Whitaker v. St. Joseph's Hospital, 415 N.E. 2nd 737 (IN, 1981).
21. Cooper v. National Motor Bearing Co., 288 P. 2nd 581 (CA, 1955).
22. Fraijo v. Hartland Hospital, 160 *California Reporter, 246* (CA, 1979).
23. Ibid, p. 251, footnote 8.
24. Kentucky Revised Statutes, §314.001 (5) (1980); Alaska Statutes, §08.68.410 (1982); Annotated Missouri Statutes (Occupations and Professions) §335,016 (1976); Maine Revised Statutes Annotated (Professions and Occupations) §2102, subsec. 2 (1977).
25. Darling v. Charleston Community Memorial Hospital, 211 N.E. 2nd 254 (IL, 1965).
26. Tarasoff v. Regents of University of California, 551 P. 2nd 334, at footnote 16 at 348, (CA, 1976).
27. Minogue v. Rutland Hospital, 125 A. 2nd 796 (VT, 1956).
28. Byrd v. Marion General Hospital, 162 S.E. 738 (NC, 1932).
29. Powell v. Fidelity Casualty Co., 185 S. 2nd 324 (LA, 1966).
30. Variety Children's Hospital v. Osle, 292 S. 2nd 382 (FL, 1974).
31. Norton v. Argonaut Insurance Company, 144 S. 2nd 249 (LA, 1962).
32. Drees, D. (July 1981). *Contact* (a publication of the Massachusetts Nurses Association), District V, *17*(3).

33. Szymczak, P. Alton woman gets $5.75 million in malpractice case. *St. Louis Globe-Democrat*, October 19, 1981. After defendants appealed the jury verdict the parties settled the case for an undisclosed amount.

34. Taylor v. Baptist Medical Center, 400 S. 2nd 369 (AL, 1981).

35. Murphy v. Rowland, 609 S.W. 2nd 292 (TX, 1980).

36. Tanner, C., & Benner, P. (Jan. 1987). Clinical judgment: How expert nurses use intuition, *American Journal of Nursing, 87*(1), 23.

37. Cline v. Lund and Community Hospital, 107 *California Reporter, 629* (CA, 1973).

38. Pigno v. Bunim, 350 NYS 2nd 438 (NY, 1973).

39. Osborn v. Public Hospital District No. 2, 492 P. 2nd 1025 (WA, 1972).

40. Favalora v. Aetna Casualty and Surety Company, 144 S. 2nd 544 (LA, 1962). See also Duling v. Bluefield Sanitarium, Inc., 211 N.E. 2nd 253 (WV, 1965) in which the nurses failed to tend to the critical needs of a teenager admitted to a hospital with a diagnosis of acute rheumatic fever.

41. Maslonka v. Hermann et al. 428 A. 2nd 504 (NJ, 1981), which overruled 414 A. 2nd 1350 (NJ, 1980).

42. See the following nursing practice statutes for examples of states specifically using the term, nursing diagnosis: Kentucky Revised Statutes, §314.011 (3-a), (1980); Florida Statutes Annotates, §464.003 (3) (a) 1 (1986); New York (Education) Law §6901, 1972; Pennsylvania Statutes Annotated, Title 63, §214 (1974).

43. Ellis v. Springfield Women's Clinic, 678 P. 2nd 268 (OR, 1984) where the court failed to convey the error in judgment principle accurately to the jury and the "good faith" factor allowed the jury to consider the physician's motivation.

The concept of safety is broad. The cases selected for inclusion in this chapter involve both usual and unusual patient care situations. A review of the case law on nursing negligence indicates that the failure to monitor and the failure to act in an appropriate or timely manner account for a substantial number of suits involving nurses. Infrequently a failure to monitor a case may involve an extreme factual situation sufficient to invoke an abandonment of care theory. The two cases that illustrate abandonment are distinguished from each other by the fact that one (*Duling*) involved a total disregard for the patient's welfare, whereas the later one (*Maslonka*) occurred over a relatively short time span and is a classic lesson in harm as a result of lack of monitoring. In both cases the end result was the death of the patient.

The section on suicide reflects a recent trend toward finding hospitals liable for harm or death because of a failure to take reasonable measures that may have prevented the destructive act. The cases involving restraint problems indicate the wide range of problems that can arise as a result of failure to apply restraints or failing to provide adequate follow-up care once they have been applied. The problem of patient identification arises most frequently in an operating room setting and for the reason that the harm may be substantial it has been included. Cases on patient mix-ups can be traced back to either a failure to comply with formulated identification procedures or reliance on a procedure that has not identified and addressed the areas of high risk.

By comparison, there are not a significant number of cases in which the theory of recovery was based on a failure to teach. The potential for liability is real and the cases included in this section indicate that such failure can have serious implications for the patient and third parties. Akin to the duty to teach is patient compliance which is a relatively new health care concept. Undoubtedly the defense of lack of compliance will appear in future malpractice cases. In any case where the defense is a lack of patient compliance it must be shown that the patient had been instructed in the management of the disease or condition and that the patient or family member comprehended the instructions.

Because physicians use a wide range of equipment in operations and diagnostic procedures most of the existing law involves them. However, with increasingly sophisticated technology and its necessary reliance on machines, many used in critical care units, the nurse has become more exposed to liability as a result of misuse. The one such case included in the chapter does not involve a complex machine. When wheelchairs collapse and bed rails fail to stay in a locked position the critical question becomes, Why?

The chapter concludes with a brief section on transcribing orders. Whether transcribing is done by the nurse or a unit secretary the ultimate responsibility for assuring that the order is accurately transcribed rests with the nurse. The *Norton v. Argonaut* case (excessive digoxin) which is discussed in Chapter 2, is a classic case of a transcribing error. Indubitably, liability would have been found on the part of the nurse, as transcriber of a patently erroneous medical order, even if someone else had administered the Lanoxin overdose. The transcribing error was based on a lack of nursing knowledge. If, however, a nurse transcribes an order that indicates that a drug, new to the market, is to be given twice a day and the physician intended to write once a day, it is unlikely that any liability would fall on the nurse because the law would not hold the nurse to a medical standard.

While the facts of many of these cases are intriguing, most of the court decisions are expected. This is because the courts rely on professional standards familiar to every practicing nurse.

ABANDONMENT OF THE PATIENT

Traditionally the legal theory of patient abandonment has been based on two activities associated with the physician–patient relationship. One is where the physician unilaterally elects to terminate the contractual relationship with a patient who continues to require medical attention and where no provision has been made to accommodate the patient during the transition. The other situation arises when the physician lacks diligence in providing necessary care. Malpractice cases that have applied the abandonment theory to nursing situations are uncommon. This is because the facts necessary to show abandonment in a nursing care context must be unusual or reflect a total disregard for the welfare of the patient. Conceivably with the expansion of nursing practice, particularly in care given by a nurse practitioner, nurses will be exposed to allegations of patient abandonment because of the primary services being provided.

A recent New Jersey case, *Maslonka v. Hermann*, held that the facts could support an abandonment allegation where the nurses failed to monitor a postpartum patient.[1] It is worth noting that the time period over which the negligence occurred was relatively short. The woman died as a result of hemorrhaging within several hours of giving birth and at the trial it was shown that no postpartum monitoring had been done. The case is covered in depth in Chapter 3 on Nursing Judgment.

The most famous case *Duling v. Bluefield Sanitarium*, involving patient abandonment by nurses, resulted from a failure to properly assess the patient's condition and a failure to communicate patient findings to the physician.[2] A 13-year-old child was admitted with a diagnosis of acute rheumatic fever. After the physician had examined her he informed the mother that he was concerned that she might go into failure and if so she would need immediate medical treatment. The events that gave rise to the suit occurred over a period of several hours on the day she was admitted to the hospital. The mother alleged that on one occasion she asked the nurses for some fluids to relieve the child's cough. No one assessed or even visited the child and the mother was told to get the fluids from a machine. When the child exhibited signs of fever the nurses told the mother to sponge her with a wet towel, but no staff member checked her temperature. The mother testified that the child's heart was pounding noticeably. At 9 P.M. the mother reported that the child's nailbeds were blue and she was told to return to the child's room. When the mother asked an aide who was passing juices to check the child she was told that it would be done later. At 11 P.M. a nurse came to the door of the room and said that the child's coughing would not permit her temperature to be taken. The mother appealed to the nurse to come into the room and check the child, but to no avail.

At 11 P.M. the mother spoke to the night nurse and was told: "I know all about Nancy. All she needs is a night's rest, and if you will sit down and be quiet she will get it." Although the child's lips were cyanotic the nurses would not telephone the physician and told the mother that if anyone called the physician it would be the nurses. Finally, the night nurse called the physician when the mother yelled, "My daughter is going to die. Nobody will come and help her." The mother asked the nurse to tell the physician that she thought the child was in heart failure, but the nurse turned her back to the mother and she could not hear what transpired. The physician later testified that none of these findings were communicated to him. After this conversation the child was given an injection for her cough, but no nurse made a proper assessment of her status. After noting that blood was coming from the child's nose the mother demanded that a hospital resident be called. The nurse obtained an order for cough syrup, but the child was unable to swallow it. Finally a nursing supervisor was called and she notified the physician who came in immediately. He was extremely upset and inquired as to how the child had been allowed to progress to such a critical condition. He found the dyspneic child in pulmonary edema with blood-tinged frothy sputum, cyanotic with a heart rate of 162. In spite of emergency care the child died the following day.

The court held that there was sufficient evidence for a jury to find the nurses negligent. Experts testified that the child's life could have been saved if the nurses had performed their duties in a proper manner. It was ascertained that the proper standard of care required the nurses to personally check the child if the nurses were informed of the mother's observations. An expert for the plaintiff testified: "The standard of procedure for the nurses at the defendant hospital would be to investigate these symptoms related to them and proceed accordingly to what they find. If such symptoms and signs are confirmed upon their observation, a physician would be notified; not necessarily the attending physician, it may be the resident. If the symptoms were not verified, I think the nurse would use her own judgment."

The events that support an abandonment theory need not be as dramatic as the rheumatic fever case and it need not involve an extended period of time. Any factual pattern that demonstrates a complete disregard for the patient's welfare, coupled with evidence of unreasonable nursing practice will raise a legitimate question of patient abandonment.

DUTY TO MONITOR

The *duty to monitor* concept has wide application. It includes both a duty to follow the orders of a physician, such as hourly neurologic checks in a head injury case, and a duty to make a judgment that closer monitoring is in order, as in situations where a patient manifests a sudden, unexplained change in physical or emotional status. A nurse does not need to demonstrate extraordinary vigilance in monitoring, but does need to demonstrate a level that is reasonable.

A recent case, *Morreale v. Downing,* allowed the issue of whether a nurse was negligent in failing to discover a hip fracture to go to the jury.[3] A 13-year-old boy suffered a severe brain stem contusion in an automobile accident and was in a coma in the intensive care unit for 3 weeks. Shortly after physical therapy was begun his mother noted a discrepancy in the length of one leg. The physician was notified and subsequent x-ray films revealed a fracture of the acetabulum. The father alleged in his complaint that nurses and other personnel should have noted the injury because they rendered frequent care and had ample opportunity while ambulating the child to observe him and notify the physician of unusual findings.

While it may seem obvious, the duty to monitor pertains to both the physical aspects of the patient's condition and the medical record.

A recent article discussed how the management of a complex ectopic pregnancy illustrated the necessity of monitoring fluid balance.[4] The woman's intake and output was meticulously noted. The medical record indicated the hourly output figures, the identity and amount of all intravenous substances and was, except for one major detail, a complete record. The nurses failed to add up and tabulate totals at critical times and a 7000-ml discrepancy of intake over output during a 30-hour period was not noted by either the nurses or the physicians. The patient's condition, complicated by a number of factors, had required large amounts of fluid and blood. The author of the article concluded by indicting the nurses for failing to provide total fluid-balance figures and the physicians for failing to seek out the figures. Although the author concluded that the patient's severe alcoholism played a major part in her death the article served to illustrate neglect on the part of both the nurses and the physicians. When neglect is coupled with causation the stage is set for litigation.

In another recent case, *Rogers v. Kasdan,* inaccurate intake and output records were a key issue when death resulted from excessive cerebral fluid buildup.[5] These cases deal with a nursing procedure which has not been the subject of litigation in the past and may well reflect a keener understanding by plaintiff attorneys of the intricacies involved in managing critical medical and nursing needs. Intake and output records serve as a basis for therapy and when they are incomplete or inaccurate may preclude instituting appropriate therapy or result in a missed diagnosis. Where a diagnosis is missed or therapy is not instituted and where harm results liability may well be traced back to the nurses who prepared the record.

The monitoring of patients necessarily includes the monitoring of equipment. There are cases in which infants placed in hospital incubators have died as a result of excessive heat.[6] Liability is found on the theory that the nurses failed to monitor the heat gauges in a reasonable manner and did not detect the malfunction in sufficient time to prevent the death of the infant. Liability may also rest with the manufacturer of the incubator.

One case, *Jones v. Hawkes Hospital,* held the hospital liable for the nurse's negligence in leaving a woman in active labor for a period of from 2 to 5 minutes.[7] The woman was restless and under sedation and had repeatedly tried to climb over the bed rails. The nurse had knowledge of the woman's tendency to climb over the rails and the husband who had been with his wife earlier, asked the nurses to watch her so she would not fall. The nurse left the patient to write in a record and was requested by a physician to accompany him while he examined a patient. The court held that no expert testimony was necessary to aid the jury in determining whether the nurse's action constituted negligence as a lay jury could determine whether their actions constituted reasonable care.

Sometimes it is difficult to determine whether the court placed greater weight on nurses' failure to monitor or on the failure of nurses to act. Frequently the two overlap, but each can independently result in a finding of negligence. The following three cases have as much implication for a breach of a duty to act as for a lack of monitoring. The first one illustrates a blatant disregard in monitoring a fresh postoperative cervical laminectomy, whereas the other two demonstrate adequate monitoring, but a failure to process the findings and establish a diagnosis that a reasonable nurse knows would indicate a need for immediate intervention. Two of the cases, *Sanchez* and *Perkins*, resulted in "vegetative" states and subsequent death.

In *Sanchez v. Bay General Hospital* the court held that the nurses deviated from accepted and recognized nursing standards in the following areas: observation, timely and responsive action, and communication.[8] Additionally, the hospital was liable for the failure to have staff competent in cardiopulmonary resuscitation. The 37-year-old mother of four underwent a cervical laminectomy as a result of injuries sustained in an automobile accident 2 years previously. The surgery was uneventful and the woman remained in the recovery room for approximately 2½ hours. Her transfer blood pressure was 120/80. Although she had been vomiting in the postanesthesia room her recovery went well. At 3:15 P.M. she was transferred to the ward. Considering the ensuing events it may have been significant that she was transferred during the change of day shift. No vital signs or other neurologic assessment were taken when she was returned to the unit. No transfer report was given or requested and the floor nurses did not review the medical record. No suctioning equipment was in place in her room.

Fifteen minutes after her return to the ward a nurses' aide took her vital signs. Her blood pressure, pulse, and respiratory rate was 96/60, 80, and 18, respectively. The aide did not report the vital signs to any nurse and no professional judgment was made to notify the physician or to continually monitor her status. The evening shift nurses were not informed of her status when they received the day report. A friend who was at the bedside reported that she was in pain and vomiting continuously. A nurse at the nurse's station told the visitor that the woman could have water although the postoperative orders indicated that she was NPO. The nurse did not look at her postoperative orders. The aide took a second set of vital signs 15 minutes after the first ones and recorded them as 90/50, 68, and 16. The aide reported the fact that the patient was vomiting and a team leader checked her vital signs. No one was informed or did anything about her deteriorating condition.

Ten minutes later the patient had a seizure and arrest whereupon the visitor went for assistance. The aide who responded to the visitor ran out in panic and failed to initiate any emergency measures. The responding team leader checked the patient's pupils, pulse and blood pressure, but did not check the airway or initiate any other cardiopulmonary resuscitation (CPR) measures. In fact neither had any CPR training. A few moments later the emergency room physician appeared and managed the resuscitation. The patient was declared "brain dead" that evening and subsequently died while on a respirator 2 months later when her innominate artery eroded causing exsanguination. Exsanguination was listed as the "actual" cause of death and the defendants failed to rebut the plaintiff's allegation that it resulted from nursing mismanagement of the tracheostomy tube cuff. In the absence of evidence to rebut the plaintiff's allegation the court characterized this as "no less than gross neglect."

The surgeon testifying about the immediate postoperative care said, "a grave event was going on and there was virtual paralysis in response to it" and that the standard of nursing care received was below the standard of care which should be given anywhere in the United States. Nursing experts testifying for the plaintiff acknowledged that the care reflected a total lack of adherence to basic nursing principles. After reviewing the medical records one expert testified that they did not indicate a complete assessment or that appropriate actions were taken at a critical time. One nursing expert was allowed to testify that a patient released from the postanesthesia room in satisfactory condition does not normally suffer brain damage and subsequent death in the absence of negligence.

The other case, *Variety Children's Hospital v. Perkins*, which resulted in brain death involved a 4-month-old child who had a tracheotomy.[9] Liability was found against both the nurse and the resident. The boy had been admitted for correction of a congenital tracheal condition. The surgery which was uneventful was done early in the evening and the child's surgeon last saw the child at 11 P.M. in the intensive care unit (ICU). Around 4 A.M. the child stopped breathing and suffered irreversible brain damage. The cause of the arrest was a massive pneumothorax from the gradual accumulation of trapped air beneath the skin. Experts determined that the child exhibited signs and symptoms of the complication, known as subcutaneous emphysema, for almost 2 hours before the pneumothorax occurred. The court held that the physician failed in his duty to diagnose the complication. Liability on the part of the nurse resulted from her failure to make a judgment that the signs and symptoms signaled a possible postoperative complication. While the opinion did not use the term, nursing diagnosis, the fact pattern clearly falls within the realm of nursing diagnosis and the failure of the nurse to establish a diagnosis was substandard nursing care. The length of time the child presented with the symptoms was an important factor in finding liability.

The next case, *Long v. Johnson*, involved harm which resulted from the nurse's failure to discontinue a pitocin infusion.[10] The harm was severe neurologic impairment suffered by the neonate. The mother had 13 prior pregnancies, all delivered vaginally and without complication. The mother, who was 43 years old, was admitted at 5 A.M. and was examined by an obstetrician who ruptured her amniotic sac. The fluid was clear. Two hours later the nurses reported a meconium discharge and the physician did another vaginal examination. No other significant findings were noted. An hour later the nurses noted irregular contractions and another vaginal examination was done. The woman felt "comfortable" and the fetal heart tones were good, however, she had not progressed beyond her admission dilatation measurement of 4 cm. Pitocin was begun right after the last vaginal examination. The hospital bylaws required that a physician begin the pitocin, but need not personally monitor the patient so long as the physician remained in the hospital. The mother later testified that no one felt her abdomen and although she drifted in and out of sleep she always awoke to the touch. The record failed to reflect that any monitoring was done during this period. When the nurses testified, none had any independent recollection of the sequence of monitoring.

At 9 A.M., 40 minutes after the pitocin was begun, an attempt at vaginal delivery was done, but without success. At 9:50 A.M. the patient complained of severe pain and the uterus visibly took on the shape of an hourglass (Bandl's ring). At 10:20 A.M. she was delivered via cesarean section. The hospital record indicated that the pitocin continued to infuse 30 minutes after the section was begun. Experts for the woman testified that the abdominal contractions could have been quickly halted by stopping the pitocin and that the uterine complication warranted stopping it. The nurse's testimony that the pitocin was discontinued before beginning the cesarean was not in harmony with the record as it was introduced at the trial. The case illustrates that very little time should have elapsed between the occurrence of the problem and the medical or nursing intervention.

The physician was not held liable. Each time the nurses informed him of their findings he examined the patient. The fact that the bylaw did not require the continual presence of the physician was significant. The case held that the nurses had an independent duty to stop infusion of the pitocin when they observed the Bandl's ring and that no such duty rested with the physician. In essence, he should have been able to rely on an appropriate nursing action.

DUTY TO TAKE MEASURES TO PROTECT THE PATIENT

The duty to take measures to protect the patient means that there is a duty to act in a reasonable way. In the law of negligence, reasonableness is a critical principle. Thus, lack of reasonable care is a key factor on which a negligence suit relies. Legally a failure to take measures or actions when the law imposes such a duty will incur liability when it can be shown that an individual suffered harm as a direct result of the failure to take reasonable action. There are a significant number of cases in which liability was found for failing to put up bed rails, leaving rails in a down position, and not replacing broken or inadequate rails. The law has consistently imposed liability when it is shown that the individual was infirm as a result of medication, disease process, age, or mental impairment. Liability may be imposed even when the infirmity, such as confusion, is short-term.

Bed Rails

There are a number of cases involving children in which the harm resulted in the tragic death of the child.

In one case, *Campbell v. Thornton,* no liability was found where a young child who was "posied" in her crib was found hanging over the side of the crib shortly after the mother left the child.[11] Testimony indicated that the mother left the side of the crib down and did not inform the nurses that she had done so. A significant factor involved in the case was the short time span between the time the mother left and the infant's strangulation. Liability may have been found against the staff if a lengthy time had elapsed during which they should have detected the mother's oversight.

In another case, *St. Luke's Hospital Association v. Long,* liability was found against the hospital for the negligence of a nurse when she placed a 3-year-old postoperative tonsils and adenoids patient in an adult-sized bed.[12] Although the bed had rails on each side the child's body slipped through them and he strangled. The mother had informed the nurse that the child tossed and turned and might fall. The court found that the nurse failed in her duty to furnish the proper equipment as well as failed to give adequate attention to the needs of the child.

A case involving an elderly woman decided in 1981 is particularly instructive because of the multiple factors involved in the fact pattern.[13]

In *Polonsky v. Union Hospital,* an 80-year-old woman was admitted to the special care unit after suffering a heart attack. She was transferred to a semiprivate room 10 days later. Her first night on the unit she was given Dalmane at 11 p.m. She had four bed rails, a set for the upper bed and a set for the lower part. Around midnight she awoke and needed to go to the bathroom. In her confusion she thought that she was in her own home. She did not ring for the nurse, but climbed out of bed. The upper rails were elevated, but the lower rails were not. She fractured her hip when she fell in the hospital corridor. Because of her poor general condition the surgery had to be delayed which significantly impaired her healing process.

Two important factors were introduced at the trial. The first was the hospital policy which read: "Bedside Rails. With confused or disoriented patients, beds should be in low position at all times with side rails up, except when nursing care is being given. If patient objects to the side rails being raised, a note to that effect should be included in the nursing notes or the doctor may indicate on the order sheet that he does not want the side rails raised." The court acknowledged that in some jurisdictions expert testimony would be required because the bed rail question involves matters of medical or professional judgment.[14] Those jurisdictions hold that the question is beyond the common knowledge of the jury. However, other jurisdictions hold that the question involves routine custodial care of the patient and is within the knowledge and experience of the jury.[15] The court held that no expert testimony was required because the hospital policy served to show negligence which the jury could deliberate upon.

The second significant factor in the case was the introduction of the drug manufacturer's warnings into evidence. One section of the warning stated, "Dizziness, drowsiness, lightheadedness, staggering, ataxia, and falling have occurred, particularly in elderly or debilitated persons." Thus, the court held that the jury could properly infer that the elderly woman was "debilitated" and that the nurse should have anticipated that she would probably become confused or disoriented and be subject to the bedrail policy. A reasonable *inference* could be drawn from the nurse's failure to raise the lower rails after administering Dalmane.

A Louisiana court in *Hunt v. Bogalusa Medical Center* held a hospital liable for failing to provide full bed rails.[16] The patient fell from a bed that had only half rails. He was a fresh postoperative patient and was confused and sedated heavily when the fall occurred. The court stated: "A hospital is bound to exercise the requisite amount of care toward a patient that the particular patient's condition may require. It is the hospital's duty to protect a patient from dangers that may result from the patient's physical and mental incapacities as well as from external circumstances peculiarly within the hospital's control."[17]

Another Louisiana case, *Smith v. West Calcasieu-Cameron Hospital*, dealt with the question of liability of the physician for failing to specifically order bed rails.[18] The court held that no liability would attach to the physician for failing to order bed rails. The court said that the particular patient care issue was properly left to the hospital staff. Liability was found against the hospital for the negligence of the nurse. The patient, who had bronchitis, was admitted in the early evening. He was given a pain medication and shortly thereafter Carbrital. Within an hour after receiving the sleeping pill he fell from the bed. The bed either did not have rails or they were not elevated. A review of previous hospital records indicated that narcotics made the patient confused and groggy. He had also fallen in the hospital during a previous admission, but did not injure himself.

The plaintiff introduced the nurses' procedure book into evidence which contained the statement, "Side rails are always applied in the following instances: (1) Patients under sedation. . . ." In addition, the hospital director testified that elevation of bed rails was not normally a matter of a medical order, but was instituted when necessary by hospital personnel. Liability resulted because the nurses violated hospital policy as well as generally accepted nursing practices.

Burns from Smoking

The problem of patients who smoke in bed frequently confronts nurses. Many hospitals have adopted the policy that patients who can ambulate may only smoke in designated areas, away from patient rooms and that visitors may only smoke in designated areas. The policy is communicated to the patient via informational booklets which are provided on admission. In view of the risk of smoking in bed and the many distractions which can occur in a hospital setting the policy is very sound. Patients who are confined to bed are instructed that smoking is permitted if they have someone in attendance. This is especially important if the patient is receiving a drug or treatment that foreseeably may result in drowsiness. In extreme circumstances, that is, where the patient has previously burned holes in the bed garments or furniture or has been seen sleeping while holding a lighted cigarette, the staff may take away the matches or the cigarettes. Such measures under the proper circumstances are reasonable to protect the welfare of other patients and prevent a catastrophe.

One court, in *Brown v. Decatur Memorial Hospital,* held that where a patient voluntarily intoxicated himself and secured matches and cigarettes whereby he subsequently burned himself a jury may find that he was contributorily negligent.[19] The court held that intoxication was no excuse for failing to act reasonably.

No liability was found against an Illinois hospital when a patient in traction severely burned herself when her nightgown became ignited by a match she dropped which was not completely extinguished.[20] The hospital in *Seymour v. Victory Memorial Hospital* successfully argued that the patient was contributorily negligent. The woman had been in the hospital for 3 days. Because she was heavily sedated with Demerol and Valium the nurses removed her cigarettes and lighter and told her to call for a nurse who would attend her while she smoked. The woman was an addictive smoker and requested supervision up to 20 times per day. She had been known to secure cigarettes from persons passing by in the hall. Evidence was not clear as to how the woman secured the cigarettes and matches. There was testimony that a volunteer sold a package of cigarettes to either the patient herself or to the woman's roommate who, in turn, gave the plaintiff a cigarette. There was no note anywhere within the semiprivate room indicating that the patient should not smoke alone. The plaintiff's theory of negligence was that an employee of the hospital had supplied her with the cigarettes and matches. However, this could not be substantiated.

A nurse testified in the case that she daily checked the patient's drawers and removed any cigarettes she found. From the testimony elicited during the trial it was clear that the patient understood the nurses instructions regarding the nature and need for supervision while smoking. The court stated: "The hospital nurses had responsibility up to a certain point because of their awareness of the plaintiff's vulnerability to falling asleep suddenly and involuntarily and for that reason they imposed supervision on her smoking. She was fully aware of this and while the evidence may have tended to show that she was physically impaired, there was no evidence that she was not rational. Thus, she was fully capable of appreciating the danger to which she was subjecting herself in evading the stricture as to supervision of her smoking."

Infirm Patients

Just as the law imposes a greater duty when caring for unconscious patients, so it imposes a greater duty when rendering care for individuals who are infirm. The underlying principle is that such individuals are less in control of their welfare than those in a noninfirm condition.

The effect of medications is a significant factor in injuries occurring in hospitals. A federal court in *Thompson v. U.S.* held that a licensed practical nurse was negligent in sending a patient to the laboratory without the aid of a wheelchair or via stretcher.[21] The patient had been admitted ambulatory the day before the injury for evaluation of a knee disability which had existed for 14 years. The physician testified that he left verbal orders for bedrest, although the nurse denied it. The patient received a narcotic during the afternoon and evening, along with a sleeping pill. He also received Vistaril and Aminophylline when he awakened during the night with dyspnea and chest pain. At 7 A.M. the nurse handed the patient a laboratory slip and instructed him to go for tests. The patient testified that there was a sign posted over his bed indicating that he was on bedrest and he objected to the nurse. While standing in line in the X-ray department he fainted and injured his finger. After three unsuccessful operations it had to be amputated. The court held that even if no sign was present liability would still be found. The nurse testified that she examined his record when she came on duty and was aware of the administered medications and the episode of chest pain.

Liability was found in another case, *Block v. Michael Reese Hospital*, involving the transport of a patient to her room after laboratory tests.[22] The patient, an 87-year-old woman, had been in the hospital for 13 days for investigation of gastrointestinal pain. In preparation for colon studies she had been on a liquid diet for 2 days and was NPO the day of the x-rays examination. She was escorted back to the unit in a wheelchair, however, she testified that the attendant left her at the nurses' station and took the chair away. The woman fainted and injured herself in the fall. The nurses contested the woman's version of events. Hospital regulations stipulated that patients were to be escorted to and from their hospital room and on their return, the escort was to notify the ward secretary at the nurses' station and then return the patient to the room. Case law in the state held that hospital regulations alone did not conclusively establish the standard of care owed. However, it was clear that the hospital did have a duty to safely return the woman to her room. The hospital did not present any testimony of the attendant, the ward secretary, or others who may have safely situated the patient. Reasonable care would require that a fasting elderly patient should be returned to her bed or, at a minimum, directions sought from the nurse who was familiar with the woman's situation. The hospital regulations, although not absolutely standard setting, served to indicate that they existed for the purpose of patient safety.

It is clear that the mental and physical state of the patient at the time of the injury is an important factual issue. The court will look to the degree the patient is dependent on health care providers to protect and guard him against harm. However, where it is shown that the patient was on notice of a particular hazard, such notice coupled with the patient's physical ability and mental alertness to ward off such harm may bar recovery or reduce the amount of money damages. Evidence of impaired judgment or severe motor deficit on the part of the patient will transfer liability to the care providers.

In a substantial number of cases defense attorneys will raise the defense of comparative or contributory negligence. At one time the legal doctrine of contributory negligence was recognized to partially or totally defeat the plaintiff's allegation of negligence. The doctrine meant that if the plaintiff "contributed" to his injury it would bar recovery of damages either completely or partially. In the majority of states the doctrine of comparative negligence has been adopted in lieu of the contributory negligence doctrine.

In finding comparative negligence the jury will assess the amount in percent from any recovery the plaintiff would have received. For example, if the total liability is worth $100,000 and the plaintiff's negligence is assessed at 25 percent, he will recover $75,000. No recovery of damages will be obtained if the plaintiff's negligence was greater than the defendant's. Comparative negligence is the failure of a plaintiff to use reasonable care to avoid injury to himself.

In an early 1970s case, *Memorial Hospital of South Bend v. Scott,* in which the defense of contributory negligence was raised, the court held that an impaired person owes ordinary reasonable care in light of the circumstances integral to the situation.[23] This standard is less stringent than the standard that an unimpaired individual would be held to.

The case illustrates, among other things, the necessity of taking a complete history and establishing a patient needs assessment. The patient had multiple sclerosis with impaired vision, impaired motor ability, including equilibrium, and other major sensory deficits. An hour after receiving Thorazine for a spinal tap he asked to use the bathroom. He was never instructed or warned about the bedpan flusher which was located near the toilet flushing apparatus. In fact, the hospital was on notice that the bedpan flushers were dangerous, and it was known that a staff member had

been burned when he inadvertently activated the bedpan flusher instead of
the correct handle. The head nurse had reported the incident and thought
all the flushers had been deactivated, but in fact only some of them had
been deactivated. The patient was severely burned when, seated on the
toilet, he inadvertently pressed the bedpan flusher and was inundated by
the scalding water.

At the time the case was brought, Indiana law held that a person who
contributed to the negligent act was barred from recovery for his injuries.
Finding liability on the part of the hospital, the court held that the patient's
physical infirmities were important factors in finding no contributory negligence on his part. In essence, the reasonable care standard was modified
to include the patient's disabilities. The two important factual findings on
the issue of contributory negligence were the lack of awareness on the part
of the patient that the flusher represented a potential danger to him and the
extent of impairment he suffered. Extending the disability concept further
it has been held that the standard of care which a child must prove is more
flexible than that which an adult must meet.[24] The law recognizes that
both a child and a severely impaired individual are under a disability that
affects their ability to recognize or respond to the threat of harm.

There are a number of cases that hold that where the patient's
request for assistance went unheeded and the patient resorted to self-
help and was injured, liability exists.[25]

In *Leavitt v. St. Tammany Parish Hospital* the hospital was negligent for
having less than adequate staff available to meet the patient's needs.[26] The
case is particularly noteworthy because it is one of the few cases which
issued an opinion specifically addressing the lack of adequate staff issue. A
number of other cases raised the issue, but did not incorporate it into the
case holding.[27] In *Leavitt* the court held that the hospital owed a duty to
respond promptly to the patient's call for assistance and that it breached
its duty by having less than adequate staff available.

The patient, who was 57 years old, was admitted for treatment of severe
congestive heart failure and diabetes. The nurses appropriately instructed
her to call for assistance when she needed to get out of bed. She was in a
weakened state and several of the drugs she was taking impaired her mental clarity. The woman alleged in her complaint that she put on the call
light and waited for at least 15 minutes. Receiving no response, she got out
of bed to walk down the hall to the bathroom. She fell as she was attempting to get back into bed. The orderly who first noted her fall and who
helped her back to bed later testified that there was urine on the floor at the
side of the bed. The court regarded this as indicative of her critical need to
get to the bathroom. In allowing recovery the court said that in addition to
the inadequate staffing the hospital breached its duty to respond promptly
in failing to at least verbally answer the assistance light to inquire into her
needs.

The issue of staffing was again raised in *Koppang v. St. Paul's Church
Home*, a case against a nursing home and its administrator for the alleged

failure to maintain an adequate nursing staff and negligent failure to observe and treat an 88-year-old resident.[28] The case was settled out of court and thus there was no legal holding on either issue. The resident had been in the nursing home for several years when she developed decubitus ulcers over her hip and coccyx. Her condition deteriorated over a 3-month period and she was finally transferred to a hospital which also found that she was suffering from malnutrition. She required pedicle skin grafts to cover the ulcers.

The staffing issue is most apt to arise in situations involving infirm patients, young children, and those otherwise not responsible for their own safety.

In a widely reported New York case, *Horton v. Niagara Falls Medical Center*, the court again addressed the staffing issue and held that reasonable care under the circumstances required greater supervision of the patient.[29] The issue was not the adequacy of the available staff, but rather the inappropriate use of available staff. The nursing staff was aware that the patient, admitted in an acute state for treatment of pneumonitis was confused, lacking in coordination, weak, and had difficulty seeing. He was admitted to a room on the second floor of the hospital with an adjoining balcony. His wife was with him during much of the early afternoon during which time he was vague and unresponsive to her questions. Shortly after his wife left, construction workers saw the man on the balcony at which time he was calling for a ladder. The workers notified the unit and he was placed in a Posey restraint and cloth wrist restraints were applied. When the physician was called he instructed the nurse to "keep an eye on him" and that if further trouble developed the physician would transfer him to a secured room. The nurse telephoned the wife and suggested she return to the hospital to sit with the husband. She was told that the staff was not free to sit with him. The wife, who lived approximately 20 minutes away, replied that she would have her mother go to the hospital immediately. Her mother lived only five minutes from the hospital. The wife requested that someone sit with the man while the mother was in transit. She was told that they were "understaffed and we can't possibly do that." The mother arrived to see the workers gathered around the patient who had fallen to the ground.

The court applied the principle that the hospital was required to exercise reasonable care and diligence in safeguarding a patient and that such care is measured by the capacity of the patient to provide for his own safety. The court considered the number of persons available either by way of staff, private duty nurses, or relatives. At the time of the incident there were 19 patients on the unit, all but 9 in an open ward. The man was in one of the private rooms. Just prior to the fall an aide who was assigned to the man's room was allowed to go to supper and the remaining staff were carrying out routine duties, taking afternoon temperatures or reviewing records. No evidence was submitted that any more pressing need or emergency existed on the unit. The entire staff consisted of a charge nurse, a practical nurse, an aide, and a registered nurse being oriented to the hospital. Hospital orderlies working throughout the hospital were also available. The court found that there was sufficient staff to provide one-to-one supervision for the short time necessary.

Two years later a federal court *Northrup v. Archbishop Bergan Mercy Hospital* held that a hospital had not exercised reasonable care in light of the fact that the decedent had previously freed himself from restraints.[30] His wife alleged that the hospital was negligent in failing to install window locks, failing to adequately restrain, failing to supervise, and failing to keep the physician sufficiently informed of the man's mental state. The man had manifested confusion, disorientation, and combative behavior after surgery which persisted off and on for a number of days. During these periods the staff had used bed rails, a vest restraint, a locked Posey waist restraint, and Librium. They did not use wrist restraints as they were not ordered. The record showed that 24 hours before his death he became very restless, tore his vest restraint apart, and shouted that he was going home. Approximately 1½ hours before his death a nurse recorded having difficulties with the patient. At the 11 P.M. shift change he appeared to be resting quietly and at 11:25 P.M. an aide who was sitting with him left to go home. Fifteen minutes later a night aide discovered he had broken from his restraints and was hanging from the window. He died in the fall from the window.

Reasonable care means that there is a duty to act when life-threatening events occur.

In *Soto v. State*, the state of New York was sued for the failure to timely transfer a resident from a state mental health facility to an acute care facility.[31] The wrongful death suit was brought by the mother of an 8-year-old child admitted for schizophrenia. There was testimony at the trial that it was routine to take temperatures twice a day and record them. The medical record reflected that the child had a temperature of 101.8°F. on March 14. The next day she was given penicillin for a temperature of 100°F. On March 16 her temperature was 104°F. and 102°F. On the day of her death her 6 A.M. temperature was 106.8°F. She had been given aspirin and an alcohol sponge bath during the night. She was given oxygen and seen by a priest. Just prior to being transferred her vital signs included a temperature of 107°F., an apical pulse of 176, and a respiratory rate of 34. She died of respiratory arrest shortly after being transferred. An autopsy showed that she had atelectasis and congestion of her brain, lungs, kidney, and liver.

A supervisor testified that she was not called to see the child until the day she died. At that time she was moribund and the supervisor ordered her removed immediately to an acute care facility. She testified that it was her responsibility to make rounds twice per shift and that she visited patients as requested by the nurse in charge of a unit or when a particular shift report warranted it. Finding against the hospital, the court held that the state had a duty to take every reasonable precaution to protect its patients from injury. The court stated that the required degree of care for patients in institutions for the mentally ill is such reasonable care and attention for their safety as their condition may require, and that when the patient is mentally retarded this obligation is imperative.

In cases of severe hemorrhage a patient is entirely dependent on others to diagnose and manage the crisis.

In *New Biloxi Hospital v. Frazier,* an early 1960s case, a jury held that negligence on the part of emergency room nurses caused a patient to bleed to death.[32] Although the court did not introduce the concept of abandonment the facts would support it. The patient, a 42-year-old man, was brought to the emergency room around 11 P.M. after being shot in the arm. The blast tore away the brachial artery and he bled considerably at the scene before being transported via ambulance to the hospital. No one examined him in the emergency room although one nurse observed him and walked away. Blood was gushing from his arm and a large puddle had formed on the floor. Twenty minutes later another nurse looked at him and she also walked away. He remained on the ambulance stretcher and was thrashing about and cursing. Finally, at the insistence of the ambulance drivers he was placed on a table and a nurse took his blood pressure and pulse and contacted a physician who arrived about 30 minutes later. The nurse placed a towel over the bleeding area but did not attempt to stop the bleeding. After looking at the wound the physician recommended that the patient, whom he had learned was a veteran, be transferred to the Veterans Administration hospital for surgery. It took a long time to make transfer arrangements. During this time neither the nurse or the physician attempted to stop the bleeding. Throughout this time the patient was perspiring, restless, and thirsty and his blood pressure decreased while his pulse rate increased.

The physician testified that he relied on the nurse to observe the patient and advise him of changes and that he would have treated the patient before transferring him. Two hours after arriving in the emergency room the patient was taken to the VA Hospital which was a 10-minute ride away. Upon arrival he was moribund and was pronounced dead in 25 minutes.

The physician was also found liable. The court held that the nurses were negligent in several respects including failure to make any inquiry of the ambulance drivers concerning the length of time the man had been wounded and the amount of bleeding which occurred at the scene, leaving him on the ambulance stretcher for an excessive length of time, failure to immediately examine the wound, failure to take even reasonably simple measures to diminish bleeding, failure to communicate essential data to the treating physician (including data they should have obtained), failure to observe the patient after the decision had been made to transfer him.

The court held that the "degree of care exacted of a hospital toward its patients is such reasonable care and attention for their safety as their mental and physical condition, if known, may require. It should be in proportion to the physical or mental ailments of the patient rendering him unable to look after his own safety." At the time the case was brought there was little case law on the duty owed emergency room patients.[33] In *New*

Biloxi Hospital the court held that "a victim should be permitted to leave the hospital only after he has been seen, examined and offered reasonable first aid." This aid must be rendered in the exercise of due or ordinary care and the almost total inattention to the patient in this instance failed to meet the ordinary care standard.

In a recent Louisiana case, *Booty v. Kentwood Manor Nursing Home,* an appeals court upheld the jury verdict for the next of kin of a 90-year-old nursing home patient.[34] The family alleged that the man fell and fractured his hip because the nursing home failed to adequately supervise and provide for his safety given his confused mental state and frail physical condition. The man and his wife had been living in the nursing home about 1 year before the accident. At the time of admission the man had cerebral vascular arteriosclerosis with resultant advanced senile dementia. He was ambulatory and a "wanderer" especially in the nighttime. Each patient admitted to the home had to be certified by a physician that he was incapable of caring for himself before he would be admitted. The entire staff knew of the man's propensity for attempting to leave the facility. Although the man did not like being physically restrained and had a decreased tolerance to sedation the nursing home physician had left "standing" orders that any patient could be restrained as necessary (PRN) for their own protection. The record indicated that the patient had been briefly restrained on one or two prior occasions.

At the time of the injury the facility was caring for 121 residents. It had a total of seven exterior doors which were easily accessible to patients and two less accessible exterior doors. All, but one of the doors was attached to a buzzer alarm system. This door was used by visitors entering and leaving the home. A nurses' station near this latter door was staffed to prevent a patient leaving through that door. When any door was opened from the inside the alarm system indicated which door had been opened. However, during the day and evening the doors were propped open for the convenience of the staff. The alarm system was not activated until the 11 P.M. to 7 A.M. tour of duty. The front door which was not connected to the system was kept open until 11 P.M. and after that time a key had to be used to open it from inside and outside the home.

The man had returned to the facility in the early evening after visiting his wife who was in a hospital. On two occasions after his return the staff had to retrieve him from outside the building. On these occasions he told the staff he was going to chop wood or was fleeing from someone. Approximately 15 minutes before the accident an aide at one of the nursing stations saw him walking near the unlocked front exit door. She testified she told him to go back to the patient rooms area, but did nothing to restrain him or to return him to his room. She said that an emergency took her and the other staff back to the patient rooms section, leaving the nurses station near the front door unattended. An LPN testified that about this same time she also told the patient to return to his room. A short time later the LPN heard someone shouting for help and she checked some of the patient's rooms, but found nothing. Shortly after that the patient was discovered lying on the steps leading to the front door. It was not known which door the man used to exit the facility. He died 12 days later from surgical complications.

In upholding the jury's verdict the appeals court said that a nursing home is not the insurer of the safety of its patients, however it was required to take reasonable steps to prevent injury to patients in conditions similar to the decedent's. Further, it found that although the home had an effective alarm and patient security system it inactivated the system for the convenience of the staff.

Summary

Measures taken to protect patients in hospitals and nursing homes include physical means, such as restraints and bed rails, and equally important, the system of monitoring an individual who is at increased risk for injury. For example, many elderly patients are physiologically unable to detoxify drugs and this may result in a cumulative effect which can cause impaired judgment. This fact, coupled with a strange environment, and visual and auditory problems may increase the risk.

An individual's history, both medical and social, is important in identifying potential problem areas. For example, a patient who is used to getting up once or twice during the night to use the bathroom will have the same need in the hospital. The courts have been consistent in finding liability where an individual rang the bell for assistance which went unheeded for an unreasonable length of time.

The law expects that protective measures will be in place to protect the patient from harm which is foreseeable. Such forseeable harm includes falls when patients have a history of dizziness or where the patient has been NPO for tests. Some of the more recent cases have addressed the inadequate staffing issue and incompetent staffing issue. The U.S. Supreme Court in one of its abortion cases took note of the staffing issue when it held that one of the state interests in the regulation of abortion facilities was a requirement that the facility "possess all the staffing and services necessary to perform an abortion safely."[35] Lack of staffing is rarely a viable defense because there is a minimum nursing standard below which no nursing activity should fall.[36] The duty to protect the patient runs parallel with the needs of the patient.

PHYSICAL RESTRAINTS

Because nurses are in a position of providing continuous care over a 24-hour period they are uniquely suited to determine when a patient should be placed in physical restraints. Nurses frequently make judgments with respect to when PRN chemical restraining drugs should be administered, but these require a physician's order. Previously, the general rule with respect to the application of physical restraints was that it required an order from the phsyician. However, today the standard is that a nurse should take reasonable measures to protect the patient from harming himself or others and such measures include applying restraints. This is particularly important when delay would increase the risk of harm to the patient or others. Equally important is the duty to monitor a patient closely to assure that the restraints themselves do not harm the patient. The extent of the duty to monitor varies with the circumstances of the patient. A patient placed in wrist restraints who has a history of impaired circulation of the arms needs to be monitored more closely than a patient who does not have such an impairment and if the impairment is significant and other restraint options are available then wrist restraints may arguably be inappropriate means to protect the patient.*

A caveat is in order with respect to the selection of restraints. Leather wrist and ankle restraints if used mandate close monitoring. Leather restraints may increase the risk of harm because they are more constraining than other types of restraining devices. When a patient fights against the restraints or becomes awkwardly positioned there is risk of swelling or direct physical injury. These types of restraints are used mostly in psychiatric wards or facilities. Another caveat is that it is unwise to wet the knots of restraining ties because of the difficulty in releasing the knot in an emergency when time may be of the essence. The emergency caveat also calls into question the use of locking devices on some restraints. This is because of the risk that the key will not be available when the device needs to be unlocked quickly or that the time lost in unlocking the device puts the patient at increased risk.

The extent of the duty to inspect the limbs or part of the body restrainted also varies depending on the patient's history. Before the patient is placed in restraints the condition of the limb or part should be assessed so that it will serve as a baseline. The patient's record should reflect the baseline and indicate that monitoring of the limb or part has been done on a regular basis. One court held that restraints should have been removed at 4-hour intervals to exercise the limb.[37] The patient in *Richmond County Hospital v. Haynes* was in a diabetic coma and had leather wrist restraints in place for a total of 30 hours without their being removed. Ordinarily courts are reluctant to impose so specific a standard, but the unreasonable length of time the patient had to endure the restraints was a factor. In addition, his inability to communicate his needs of discomfort was an important factor.

When nursing policies are being established or evaluated, attention

---

* See Appendix A on Nursing Guidelines for Use of Restraints in Nonpsychiatric Settings (at back of book).

should be given to the "reasonableness" element when specifying the time spans for monitoring or removal for inspection or exercise. If policies exist and have not been complied with they will find their way into the courtroom. Sometimes inspection of the part can be accomplished without disturbing the restraint, however, reasonableness would require the unwrapping or complete removal of restraints when a patient has been "fighting" them. Policies should distinguish monitoring the restrained limb for adverse effects from releasing them to exercise the part, especially where the policy sets out time periods.

Restraints should be used judiciously. If the facility has an up-to-date policy on restraints it should be complied with. When a nurse makes a judgment that a patient needs to be restrained and there is no order the patient's physician or other medical person should be put on notice of the necessity for restraints. The frequent assessment of color, sensation, and motion of the restrained limbs should be indicated in the patient's record. Most states have regulations relative to the use of restraints in psychiatric facilities and nursing homes. These regulations, internal policies, and guidelines or standards adopted by recognized nursing authorities or groups are important sources of evidence in helping a jury determine whether reasonable care under the circumstances was rendered.

In summary, reasonable care requires frequent monitoring of the restrained part and this may, but not necessarily, require removal of the device. With respect to removal of the device for the sole purpose of exercise, reasonableness (as a *minimum*) would require that it be done at least once every 8-hour period. Important factors to consider are whether the device restrains the entire body, such as chest jacket, or a part, such as the hand to prevent removal of a dressing. Where the device acts to restrain most body movement, reasonableness would require more frequent release to preserve the integrity of the body systems. The patient's history of an impaired system also plays a significant role in deciding how frequently exercise is necessary for the whole body or a part.

Physical restraint problems can occur as a result of restraining during operative procedures.

> In one early case, *Palver v. Clarksdale Hospital*, the patient alleged that gangrene resulted from being strapped around the feet.[38] He said that the 45 minutes they were on the weight of his body caused swelling and impaired his circulation. In a later case, *Koepel v. St. Joseph's Hospital*, a patient alleged that severe damage to his ulnar nerve resulted from placement of the operating room table strap.[39] The patient had complained of the placement of the strap while in the operating room and before anesthesia was given. On regaining consciousness he complained of pain and numbness of his arm. Both cases illustrate the need to select reasonable restraining devices and positions, as well as a duty to monitor their effect.

A Florida court, in *Moore v. Halifax Hospital*, held that there was sufficient evidence for the jury to decide whether a child's injuries resulted from negligence in securing the child's arm to a restraining device or by the nurses failure to prevent the child from struggling against the intravenous boards tightly strapped to the child's arms.[40] The 6-year-old child had eye surgery on both eyes. Initially the child had one board taped to each arm to prevent her from touching or dislodging the dressings. Later that evening a nurse changed the restraining device and applied two boards to each arm and secured it with adhesive tape. Evidence indicated that the evening nurses monitored the arms frequently and the child did not complain of the boards during that shift. The mother, who remained with the child, testified that the child began to show discomfort during the night shift and that she asked that the arms be checked. The nurses checked the child's arms but did not remove the boards although the child complained about the boards and continued to struggle against them. When the boards were removed the child had suffered injuries to both elbows.

The court held that it was a jury question whether there was negligence in securing the boards too tightly or whether the staff was negligent in preventing the child from struggling. The fact that the mother had reported that the child was in distress and otherwise called attention to her arms served to put the nurses on notice of the possibility of harm. A previous Florida ruling had established that a greater standard of care should be exercised in the treatment of the very young or very old, particularly if they are under sedation or other physical impairment.[41] Both cases adopted the principle that the amount of care is measured by the capacity of a patient to care for himself.

Negligence may also be based on the nurse's failure to apply restraints. However, the courts have consistently held that a hospital is not an insurer of the safety of its patients. Just because a patient falls from a bed or chair does not necessarily constitute negligence.

In *Clark v. Harris Hospital* a Texas jury found that the nurses were not liable for failing to place an elderly woman in a Posey restraint.[42] The woman had been in the hospital for 8 days and fell. She subsequently succumbed to the injuries associated with the fall. The woman's daughter sought to show that the nurses failed in their duty to restrain her and that she either fell out of bed or was not refrained from climbing out of bed. The daughter failed to show that the nurses were on notice or should have been on notice that the woman might harm herself in a fall from the bed. The case illustrates the burden on the party bringing the suit to prove, to the satisfaction of a judge or jury, that something a nurse did or failed to do was causally connected to an injury sustained by the patient. The outcome may have been different if the woman had proved that the nurses knew or should have known that the woman had a recent history of climbing over the bed rails or that she was unable to maintain an upright position when placed in a chair. Liability in these types of cases requires notice. Liability will not be based on hindsight because such a test would be overly harsh.

SUICIDE

As in all negligence cases the legal maxim, "reasonable care under the circumstances" applies in suits where an individual has committed suicide or has suffered bodily harm in a suicide attempt. The circumstances of a case may be quite variable. For example, whether a patient was in a psychiatric hospital or a general hospital and if in a general hospital, whether it had psychiatric facilities and staff knowledgeable in acute psychiatric care management. There are a number of cases in which a patient admitted for a medical or surgical condition became depressed sufficiently so as to become a potential suicide risk. The more recent concept of "open psychiatric wards" has had an impact on the suicide cases and the courts have not been uniform in their decisions.

The number of recent cases finding for the patient or next of kin do not support the old maxim that if a patient intends to commit suicide nothing can be done to deter the patient. In determining whether liability should be incurred the courts take notice of what the staff knew or should have known about the patient's mental condition. In determining whether "reason to know" exists, the courts look to whether the hospital knew about the patient's history of previous suicide attempts or manifestation of suicide tendencies prior to admission or from the patient's behavior since admission.

There is dicta, that is, judicial comment, but not the judicial holding of a case, in some cases suggesting that a patient's suicide may constitute a "new and independent cause." Such arguments are made in an attempt to break the chain of causation in certain situations. The argument is strongest where the hospital remained ignorant of the risk of suicide.[43]

> An early California case, *Wood v. Samaritan Institute*, held that where the evidence supported a lack of due care on the part of the staff when a voluntarily admitted alcoholic patient jumped from a window it was a question for the jury to decide whether liability would be found against the hospital.[44] The physician had left orders to restrain "as the occasion requires." The patient had behaved delusionally while in the facility.

To date, the courts have not held a general hospital to the same standard of care as a psychiatric facility. However, where a general hospital has a psychiatric unit, presumably with staff equally skilled and knowledgeable as those employed in a psychiatric facility, the standards would be on a parity. It is not known what impact the concept of deinstitutionalization may have in patients seen in emergency rooms in acute crisis. Undoubtably, some may be there because of attempted suicide and the degree of risk of further attempts should be evaluated. How long strict suicide precautions continue is a medical judgment.

However, whenever a nurse assesses that circumstances point toward acute suicide ideation, she is under a duty to take reasonable measures to safeguard the patient, even if this means going beyond the physician's orders in providing seclusion, restraints, or constant monitoring.

A Montana case was sent back to the trial level to determine whether the nurses exercised good judgment when they failed to contact the physician to inform him that the patient's condition had changed.[45]

> The court, in *Hunsaker v. Bozeman Deaconess* said, "Nurses are to carry out instructions of attending physicians except in cases of emergency. When an emergency arises, it is, of course, incumbent upon the nurses to exercise their own judgment until a report can be made to and instructions received from the attending physician."
>
> The patient had been admitted for "emotional strain." The day after he was admitted a consulting psychiatrist transferred the man from the first floor to a secure unit on the second floor with screened windows and locks on the door. He ordered that the door be locked if the man was unattended. Although an aide was in the room the man ran out the unlocked door and jumped out a window, seriously injuring himself.

General Hospital Versus Psychiatric Facility: Some Distinctions

A majority of the early cases dealing with suicide made a distinction between suicides occurring in psychiatric facilities from those occurring in general hospital settings. As in all cases of negligence the exercise of reasonable care under the circumstances prevails. The concept of "independent" nursing judgment has been cited in a number of cases. Independent judgment applies in cases where a physician has left an order based on a prior assessment and which no longer constitutes reasonable care because the patient is manifesting behavior requiring a more secure environment.

> A 1972 case, *Johnson v. Grant Hospital*, held that a general hospital which ordinarily does not treat and is not equipped to treat mental patients should not be held to the same standard of care as a hospital which is equipped to provide care for patients who display a tendency to commit suicide.[46] The patient, who had a diagnosis of schizophrenic reaction or acute anxiety reaction, had twice attempted to leap from the window of her ninth floor hospital room. These attempts occurred the evening before her actual death leap. The court placed considerable reliance on the fact that the nurses complied with the physician's order. His order was that the door to her room was to be locked at night. It was opened in the morning at the patient's request and 45 minutes later she committed suicide. The woman's husband argued that a jury should have had the opportunity to decide whether the hospital had complied with its duty to protect against a reasonably forseeable risk of injury or death. The trial court would not allow

the case to go to the jury because it held that the staff had provided all protective measures directed by the attending physician. When the plaintiff appealed the trial courts decision, the court held that the hospital was required to do no more to protect the deceased from self-inflicted injury than was ordered by the physician. In affirming the decision in favor of the hospital the appeals court gave considerable weight to the fact that the prevailing hospital practice was that nurses act only on specific physician orders. However, one appellate court judge said that although the case holding removes from a general hospital all responsibility except obedience to the orders of the attending physician, there may exist a special situation in which the hospital personnel should exert an independent judgment in the expertise of reasonable care for the patient's safety.

An early Minnesota case, *Clements v. Swedish Hospital,* also held a general hospital to a less stringent standard than a psychiatric facility.[47] The patient was admitted after an automobile injury and became depressed. Her depression was known to the staff and attending physician. No specific medical treatment was ordered for her depression. The court held that there was nothing to indicate that the patient was contemplating suicide and the physician had not placed the patient on any type of suicide precautions. The court said that it was too heavy a burden to hold the hospital liable for not applying restraints or taking other steps to restrict or confine the woman upon its own initiative. In dicta, the court said that if the facility was a psychiatric facility, failure of the employees to restrain a patient confined for a mental disorder or developing mental disturbance and manifesting suicidal behavior, liability might be found.

However, another early court, in *Rural Education Association v. Anderson,* held that the test is the extent of notice that a patient has given and held that the hospital was liable for the negligence of the nurses.[48] The physician had requested that the patient be kept on the ground floor of the general hospital and the nurses allowed him to wander through the hospital. The man had been admitted for treatment of emphysema but was known to have delusions. He was fatally injured when he jumped from an unsecured window on a surgical unit. The court held that the staff was on notice of his irritational behavior. They had testified that he reported receiving a telegram from his dead father and that they had been unable to manage him. The court said that the hospital owed a duty to provide an attendant or take other protective measures that would be deemed necessary in view of the patient's symptoms and the physician's request. The court went on to say that the fact that the wife did not obtain the services of a private duty nurse as argued by the defendant would not relieve the hospital of its duty to see that the patient was given the special attention that his mental state warranted.

Courts are not likely to find negligence where the patient only exhibited signs of mental instability, but without some demonstrated or expressed suicidal ideation.

No liability was found in *Mesedahl v. St. Luke's Hospital Association.* In this case, a patient was routinely admitted to a general hospital.[49] No history of the patient's past or present illness was made available to the staff by the family or the attending physician. Although the nurses had observed that the patient had a "wild glare" in her eyes the court said that no duty existed to anticipate the patient's suicidal thoughts or take more elaborate measures. The woman jumped through the glass of a partially barred window.

A recent case, *North Miami General Hospital v. Kraskower* found liability on the part of the hospital for the negligence of its nursing staff where notice of the patient's needs had been given, but were not communicated to all essential parties.[50] The decedent, a man with known suicidal tendencies and who had been under the care of a psychiatrist for many years, was admitted as a psychiatric patient. While he was out of the hospital on a temporary pass to get a haircut he attempted suicide. When he returned to the hospital via the emergency room he was transferred to an orthopedic unit because of his injuries. The emergency room physician ordered "suicidal precautions" which in that facility meant that an attendant be with the man 24 hours a day. The nursing staff failed to note the order or otherwise communicate it. A nurse secured from a registry left the patient unattended whereupon he jumped from a hospital fire escape. The nurse had not been informed of the patient's potential for suicide and was on an errand for the patient at his request when he jumped to his death.

In an early New York case, *Santos v. Unity Hospital,* the court held that the question of negligence should have been allowed to go to the jury for their deliberation.[51] A woman in labor who had an intrapartum psychosis died after jumping from an unsecured hospital window. The nurse who was assigned to 12 other patients had briefly left the woman unattended. The court held that the hospital owed a duty to the patient to safeguard her from self-inflicted injury or death in proportion to her needs.

The last two cases in this section emphasize the concept of notice and illustrate its importance in aiding a jury in its deliberation.

In *Harris Hospital v. Pope,* a woman who was hospitalized after an automobile accident jumped out a hospital window the night before her operation.[52] She had been in the hospital for 4 days but gave no indication of suicidal behavior. In fact, she had a history of a previous suicide attempt, but this fact was not communicated to the hospital staff prior to the jump. The automobile accident had been a suicide attempt. The woman had been checked by a nurse just a few minutes before she jumped. No liability was incurred.

However, sufficient notice of a patient's intent to commit suicide existed where in *Eady v. Alter* the patient was acting nervously.[53] The man, who had been admitted for bronchitis, had attempted to induce another patient to jump from the window with him. The other patient was then transferred to another room because of the decedent's attempt to get him to jump with him.

Judgment

A recent Massachusetts case which was ultimately settled out of court raised a number of important practice issues.[54]

> In this case, *Delicata v. Bourlesses* the nurse was sued individually for the alleged malpractice and although the case did not proceed to trial it is instructive because it raises a nursing judgment issue. In Massachusetts the plaintiff must prepare an offer of proof before the case can proceed to trial. A number of states have similar screening statutes. The case was appealed when the tribunal found that the plaintiff's offer of proof was insufficient. On appeal the court held that the suit had satisfied the statutory requirements and should have been allowed to go to trial.
>
> The decedent, a 39-year-old woman, had cancer which had metastasized to the bone. When she learned of the metastasis she became depressed over her condition and attempted suicide in the presence of her daughter by choking herself with a towel. She was initially admitted to a general hospital, but was transfered to a Boston hospital that had an acute psychiatric unit. During the 5 days she was at that hospital the medical and nursing notes reflected her depressed mental state. The psychologist's progress notes indicated that she was experiencing a moderate depressive reaction and noted her "very depressed" state the day before her death. The day after her admission a nursing notation indicated that she was very depressed and wanted to die. At one point she asked the staff to assist her in committing suicide. Originally the staff supervised her constantly, but both a psychiatrist and psychologist felt that suicide precautions were not necessary. Three days before her suicide she tried to refuse her chemotherapy and stated that she wanted to "give up." The nursing notes for the last 3 days of her life indicated that she was depressed and angry. The evening of her suicide her husband noted her mental distress and informed the nursing staff of her severe agitation as he left the ward. When evening visitors hours were over the woman left the ward and locked herself in the tub room. Forty-five minutes later the nursing staff went in search of the patient. They had to get a master key to unlock the door. The woman was submerged fully clothed in the water-filled tub. In spite of resuscitation she was pronounced dead 30 minutes later.
>
> In a sworn affidavit the nurse expert for the plaintiff offered the opinion that the nurse was on notice that the woman was severely depressed and that her statements and behavior demonstrated a worsening clinical condition and that such condition required a monitoring schedule of at least every 15-minute checks. On appeal of the tribunal decision the court held that the hospital records available to the nursing staff would alert a reasonably competent nurse in a similar situation that measures should be taken to protect her. Further, the opinion stated that the woman was left in a

"potentially dangerous situation unattended and unobserved for an unreasonably lengthly period of time." Plaintiff's expert concluded in her offer of proof "that, despite the psychiatrist's finding three days before that suicidal precautions were unnecessary, a reasonably skillful nurse in the defendant's position would, at a minimum, have monitored Mrs. Delicata during the bath, based on the patient's condition that evening, or should either have instituted closer supervision on her own initiative or sought permission from a staff physician to implement stricter controls."

Finding sufficient evidence to show possible malpractice on the part of the nurse, the tribunal erred when it exonerated her from responsibility on the basis of perceived negligence on the part of other medical personnel charged with the woman's care. In essence, the court said that the concurrent negligence of other alleged wrongdoers would not relieve her of liability for her part in the patient's death.

Although the case against the nurse did not proceed to trial, it demonstrates that courts are taking notice of advancements in the nursing profession. It relied on the expertise of a nurse in establishing the duty owed. In the past, physicians were chosen to testify about nursing care. The facts of the case may be intimidating because it ostensibly required the nurse to modify the judgment order of the psychiatrist and the psychologist. From a professional perspective the case reflects the changing view of the courts that nursing as a discipline is now considered distinct from the medical profession, although it is recognized that the two share some overlapping functions. Both require that judgments be made. This case required the evening nurse to make a judgment, based on patient knowledge, that the patient was at substantial risk to cause herself harm. This came in the form of a request to go to a locked tub room. The opinion inherently recognizes that nurses receive patient reports, review patient records, establish plans of care, and are in a unique position, by virtue of their proximity to the patient, to make critical decisions regarding the patient's care.

Establishing a medical diagnosis is both an art and a science, and establishing a precise and certain diagnosis of a mentally ill patient is perhaps more complex. A depressed psychiatric patient may be classified a suicide risk somewhere between a range from high to low. A patient properly classified as a low risk does not require the same supervision and monitoring as a high-risk patient. In the case just presented the plaintiff's nursing expert said that as a minimum the woman should have had constant attendance during the bath and checks every 15 minutes otherwise. The law does not require absolute certainty in classifying the patient, but it does impose a standard of care as established by reasonable and competent psychiatric practice. Some recent cases have had to deal with the modern psychiatric practice of caring for patients in the least restrictive alternative setting. The law recognizes that classifying the risk on which to base the extent of restriction is a matter of judgment.

Reasonable and competent psychiatrists may differ in matter of judgments so long as they conform to prevailing standards.

A recent case brought under the Federal Tort Claims Act, *Abille v. U. S.*, allowed a widow to recover for the negligence of a psychiatrist and nurses caring for her husband.[55] One of the lessons in the case is that even where treatment may include the least restrictive alternative doctors and nurses are not thereby relieved of their obligation to exercise due care for the safety of the patient.

In *Abille*, the patient voluntarily admitted himself to the psychiatric unit of an Air Force hospital on April 26, 1977. His admission notes indicated the following, "obsessive preoccupation with suicidal ideas for 3 weeks." He had no prior history of depression and there was some indication that it was associated with an antihypertensive drug he had been taking for several years. The drug was discontinued several days before his admission. There were no further notes on the physician's progress notes while he was alive. As was the department policy he was automatically assigned to an "S-1" category because of his newly admitted status. An S-1 status meant that he was not allowed to leave the psychiatric unit without a staff escort.

The nursing notes indicated that the patient had difficulty in sleeping and was nervous. A psychiatric technician noted that he was depressed and concerned about his suicidal thoughts. Sometime between his admission and April 30 the psychiatric nurse responsible for his care treated the patient as having been assigned to an S-2 status which the nurses understood to mean that a patient could leave the unit escorted by a staff member or unescorted with the approval of the charge nurse providing the patient sought to go to a specific place within the hospital and for a specific purpose. A government memorandum was admitted into evidence which stated, "S-2 level was assigned to patients who had been an inpatient for at least 24 hours, were not considered suicidal. . . . did not exhibit behavior that might be harmful to himself or others."

On Saturday, April 30, the charge nurse allowed the patient to attend mass unescorted. Early the next morning the charge nurse permitted the patient to go to breakfast unescorted. Shortly after leaving the ward his body was found on the ground, beneath a window of a seventh floor unsupervised lounge. The death certificate listed suicide as the cause of death.

The nurses testified that they allowed the patient to leave the unit unescorted the last two days of his life because they assumed that his status had been changed from S-1 to S-2. Neither charge nurse could remember how or when the status change was made, or by whom. His physician testified only that he authorized it, but there was no record of the order. A medical order, written on April 29 did not change his status, however, a reference to that effect was added by a nurse on May 1, after the patient was pronounced dead. The court held that the plaintiff's evidence supported a finding that the physician had not left an order changing the patient's status for monitoring and supervision, thus, the nurses in allowing the patient to leave the unit unescorted constituted a breach of the standard of care under Alaska law. The plaintiff's expert testified that the patient remained suicidal until the time of his death and further, that a suicidal disposition continued to be displayed by the patient and was recognized by the staff as such.

As to the physician, the court recognized that as a matter of medical judgment reasonable and competent psychiatrists, acting within the standard of care could differ as to treatment orders. However, the fact that the physician could have changed the man's status was not in issue, but rather, that he did not change his status in a manner which was consistent with an acceptable standard. The physician's "failure to keep contemporary progress notes reflecting his exercise of judgment, and the basis for it, was below the standard of care."

Nurse's Failure to Act on and Convey Patient Information

In *Adams v. State*, a woman admitted to a psychiatric facility was diagnosed as being in an acute depression.[56] While hospitalized she attempted suicide twice. After her second attempt her physician gave the head nurse a verbal order that the patient was not to leave the unit. The nurse failed to write the order and the patient left the hospital during the next shift and ran in front of an automobile. Liability was held because of the nurse's negligence.

The next of kin of a New York man, in *Cohen v. N.Y.*, who had been diagnosed as a paranoid schizophrenic recovered damages when the man left the ward and committed suicide.[57] He had been on a psychiatric unit with an open door policy. When the man voluntarily admitted himself 4 months before the suicide he manifested a potential for suicide which was documented in his record. At the trial the attending psychiatrist testified that she had not been informed as to his potential for suicide near the event. The psychiatrist also testified that the man should not have been allowed off the unit because the nurses were aware of his current suicidal ideas. The court stated that the facility lacked a definitive policy with regard to the authority of the unit nurses to independently decide to restrain a patient's freedom when there were indications that suicide was a distinct threat.

By way of contrast, another New York court in *Lichtenstein v. Montefiore Hospital* found no liability where a patient was in an "open" psychiatric unit.[58] The patient's psychiatrist ordered that the man's whereabouts be checked every 15 to 30 minutes. A nurse whose duty it was to see that no unauthorized person left the unit was stationed near the exit door. The patient was legally free to leave the hospital at will. He left the hospital without telling anyone and while the hospital staff were trying to locate him they were notified that he had been killed by a subway train. The state high court held that absent other evidence of negligence the hospital could not be liable for his leaving. The court held that where a patient is admitted to a psychiatric unit with an open door policy the fact that he left without authoritzation will not be sufficient to constitute negligence on the part of the staff. It continued on to say, "the nurse was . . . not a sentinel . . ." and any patient on an open unit, dressed in his clothes could get by the nurse. The second New York case differs from the first in that there was no evidence presented at the original trial that the patient had put the staff on notice that he intended to harm himself, nor was there other facts which would support the negligence allegation.

Sufficiency of Monitoring

Once it has been established by the evidence that the hospital staff had notice that a patient was a high suicide risk the issue then revolves around the measures which were taken or should have been taken to protect the patient.

In an early Washington case, *Kent v. Whitaker*, the court found for the family where it was shown that the patient had not been adequately monitored.[59] The decedent, a 41-year-old woman, had attempted suicide in her home and was brought to the hospital by her son. She had her stomach lavaged and was admitted to a private room void of furniture. The hospital did not have separate facilities for acute psychiatric patients. The hospital employees denied a request by the family to stay with the patient. They assured the family that she would be watched closely. The door to the room was locked and the woman was observed from time-to-time through a peephole. The nurse responsible for her care had at least 12 other patients under her care. The woman was receiving intravenous fluid. Later that day the staff found the woman dead with the plastic intravenous tubing wound around her neck.

By way of contrast, a court in a later case, *Hartman v. Memorial Hospital of South Bend*, determined that the facts would not support a decision against the hospital. The wife of a man who committed suicide within a day of his admission to a general hospital for acute depression alleged that the nursing staff failed to exercise due care in the care and supervision of her husband.[60] Finding in favor of the hospital, the court ruled that the wife failed to demonstrate that the nurses owed any duty greater than the measures undertaken. The husband had been admitted to the psychiatric ward for acute depression. During the immediate hospitalization period his mood ranged from periods of calm to distress. He received drugs for his distress. The orderly assigned to care for him on the second day of hospitalization received a report from the night attendant which indicated that he had been distressed during the night. The orderly went to the patient's room and spoke with him. He did not appear to be in any distress. About 10 minutes later a nurse visited the patient and spoke reassuringly to him. Several minutes later the staff found the patient in bed, cyanotic and without vital signs. Attempts at resuscitation failed. Further examination revealed that he had asphyxiated himself by wedging a small plastic medicine cup in his throat.

The wife's principal allegation was that the hospital should have maintained continuous, "one-on-one" monitoring of the decedent. Two nurse witnesses, one for the plaintiff and the other for the hospital, testified that a suicide could, in fact, occur in the presence of constant observation. Equally persuasive was the testimony of two psychiatrists that the man's death could not absolutely be prevented. The court held that an instruction to the jury which stated, that the man's suicide would have occurred no matter what nursing and hospital care was rendered, was proper.

Factually the case illustrates that the legal concept of foreseeability need not specifically identify the exact means by which one may commit suicide. The concept of foreseeability is satisfied where the individual has given notice that serious thoughts of suicide are presently being entertained. The law does not impose a burden to absolutely prevent suicide; it mandates only that reasonable measures be taken to try and prevent it, as long as the patient remains at high risk. Although the patient committed suicide by a means which no nurse could have foreseen it was the fact that the duty to monitor the patient was met which resulted in no liability.

A significant number of the suicide cases occurring in both psychiatric and general hospital settings have been by means of jumping from unsecured windows.[61] For this reason some general hospitals have a policy requiring that high suicide risk patients be located away from the high story units. However, this measure alone will not satisfy the legal duty. Some attention must also be given to the security of the room itself, especially with regard to locks on the windows and door. These security measures coupled with reasonable supervision in light of the circumstances are the best protection against liablity. Many of the measures that should apply to suicides also apply to protecting confused and disoriented patients who have manifested signs of unsafe behavior.[62] In a large percentage of patients, confusion and disorientation will disappear. So too, will the acute suicide risk phase as the patient responds to drug management. The law requires that the providers of care do that which is reasonable to protect the patient during this vulnerable phase.

In the case, *Psychiatric Institute of Washington v. Allen*, the parents of a 13-year-old boy successfully sued after the child was found unconscious with a belt around his neck.[63] He died without regaining consciousness. He had a history of serious psychiatric problems and at the age of 12 years, after 3 months of treatment by a private psychiatrist, the child was referred to a children's hospital where he was treated for 6 weeks on an emergency basis for fire-setting episodes with suicidal ideation. That hospital developed a plan of care based upon his psychiatric needs. One of the stated goals was the prevention of suicide. He was transferred to the defendant institute in June 1980 where the reasons for his admission included immediate threat of suicide, significant deviant behavior which is unacceptable to patient and society, and plan to institute a treatment plan not previously tried by referring hospital. He remained at the institute until October 1980 when he was discharged for eye surgery. At that time he had shown some improvement but required further extended psychiatric treatment. He returned to the institute on August 12, 1981 and his treatment plan included monitoring of "self-destructive behavior." During the next month his condition deteriorated and he failed to respond to the treatment plan. Immediately before he killed himself he asked two nurses if "it hurt to starve yourself." His behavior over the previous several days was angry and defiant and he was caught removing putty from the safety windows. One of the nurses responded that it "hurt to starve yourself and wouldn't be a good idea." Within moments after leaving the nurses he was found unconscious.

The plaintiff's expert testified that the care and treatment provided failed to meet the standard of care required of an in-patient psychiatric facility. Part of his opinion was based on the fact that the institute had failed to obtain his medical records from the referring hospital in 1980 and had failed to inform the staff fully of the child's psychiatric history. He said that it was the "responsibility of a psychiatric hospital and the staff of that hospital . . . to be fully informed of all relevant history, to be aware of what needs to be communicated to the staff and to see that the staff is cognizant, is knowledgeable about the pertinent history." Further, he said that the staff, based on the behavior the child was demonstrating, should have taken more seriously his question as to whether "it hurt to starve yourself." They should have made an effort to counsel him and should have placed him on suicide precautions. The nurse thought the question was asked in a "joking manner." In a footnote, the court noted that curiously, at the time of his readmission the day before he killed himself one of the staff when filling out a form captioned "Likelihood of Serious Harm" checked a box indicating that the child did not have a "history of attempted suicide or self-destructive behavior."

Summary

One of the most important questions in suicide cases is whether the nurses had reason to know that the patient was at high risk as a potential suicide. Without this threshold finding it is unlikely that liability will be found. Nurses caring for a high-risk patient who ultimately harms himself can expect to be involved in a suit because of their contact with the patient over the 24-hour period.

In recent years the next of kin have been successful in bringing suicide suits. That nothing can be done to prevent suicide is a misconception. The test is what could have been done that was not done once the immediate threat of potential suicide was diagnosed. The defense argument that a patient can commit suicide right in front of the caretaker will be matched with the argument that in *this* case it should not have happened because of the facts. As in all negligence cases the patient's immediate history as documented in the record is important in determining what observations were made and what actions were taken in response to the observed patient need.

DUTY TO TEACH

Teaching, instructing, and counseling have long been identified components of nursing practice. While most states specifically identify such a role via state statute it is inherent in the practice of nursing. Although the number of reported cases in which a failure to teach theory of liability is raised are not as extensive as the number of other liability theories, there is, nonetheless, considerable potential for liability. Nurses generally make time for and excel in such areas as the teaching of diabetics, postoperative care and self breast examination. However, the following cases indicate the wide range of potential liability for failing to teach the patient or family members. In several cases the suit was brought by a third party who was injured as a result of a teaching failure.

The need to provide necessary instructions when prescribing medications is illustrated by cases in South Carolina and Washington.

The legal question in the South Carolina case, *Whitefield v. Daniel Construction Company*, was whether the death of an employee who died in an automobile crash arose out of and in the course of his employment.[64] The court held that the decedent's family was entitled to compensation. The man had suffered a scalp laceration on the job. He was sent to a physician who stitched the wound and gave him a prescription for six $1\frac{1}{2}$-grain capsules of Nembutal. The physician gave no instructions except, "take when necessary for pain." He did not warn him of the consequences of taking the capsules in excess. The man filled the prescription and took one capsule and there was evidence that he may have taken a second capsule.

After leaving work the man rode with a co-worker a distance of 20 miles. He then took the wheel and continued to drive to his home which was 50 miles further. A few miles down the road he ran off the road and was assisted by a farmer to a nearby garage for repairs. The farmer later testifies that he did not appear to be in control of his faculties, but he was not drunk. The man crashed into a bridge 2 miles from the garage, killing himself.

State law dealing with compensation provided that the consequences of any such malpractice would be considered as part of the injury resulting from the accident. Evidence was introduced that the employee should have received a narcotic for pain and not a sedative. The physician was prohibited from prescribing narcotics because of a prior infraction. There was evidence that the sedative had different effects on different individuals, sometimes causing confusion, excitement, delirium, and an appearance of inebriation. There was testimony that one capsule would not have impaired his abilities, but two would.

In the Washington case, *Kaiser v. Suburban Transportation System*, the original trial held that a bus driver and the bus company were liable for injuries to a passenger when the driver dozed at the wheel.[65] When the case was appealed the court sent the case back for a new trial. In sending the case back, the court instructed the trial judge to instruct the jury to find against the physician and/or the pharmacy if it found no warning was given to the driver relevant to drug side effects. However, if the jury found that the physician did provide a warning then the verdict should be against the driver and the company.

The driver received a prescription for an antihistamine for a nasal condition. At the original trial there was evidence that the physician did not inform the driver of any of the drug's side effects. The physician was aware that the man drove a bus for his livelihood. The pharmacy where the prescription was filled did not give the man any of these warnings. The prescription label indicated that he was to take 1 tablet four times daily, before meals and at bedtime. The man took one pill at 5:20 A.M. and began his bus route at 7 A.M. A few miles from the accident scene the driver noticed that his eyes had become heavy and he was drowsy. He continued to drive and a short distance later he hit a telephone pole injuring the passenger who sued.

There was evidence that reasonable medical care required that a warning be given when a prescribed drug possesses known danger. It was also shown that 20 percent of those taking the drug experience undesirable side effects. The physician unsuccessfully argued that even if he was negligent the fact that the driver continued to drive, although groggy, was an intervening factor which should absolve him. The court held that one who innocently takes prescribed pills could not be negligent unless there was knowledge of the pills' harmful effects.

In another automobile accident case, *Freese v. Lemmon*, the court held that a pedestrian could sue both the motorist and his physician for injuries when the motorist lost control of his automobile.[66] The driver had an epileptic seizure 3 months before the accident and consulted the physician for diagnosis and treatment. The court held that a viable cause of action existed against the physician because he knew of the first seizure, but failed to diagnose its cause and failed to advise the patient of the dangers involved in driving. Additionally, he advised the man that he could drive.

These three cases have particular implication for nurses who have authority to prescribe. They also have direct implication for nurses working in a physician's office or a clinic setting. It would be important factually to know whose responsibility it is to do essential health counseling and teaching, especially in situations where there is a team or collaborative approach in rendering patient care. It is unlikely that courts will accept the argument that time does not allow patient teaching, especially where the failure to teach foreseeably would put the patient at risk.

In *Kirk v. Michael Reese Hospital and Medical Center*, a passenger in a vehicle driven by a man who hit a tree because of side effects of Prolixin Decanoate and Thorazine sued the two drug companies who produced the drugs, the prescribing physicians, and the hospital.[67] The plaintiff suffered severe and permanent injuries. The drugs had been ordered by the two defendant physicians and was given by hospital personnel. The patient was then discharged from the hospital. The same day he was discharged he consumed an alcoholic beverage which combined with the drugs impaired the man's mental and physical abilities. All the defendants argued unsuccessfully that the consumption of an alcoholic beverage constituted a superseding intervening cause for the accident—in essence, that the alcohol ingestion was unforeseeable and was a factor which caused the accident. The plaintiff argued that the drug manufacturers failed to provide adequate warnings of the adverse effects of their drugs and the doctors, as well as the hospital, failed to warn their patient before he was discharged and no longer under their control that the drugs would impair him both mentally and physically. He alleged that all the defendants knew or should have known of the adverse effects of the drugs.

The court finding for the plaintiff said that all the defendants owed a duty to the patient to warn of the side effects and the duty to warn included a duty to "adequately warn." Further, it was foreseeable that this failure to warn may harm innocent victims such as the plaintiff. The hospital sought to defend itself by arguing that the prescribing of drugs was a medical question entirely within the discretion of the treating doctors. In sum, that the hospital cannot be held for practicing medicine negligently because only physicians can practice medicine. However, the court said that the hospital's own negligence for a failure to warn applied. Citing *Darling* the court said,

> Moreover, the old conception that a hospital does not undertake to treat the patient no longer reflects reality. Plainly, hospitals do far more than merely furnish an edifice for treatment. Rather, they regularly employ on a salaried basis a staff of physicians, nurses, pharmacists, technicians, and medical administrative professionals. . . . It follows that hospitals must assume certain responsibilities for the care and treatment of their patients.

The court said that within this care and treatment context

> before a patient is discharged the hospital has a duty to warn the patient of the adverse effects of drugs that were administered by the hospital if the hospital knows or should know that the drugs will impair the patient's mental or physical abilities, or will be potentially dangerous in combination with particular foods, beverages, or other drugs.

In a footnote the court said the hospital is not discharged of its responsibilities just because the attending physician has the same responsibility (citing *Darling*).

In a Minnesota case against an attorney for failing to file a malpractice suit against a physician within the statute of limitations, the court ruled in favor of the patient's family.[68]

There was evidence in *Christy v. Saliterman* that the man suffered second and third degree burns when he fell asleep in a chair after taking paraldehyde which had been prescribed. The man had a long history of depression and an immediate past history of treatment for alcoholism. He was also drug dependent and a heavy smoker. The allegations against the physician included discharging the patient before establishing suitability for discharge and for failure to instruct the family about the properties and characteristics of paraldehyde and other drugs.

The man had seven electroshock treatments over a period of 7 days, just before his discharge. Although the man had been scheduled for electroschock treatment the next day the psychiatrist discharged him when the hospital billing department notified him that the man's insurance coverage had expired. It was shown that the electroshock treatment impaired his memory and ability to assume responsibility for his own welfare. During the 23-day course of hospital care and treatment the man had received substantial amounts of medicine including barbiturates, sedatives, and tranquilizers. It was also known that he had requested excessive doses of medication in the past.

There was expert testimony that this was a situation in which the patient and his family should have been warned about the medication dangers, including the deep sleep effects of overdosing with paraldehyde. There was evidence that the man may have taken an overdose. On the day of his discharge he received two doses of paraldehyde while in the hospital for extreme agitation. Experts testified that the wife, in view of the man's condition, should have received information from the psychiatrist concerning the use of paraldehyde, including the reason for giving it, its possible side effects, and the dangers of an overdose. The drug has cumulative effects when taken in more than prescribed doses and there was knowledge that the man had requested excessive doses in the past. The court held that even though the wife knew of her husband's past dependence on drugs, his propensity to take excessive doses would not relieve the physician from the duty to give suitable warnings and instructions about the medications he prescribed. The court held that it was well established that a physician has the duty "to give the patient or his family or attendants all necessary and proper instructions as to the care and attention to be given to the patient and the cautions to be observed, and a failure to give such instructions is negligence which will render him liable for resulting injury."

In a later case, *Lea v. Family Physicians* the court held that there was insufficient evidence upon which a jury could determine whether a physician had breached his duty to instruct an elderly woman to report any worsening of her physical condition.[69] The plaintiff, a 72-year-old woman lost her leg due to an arterial embolic blockage. She alleged that the physician's failure to warn her of such a complication and the need to act promptly in the presence of certain signs and symptoms constituted negligence.

The woman, who was energetic and active, had been treated for a newly diagnosed atrial fibrillation. She had been cleared by her regular physician to make a 500-mile journey to visit her daughter who was a practicing nurse. The physician forwarded the woman's history to a designated physician in the daughter's area. That physician found the woman to be in digoxin toxicity and hospitalized her for several days, discharging her on Inderal. He saw her 10 days later when she complained of severe leg pain. He checked all her pulses and found no obstruction. He ruled out a stroke or obstruction and diagnosed Inderal toxicity. He reduced her dose by half. A few days later the daughter noted that the veins in the woman's legs were distended. Medical testimony established that this was not indicative of occlusion. During the early evening and night in question the woman had severe pain, but assumed that it was from the Inderal. The daughter spoke to the physician in the hospital at 11 P.M. and he said he would see the mother at 8 A.M. She was examined at 8 A.M. the next morning by the same physician and at this time he found weak peripheral pulses in the involved leg and discoloration of the toes. Her atrial fibrillation had increased. An attempted bypass operation was unsuccessful and her leg was amputated.

The mother and daughter alleged that the physician breached a duty to tell the woman she should call the physician or return for further evaluation if her signs and symptoms worsened or she had new ones. They testified that the physician said the drug caused the pain and that it would cease when the dosage was decreased. The physician testified that he instructed both the woman and her daughter to notify him if her symptoms worsened. All parties agreed that duty and the woman's situation required that the physician should instruct the patient to monitor her signs and symptoms and seek medical care in the event of serious findings. The court held that the physician was in touch with the patient via the daughter and that she provided him with no symptoms which would indicate occlusion. There was no liability on the part of the physician for relying on the daughter's report.

The facts involved in an Indiana case, *Chamberlain v. Deaconess Hospital,* can be somewhat intimidating because they involve an allegation that a nurse failed to instruct the patient in the proper procedure for collecting a 24-hour urine specimen.[70] This case serves to put nurses on notice that even the most routine diagnostic procedures involve teaching. The man was admitted for the treatment of ulcers and diagnostic tests and for other complaints. The legal issue in the case was whether the nurse properly taught the patient how to safely save his urine and pour it into a gallon jug by using a funnel and if so, whether the man acted in a prudent manner in giving the specimen. The nurse alleged that the patient did not follow her instructions and the patient disclaimed that he was taught how to save the specimen. Under Indiana law at that time if it was shown that the patient was contributorily negligent, then he was barred from recovery of damages even though the nurse was negligent. Thus, both the nurse and the patient were under a duty to exercise reasonable care under the circumstances.

The man suffered severe and painful burns and scarring of his penis when he voided directly into the mouth of the jug and a chemical reaction of the urine with the hydrochloric acid occurred. The jury held in favor of the hospital and no liability on the part of the nurse attached.

a short-term or a long-term health problem teaching is an essential part of care. It is also important to remember that learning needs and the level of comprehension may differ according to the phase the patient is in. Where the patient is unable to manage the problem, family members or other designated individuals should be instructed. To provide continuity of care, especially in regards to major health needs, such as diabetes, the patient's discharge records should include documentation of the learning need, how and to what extent it was achieved, and any necessary follow-up after discharge. Most hospitals and agencies have developed a patient teaching form which is an integral part of the medical record.

In a recent wrongful death action, a Louisiana mother in *Crawford v. Earl Long Memorial Hospital* alleged that she was not instructed by the emergency room nurses to watch her son for latent head injuries.[73] The son had been taken to the hospital after being hit on the head. On examination there was no change in his level of consciousness and he had no other signs of intracranial bleeding. The nurse was instructed to telephone the mother to take the son home. The nurse testified that she instructed the mother to awaken the son at regular intervals to determine his level of consciousness. The mother testified that she received no such instructions. The next morning the son was found dead in his bed.

The jury found for the hospital after the nurse testified that she specifically requested the mother to come to the hospital so that instructions could be given in person. The mother asked that the son be put in a taxi and sent home. A footnote to the opinion states that the hospital now requires that all instructions for head-injured patients be formalized in writing. The lesson to be learned from this case is that when the teaching or instruction involves a complex or intricate principle it should be in writing.

One caveat about written discharge instructions given to the patient or family should be made. The signs and symptoms of an insulin reaction or diabetic acidosis remain constant whereas the times and doses of drugs prescribed at the time of discharge are apt to change. It should be stressed that instructions given in preparation for discharge may be changed by the treating physician for a number of reasons. Patients should always be directed toward a responsible person in the event they have questions.

Summary

The numbers of cases involving the issue of a nurse's failure to teach a patient critical information are increasing although the number of reported cases is not as high as one would expect. Patient teaching involves preoperative situations, as well as less immediate teaching related to treatment objectives. Arguably, merely telling a patient to do something or not do something is insufficient. Nurses must assess the patient's ability to understand and provide an adequate explanation of why compliance is necessary. Basic learning and teaching principles apply to patient or family instructions.

Thus far, the majority of cases involve a failure on the part of the physician to instruct the patient about the effects of drug therapy. The harm caused can affect a third party such as a pedestrian run over by a patient on drugs that caused him to fall asleep. There is real potential for liability for nurses working in offices, clinics, and day surgery facilities, as well as in any setting where the patient contact is for a short period such as the emergency room. The medical records of a patient who is hospitalized for a longer period should include sufficient documentation in the nurse's notes or in a flow sheet which includes a teaching category that the teaching extended over a period of time. Documentation or formal written instructions should be done when the patient contact is limited.

IDENTIFICATION OF THE PATIENT

There are not a significant number of reported cases dealing with patient identity problems. There may be a rational explanation for this. That is because such cases may be settled out of court and never reach the trial stage because of the limited defense theories available to the defendant. Another reason is the practice of identifying a patient via an identification band secured to the patient's wrist which remains in place throughout the entire hospitalization period. This system has made the practice of "identifying the bed," but not the patient, obsolete. Some hospitals subscribe to the informal practice of not putting patients with the same or similar name on the same unit. Although there may be a unique situation where two patients with the same last name are located on the same unit it is not a good practice and forseeably patient mix-ups with medications, diagnostic tests, documentation, and patient reports may occur. Stamping the name of the wrong patient on requisitions is an added problem when similarly named patients are assigned to the same unit. When patients with similar names go to the operating room or for x-ray examination there is increased risk of mix-up. Daily diagnostic and surgical sheets should be reviewed beforehand to identify potential problems and extra caution taken to prevent mix-ups.

Lost or obliterated name tags should be replaced as soon as their absence or unrealiability is noted. Patient identification problems are most apt to occur in situations where patients cannot acknowledge

situation requires that the incident be reported immediately in order that it can be retrieved as quickly as possible. This is especially true when the risk of needle migration or travel to another part of the body is great. In such situations the patient should be instructed to immobilize the part, and if possible restraining devices should be applied to prevent unnecessary movement.

The concept of notice is important. Liability will exist where the nurse had notice or should have been put on notice that a piece of equipment was malfunctioning. Liability will be incurred where a patient was injured because of a broken bed rail which was known to be broken or where an unreasonable amount of time lapsed before it was repaired or replaced. Notice is present where evidence exists that the wires of a piece of electrical equipment were frayed or exposed.

One of the leading cases dealing with liability for equipment failure is a Texas case, *Bellaire General Hospital v. Campbell*, in which the hospital, as a corporate entity, was found liable for failing to have emergency equipment ready for use.[80] The court concluded that the failure was causally connected to the death of a 4-day postoperative patient. The diagnosis of acute pancreatitis was established after an exploratory laporatomy. Postoperatively the woman was cared for in the intensive care unit, but was moved to a semiprivate room. On the afternoon of her death she experienced dyspnea and became cyanotic and her physician ordered oxygen delivered by positive pressure. This, to some extent alleviated her respiratory distress. The exact cause for the distress was never identified. Three hours after the initial distress she experienced another acute episode which was relieved by increasing her oxygen intake although she remained restless. At the request of her husband and the approval of her physician she was transferred a short distance to a private room. She was disconnected from her wall oxgyen source and was transferred without portable oxygen. The woman, who experienced air hunger throughout the transfer, ceased breathing. A nurse attempted to engage the oxygen hookup into the outlet in the new room, but was unable to because a light fixture prevented insertion of the hookup. Valuable time was lost in obtaining a portable oxygen unit and CPR efforts failed.

The hospital agreed that it was negligent in not having a properly functioning supply of oxygen in the room the patient was being transferred to and for not having a portable oxygen supply available during the period of transfer. However, it argued that these two negligent acts were not causally connected to her death. Her death certificate listed cardiac arrest as the cause. Although her physician testified that he considered it unlikely that the woman would have recovered from the acute pancreatitis, the court held that proof of "reasonable probability" of causation would suffice and that the plaintiff had presented sufficient proof of medical probability.

A municipal hospital, in *Jones v. City of New York*, was held liable for the death of a young man when it was determined that the insertion of defective chest tubes resulted in bilateral pneumothorax within 12 hours of the surgery.[81] Although the boy had been very ill when he underwent a liver transplant and may have ultimately died the court said that the fact that he might well have died sooner because of his debilitated condition could not exculpate the hospital from its negligence.

A man recovered damages for pain and suffering incurred when he fell from a Circolectric bed while being rotated.[82] The young man in *University Community Hospital v. Martin* was a paraplegic as a result of a gunshot wound and fell when the nurse who was responsible for checking the bed failed to check on the position of an essential bolt.

A Pennsylvania court in *Hamil v. Bashline* held that a jury should decide whether the failure to take an electrocardiograph test substantially contributed to the death of a patient.[83] The defendants unsuccessfully argued that although they were negligent, such negligence did not cause the decedent's death. The decedent's wife called the hospital around midnight and told the night supervisor that her husband was suffering from severe chest pains. The supervisor advised the wife to bring the husband to the hospital. The physician assigned to the emergency room could not be found and another physician ordered an electrocardiogram. The electrocardiograph machine failed to function and he ordered that another machine be obtained and then he left the hospital. However, the staff was unable to find a second machine and the wife took her husband to the office of a private physician. The decedent did not receive any pain medication or oxygen while in the emergency room. He died while the EKG was being taken.

The legal issue was whether liability should be imposed in the face of testimony that defendant's expert said that death was imminent when he arrived at the hospital and that the man would have died regardless of any treatment. Plaintiff's expert testified that a substantial chance for survival was lost by the failure to receive prompt treatment and his testimony was held to be sufficient for a jury to deliberate on.

In a case, *Green v. U.S.*, which involved coronary bypass machines a physician's assistant, surgical fellow, and primary surgeon were held liable when a 54-year-old woman was deprived of oxygen and suffered severe and irreversible brain damage.[84] Two negligent acts were identified, one being the reversal of the arterial and venous lines and the other being the fact that it was allowed to continue for 20 minutes into the operative procedure.

A perfusionist, who was not found negligent, prepared the heart-lung machine and handed the tubing to the physician's assistant whose task was to straighten the arterial lines, place connectors on two venous lines (but not on the arterial line) and clamp the lines to the operating table with the arterial lines closest to the patient's head. However, the assistant placed the connector on the arterial line and clamped the venous line closest to the patient's head. The court held that without the physician's assistant's initial acts of negligence,the woman would not have been rendered brain dead. However, the two physicians should have detected his errors.

All the lines were the same diameter, texture, and color. Since the incident, a marked-lines system has been used. However, at the time of the

and will automatically question an unusual treatment modality. Such diligence in transcribing orders serves the patient, the facility, and the physician well and reflects a professional attitude. When a physician's order does not make sense the reasonable, prudent nurse will necessarily take some measures to clarify it.

SUMMARY

The concept of safety has broad application to every nursing activity. Although this chapter deals with some specific concepts, the materials in several other chapters inherently deal with safe practice issues. One of the newer liability themes used by plaintiff's attorneys and traditionally associated with medical care is that of abandonment of the patient. The use of the term itself conveys a careless disregard for a patient's well being. Its application in nursing situations has thus far been limited. The duty to monitor theme appears in a significant number of cases and frequently the harm suffered because of the nurse's alleged negligence can be considerable. These include paralysis and loss or substantial impairment of a limb. The duty to monitor is increased when factors such as a complex past history exist. Such a fact will be a significant finding in proving liability. Coupled with a duty to monitor is the duty to take appropriate measures to minimize any harm which the patient may suffer. Inherent in this duty is the need to report complications and findings quickly. The facts of a case will determine what was an unreasonable delay. The case law which deals with the use and misuse of bedrails is considerable, particularly as it relates to the need to protect vulnerable patients such as young children, the elderly, and unconscious patients. There is a large body of case law which deals with the use of physical restraints. The courts have adopted the legal maxim that neither hospitals or nursing homes are the absolute insurers for the safety of their patients.

Liability for a patient's suicide has been developing in the past two decades. With the advent of the newer drugs available to treat mental illness the courts have dispelled the idea that suicide cannot be prevented. The courts and juries are aware that suicide may be prevented in some instances if the patient is physically protected by the use of the newer drugs and close supervision and monitoring until the patient has passed the crisis phase.

The liability theme of a failure to instruct the patient or his family has recently begun to appear in reported decisions. This liability concept or theme has special significance for nurses because of the amount of teaching and health counseling they do in all practice settings. Patient identification problems can occur more frequently in a hospital setting because of the large number of patients that use such facilities and the many kinds of diagnostic procedures that are done. Injuries which result from patient mix-ups can be severe, especially if they occur in the operating room. Conceptually, problems with equipment can result from a malfunction of the machine itself, or misuse of it. Almost always, the user of the machine and the manufacturer will, at least initially, be sued if harm occurred. Many of the cases cited in this chapter involve a breakdown or absence of an effective system to prevent unsafe practice. One of the goals of an effective system is to minimize human error and identify and eliminate unsafe practice. As in all injuries the system should be reviewed to see if it can be improved upon or communicated to health care providers in a more effective manner.

REFERENCES AND NOTES

1. Maslonka v. Hermann, 428 A. 2nd 504 (NJ, 1981) which overruled 414 A. 2nd 1350 (NJ, 1980).
2. Duling v. Bluefield Sanitarium, 142 S.E. 2nd 754 (WV, 1965).
3. Morreale v. Downing, 630 F. 2nd 286 (1980).
4. Jewett, J. (Sept. 2, 1982). Report From The Committee on Maternal Welfare—"Alcoholism, ectopic pregnancy, and cardiopulmonary failure." *New England Journal of Medicine, 307*(10), 621.
5. Rogers v. Kasdan, 612 S.W. 2nd 133 (KY, 1981). See also, *Beardsley v. Wyoming Community Hospital* in Chapter 5.
6. Davis, M. Nurses are suspended after baby dies from hospital incubator heat. *Washington Star* (Washington, DC), July 17, 1981.
7. Jones v. Hawkes Hospital of Mount Carmel, 196 N.E. 2nd 592 (OH, 1964).
8. Sanchez v. Bay General Hospital, 172 *California Reporter, 342* (CA, 1981).
9. Variety Children's Hospital v. Perkins, 382 S. 2nd 331 (FL, 1980).
10. Long v. Johnson, 381 N.E. 2nd 93 (IN, 1978).
11. Campbell v. Thornton, 333 N.E. 2nd 442 (MA, 1975).
12. St. Lukes' Hospital Association v. Long, 240 P. 2nd 917 (CO, 1952).
13. Polonsky v. Union Hospital, 418 N.E. 2nd 620 (MA, 1981).
14. Citing, Carrigan v. Sacred Heart Hospital, 178 A. 2nd 502 (NY, 1962); Mossman v. Albany Medical Center, 311 N.Y.S. 2nd 131 (NY, 1970).
15. Citing, Louis v. Chinese Hospital Association, 57 *California Reporter, 906* (CA, 1967); Norris v. Rowan Memorial Hospital, 205 S.E. 2nd 345 (NC, 1974); Cramer v. Theda Clark Memorial Hospital, 172 N.W. 2nd 427 (WI, 1969).
16. Hunt v. Bogalusa Community Medical Center, 303 S. 2nd 745 (LA, 1974).
17. See also Kaunitz, K. K. (Dec. 1981). What is the status of the law on the use of bed rails and side rails to restrain patients? *Hospital Medical Staff, 10*(12), 11.
18. Smith v. West Calcasieu-Cameron Hospital, 251 S. 2nd 810 (LA, 1971).
19. Brown v. Decatur Memorial Hospital, 367 N.E. 2nd 575 (IL, 1977).
20. Seymour v. Victory Memorial Hospital, 376 N.E. 2nd 754 (IL, 1978). See also Snelling v. Middleton, 706 S.W. 2nd 891 (MO, 1986) where suit against nurses was dismissed.
21. Thompson v. U. S., 368 F. Supp. 466 (1973).
22. Block v. Michael Reese Hospital and Medical Center, 417 N.E. 2nd 724 (IL, 1981).
23. Memorial Hospital of South Bend v. Scott, 300 N.E. 2nd 50 (IN, 1973).
24. See, for example, Perry v. Fredette, 261 A. 2nd 431 (NH, 1970).
25. See, for example, Newhall v. Central Vermont Hospital, 349 A. 2nd 890 (VT, 1975).
26. Leavitt v. St. Tammany Parish Hospital, 396 S. 2nd 406 (LA, 1981).

MEDICATIONS

Most patients are aware that all drug use involves a risk of some sort. However, the higher the known risk of drug therapy the greater the duty owed by the nurse or physician in protecting the patient against such risks. There is, of course, a known risk with any injection, but a risk cannot be equated with a negligent act. For example, while there is a risk of infection with an injection, that fact alone will not impose liability. Liability is most likely to be found where the nurse was put on notice, or should have been put on notice, that the injected substance would not be absorbed. The nurse must use reasonable judgment in selecting the injection site.

There is also a risk with IV medications, especially if they are given by continuous infusion, that they may leak into surrounding tissue. Under that circumstance liability may be imposed for failing to monitor the infusing medication. Not all injuries associated with the use of the intravenous route incur liability. For example, in *Sugulas v. St. Paul Insurance Company* the court exonerated a physician who missed a vein and punctured an artery.[1] It was shown that the procedure followed by the physician was correct. The physician had done between three and eight similar procedures each day for approximately 8 years. The physician's expert testified that a mishap of this kind is bound to happen occasionally even to the most skillful

tency, either in terms of clinical skill or nursing knowledge, to administer a prescribed drug, this fact should be communicated to her superiors and the physician. In a suit in which it is alleged that a nurse caused harm to a patient, the nurse would have to show a number of things including that she was executing precise orders, followed any existing protocols, and was skilled in the technique of administering the medication in the manner in which it was given.

A number of pharmacist groups have actively sought to increase the role of the pharmacist, and in particular, the hospital pharmacist in becoming a more active member of the health care team. These groups view the role of the hospital pharmacist as requiring affirmative action to prevent hospital medication errors. They also believe that hospital pharmacists should play an advisory role to nursing staff. In 1979 a joint committee of the American Nurses' Association and the American Society of Hospital Pharmacists (ASHP) approved the Guidelines for Collaboration of Pharmacists and Nurses in Institutional Care Settings.[4]

The need for collaboration is based on the premise that the complexity of drug therapy requires consultation between nurses and pharmacists on a regular basis. In order to promote the exchange of information between both disciplines, the Guidelines proposed that facility orientation of both nurses and pharmacists should include the hospital pharmacy and patient care units to appraise both groups of the workings of the other. The Guidelines encourage collaboration whenever there is overlap of professional roles, such as monitoring adverse drug reactions and patient education. The Guidelines include a list of the ways in which the pharmacist would serve as a resource for the nursing staff. These include: information on investigation drugs used in the institution, drug computations, drug side effects and therapeutic risks, drug interactions, and the effect of patient age and pathophysiology on drug action. While some facilities may view such collaboration as time consuming and more costly, it is likely that the benefits far outweigh these two factors.

The courts have held that while nurses are not required to watch each patient 24 hours a day they are responsible for hazards reasonably to be forseen and risks reasonably to be perceived. A New York state facility was liable for failing to monitor a patient after he was given Thorazine.[5]

In *Brown v. State of N.Y.*, a young man who was recently admitted in a withdrawn condition to a state hospital suddenly became violent and assaultive. He was given 200 mg of Thorazine and transferred to a seclusion room unattended. One hour later he was found in an apneic state and subsequently died. The court said the failure to observe the patient in the presence of known serious side effects, including shock and arrhythmia, was the proximate cause of death.

MEDICATION ERRORS IN GENERAL

There are six common types of hospital medication errors.[6] These include (1) *omission*—drug ordered but not administered; (2) *unordered drug*—drug not ordered but administered; (3) *incorrect dose*—a dose administered either above or below the correct dose; (4) *extra dose*—a dose given in excess of total number of times indicated in physician's order; (5) *wrong form*—drug administered in dosage form not included in the generally accepted interpretation of a physician's orders, i.e., oral administration when order or manufacturer states other route; (6) *wrong time*—drug administered 30 minutes prior to or after scheduled time.

Of these six types of errors, two warrant further comment. The error of *omission* also includes an unreasonable delay in implementing a new or changed order.

> In a recent Connecticut case, *Pisel v. Stamford Hospital,* one of the findings of fact was that the nurses delayed in transcribing an order for an antipsychotic drug for a patient and when it was finally transcribed it was out of stock.[7] The nurses failed to inform the physician of this fact and the patient's agitation consequently increased and she subsequently seriously injured herself.

> In another case, *Gasbarra v. St. James Hospital,* an expert testifying on behalf of the plaintiff testified that, among other negligent nursing acts, nurses unreasonably delayed administering a medication ordered by the physician of a critically ill 14-month-old girl who subsequently died.[8]

The fact that the plaintiff alleges delay in implementing a medication order is a significant factual issue. The courts will look at the circumstances surrounding the delay and the resultant harm. Where it is shown that the delay was not in accordance with accepted nursing standards and serious harm results, liability is not unlikely.

Some facilities strictly adhere to the "30-minute extension rule" which permits administration of a medication 30 minutes prior to or after a scheduled time. Thus, a medication due at 9 A.M. may be given between 8:30 A.M. and 9:30 A.M. In facilities which strictly adhere to the 30-minute extension rule a 9 A.M. medication given at 9:45 A.M. would be regarded as a "wrong time" medication error. Of course, some drugs must be given at a precise time notwithstanding the 30-minute rule. The flexible time limit was established a number of decades ago. Since that time the number of drugs on the market has increased substan-

hospital system or routine is indicated. For example, a recent journal article reported an incident in which an adult dose of Ergonovine, a drug given to increase uterine muscle contraction, was accidently given to a newborn in the delivery room. The intended drug was vitamin K.[11] The infant suffered respiratory failure, convulsions, and acute renal failure. The authors suggested that such errors would be avoided if the hospital adopted the practice of administering the vitamin K in the neonatal nursery, instead of in the delivery room.

By carefully reviewing medication incident reports, human error, system failure, and poor or absent policies can be identified as the cause. The emphasis should be on correction of the system or changing unsafe nursing practices, rather than punishing the "wrong-doer." There are, of course, some errors that cannot be neatly categorized. A nurse with a flawless performance record may commit the most unpredictable error, but this is perhaps more the exception than the rule. Fatigue may also be an important factor where a nurse works back-to-back shifts or where the rotation schedule causes nurse fatigue.

Some factors militate against nurses committing medication errors. The majority of nurses are highly conscientious when preparing and administering medications. Also, the system whereby multiple nurses administer medications limits serious violations because one nurse's error or unsafe practice is easily noticed by another nurse. This system prevents repetition of the error if it occurred because of a transcription mistake. Nursing, like medicine, is a dynamic profession, and nursing demands in terms of theoretical and clinical knowledge are significant. Nurses are spending more and more time updating their scientific knowledge about medications, and this will be increasingly true as new medications are introduced and medical and nursing knowledge related to them evolves.

INJECTIONS

There is a significant body of law dealing with injury as a result of an injection. It is, of course, true that any injection carries with it some risk. However, risk from an injection is distinct from an injury that results from a negligently administered injection. The early injection cases held that the doctrine of res ipsa loquitur would not be applicable to these types of cases. The doctrine, which translates into "the thing speaks for itself," transfers the burden of proof from the plaintiff to the defendant. Thus, the defendant must demonstrate that he was not negligent.

Infections and other adverse reactions might result from injections and, in and of itself, this does not imply negligence or liability. Most injection cases deal with injury to a nerve. Some deal with deterioration of surrounding structures. The reason most courts refuse to allow application of the res ipsa loquitur doctrine is because an injury may occur in the absence of nursing negligence. The legal concept of strict liability or liability without fault is inapplicable to the injection cases. The types of injuries that may result from an injection, most frequently gluteal, occur when the needle directly strikes the nerve or where the substance injected causes congestion in close proximity to a nerve. The problem may result from faulty site selection, improper needle length, or improper route of administration. The site selection problem arises when the nurse fails to rotate or use different sites or selects a site that a reasonable nurse would know would probably present absorption problems. There are a few cases in which the judgment of a nurse was called into question when the length of the needle was inadequate and the medication was delivered into the wrong area. Another legal theory that has been argued by the plaintiff is that the physician has a duty to instruct the nurse in the injection technique. Although a viable theory of liability making the physician responsible for the nurse's action, currently the theory has limited application because nurses are presumed to know how to administer injections. In addition, a hospital's continuing education program assumes the responsibility of teaching its nurses any unusual techniques associated with the newer medications. This concept of making the physician responsible for the injury which resulted from the nurse giving the injection evolved because the doctrine of charitable immunity precluded the plaintiff from suing the hospital. The doctrine held that an individual could not sue a hospital because one of its purposes was to provide charitable hospital care. This doctrine has been either abolished or modified to permit suit against the hospital.

Nerve Injury

Where it is shown that the paralysis occurred in the absence of neligence the courts have held in favor of the individual who gave the injection. Thus,

in *Lamb v. Oakwood Hospital*, where a 6-year-old child who underwent a tonsils and adenoids operation developed paralysis in the leg in which the preoperative medication was given, the court held there was no liability.[12] The court found that the evidence warranted a finding that the nurse gave the injection according to recognized and accepted nursing standards. The child did not exhibit any impairment until after discharge.

In another case, *Evans v. U.S.*, involving an injection given to a young child the court held that the nurses were not liable for a 13-month-old child's leg paralysis which occurred after receiving one of many gluteal injections.[13] The defendants succeeded in persuading the jury that the inju-

medication after the patient put the nurse on notice of pain. It is a fundamental nursing principle that the administration should be halted when the nurse is put on notice of a possible problem. There are, of course, some medications that will "sting" or cause "cramping" if injected too rapidly. Injections are not without some inherent risk to the patient.

Summary

In summary, there are a significant number of suits for injury as a result of nerve injury.[19] A large percentage have found in favor of the injured patient. It is only recently that the defense has been successful, in some instances, by showing that the injury may have been caused by means other than directly piercing the nerve. The law requires that the plaintiff prove that the nurse was negligent in site selection, administration technique, drug knowledge, or in preparing the injection. Coupled with a showing of causation between the negligence and the injury, recovery of damages for the resultant harm will be allowed.

Broken Needles

Prior to the use of disposal syringes and needles the problem of broken needles was greater. The mere fact that the needle broke does not in and of itself establish negligence. Broken needles can occur when the patient moves, with improper usage or mishandling of the syringe, or from a defect in the product itself. Perhaps the greatest potential for liability is a failure to institute emergency measures to retrieve the foreign object as quickly as possible. At a minimum, the patient should be instructed to remain immobile to prevent the needle from becoming more imbedded in muscle or tissue. This is particularly important when the needle breaks while inserted in a vessel where the potential for needle migration to another area of the body is increased. A needle can travel in the blood vessel to another part of the body, e.g., lodge in the heart. An incident involving a broken needle should be reported immediately.

> In *Barber v. Reinking*, a licensed practical nurse (LPN) gave a polio booster injection to an infant in a pediatrician's office.[20] While holding the child over her lap the nurse held him down with one hand and administered the injection with her free hand. The needle broke off in the gluteal muscle when the child suddenly moved. A statute existed which provided that inoculations were to be given only by licensed registered nurses. The trial court dismissed the suit in favor of the defendants, however on appeal the case was sent back to the trial court to be retried. The appeals court held that one who undertakes to perform the services of a licensed registered nurse must have the knowledge and skill possessed by a registered nurse. The court said that the plaintiff was entitled to have evidence of violation

of the statute prohibiting one who is not a licensed registered nurse from administering inoculations submitted to the jury for their deliberation. In addition, at the trial the defendant had raised the defense that the infant contributed to the breaking of the needle when he moved. The appeals court held that the conduct of the infant was germane to the case only in determining whether the LPN was negligent in failing to anticipate the sudden movement of the child and to take measures to guard against it while administering the injection.

Physician's Failure to Instruct the Nurse

As previously mentioned, plaintiffs sometimes sue the physician to get around the charitable immunity doctrine in the injection cases. The majority of decisions have held that, in the absence of unusual circumstances, a physician has a right to rely on the fact that a nurse is competent to administer injections. Where, however, the route or administration technique is unusual, a jury may find that a duty to instruct the nurse in the procedure existed. In some circumstances, good and accepted medical practice may require the presence or direct supervision by a physician. This is particularly true when the physician knew or should have known that the technique was unfamiliar to the nursing staff. In order to show that the physician is liable, the plaintiff must show that the failure to instruct or personally supervise the administration of a medication was negligence and such negligence was a proximate cause of the patient's injury. For example, where it is not usual to administer medication directly into the cerebral ventricles a court may find that specific instructions should have been left by the physician when such an order is written. This, of course, does not mean that a nurse who undertook to administer medication into the ventricles according to an order would be absolved from responsibility in the event of harm. It only means that the plaintiff has two viable defendants.

The duty to instruct may involve the actual administration of a specific medication or it may involve necessary monitoring that is unique to the drug. In recent years the use of subarachnoid or intrathecal narcotics has proved effective in managing pain in postoperative patients and terminal cancer patients with intractable pain. However, intrathecal morphine has potential for long-term aftereffects. When used as an analgesic, even at low dosages, it can effect the patient up to 30 hours. There are reported cases of delayed onset of respiratory arrest which may be caused by the slow movement of the narcotic in the cerebrospinal fluid as it passes the medullar respiratory center on its way to the choroid plexis where the spinal fluid exits from the central nervous system.[21] A persuasive argument can be made that there is a medical duty to alert nurses caring for patients being managed by intrathecal narcotics that frequent respiratory monitoring should be done.

ister. The administration of intravenous medications requires no more mental concentration than administration by any other route, but the nurse must necessarily be aware that the intravenous route is rapid-acting. There is, of course, nursing knowledge that deals specifically with the administration of intravenous drugs. For example, it is essential that the nurse know that some drugs such as phenobarbital must be injected slowly, at a rate not to exceed 50 mg per minute.[26]

There are drugs that are administered intravenously by nurses in clinical areas such as the recovery room, special care units, and the emergency room that are not generally administered by nurses in other patient areas. It is essential that nurses working in these settings receive special instruction; they must also be certified by the nursing department. In addition, drug protocols and policies relevant to the administration of such drugs must be developed. The policies should identify those practice settings in which nurses are permitted to administer intravenous medications, and the names of certified nurses should be kept on file. The policies should identify those drugs that may be given by intravenous push therapy and indicate that unless a drug is identified it will not be a nursing function to administer it. Such policies must be reviewed frequently by both medical and nursing departments. It is not uncommon to find that nurses who have practiced in an ICU setting to be assigned as "float critical care" nurses to other clinical units. They are, of course, competent to function as ICU nurses.

Much of the case law relevant to intravenous medications deals with failing to monitor the patient and the effect the intravenous additive has on that patient. These cases tend to arise where the solution has gone into the tissue for a prolonged period and has caused an injury necessitating subsequent grafts.

A New York case illustrates the duty that attaches to the intravenous fluid procedure, whether medications are added or not.[27]

In *Beardsley v. Wyoming County Community Hospital*, a 6-year-old boy suffered brain damage from cerebral edema when the nursing staff inadvertently gave double the amount of salt-free fluids ordered by the physician. The plaintiff also said the hospital staff was negligent for failing to monitor the child's electrolytes. On the first postoperative day his intake was 2400 cc in contrast to an output of only 250 cc. The nurses should have monitored the child's intake and output levels over the 24-hour period, judged that they were not acceptable levels, and reported the findings to the physician.

Nurses should be conscientious about following the manufacturer's instructions in preparing intravenous medications. Any inconsistencies between the package-insert instructions and preparation directions developed by the IV department should be resolved before a problem arises. The nurse should comply with the manufacturer's recommendations relative to the amount and type of dissolving solution. Where the nurse has used less than the recommended amount of diluent the defense would be placed in a position of having to show that the harm was not causally connected to the less than recommended amount.

In addition to the general information contained in the package insert which accompanies the intravenous drug, it would be argued that the nurse should be aware of information contained in the special "black box warnings." These warnings are contained in the insert pamphlet in a special warning section. For example, the special warnings for kanamycin sulfate state that it is a potentially nephrotoxic and ototoxic drug. Therefore, nurses would need to assess and monitor for these serious effects. Failure to do so would constitute evidence of less than accepted nursing care. Where the patient is receiving an unusually high dose or where the patient is on prolonged therapy the duty to monitor is increased.

DRUG MODIFICATION AND UNUSUALLY HIGH DOSES

Three questions frequently confront nurses who are transcribing or administering prescription orders. One is whether a drug that is ordered in an unusually high dose may be given. The second question is whether and under what circumstances a nurse may modify a drug order. The third question is whether a range-of-dose order is a proper order.

Unusually High Doses

When a physician orders an unusually high dose it is generally picked up by the transcribing nurse or by the first nurse who is scheduled to give it. Nurses and pharmacists frequently become involved in the high dose dilemma because nurses administer the drug and the hospital pharmacist dispenses the drug based on the order. Some orders present no nursing judgment problem because they are patently incorrect. These present little problem and can be managed efficiently by contacting the physician who rewrites the order. However, it may be that the physician intended to write such a high dose.

In order to assess the legal implications of the order the nurse must have some knowledge of the system for Food and Drug Administration (FDA) approval. When the FDA approves a drug it is verifying it to be safe and efficacious for specific use and in specific doses.[23] In 1961 the FDA promulgated a regulation that required a package insert for all prescription drugs. The insert which must be FDA approved provides information about indications for use, effects, dosages, routes, hazards, side effects, and contraindications. However, it is important to know that the FDA did not intend the regulation to interfere with the practice

attention to the order so that associated medical monitoring needs will be flagged.

The decision to order a drug, including the specific dose, belongs to the treating physician. The determination of what is a medically correct dose is considered a medical judgment. The manufacturer's recommended dose for a specific disease or condition may be used as one means of measuring whether a physician complied with recognized and accepted practice standards, but it may not establish the definitive standard of care. The law will not automatically impose liability on the physician if harm occurs to a patient as a result of the unusually high dose. However, the law will impose an increased duty to monitor and otherwise protect the patient. In some situations, depending on the facts of a case, the law may find that the physician owed a duty to leave instructions for the nurse if the medication dose will yield a problem not generally within nursing experience or knowledge. In sum, if the recent medical literature supports the physician's medical decision to order an unusual course of therapy and the physician is skilled in managing the therapy, the law will not hold the physician liable unless unusual circumstances exist.

> An unreported Texas case, *St. Anthony's Hospital v. Bullis*, demonstrates the potential for liability for the hospital, as well as for the physician in these types of cases.[29] The physician, who was a general practitioner, was sued when he ordered an excessive dosage of digitalis for a 28-year-old woman who had tachycardia. The woman's electrocardiogram (EKG) was abnormal, and she failed to be controlled for a number of days. The physician did not consult a cardiologist. The hospital was also sued for the alleged negligence of its hospital pharmacist for failing to recognize the excessive dose order and its nurses for the failure to note the symptoms of digitalis intoxication. The woman suffered a cardiac arrest and was in a coma for 3 years before dying. All the defendants settled the case before it went to trial.

Drug Modification

Under ordinary circumstances, nurses do not have specific or implied authority to modify a physician's order. *Drug modification* is defined as those instances where a nurse gives less than the ordered dose. The most common situation that may permit a nurse to modify a drug arises when the patient findings indicate that the ordered dose would be excessive under the circumstances. This exception is based on nursing knowledge and patient observations and should not be confused with drug management. The drug modification concept is generally limited to the administration of narcotics, sedatives, and tranquilizers. There are no instances where a nurse should give more than the ordered dose. When a facility permits drug modification, the nursing policy should, wherever possible, specify the limits in written formal policies. No nursing practice statute acknowledges the drug modification concept. However, it is frequently done in practice and should be acknowledged by policy if the nursing and medical departments agree on situations or drugs that would warrant modification.

If a facility decides not to permit nurses to modify a drug, this, too, should be communicated via formal policy. Such a policy provides some assurance that nurses who have worked in facilities that permit nurses to modify a drug dose will be on notice that it is not permitted in every facility or setting. Where a facility does not permit any drug modification the nursing policy should indicate what steps the nurse is to follow when a nursing judgment is made that the patient should not receive a full dose. The policy may indicate that the nurse is to consult with a nursing supervisor or contact the patient's physician. Where a policy permits modification the policy should also indicate how the fact of the modified dose should be communicated to the physician. Merely charting the administered modified dose on the medical record and in the nursing notes will not be sufficient because it is generally admitted by many physicians that they do not read nursing notes. Many of the rules applicable to modifying a drug also apply to a situation in which a drug is omitted altogether. The treating physician must be appraised of the fact in order to assess the situation and make any changes in the medical plan of care.

> While not specifically a drug modification situation, *Rowland v. Skaggs Companies* illustrates the principle that reasonable care requires a proper investigation of the situation.[30] Inadvertently, a pharmacist labeled 150-mg capsules of Elavil as 25-mg capsules. The patient called the prescribing physician's office for advice and spoke to the nurse. The nurse instructed the woman to take six of the 25-mg capsules to equal the prescribed 150 mg. The woman was hospitalized because of the overdose and sued the pharmacy. The pharmacy in turn sued the nurse for negligence.
>
> The nurse should have instructed the patient to take the bottle back to the pharmacy. Even assuming that the nurse could have had the patient describe the color, shape, and numbers on the pills she received, thus permitting the nurse to identify the exact dose by referring to the Product Identification section of the *PDR*, the patient would then have to change the label on the prescription bottle herself. Having the woman write over the pharmacy label arguably would increase the potential for error further down the line.

Range of Dose Orders

It is not uncommon for physicians to order narcotics, especially for the management of postoperative pain, in a "range of dose" form. Such an order may read, "Demerol 50–100 mg q. 3–4 hours p.r.n. for pain."

Such orders are recognized and accepted medical practice. It is implicit in the order that the nurse will make a nursing judgment with respect to both the time and dose limit. These types of orders generally do not present a practical or legal problem. Practically, if the nurse gives the 50-mg dose rather than the maximum dose of 100 mg, she should assess the patient soon after administering the lesser amount to make sure that the patient obtained relief. If the lesser amount does not relieve the pain then the patient can be given additional medication to the maximum dose ordered. The problem arises when the narcotic loses its effect an hour or 2 after the smaller dose is administered. Then a decision must be reached whether to give the remaining dose or have the patient wait until a reasonable time has elapsed and give the maximum dose. The potential for liability is in failing to monitor the patient closely for respiratory depression or giving a full dose too soon after the reduced dose.

A range of dose order for other drugs would not be accepted medical practice and should not be implemented in the absence of a clear, precise medical directive. For example, an order for "Lasix 40–80 mg daily" would not be a precise order and thus, does not come within the limited exceptions to the precise order rule. The narcotic order calls for a judgment based on immediate patient findings. In addition, the medication is given to relieve a transient finding, pain. In contrast, drugs that have a therapeutic effect require medical judgment. If the physician is unable to write a precise order until the daily findings are communicated to him the procedure similar to the ordering of daily anticoagulants should be followed. That is, having the nurse communicate the daily laboratory results and then implement the physician's precise order.

The only reported case dealing with a drug given in a range of dose form is a 1974 case, *Davis v. California*.[31] The case dealt with a question of eligibility for unemployment compensation and arose when a nurse was discharged from her hospital position. The nurse alleged that the discharge was not for "just cause" whereas the hospital claimed that the discharge was for work related misconduct, making her ineligible for compensation.

The hospital at which the nurse had been employed for 12 years had a known policy and procedure to be followed in the event a nurse wanted to give less than an ordered dose. The surgeon had left orders that a postoperative cholecystectomy patient was to be given 100 mg of Demerol as needed for pain. The nurse testified that she gave 50 mg because the patient appeared drowsy and that she had consulted with the charge nurse who concurred with the smaller dose decision. The charge nurse subsequently testified to that effect and another nurse testified that although it was theoretically wrong to halve the narcotic she would probably have done the same thing under the circumstances. The surgeon also said that many nurses do this and he had no objection to the nurse making a judgment to give a lesser dose of narcotic. Ruling that the discharge was for misconduct the state agency said that the claimant's action was a "willful disregard" of her employer's interest when she disregarded the known policy. The hospital protocol required the medication nurse to obtain authorization from the patient's physician or his designated standby. It was established that a medication nurse has a responsibility to obtain the necessary permission to change the order or to obtain any needed clarification relating to it. The nurse was unsuccessful in arguing that although she knew the policy existed her disregard was a good faith error in judgment rather than misconduct because she believed that the hospital knew that nurses deviated from the policy and, in effect, accepted the practice. Thus, the nurse was faulted, not for doing what might be regarded as customary practice, but for disregarding an internal policy.

TRANSCRIBING ORDERS

Transcription errors account for a large number of medication errors. Different policies may exist when transcribing physician's medication orders as contrasted with transcribing other patient care orders. This is because of the danger an incorrect medication may pose for the patient. One common policy is that the first nurse administering the medication must cross-reference it with the original physician's order and place her initials next to the order and the original transcriber's initials. This assures that two nurses have had the opportunity to pick up any error when the order was transcribed to the medication record. It is also good practice when checking the accuracy of any medication order to begin with the most recent order in the physician's order book and work back to the date cited on the medication record rather than immediately proceeding to the date indicated in the medication record. Subsequent decreases in doses or other orders would not be picked up if the date the order was transcribed was the only point of reference.

It is not uncommon for nurses when administering medications to pick up a transcription error made by the original transcriber. It is also fairly common for an error unknowingly committed by one nurse to be picked up by another nurse when checking the patient's medication record. This built-in double-checking tends to prevent long-term errors. Perhaps no other group of workers has such a unique error detection mechanism. It exists because of the nursing practice of continually assessing patient data.

Perhaps the most error-prone medication system involves the use of a medication card system. Medication cards are the least acceptable means of giving medications for a number of reasons. They are lost easily; if this occurs a replacement card must be written, thus increasing the margin of error. They may be placed or returned to the wrong hourly slot-box and thus omitted. The omission may not be picked up until the entire unit's medications have been completed or later. When medication cards are used they are generally cross-referenced with a medication sheet, which is itself a secondary source of information, and not with the physician's order sheet. This of course increases the possibility of error. It is important when reviewing medication errors to determine whether the potential for errors is built into the system, and to change the system accordingly.

The unit dose system, in which a copy of the original physician's order is sent to the pharmacy and the pharmacist prepares and packages each individual medication dose for the patient, is perhaps the safest method. Any method that reduces the number of secondary sheets is the preferred system from a safety perspective. One last point should be made before leaving this area; if the pharmacist does not have the ordered medication this fact should be communicated to the physician.[32]

MEDICATION ERRORS

Admittedly a significant number of wrong medications are administered. The most serious errors involve the wrong drug, route, or dose. The reported cases are particularly intimidating because they frequently result in serious harm and sometimes death. Every facility should review medication incident reports closely with an eye toward changing an outdated system or factoring out the potential for human error. No matter what the medication being administered or how long a nurse has been administering medications the procedure requires intense concentration. No nurse should deviate from the time-honored systematic procedure. The fact that a facility functions under a unit dose medication system will not absolve the nurse from liability if the nurse was on notice or should have been on notice that the medication the pharmacist prepared was incorrect. In addition, all the other judgment and skill components are not altered by the use of a unit dose system.

Incorrect Calculation

Mathematical calculations are an important aspect of all nursing education programs. New nurse employees are given a mathematics test during the orientation process and are required to achieve a passing grade. Some facilities require that designated medications be double-checked by a second individual. This is particularly important when the nurse is a student. It may be an important measure because of the fact that calculations are becoming less common. Drug computations is one of the areas identified in the American Nurses' Association (ANA) Guidelines for collaboration of pharmacists and nurses in institutional care settings.[33]

There are not a large number of reported cases in this area.

However, in one recent case, *Moore v. Dallas County Hospital*, a husband and his three children agreed to a settlement where the decedent-mother died of a respiratory arrest after receiving an intravenous overdose of magnesium sulfate.[34] The 27-year-old woman became eclamptic after delivering her third child and her physician ordered the anticonvulsive medication. After calculating the dose the nurse handed the physician the incorrect intravenous solution. The woman died within minutes after the intravenous piggyback bottles were hung. Both the hospital and the physician contributed to the settlement. The physician was included in the suit on the theory that he had an opportunity to detect and correct the nurse's mistake.

However, in another tragic drug dose case, *Dessauer v. Aetna Life Insurance Co.* the jury found against the nurse.[35] Further, the court held that neither the hospital or the nurse who administered the drug could be indemnified or receive a contribution from the emergency room physician who ordered the drug. The hospital and the nurse agreed to settle the case for $225,000. The basis for the suit against the hospital and the nurse was a lethal overdose of lidocaine.

The decedent was admitted with complaints of chest pains and the physician made a tentative diagnosis of acute myocardial infarction. He ordered lidocaine 50 mg and the nurse erroneously injected the wrong vial which resulted in the man receiving 800 mg of the drug. Directions on the vial read: "For dilution only. Not for direct injection." The nurse was the one who selected the vial. The physician handled both the vial and the syringe two or three times just before the nurse injected its contents into the patient. Two of the physician's experts testified that his failure to read the label did not fall below the standard of care. The patient arrested and was resuscitated, but suffered irreversible brain damage and was subsequently disconnected from life-support systems. The nurse had been transferred from the obstetrics department to the emergency room. Presumably, the two key factors contributing to the error were the floating of the nurse from the obstetric department to the unfamiliar and threatening emergency room, and a lack of scientific and practical knowledge of the drug.

A third-party suit was brought against the physician for negligence in his care of the decedent, as well as negligence in his supervision of the nurse. In the suit by the hospital and the nurse to recover all or part of the money they paid the decedent's estate. the jury responded that neither should recover damages against the physician. The jury, when asked by the court whether the nurse was negligent, responded in the affirmative and stated that her negligence was the sole proximate cause of the man's death. The hospital and nurse failed to present medical expert testimony to support their allegation of medical negligence. The court held that neither the "borrowed servant" doctrine or the "captain of the ship" doctrine applied. Both theories would have absolved the hospital of liability by finding that the physician controlled the actions of the nurse. The physician did not exercise any right or duty to supervise or control the nurse, he did not engage her service, supervise the method or manner in which the medication should be administered, nor did he supervise the type of vial and syringe used.

In dicta to the case the court stated: "the primary duty of a doctor in an emergency is to focus upon the serious medical problem from which a patient suffers . . . the primary duty of the hospital is to focus upon the competence of nurses to perform their duties. The doctor's and hospital's duties are independent primary duties. . . . A doctor has the right to rely upon a hospital to furnish a nurse who is qualified, competent and trustworthy in the performance of her duties."

Procedural Breaks

Every nurse knows the "five rights"; that is, the right patient, drug, dose, time, and route. Every nurse is taught the basic standard of care with respect to reading labels when preparing medications. The reading standard is that the label is read three times before the drug is administered. The readings are done at defined points in the preparation procedure. Once, when taking the drug from the shelf or the patient's individual medication box; once, when cross-referencing the actual medication with the transcribed order; and once, when returning the medication container to the shelf of the patient's box. The system provides three distinct opportunities to pick up an error. The medication procedure itself has a number of built-in cross-checks.

A federal case which involved the interpretation of an insurance policy clause illustrates several deviations from the administration standard.[36]

> In *Reid v. Aetna Life Insurance Co.*, the patient, who had uneventful surgery earlier in the day, was receiving intravenous antibiotics. While preparing his third IV dose the nurse diluted the antibiotic powder with anectine instead of normal saline. Anectine is a neuromuscular blocking agent and is used in surgery as an anesthetic agent. The patient went into respiratory arrest and died 5 days later.
>
> It is clear that the nurse failed to read the label correctly, if in fact it was read at all. Errors can occur because the size or shape of a vial or ampule resembles that of the intended drug or diluent, but the cause of these types of errors is a breakdown in the medication procedure. A risk manager reviewing this kind of incident has to determine why such a drug was found in the proximity of a medicine cart or a medicine closet. It would be highly unusual for such a drug to be kept on a patient unit. The policy in most facilities is that the drug would be kept in the operating room. It is regarded as a specialized drug. If there is a need for such a drug on a patient unit, a special procedure for obtaining it should be followed. The procedure should also require that any unused portion be signed back into the operat-

ing room medication stores. Such a procedure would not eliminate all medication errors, but it would provide some assurance that one class of drug would be in an area where its use is routine, and when it is necessary to use it in another hospital area the procedure would not structure error.

Misreading of a label caused severe and permanent damages to a patient in *Gault v. Poor Sisters of St. Frances* who was admitted for routine gastric studies.[37] Instead of injecting an 0.85 percent saline solution into the Levine tube for gastric cytology the nurse injected a 10 percent sodium hydroxide solution. The patient, who was 28 years old, required long-term esophageal mechanical dilation because of the resultant esophageal strictures. In addition he had to undergo gastric resection and a 19-week hospitalization resulted in narcotic addiction. The nurse was held liable.

Sometimes there is a breakdown in "the system" which causes a patient to receive something harmful. In a recent Tennessee incident an elderly man who was awaiting eye surgery died after drinking oil of wintergreen, an air freshener, with orange juice.[38] The nurse took the green liquid out of the refrigerator and mixed it with the juice. Both the intended medication and the oil of wintergreen were green liquids. The refrigerator was for the storage of medicines only. The tragedy was attributed to "a human error."

These kinds of human errors frequently result from a careless breakdown of a safe system or a disregard of hospital policies designed to prevent such incidents.

Incorrect Route

It is important that the nursing plan of care include the implications of the patient's drug management. Drugs administered parenterally require patient monitoring that is different from situations in which the drug is administered orally. Some drugs that may safely be administered intramuscularly cannot be given directly into the vein without an adverse response.

In *Moore v. Guthrie Hospital,* a postoperative patient whose medication order directed that he receive penicillin and Chymar via the intramuscular route, was given both drugs by the IV route.[39] The patient suffered an immediate grand mal seizure. The patient sued the physician and the hospital for the nurse's action. The suit against the physician was dismissed, but the court held that the issue of the nurse's liability was for a jury to decide.

An early 1960s case, *Larrimore v. Homeopathic Hospital,* illustrates the incorrect way to check a physician's order when a question about the order arises.[40] The critical standard of care issue before the court was whether or not the nurse should have gone back to the earlier orders to learn what had transpired during her days off. The court held that no expert was necessary to establish the standard.

The patient had been diagnosed as having chronic glomerulonephritis and his physician decided to test his response to Ansolysen with hopes that it might arrest the malignant hypertension. The patient received 1-mg doses at periodic intervals, all given parenterally to permit absolute control of the dose. The patient failed to respond and it was decided that he would be discharged home. Because an abrupt withdrawal of the drug would present complications the physician discontinued the parenteral route and on October 1 ordered that the drug be given *orally* and in a 20-mg dose. On October 2 the order was the same. On the day in question, which was October 4, the physician left the following order: "Increase Ansolysen, 30 mg at 8 A.M., 30 mg at 2 P.M., and 30 mg at 8 P.M." The orders from October 1 to October 4 were on a single sheet. On October 4, the physician handed his order sheet to a nurse who had been off duty since October 1. She had previously given the drug by injection to the patient. When the nurse read the order she inquired of the physician whether he wanted her to give the patient 30 mg of Ansolysen. He answered in the affirmative, whereupon she prepared a syringe with a 30-mg dose of the drug. Both the patient and his wife protested the injection, indicating that the physician had told them that he would not order further injections. The nurse reread the order sheet and returned to the patient's room, insisting that it be given. Reluctantly the man permitted her to inject the medication. When the nurse informed the patient that he was to receive another injection the following day the man stated he would not take any more injections. The nurse then telephoned the physician and learned that the 30-mg dose should have been given orally. Emergency measures were instituted. The patient was discharged 2 weeks later, but returned a short time later and died several days after the readmission.

The hospital was held liable for the nurse's error. It had argued that the patient gave his consent, but the court held that the consent was given only after the nurse had reassured the patient that the dose was properly ordered by his physician. The court said that the nurse had but to read all the physician's orders in order to avoid the mistake she made. "The very purpose of the order sheet is to guide the nurses in carrying out the doctor's orders." Had the nurse gone over the order sheet she would have learned what transpired during her absence and avoided the error. Her duty to go back must also be decided in light of the fact that the last entry said nothing concerning the method of administering a dose of such an unusual size. The nurse went on the assumption that nothing had been changed.

The case points out the importance of teaching the correct method of reviewing a medical order when there is a question about the order. The orders should always be read from the most recent one back to the order in question. In addition, when the nurse questioned the physician about the appropriateness of the 30-mg dose she should have fully expressed her inquiry. She merely questioned one aspect of the order, that of the dose. She did not convey to him that she was uncomfortable about the difference in a 1-mg parenteral dose and a 30-mg parenteral dose. If the nurse had sought a more extensively reasoned explanation for the order the error would have been averted.

A final point is that when a patient expresses hesitancy about any form of therapy it frequently has a basis. The patient should be asked what his understanding is and any inconsistency should be resolved. Sometimes this can be done by reviewing the medical record and other times it requires consultation with the physician. The point is that whenever a patient puts a nurse on notice that something is not as expected, whether this concerns a new medication or a different-colored capsule, the nurse should take measures to confirm the correctness of the order or medication preparation.

No Medication Ordered

There may be many reasons why a patient receives a drug that was never ordered. The mistake may be traced back to a transcription error, that is, writing the wrong patient's name on the medication card or record, or stamping the wrong name on the pharmacy requisition slip. This kind of error can be picked up when the nurse questions why the patient would be receiving the particular "wrong" medication. The only reasonable way of checking is to go directly to the physician's order to verify it.

A large number of wrong medications are given because the nurse was distracted by talking to the patient or someone else instead of waiting until after the "steps" have been completed. Assuming the transcription was correct, it is the nurse's responsibility to make the final step of matching the patient's name bracelet with the medication order iust before administration of the drug.

> In *Peltier v. Franklin Hospital*,[41] the family of the decedent settled out of court for her wrongful death when she was negligently given potassium chloride which caused an immediate cardiac arrest. The drug had not been ordered by the physician. In this type of case the only issue in dispute is how much money will be owed for the death. Most frequently the defendant will admit liability for the death.

Duty When an Overdose Is Given

When an overdose or wrong medication is given there is, of course, a duty to take whatever measures can be reasonably taken to prevent or minimize the harm to the patient. The physician must be informed so that orders may be written and existing orders reviewed in light of the error. Except when the wrong medication will not harm the patient the physician must be informed immediately. In that case it will not harm the patient to delay informing the physician until he is available. The delay period, of course, must be reasonable as determined by the facts of the case.

Some mistakes require immediate follow-up. In a case where an infant's injury was attributed to the negligent administration of Demerol to the mother while in labor, a hospital settled for a million dollars.[42]

> In this case, *Nieto v. Kurzner*, the nurses administered an overdose of Demerol which caused the fetus' heartbeat to decrease. No oxygen was given to the mother for the remaining half hour she was in labor. Narcan was not given until after the mother delivered. The infant's respirations were depressed at birth and he suffered brain damage.

In a suit brought for anoxic brain damage of a 58-year-old woman who received a massive overdose of insulin, there was a settlement for over one million dollars.[43]

> In *Clark v. Presbyterian Hospital*, a woman was admitted for a mandibular abscess following a tooth extraction. The Decadron she received caused hypoglycemia which in turn was treated with insulin. One of the defendants was the private duty nurse who, using a regular syringe gave the patient 80 units instead of the ordered 8 units. When the woman lapsed into a coma the resident was unable to find her medication sheet and the overdose was not picked up quickly. The administration of glucose was delayed for several hours.

Some hospitals have a policy that requires a double-check of some of the more dangerous drugs, such as insulin, preoperative medications, and divided doses. This is a valuable procedure, at least in situations where the nurse is new to the facility or is a new graduate trying to adjust to a less structured work climate. Special precautions should be taken when the nurse is a "learner" or has come from another institute and may be unfamiliar with both the routine and the practice setting.

SUMMARY

Not all medication errors will result in a lawsuit. If the patient doesn't suffer any harm when the nurse gives Phenobarbital grains $\frac{1}{2}$ to the wrong patient no suit will be brought. However, many medication errors are serious and some result in death. Apart from some nursing judgment cases involving the administration of medications most involve a breakdown in the procedure itself.

This chapter illustrates that errors involving the procedure of giving prescribed medications are varied, intimidating, and sometimes tragic. Because the administration of medications is part and parcel of caring for patients, both within and apart from the hospital setting, the potential for error is considerable. The time-honored system of multiple checks, faithfully adhered to, is the best protection against errors. The medication procedure is the only area in nursing which does not, and should not permit shortcuts. Few of the judicial holdings cited here are surprising. The majority of cases cited here are reported ones, that is, cases beyond the trial level. Presumably a larger number were settled out of court or are unreported lower court trials. Nevertheless, the range of incidents gives nurses a clear picture of what not to do.

The injection injury cases no longer permit application of the res ipsa loquitur doctrine as the defense frequently argues that other factors "more probable than not" caused the unfortunate result. If it can be shown that the nurse used the accepted nursing technique and procedure when giving the injection, no liability will be found. The res ipsa loquitur doctrine applies to fewer and fewer injection cases.

While any wrong medication can cause harm, nurses should be most cautious when administering fast-acting IV medications because there may be no opportunity to correct or mitigate the effect. While it may be necessary to "float" a nurse to an area such as the intensive care unit or the emergency room, some alternative should be found to having a nurse who is unfamiliar with fast-acting emergency drugs administer them.

When a unit or facility uses unusually high doses special procedures and protocols should be in force to protect both the patient and the hospital. Such procedures should be developed by the medical staff and conveyed to the nursing staff by formal policy.

The adage that "we learn by our mistakes" is important in preventing potential errors. The medication system must always be subject to evaluation and modification as it is likely to be a principal cause for errors. If nurses comply with the "five rights" the number of medication errors will be lessened, but it is imperative that the safest possible system of administering medication that will meet the needs of the facility be instituted.

REFERENCES AND NOTES

1. Sugulas v. St. Paul Insurance Co., 347 S. 2nd 855 (LA, 1977).
2. Campos v. Weeks, 53 *California Reporter*, *915* (CA, 1966).
3. Newton, M., & Newton, D. (Sept. 1977). Guidelines for handling drug errors. *Nursing 77*, 62.
4. Anon. (Feb. 1980). ASHP Report: ASHP and ANA guidelines for collaboration of pharmacists and nurses in institutional care settings, *American Journal of Hospital Pharmacists*, *37*, 253. (See Appendix B in back of book.)
5. Brown v. State of N.Y., 391 N.Y.S. 2nd 204 (NY, 1977).

6. Anon. (1967). Medication errors, §24; in *18 Proof of facts* (1st ed.). Rochester, NY: Lawyers Co-operative Publishing.

7. Pisel v. Stamford Hospital, 430 A. 2nd 1 (CT, 1980). See Chapter 2 for discussion of case.

8. Gasbarra v. St. James Hospital, 406 N.E. 2nd 544 (IL, 1980). The plaintiffs argued that the 2-hour delay proximally caused the child's death, but the physician, who was also a named defendant, testified that the nurses had already given some ordered medication. A jury found in favor of the defendants.

9. Anon. (1967). Medication errors, §26; in *18 Proof of facts* (1st ed.). Rochester, NY: Lawyers Co-operative Publishing.

10. Fink, J. (1978). Hospital medicine errors; Hirsh, H., & Schweitzer, S. (Eds.) *Lawyer's medical journal* (pp. 139–155; Vol. 6). Rochester, NY: Lawyers Co-operative Publishing.

11. Mitchell, A. (Aug. 12, 1983). Letters: Accidental administration of ergonovine to a newborn. *Journal of the American Medical Association, 250*(6), 730.

12. Lamb v. Oakwood Hospital, 200 N.W. 2nd 88 (MI, 1972).

13. Evans v. U.S., 319 F. 2nd 751 (1963).

14. Honeywell v. Rogers, 251 F. Supp. 841 (1966).

15. Southwest Texas Methodist Hospital v. Mills, 535 S.W. 2nd 27 (TX, 1976).

16. Wilmington General Hospital v. Nichols, 210 A. 2nd 86 (DE, 1965).

17. Kord v. Baystate Medical Center, 429 N.E. 2nd 1045 (MA, 1982).

18. Dixon, M. (1982). *Drug product liability*, §7.14(2) at p. 7-53. New York: Matthew Bender.

19. 45 *American Law Review 3rd* 731, § Negligent Injections.

20. Barber v. Reinking, 411 P. 2nd 861 (WA, 1966).

21. Tung, A., Maliniak, K., Winter, P., & Tenicela, R. (Dec. 12, 1980). Intrathecal morphine for intraoperative and post-analgesia. *Journal of the American Medical Association, 244*(23), 2637; Babcock, et al. (April 17, 1981). Letters to the editor—Respiratory arrest after intrathecal morphine. *Journal of the American Medical Association, 245*(15), 1528.

22. Su v. Perkins, 211 S.E. 2nd 421 (GA, 1974).

23. Porter v. Patterson, 129 S.E. 2nd 70 (GA, 1962).

24. Muller v. Likoff, 310 A. 2nd 303 (PA, 1973).

25. Barnes v. St. Francis Hospital and School of Nursing, 507 P. 2nd 288 (KA, 1973).

26. Loebl, S., Spratto, G., and Wit, A. (1977). *Nurse's drug handbook* (p. 303). New York: John Wiley & Sons.

27. Beardsley v. Wyoming County Community Hospital, No. 15073, Wyoming Cty. Supreme Court Ct., NY (Sept. 5, 1979); cited in 23 *Association of Trial Lawyers of America Law Reporter (ATLA L. Rep.), 331* (Sept. 1981).

28. Kaunitz, A. (Feb. 1982) Point of law: Legal implications of prescribing and administering FDA-approved drugs in nonapproved ways. *Hospital Medical Staff, 11*(2), 15.

29. St. Anthony's Hospital v. Bullis, No. 56,733, Potter Cty., TX. (Feb. 17, 1981); cited in 24 *ATLA L. Rep., 331* (Sept. 1981).

30. Rowland v. Skaggs Companies, Inc., 666 S.W. 2nd 777 (MO, 1984).

31. Davis v. California, 117 *California Reporter, 463* (CA, 1974).

32. See Pisel v. Stamford Hosp., 430 A. 2nd 1 (CT, 1980), in which a 3-day delay in obtaining or transcribing the medication was cited in the opinion.

33. Anon. (Feb. 1980). ASHP Report: ASHP and ANA guidelines for collaboration of pharmacists and nurses in institutional care settings. *American Journal of Hospital Pharmacists, 37*, 253. (See Appendix B in back of book.)

34. Moore v. Dallas County Hospital, District Court, Dallas County, TX. No. 77-4700-C (Aug. 31, 1978); reported in 22 *ATLA L. Rep.*, 182 (May 1979). See also Cushing, M. (1986). Drug errors can be bitter pills. *American Journal of Nursing, 86*(8), 895.

35. Dessauer v. Memorial General Hospital, 628 P. 2nd 337 (NM, 1981).

36. In Reid v. Aetna Life Insurance Co., 440 F. Supp. 1182 (1977). The policy provided that no recovery would be provided where the death was "caused or contributed to by, or as a consequence of, medical or surgical treatment." The court interpreted the clause as meaning that the death was a consequence of medical treatment.
37. Gault v. Poor Sisters of St. Frances, 375 F. 2nd 539 (1967).
38. Anon. (May 15, 1985). *Biomedical safety and standards* (p. 79). Brea, CA: Quest Publishing.
39. Moore v. Guthrie Hospital, 403 F. 2nd 366 (1968).
40. Larrimore v. Homeopathic Hospital Association, 181 A. 2nd 573 (DE, 1962).
41. Peltier v. Franklin Foundation Hospital, No. 73-142-F, St. Mary Parish, LA (Jan. 19, 1985); cited in 28 *Atla L. Rep., 182* (May 1985).
42. Nieto v. Kurzner, No. 18457/76, N.Y. County Supreme Court (Oct. 10, 1980); cited in 24 *Atla L. Rep., 41* (Feb. 1981).
43. Clark v. Presbyterian Hospital, No. 21159, N.Y. Bronx Cty. Supreme Court (Dec. 16, 1983); cited in 27 *Atla L. Rep., 186* (May 1984).

COMMUNICATION AND DOCUMENTATION

The concepts of *communication* and *documentation* are important in any discussion of nursing malpractice. Liability may be based on the legal theory of delay in communicating or failure to communicate essential patient findings or changes. The concept of documentation in a legal sense speaks to the task of proving that reasonable care was or was not carried out. Record keeping is an integral part of patient care. Its chief purpose is to provide formal documentation of what has been done for the patient and for what reason. Records also are an important means whereby the various providers of care communicate with each other in a formal way. That does not mean to imply that verbal communications play a less important part in patient care.

At a trial or other judicial proceeding the parties will have access to the patient's chart. Absence of charting in a situation where a reasonable nurse would have charted will likely place the plaintiff at an advantage. Lawsuits come to court many years after the event, and testimony based on independent (without documentation) recollection, unless the circumstances are unusual, is less credible in the eyes of a jury. Observing, reporting, and recording go hand-in-hand. Nursing notations should reflect the event and the nursing judgment, that is, the patient evaluation and the action taken. A good rule is never to record an event without some interpretation of its significance and the action taken. For example, if a nurse finds a patient, who had angiography during which the femoral artery was used, who is up and walking about shortly after being returned from the X-ray department, her notes should reflect the nursing management of the situation. The record and incident report should include the following immediate management: patient returned to bed, wound inspected, vital signs checked, assessment done of why the patient got out of bed, and reteaching of patient. The patient may not have been properly prepared, there may be a language problem, or the patient may be confused because of medications. Subsequent notes should reflect ongoing management. Under these circumstances the physician should be appraised of the event and informed of the follow-up nursing care.

Juries give considerable weight to records made at the time the care was rendered, especially if the recorders had no knowledge of pending suit. This is because the notes reflect credibility. In the eyes of the jury a lack of exactness implies a lack of attention and, in an extreme case, it could be considered evidence of neglect. Some attorneys take the position that nurses' notes "are probably the most fruitful source of proof of significant events."[1]

A final note should be made in reference to the common practice of placing notes in the front of the record. This is most frequently done when new information is obtained and the recorder wishes to call it to the attention of others. It is not uncommon for a nurse, when discovering that a preoperative patient has an elevated temperature or other vital sign, to attach a note on the front of the patient's medical record to inform the surgeon and anesthesiologist. This system of attaching notes to the front of the hospital record is also used to inform the anesthesiologist that the patient told the nurse that he had changed his mind about the type of anesthesia he wanted. Both kinds of information should be verbally communicated to the anesthesiologist and surgeon in order that they may either alter their operative plan or have a further discussion with the patient. Nurses are in a position to obtain this "late" information because they are the ones who prepare patients for surgery or a special procedure. Rather than placing notes on the front of the record, which could be lost or otherwise not seen, the information should be recorded in the record and the appropriate individual immediately informed of the new patient data. The rule is that if the information is important it should become an integral part of the record.

DUTY TO COMMUNICATE ESSENTIAL PATIENT FINDINGS

A number of malpractice cases have found the nurse liable for the failure to communicate essential patient findings or the failure to communicate information furnished by the patient or a knowledgeable third party. Additionally, a substantial or unreasonable delay in communicating findings may also incur liability. From a practical point it is important that the nurse understand that merely documenting a critical patient finding or change without appropriate follow-up, that is, informing the attending physician in a timely manner, will "more probable than not" result in liability if the patient suffers harm.

In law there is an axiom, "Time is of the essence." It is not surprising that this axiom is sometimes found in legal opinions involving nursing malpractice. A good rule to follow whenever information comes to the attention of the nurse, which if known by the attending physician would cause the physician to write new medical orders or to cancel or elaborate on existing orders, or to discontinue orders, is to verbally communicate the information to the physician. The timeliness of the communication depends on the salient facts of the situation. There is, of course, the necessity to evaluate the new patient data in light of surrounding circumstances and make a nursing judgment which is reasonable under the circumstances. Practically, the test of reasonableness may be more difficult to establish in the courtroom where the breach of duty was delay rather than a failure to communicate. This is especially true if defense experts testified that the delay was for the purpose of carrying out further nursing assessment measures. However, if the delay was inappropriate under the circumstances the plaintiff will have a less difficult time establishing reasonableness. The duty to communicate essential information is not confined to informing the physician. Communication among nurses during patient rounds and during the change of shift nursing report is critical because nursing care is based in large part on verbal reports. Communication among other health care providers is equally important.

Timely Communication

The importance of prompt reporting of critical patient changes is illustrated by an Illinois case, *Garfield Park Community Hospital v. Vitacco*, in which a 9-year-old boy had to have his right leg amputated because of ischemic necrosis.[2] The child suffered a fracture to his left femur after being struck by an automobile. He was placed in Bryant's traction July 3 and remained in it for 11 days. He was seen by his physician daily and on July 9 his legs were unwrapped and examined. The nurse's notes indicated that from July 3 to July 8 his condition was stable. A July 9 note indicated, "Dr. Vitacco here—left foot edematous." During the next 2 days the nursing notes indicated that the child complained of severe pain in both legs with swelling of the right foot. However, a nurse's note indicated that the circulation remained "good." On July 12 the physician ordered an increase in the weights. His progress note indicated that the circulation was good at that time. The first significant change in the temperature of the child's foot occurred in the 3–11 P.M. notes on July 12th. The note read, "right foot swollen and cool to touch." During the morning of July 13 an orthopedic surgeon on the hospital staff passing the room noted the child's distress and inspected his legs and feet. Finding them cold, the surgeon removed the patient from traction and told the nurses to notify the treating physician. Some 4 hours later he rechecked the boy and found the left leg had color, minimal motion, and was warm. However, the right leg lacked sensation and could not be moved voluntarily.

Both the hospital and primary physician made settlement payments and the hospital sought indemnification from the physician. The court held that negligence on the part of the nurses precluded indemnification. A physician testifying for the plaintiffs said that changes in the color, sensation, and motion (CSM) of the limb should have been noted by the nurses who should then promptly notify the physician. Another physician testified that it was "absolutely basic" for a nurse to notify the physician immediately on noting signs and symptoms of decreased CSM.

There are a number of cases where delay has resulted in the death of a patient. The position of most courts is that where the chance to live is lost because of the negligent failure of the physician to diagnose the condition or timely respond to critical patient changes that have been communicated to him, liability exists.

One court, in *Goff v. Doctor's General Hospital of San Jose*, found that the negligence of the nurses in failing to timely contact the physician was a contributing cause of death.[3] A woman delivered at 7 P.M. after receiving a labor-inducing drug. The physician did not suture an incision made in the cervix, but rather inserted pressure packs. The nurse who had attended the birth informed the physician on three different occasions that she assessed the postpartum bleeding to be excessive. He instructed her in the technique of measuring the vaginal flow and she began to test the flow at 9:30 P.M. By 10:15 P.M. she found that the pads were close to saturation, however, she did not take any vital signs. She did not call the physician because in her opinion "he would not have responded." The nurse testified that she assessed the situation as an emergency throughout the last 45 minutes of her shift. She reported her findings to the night nurse at the 11 P.M. report. She was critical of the physician's lack of concern. It was not until 11:15 P.M. that the physician was notified of the patient's condition by the night nurse who had found her in shock. The physician came within 10 minutes but attempts to treat her hemorrhage, including attempts to insert a peripheral intravenous line, were unsuccessful.

The court found that the nurse's failure to report her findings and assessment of the situation to her superior increased the woman's peril and precluded prompt measures to save her life. A physician who testified that the physician's failure to suture the cervix was a lack of due care also testified that if the nurse had completely assessed the patient and not acted on her own opinion of the doctor's attitude and qualifications the patient may have lived. He testified that both nurses had enough time to have reported the circumstances to a superior. He said, "Time was of the essence." The court also commented that if emergency measures were taken earlier the attempts to ensure blood replacement via intravenous lines may have been successful.

In another case, *Karrigan v. Nazareth Convent and Academy,* liability was found against the nurses because the court found a 12-hour delay in reporting an adverse response to the removal of a T-tube was unreasonable.[4] The physician had ordered the removal when he visited the patient early in the day. He was to be discharged the following day. Shortly after the removal the patient complained of pain and the nurse called the physician who ordered a pain medication. However, the nurses failed to communicate further with the physician although the man's pain increased and he began vomiting. When the physician visited the patient on his evening rounds he discovered his distress which resulted in an additional 3 weeks' hospitalization.

In a number of cases liability was found for the nurse's failure to contact the physician when a postoperative patient developed complications.

In *Kolakowski v. Voris,* the court held that a trial court was in error when it prematurely dismissed a suit that had been brought against several surgeons and the hospital for the negligence of its nurses.[5] The court held that there were issues of fact which the jury as the triers of fact had a right to decide.

The plaintiff had undergone back surgery for pain. In the immediate postoperative period the patient complained of the inability to bend his left leg, along with weakness and numbness on his right side. A nurse noted the fact in the record along with the patient's subsequent complaints that he could not move his legs and that they felt stiff. An hour and one half later the nurse recorded that the patient could move his right leg slightly, but could not move his left leg at all. He also had a temperature of 102°F. There was a notation in the record that the neurosurgeon was called but could not be found. There was no indication in the record that any attempt was made to inform one of the assisting surgeons. The following day the neurosurgeon found that the patient had poor hand, wrist, and leg movement, impaired sensation, and hyperactive reflexes. He diagnosed the patient as having spastic quadriparesis, which evidence indicated could be caused by either spinal cord compression or cord edema. If it resulted from compression it should have been surgically reduced as soon as possible to offer the best chance of recovery. The physician admitted that the patient's postoperative symptoms were unusual and demanded attention. The evidence showed that he treated the patient the first postoperative day as having cord edema although the factors which generally cause cord edema, trauma, and impaired circulation did not appear to be present. The court found that a jury, if permitted to decide the case, could have rendered a verdict against the hospital for the failure of its nurses to recognize the seriousness of the patient's condition and promptly inform the physician.

The court held that there was a material issue about what caused the paralysis and the plaintiff's evidence should be heard by the jury. The case illustrates that serious postoperative findings require quick attention and where an opportunity to treat the patient is lost, liability may result. In this case the tragic result of quadriplegia may have been prevented.

A Minnesota case, *Sandhofer v. Abbott-Northwestern Hospital,* deals with the issue of timely notification of a change in a patient's condition and illustrates the element of causation.[6] The evidence against the physician and the hospital was held sufficient and the jury apportioned the damages award between the two. The patient, who had sustained a comminuted fracture of the wrist, underwent surgical open reduction on June 22. The plaintiff attributed his ultimate injury to the medical and nursing care given in the immediate 5-day postoperative period. During this period impairment in circulation caused necrosis which necessitated amputation below the elbow several months later.

The physician requested the nurses to check CSM of the limb which was also in a cast. Both the physician and staff monitored the arm by "blanching" to ascertain return of blood to the fingers after local depression. The plaintiff introduced the nursing notes which covered the 5-day period from June 23 to June 27. They indicated the following: June 23—fingers very blue, cool, and swollen; June 24 (A.M.)—color and sensation good, (P.M.)—swollen and cyanotic; June 25—fingers swollen and dark blue; June 26—fingers swollen, bluish, and cool; June 27—fingers bluish and cool. The nurses later testified that they were concerned about the condition of the fingers. The observation on June 25 was made by a nurses' aide who did not notify anyone of her findings. On June 27 the physician bivalved the cast after being summoned to the hospital by a concerned nurse. No physician's progress notes existed for June 24, 25, and 26.

The physician testified that on the day the cast was split the circulation was good, but his notes indicated ischemia of the hand. The patient testified that the arm was hard and that chunks of his arm were taken out as the cast was spread. Sores were noted on the arm. Expert testimony established that such hardness was consistent with ischemia. Experts for the plaintiff testified that the failure of the nurses to notify the doctor of significant, observable changes in the patient's condition was a direct cause of the injury. The duty to notify continued as long as the man stayed in the hospital.

In circulation impairment cases, the courts have found liability where the harm occurred in a relatively short-time span, as well as over a period of several days.

In *Brannan v. Lankenau Hospital,* a case in which the court found against both the physicians and the nurses, the time span involved was 16 hours.[7] The court held that no expert nursing testimony was necessary to establish the applicable standard of nursing care, in view of the fact that the physician had left explicit orders to closely monitor the patient and the orders were clearly not carried out.

The plaintiff underwent an emergency esophagoscopy to break up meat which was lodged in his esophagus. During the procedure a screw on the grasping forceps broke and the sharp portions of the instrument came in contact with the wall of the esophagus. No evidence of perforation was seen and he was transferred to the recovery room. By 8:00 P.M. his temperature had increased to 100.4°F and the nurses promptly notified the surgeon who called in a specialist. The surgeon did not inform the specialist of the incident with the forceps and his concern about perforation. The consultant examined the patient at 11 P.M., but found no evidence of laceration. He requested close monitoring and transfer of the patient to the surgical intensive care unit. The transfer was not done until 4 A.M. at which time the man's temperature was 100.8°F. At 8 A.M. the specialist returned and found the man's temperature had increased to 101.8°F with elevated respirations and pulse. The nurses had not monitored these signs and had not informed the physician of any changes. Based on these findings the patient was diagnosed as having a perforated esophagus and antibiotics were ordered. It was not until 12:30 P.M. that the first dose was administered and by that time he manifested multiple signs of infection. Secondary to the infection he suffered a meningeal stroke. The court held that the failure on the part of the staff to monitor changes and notify the physician was a "glaring example of want of care."

Failure to Inform Physician of Patient Status

Before the practice of requiring the presence of a physician in the obstetric department of a hospital, or the influential nurse-midwive movement had come to the fore, it was routine for nurses to examine the patient, monitor their progress, and call the physician just in time for the delivery.

In one case, *Hiatt v. Croce,* the issue was whether the nurse's failure to procure the attendance of the woman's physician at her time of need constituted negligence.[8] The court held that the nurse's delay in communicating the woman's status of labor to the physician was negligent and was the proximate cause of the woman's injuries.

The woman who entered the hospital for the delivery of her second child had notified her physician that she was going to the hospital. The hospital also notified the physician when she was admitted at 7 P.M. Her progress was uneventful during the night. The defendant nurse came on duty at 7:30 A.M. at which time the woman was dilated 7 cm. The nurse instructed the husband to time the contractions and to notify her when they increased. At that time the husband informed the nurse that his wife quickly went from 7 to 8 cm during the first delivery. The husband frequently reported to the nurse, who was reading a magazine at the nurses' station. After the woman had reached 8 cm at 8:30 A.M., the husband and the woman's mother repeatedly requested that the physician be called. On one occasion the nurse told the husband that she "never lost a father yet so you just go back there and sit down." Ten minutes later the woman called out that the baby was coming. The nurse called the physician and put the patient on the delivery room table. The woman transferred herself from the bed to the cart and from the cart to the table. She placed herself in the stirrups. The nurse went to get another physician. Although the record said that the physician delivered the infant the nurse testified that she performed the delivery. The mother testified that the infant's head and shoulders were delivered while she was unattended and she fainted before the birth was completed. The physician who responded to the nurse's request for help began to suture the woman's lacerations. Her private physician came in, administered gas, and completed the repair.

The woman required over 15 sutures to repair the lacerations in her vagina and labia. She subsequently sued the hospital for pain and suffering and loss of sexual sensation. Finding against the nurse, the court stated that she was responsible for the delay in notifying the woman's physician to come to the hospital. The court said that in establishing the standard of care owed to the woman a nurse must weigh the various factors to be considered in determining the imminence of childbirth. These factors include the position of the unborn child, the dilation, the progress of dilation, and the frequency and intensity of the contractions.

Failure to Communicate Information Supplied by the Patient

When information is given to the nurse or other health care provider by a patient or other individual, the system for communicating the information should be uniform and workable. For example, a system that requires that patient allergies be noted in too many places increases the risk that the information will not find its way to all the places that hospital policy mandates. The risk is particularly great where the patient does not recall a specific allergy when initially asked the question, but remembers later and then tells someone. Ordinarily when the patient is first admitted the question, which is a part of the nursing history, is asked and the interviewer records any noted allergies in the appropriate place(s). However, when information is not given by the patient initially, there is a real possibility that it will be noted in some of the designated places, but not all, if they are too numerous.

Much of the information given by patients or family members is extremely important. It may be a vital clue in diagnosing a medical problem or it may be the basis for establishing a plan of nursing care.

In a widely reported case, *Ramsey v. Physicians Memorial Hospital*, the emergency room nurse failed to communicate the fact that a mother had removed two ticks from her child and an incorrect diagnosis was made by the physician.[9] The child died of Rocky Mountain spotted fever and liability was found against the hospital for the nurse's action. The jury regarded the tick removal as "significant data." No liability was found against the physician.

In another example, a Pennsylvania court, in *Yorston v. Pennell*, held a surgeon responsible for the negligence of his resident, a junior intern, and a nurse-anesthetist for failing to indicate on the medical record that the patient was allergic to penicillin.[10] At that time the hospital could not be sued for the negligent acts of its nursing staff because of an immunity statute.

The patient was admitted for emergency surgery after an industrial accident. He had previously been advised by a physician that he was allergic to penicillin and should not receive the drug. The doctor wrote a note for the man which he kept in his wallet and which he showed to several of the nurses and to the intern on admission. The intern testified that during the operation he told the nurse-anesthetist to record the allergy, but the information was not verbally communicated to the surgical resident who unwittingly wrote an order for penicillin. Each time the nurses administered the drug to the patient he repeated the fact of his allergy. After receiving three doses he outright refused it. His refusal was communicated to the surgical resident who immediately discontinued the drug. He subsequently suffered severe physical and personality changes as a direct result of the penicillin injections.

Documentation Without Communication

It is not unusual for physicians to say that although they read other parts of the medical record daily they do not customarily read nurses' notes. The courts tend to hold the nurse liable for failing to verbally inform the physician of negative patient findings even where the nurses have documented the findings. Although a number of courts have found against both the nurse and the physician, these decisions are not consistent enough to provide direction. The courts will consider the facts of the case and generally find liability against both providers when the case is extreme.

In *Pettis v. State of Louisiana*, a patient with a diagnosis of schizophrenia showed minimal response to chemical drugs and physicians decided to treat him with electroshock (ECT) therapy.[11] A pretreatment film revealed that the patient only had a scoliosis condition. He was scheduled for a series of ECT treatments over a 10-day period. The nursing notes indicated that after the second treatment the patient complained of back and shoulder pain. The nurses did not inform the physician. The nursing notes indicated that he was complaining of back, lumbar, and spine pain after the fourth treatment. Subsequent notes read, "complaining of pain in arms and legs," "appears completely helpless, can't move arms or legs . . . complaining of pain in arms and legs," "has old bruise on right shoulder—down arm to elbow—shoulder swollen and tender to touch. May have fracture."

The physician did not examine the patient until after four of the treatments had been completed. At that time he discontinued any further treatments and ordered x-ray films of the patient's back. The findings were not known until 3 days later when the report revealed fractures of the bodies of three thoracic vertebrae. He was transferred to a medical unit at which time it was found he had fractures of both humerus and both femoral necks. He had hip surgery but remained severely debilitated.

The court held the nurses liable for failing to inform the physicians of the patient's complaints of pain. If they had informed the physician additional injury would have been prevented. In addition, the hospital was found liable for failing to include the patient's findings on a "24-hour report." The report was designed to accommodate the physicians who said they did not have time to read the patient's chart before treatment. The procedure was that the chief nurse on the day shift completed the report and forwarded it to the clinical director by 8 A.M. The report contained "unusual things."

The physicians who gave the treatments were also found liable. The court said that the case did not involve an error of judgment or want of skill, but rather was a situation where the physicians failed to exercise reasonable care and diligence. The court determined that the physicians had an independent duty to determine if the patient had experienced pain after the treatment. Testimony established that from 2 to 30 percent of patients who do not receive a paralyzing anesthetic sustain fractures. Although the doctors testified that they did not have time to read the nurses' notes the court noted that the nurse's entries were contained in three lines and would have taken only a moment to read just before giving the treatment. With respect to the 24-hour report the court said the omissions by the chief nurse were not sufficient to relieve the physicians of their duty.

In a recent legal publication, an attorney wrote that generally, doctors skip over nurses' notes because they consider them time-consuming and redundant. He also stated that when making hospital rounds, doctors are supposed to read the notes, but most prefer to get an abbreviated oral report from the nurse, rather than spend the time required to read the handwritten entries of several different nurses (Conversely, it should be noted, plaintiff's lawyer takes the time to read every entry in each page.[12])

Communications Between Health Care Facilities

When a patient is transferred from one health care facility to another the law may impose a duty to inform the successor facility of special patient problems. This duty is probably less a problem where the patient has been transferred fairly quickly and before the staff has obtained "unusual" information. Such would be the case where the transfer was necessary because of the inability to medically manage the patient's condition. However, where it is known that the patient adversely reacts to a combination of drugs there would be a clear duty to appraise the second hospital of this fact. When patients are transferred from hospital care to community nursing management or where a nursing home resident is transferred from the home to a hospital, a nurse ordinarily completes a nursing referral form which is intended to provide information and direction.

> In *Keestview Nursing Home v. Synowiec,* a Florida nursing home was held liable for the death of a man who had recently been transferred from their facility to an acute care facility.[13] The man was admitted for medical treatment and the nursing home did not provide information which would have alerted the hospital to the fact that he had organic brain disease. When the nursing home nurses later testified, they said that they recognized that these types of patients required special supervision because of their tendency toward wandering, forgetfulness, and loss of mental acuity. The man wandered away from the hospital and was found dead several days later.
>
> The nursing home was not successful in its argument that the widow presented no proof that the decedent had exhibited a tendency to wander while he resided at their facility. The widow presented the following arguments: (1) the elderly man was known to be suffering from senility, (2) his mental state had deteriorated to a point where he had to be put in a secure facility, (3) he was known to have ailments that render a person incapable of caring for himself and that often involve wandering, (4) he was recognized by the nursing staff as a man who had at least a minor tendency to wander, (5) the nursing home knew that the wife placed him there because she had been unable to curb his wandering from their home into the street, (6) his condition required the nursing home to identify him as a "watch patient," and (7) he was the type of patient that required constant care and observation. The court said that although the nursing home did not send accompanying medical data to the hospital in regards to his senility, experts testified that it would have been good practice to do so because such information should accompany any patient who has a tendency toward wandering, forgetfulness, and loss of mental acuity.

Failure to Communicate Physician's Instructions

The system for writing and transcribing orders on the hospital unit is well established. Most legal authorities discourage the taking of verbal orders because of the potential for error. Unfortunately, nurses too frequently disregard the risk associated with verbal orders by permitting physicians to leave verbal orders when the situation does not warrant it. Most hospitals have a policy or bylaw requiring that all telephone orders be confirmed and co-signed within a specified time, generally 24 hours. Not all hospitals require the physician to co-sign orders given verbally during patient rounds or at other times when the order is dictated to the nurse. If a hospital has incidences of incorrect medical orders being implemented or orders not being implemented, the method of leaving orders should be reviewed first. If the incidences involve a substantial number of unnecessary verbal orders the practice should be discontinued and periodic follow-up review should be conducted to ensure that the practice is not continuing.

In the following case, *Childs v. Greenville Hospital*, the court held that the issue of whether the nurse communicated the precise instructions of the physician was one for the jury to decide as triers of fact. There was dispute between the physician and the nurse as to what was said over the telephone in the emergency room.[14] The patient, who was 7 months pregnant, bleeding, and in labor went to the defendant hospital's emergency room. The woman was vacationing in the area. The hospital was a private facility. The night supervisor examined her and telephoned the physician on call. In the pretrial discovery the supervisor testified that the doctor said, "Tell the patient to get in touch with her own doctor." The physician's affidavit said, "I told the nurse . . . to have the girl call her doctor at Garland and see what he wanted her to do." The woman testified that the supervisor told her that the doctor had told her to go see her own doctor, whose place of practice was in her home town of Garland, and find out what he wanted her to do. The woman testified that she was hesitant, but left when the supervisor assured her that she would have sufficient time.

She delivered in the car. An earlier suit against the physician held in his favor because it was not established that a patient–physician relationship existed. The court held that such a relationship was necessary to establish that he owed her any duty of care.[15] However, in the suit against the hospital the court held that there was a clear duty owed by the nurse to communicate the physician's information accurately, but the credibility to be affixed to the nurse's testimony was to be determined by the jury. Conversely, the jury could conclude that the testimony of the woman, if believed by them, was a violation of the duty owed. The woman's testimony would be that she was told she would have sufficient time to make the trip to the neighboring town rather than telephone her physician for instructions. In cases like these the jury must weigh all the evidence in order to resolve the conflict in testimony.

Summary

The concept of communication embraces both verbal communication and written communication. Broken down further, the concept includes both a delay in communication and a failure to communicate at all. The documentation part comes into play either when there is a conflict in testimony during a trial or essential patient data is not recorded in the hospital record.

The communication of essential patient findings must be made in a timely fashion. This means that the time span must be reasonable under the circumstances. Delay may deprive the patient of the chance to live. Frequently the physician defends the suit against him by saying that the nurse failed to communicate the information in time to save the patient's leg or his life. There are other ways in which communication of patient findings is vital. For example, in a few cases liability was found against the nurse for failing to tell the physician what the patient or family member told the nurse. Where the nurse documents important information, but fails to verbally inform the physician, liability will exist. Caution should also prevail where a patient is being transferred from one facility to another. It is important that essential patient data be communicated to the receiving facility.

DUTY TO DOCUMENT ESSENTIAL PATIENT FINDINGS AND CARE

Documentation of nursing care and events relevant to care and treatment is an important professional activity. A Joint Commission on Accreditation of Hospitals (JCAH) standard states that: "Documentation of nursing care shall be pertinent and concise, and shall reflect the patient's status. Nursing documentation should address the patient's needs, problems, capabilities, and limitations. Nursing intervention and patient response must be noted. . . ."[16] In litigation it is essential to establish the extent of care that has been provided in order to indicate to the jury that the recognized and accepted medical or nursing standard was met or was not met. This is done by evidence such as the medical record and hospital policies. The medical record may also give evidence that the standard of care was not met because the record does not indicate what was done for the patient. Where the care is routine the nurse will testify that such routine care is not generally documented. However, this may not be persuasive when the facts surrounding a case are unique or where the plaintiff has evidence other than the medical record that is more credible to the jury. One practice may pose a unique problem for both parties; that is when the defendants testify that the patient was monitored and appropriate care given, but hospital policy requires that the notations be discarded or destroyed. Such a practice, especially if it includes day-to-day nursing progress notes, may be harmful to both the defendant's and plaintiff's case because potential evidence is lost.

Significance of Omissions

Parts of a hospital record may be used effectively to establish the plaintiff's case or to defend the position of the defendants. Because the role of the jury is that of triers of fact it is not possible to generalize about whether a given record will help or hinder the defendant. The jury looks to the surrounding facts in attaching credibility to the different sources of evidence. This point is well illustrated in cases that involve monitoring and subsequent reporting of the circulation status of limbs after trauma.

In an Illinois case, *Collins v. Westlake Community Hospital*, the court held that the question of liability was to be decided by the jury because the sequence of events as appeared in the medical record could have led them to draw a conclusion that the nurse caring for the child during the night shift did not monitor the toes.[17] The young child in this case fractured his left leg when he was struck by an automobile. He was placed in immediate traction and the doctor orders included, "Watch condition of toes." The physician testified that it was routine nursing care for the nursing staff to check circulation, but he said, "I wanted to be sure that it was understood that they should watch the toes very closely." Forty-eight hours after the accident the child developed a clot in the femoral artery and underwent an emergency embolectomy, but had to have the limb amputated the following day because of ischemia.

One of the hospital nurses charted a 10:30 P.M. note which said that the toes were cool to touch, but were "being observed closely." The physician visited the patient at 11 P.M., performed certain circulatory tests which indicated to him that the circulation was adequate. The foot and leg were not swollen and the temperature was normal. However, he did note a loss of sensation in the foot and consulted a neurosurgeon because he was concerned that there might be nerve damage. The notes written by the nurse during the 11 P.M. to 6 A.M. period were as follows: "12:30 Unable to sleep. Milk given. 1:30 Awake—med. given for pain. 6 A.M. A good night—states he feels better. Left foot is cold—color is dusky—appears to have no feeling in foot. Dr. Hubbard notified." The doctor went to the hospital immediately, removed the traction and prepared for immediate surgery.

The nurse who had been on duty the previous shift testified that normally a nurse does not always record on the chart the observations every time the patient is checked and that only abnormal findings are charted. The physician testified that in his opinion the nurses kept him adequately informed of the child's condition. However, citing *Darling* the court held that sufficient evidence was presented by the plaintiff on whether the nurse exercised due care in observing the leg during the night when the circulation apparently ceased.[18] In *Darling* the court said, "On the basis of the evidence before it the jury could reasonably have concluded that the nurses did not test for circulation in the leg as frequently as necessary, that skilled nurses would have promptly recognized the conditions that signaled a dangerous impairment of circulation in the patient's leg, and would have known that the condition would be irreversible in a matter of hours."

However, another case, *Glen v. Kerlin*, decided in a different jurisdiction at about the same time as *Collins* reached a different conclusion and held for the hospital. Among the allegations against the nurses was their failure to discover the decubitus ulcers earlier when treatment would probably have been more effective. The plaintiff unsuccessfully argued that it was error for the court to allow the nurses to testify about the care they gave when the nurses' notes did not contain corresponding entries to corroborate their testimony.[19] The man, who had been paraplegic for 6 years, entered the hospital for a cystectomy and bilateral cutaneous ureterostomy. He was hospitalized for 29 days during which he underwent a second procedure to anastomose one ureter to the other because it had become gangrenous. The patient alleged that he developed decubitus ulcers on his right ankle, at the outside of his right foot, both buttocks, lower back, and the top of his left foot. They failed to heal and ultimately he had to have his right leg amputated.

The patient's physician, who was also a defendant, testified that he was concerned that the anastomosed left ureter would separate and spill its contents in the peritoneal cavity, therefore he ordered "no unnecessary movement." He did not prescribe any decubitus care. The physician testified that he first noticed the red pressure areas 8 days before discharge and ordered frequent rotation. On discharge he instructed the patient's wife in the care of the areas. The physician testified that he believed the sores would heal as they had in the past.

The wife presented no evidence to contradict the physician's testimony that the decubitus ulcers were present prior to the week before discharge or that they were in an advanced state when the patient left the hospital. The defendant hospital presented evidence that, if believed by the jury, showed that the man received the maximum nursing care under the circumstances. In explaining the absence of notes indicating the care given, the nurses testified that not all of the attention provided a patient is necessarily recorded and that a minor activity such as position changes would not be detailed. The court held that the absence of such detailed entries did not lessen the credibility of the nurses' testimony. An orderly who attended the patient recalled seeing bed rolls and "doughnuts" on the occasions he bathed the man. On balance the wife's evidence did not outweigh the defendants. There was no evidence that she made complaints or requests of the staff.

Record Omissions as Evidence of Lack of Care

When the medical record includes evidence that is consistent with the testimony given at a trial the jury gives it considerable weight. Of course, this advantage may be rebutted by the opposing party. In addition, the facts surrounding the case may lessen the impact of testimony even where there is corroboration in the records. However, where the medical record omits an entry, this point will be stressed by the party seeking to have the jury consider the lack of the entry as evidence that such care was not given.

In a case in which the plaintiff alleged that a premature infant had received excessive oxygen which resulted in retrolental fibroplasia, the plaintiff's attorney sought to have certain instructions included by the judge in his charge to the jury.[20]

The physician in *Siirila v. Barrios* had ordered the oxygen to be run at specific concentrations during the 41 days the infant was receiving it. Sometimes the nurses ran the oxygen at higher levels than ordered. The record was lacking in details. During the trial the plaintiff's attorney was allowed to present testimony on the alleged failure to record information on the infant's charts and records. He also addressed the issue in his closing argument to the jury. When he lost the suit against both the hospital and physician, he based one of his appeal issues on the fact that the judge would not give the following charge: "I charge you, that you may consider as evidence the matters contained in this hospital record, and also concerning the lack or absence of an entry in said hospital record, which should have been entered if such act, occurrence or event had taken place, can be considered as evidence by you that such act, transaction, occurrence or event had not taken place."

Applying a state statute and a court rule, the court held that the instruction was unnecessary because the jury had heard the evidence during the testimony phase of the trial and would give it its weight. The lesson illustrated in the case is that omissions in a record can be used as evidence of lack of care that may be sufficient to establish negligence.

In another case, *Stack v. Wapner*, the court held that where the physicians did not make any notations in the records of a woman in labor the jury could conclude that no monitoring occurred.[21] The woman was admitted to a teaching hospital for the birth of her fourth child. She was started on Pitocin at 2:45 A.M. There were no chart entries until 5:15 A.M. In fact, throughout the labor there were only three notes, and only one that gave evidence of the quality of monitoring. Following her delivery at 8:30 A.M. she began to bleed which necessitated a total hysterectomy and the administration of 6½ pints of blood. She had to be readmitted because of infectious hepatitis which was secondary to the blood transfusions. She subsequently had a partial hearing loss in both ears from the medications given to treat the hepatitis.

The defendants sought to justify the omissions by presenting evidence that a blackboard was posted in the labor room hall which indicated the status of each woman in labor. Relying on the testimony of one of the defendant physicians and another witness, the defendants argued that the "positive" evidence provided by their testimony could not be outweighed by the "negative" evidence of the absence of entries on the woman's chart. However, the court held that the "negative" evidence was a kind of evidence from which the jury could draw an inference that monitoring was not done. The plaintiff had also presented evidence of a hospital policy requiring that its charts contain a reference to all observations and treatment.

In a more recent case, *Wagner v. Kaiser Foundation Hospital*, an Oregon court put the negative aspect of record omissions in a different legal light.[22] The court held in favor of the plaintiff. The defendant hospital argued that the negative evidence (chart omissions) should not have been admitted because the plaintiff had no positive evidence to support his allegation that the nurses did not monitor postoperative respirations. Specifically addressing the negative evidence issue, the court said that use of that term confuses, rather than aids, the jury's deliberation. The question is whether affirmative indirect or circumstantial evidence was offered so as to provide a basis from which the jury could properly draw an inference that there was a lack of monitoring.

According to testimony on behalf of the plaintiff, he had been given an excessive dose of narcotic by the nurse-anesthetist and had not received a sufficient antagonistic dose at the close of the procedure. As a result of not being given a sufficient antagonistic dose the patient could have "forgotten to breathe." The analgesic drug would have stayed in the patient's system for approximately 5 hours. There was also testimony that it looked like "the patient could breath, but then 30 minutes later the respirations may have slowed way, way down again because of the tremendous (amount of) narcotic aboard" and that the probable respiratory depression could have dropped to two to three breaths per minute which would not have insured an adequate amount of oxygen to maintain cerebral integrity. The patient sustained significant brain damage including severe memory loss. The man, who was in his mid-forties, had been employed as a teacher and was ultimately discharged because he could not function in the job.

The recovery room nurses notes demonstrated that his blood pressure and pulse were recorded at 15-minute intervals. However, in spite of the fact that the chart had a section for charting the respirations there was no documentation that this specific sign was monitored. The notes, which were written during a 2-hour period, stated that the patient was "doing well." The recovery room nurses had no independent recollection of the man or events surrounding his care. There was testimony on behalf of the nurses that depressed respirations might not be noticed by reasonably trained competent nurses even if they were properly monitoring a patient. The court concluded that the jury had sufficient evidence to find against the defendants. The court said, "if defendants' recovery room nurses had properly monitored the rate and depth of plaintiff's breathing they would, in the normal course of events, have discovered what was then happening in time to give him oxygen so as to prevent the brain damage."

In a New York case, *Topel v. Long Island Jewish Medical Center*, decided several years after the "blackboard case,"[21] the court held that where a hospital presented other evidence to support its position that a patient was adequately monitored no liability would exist against the hospital for the negligence of its nurses.[23] The next of kin brought suit against the hospital after a psychiatric patient hung himself with a belt he had been permitted to wear throughout his 5-day stay. On the day he was admitted he had tried to commit suicide twice. His diagnosis which was established when he was admitted to the emergency room was psychotic depression. The day after his admission he was placed on three different drugs and ECT therapy was planned. His psychiatrist instructed the nurses to see that the "patient was followed and seen every 15 minutes" to prevent the man's acting out his suicidal ideation. One nursing note said that the patient was trying the windows. It was known that one of the means of suicide verbally expressed by the patient was jumping out a window. His symptoms did not abate and on the third hospitalization day a nurse, on her own initiative, placed the man under "constant observation." Quotes by the patient which were included in the notes indicated that he was severely depressed and suicidal. Two days before his suicide the nurse returned him to the 15-minute monitoring schedule.

The nurses testified that they checked the man every 15 minutes. The man's wife argued that the hospital record did not bear out its contention that the decedent had been in fact observed at 15-minute intervals as the psychiatrist ordered. Specifically addressing that issue, the court said that the absence of a written record of such observation was explained when the hospital presented evidence that such notations were made on worksheets which were kept separate from the permanent medical record and destroyed at the end of each week. Further, the court said that the wife had presented no evidence that the worksheet procedure constituted an improper hospital practice.

Several observations may be made about the decision. Under the facts of the case the hospital could not be held liable for carrying out the course of treatment prescribed by the patient's attending physician. Recent cases have held the hospital, as a corporation, is liable if it fails to institute a process whereby the qualifications of its medical staff are not adequately reviewed at the time of appointment. The wife also sued the psychiatrist, but the court held that his judgment was compatible with good practice.

Another significant aspect in the case is the fact that the wife did not produce any evidence attacking the hospital's practice of destroying the worksheets. The worksheets would have been the only physical evidence showing that the 15-minute checks were done. Some argument can be made that the practice of discarding them, especially in that no summary of them was made, was not in the best interest of continuity of care. Conversely, the hospital could argue that the worksheets were similar to the intake and output notes which are not part of the permanent record and are discarded on discharge. However, the daily intake and output totals do become a permanent part of the record because there is a space to record 24-hour totals. The reason given for discarding the daily suicide monitoring worksheets was that the need for them was transient and they would occupy considerable space if maintained as part of the permanent hospital record. However, if the worksheets had contained a comment section, arguably a summary of the comments should have been prepared.

Poor Records

The central issue in a recent Kentucky case which was appealed was whether the poor quality of the records maintained by the nurses was a substantial factor in causing the death of a woman who had sustained a head injury in an automobile accident.[24]

The trial court in *Rogers v. Kasdan* found for the plaintiff, but an intermediary appeals court overturned that verdict and found for the defendant hospital. The plaintiff appealed that decision to the state supreme court which held that although the plaintiff had presented sufficient evidence warranting the jury verdict in favor of the plaintiff, the supreme court could not reinstate a plaintiff's verdict because there was a flaw in the judge's instructions to the jury. The court ordered that a new trial be held because the plaintiff's jury instructions were too prejudicial.

The decedent was admitted to the hospital after being seen in the emergency room. She was under the care of a plastic surgeon and 7 days after admission died from untreated water intoxication brought on by excessive fluid buildup. Experts testifying on behalf of the woman's estate said that the impact sustained should have alerted the surgeon to the possibility of brain injury. In addition, he prescribed a drug (later discontinued) which masked the signs of increasing intracranial pressure. There was more than sufficient evidence that the nursing staff did not follow rules adopted by the hospital. The evidence showed that intake and output records were not accurately compiled or tallied and that the nurse's notes did not agree with the medication records. There were disparities between the physician's written orders and the progress notes, in addition to discrepancies among the various sets of records, many of which were illegible and incomplete.

The plaintiff's attorney submitted substantial evidence which, if believed by a jury, could cause them to properly find that the hospital failed to establish appropriate procedures to determine whether the nurses were maintaining adequate medical records. Such records would have helped the patient receive effective continuing care sufficient to enable a physician or other medical practitioner to assume the care of the patient. The plaintiff also alleged other acts of negligence including the failure of the nurses to comply with rules pertaining to the administration of drugs.

Summary

As the number of suits has increased, documentation of care, both medical and nursing, has taken on new importance. The record is an important source of evidence during the trial. Where the nurse documents that a certain event took place the jury will attach considerable credibility to it because it was recorded at the time of the event and not afterward when suit was filed. Of course, juries may believe a nurse's testimony in the absence of documentation, but the facts of the case and the demeanor of the nurse during her testimony will influence how much is to be believed. Omissions can be a problem.

In some instances, omissions can be evidence of neglect and the jury may be so instructed by the judge. If the patient event is very unusual the jury is likely to attach more to an omission. Also, if a chain of "serious" events occurred, a reasonable person would expect to see documentation of the events. Once it is explained to the jury that the purpose of a medical record is to communicate to all persons caring for the patient necessary information, it is difficult to explain a blatant omission. The record, after all, exists to provide a permanent record for those caring for the patient so that they can refer to it when evaluating response to care and treatment.

The problem of the lost page or the altered page may be very problematic for the defense attorney. A lost page, alone, will never win a case, but it certainly will strengthen the plaintiff's case. Where a notation is missing the nurse may be able to supply the information if the event in question was so unusual that she can remember it by "independent recollection." A jury will understand that the nurse is unlikely to forget the birth of triplets on New Years Eve. However, it is unlikely that a jury will believe the nurse when she testifies several years later that she gave a noon medication when it has not been recorded.

NURSE'S DUTY TO REPORT QUESTIONABLE CARE

In 1965 the *Darling* case established that nurses owed a duty to inform their superiors if the medical care being administered did not conform to the prevailing medical standard of care. The circumstances of the case made it clear that the courts did not expect that nurses would take the place of the primary physician. Rather, that where it was known or should have been known that the quality of medical care was lacking in fundamental principles, there was a duty to act.

In a Virginia case, *Utter v. United Hospital Center*, the court upheld a jury verdict against both the hospital and the physician.[25] It is likely because of the facts that the decision would have been upheld even if the hospital did not have the following policy which was published in the hospital nursing manual:

If a registered nurse has any reason to doubt or question the care provided to any patient or feels that appropriate consultation is needed and has not been obtained, she shall direct such question of doubt to the attending practitioner. If, after this, she still feels that the question has not been resolved, she shall call this to the attention of the department chairman. Where circumstances, in his opinion are such as to justify such action, the chairman of the department may himself request the consultation. In such cases, two consultants shall be named by the president of the medical staff. If both of said consultants are in agreement, the attending practitioner will be expected to accept their recommendations.

The plaintiff was admitted to the hospital after the defendant physician applied a cast to his arm in the emergency room. The professional breach occurred during the third day of hospitalization. The hospital record revealed in detail that the patient's condition was critical and deteriorating. Several of the nurses testified that the man's arm was black and very swollen. His temperature was very high and there was a foul-smelling drainage from the cast. At times the patient was delirious. The charge nurse called the physician and informed him that the patient could not retain his oral antibiotics. The treating physician testified that he did not recall the nurse reporting any sign of drainage or delirium. He said that knowledge of these signs would have been very important and that the nurse's failure to provide this information would be at variance from usual and normal nursing practice. No nurse acted on the policy to obtain the opinion of a consult.

On the fourth day the patient was transferred to a facility where he received hyperbaric chamber treatments for the infection. He had to have his arm amputated at the shoulder joint. The physician who treated him at the second hospital said that the patient's life was saved "by the skin of his teeth." He subsequently testified on behalf of the patient that the nurses should have realized the urgency of the situation because of the deteriorating condition.

In response to the hospital's argument that the nurses did all that their duties required, the court said that the nurses should be charged with the obligation of taking some positive action. "Nurses are specialists in hospital care who, in the final analysis, hold the well-being, in fact in some instances, the very lives of patients in their hands."

The following case illustrates that if support is given to the nursing staff when they raise legitimate questions involving care and treatment, and the situation is reviewed according to hospital bylaws the best interests of all parties is served well.

The legal issue in *Scappatura v. Baptist Hospital* was whether the surgeon had due process protection when the hospital invoked its emergency bylaws in suspending his privileges.[26]

The bylaw stated that in cases of an emergency which involve danger to the health of patients or hospital personnel, a physician's privileges may be temporarily suspended by the chief of staff. The patient incident involved elective major vascular surgery on a 68-year-old man. The patient had chronic heart and lung disease and preoperatively he had an abnormal electrocardiogram (EKG) reading. On the morning of the operation, which was a Friday, he had a fever which was associated with an upper respiratory tract infection. There was no allegation that the operation was performed in less than a satisfactory manner. However, the patient developed serious immediate postoperative complications and deteriorated quickly. The nurses who assisted the surgeon during the management of these complications said that the measures taken were "extreme, unusual, and perhaps unsafe." The patient died during the postoperative night.

The nurses promptly informed a nursing supervisor who reported the incident to the nursing director on Monday morning. The nursing department discussed the matter with the medical director for the intensive care unit. A written memorandum of the incident was sent to the medical director who consulted with the hospital administrator and the chiefs of surgery and staff. That group informed the surgeon of the complaint, reviewed the patient's chart, and interviewed the nurses. The review committee voted unanimously to suspend the surgeon pending a thorough investigation. He was later reinstated with restrictions.

The court held that the emergency suspension, done without a formal due process hearing, was in compliance with the emergency provision. The chiefs and the administrator testified that the reasons for the emergency suspension were (1) failure to have a consultation preoperatively in view of the significant surgical risk to the patient, (2) questionable judgment shown by the physician in wasting time on unnecessary procedures and in the manner in which they were carried out, and (3) the surgeon had a similar case the next day in which the same errors or judgment might be repeated. The court also held that the procedure of conferring with others was in the spirit that the legislature encouraged by enacting the Professional Standards Review Organization (PSRO) statute.

INTEGRITY OF THE MEDICAL RECORD

Many states have enacted statutes mandating the length of time hospital records must be retained. Statutes indicate the length of time hospital records must be retained and some spell out what specific parts of a record must be kept. In 1975, Massachusetts enacted a statute requiring that nurse's notes must be retained as part of the permanent hospital record.[27] Some states by regulation spell out what must be included in the hospital record.

In addition to the use of the medical record in civil suits it is frequently used in criminal cases and judicial hearings, such as child abuse cases. One problem which may surface or be a critical issue during a negligence suit is the credibility of the record itself. The plaintiff may allege that there have been alterations in the form of additions or deletions in the record. Another problem is the "lost" page or other physical evidence, such as a tissue slide or x-ray film. Loss of the entire hospital record is uncommon, but loss of office records is a problem.

Because of the importance of the medical record to both the plaintiff's and defendant's case it is worth including case law and commentary on the issue of record credibility and integrity. If an attorney has been consulted by an individual who believes that negligence was involved in the management of his case the attorney obtains the record and reviews it. When a record is reviewed for the purpose of identifying and developing a legal theory it takes on an entirely different light. The focus no longer is documentation for the purpose of care and treatment. The attorney pays particular attention to the sequence of orders, notations, and reports. Some legal commentators take the position that the recordation of incidents of care and treatment in chronological sequence is essential.[28] "Any attempt, for whatever reason, to alter the sequence will give rise to a prejudicial inference in the minds of jurors."

The experienced attorney, just as the experienced physician and nurse, has developed skill in abstracting essential information from the record. While the physician and nurse develop the ability to review a record, abstracting the salient information quickly, the attorney labors over each page and scrutinizes the record as a whole. Nurses and physicians do not look at the record as a whole. The means by which corrections are made in medical records is important. It is not uncommon for plaintiff's attorney to have a handwriting expert evaluate the record when there is a legitimate question as to the signature or recording of information. They are frequently consulted where the handwriting is changed, erased, or obliterated. Juries resent, and will penalize, any attempts to deceive or conceal the truth.[29]

Correcting the Medical Record

In 1973 the report prepared by the Secretary's Commission on Medical Malpractice acknowledged that the practice of altering medical records to cover mistakes was done and went on record to say it was an "intolerable" practice.[30] The commission recommended that legislatures enact statutes to prohibit modification, alteration, or destruction where the intent is to mislead or misinform. Arguably, the act of changing medical records is a risky procedure, but there does not appear to be law outright preventing inaccurate notes from being changed.[31] In California, the altering or modification of medical documents, if done with the specific intent to avoid liability or to misrepresent the true state of facts, is a crime. The relevant statute states: "Any person who alters or modifies the medical record of any person, with fraudulent intent, or who, with fraudulent intent, creates any false record, is guilty of a misdemeanor".[32] The statute requires an intent to defraud coupled with the alteration or creation. It is clear from the wording in the statute that mere alteration does not present a prima facie case that it was altered to deceive, misrepresent, or escape liability. Some legal commentators have written that the problem of medical alteration is sufficiently widespread and should not be overlooked in trial preparation.[33]

It is not uncommon for a nurse to make a mistake and chart information pertaining to one patient in the record of another patient. Nor is it uncommon for a physician to write notes on one patient's progress sheet that pertain to a different patient. Most frequently the error is picked up by the recorder near to the time of the writing. There should exist a standard procedure in the facility as to the method of correcting such mistakes. Perhaps the best procedure is to write an addendum referencing back to the original error. This should be done, even where there are several days separating the notations. All legal commentators agree that the practice of erasing, obliterating, or defacing to correct a mistake creates too great an impression that it was changed for a dishonest reason. Plaintiff's attorney will argue that such alteration demonstrates the defendant's consciousness of wrong-doing. Thus, the attorney will seek a jury instruction that the spoliation of the record demonstrates a "consciousness of guilt." At the least an alteration will give rise to an inference of guilt.

The system of recording patient notes varies somewhat with the individual hospital. A hospital should have a formal policy informing the nursing staff as to the minimum number of times a nurse must write notes during a single working shift unless it is accepted that the custom requires charting at the end of the shift. Of course, unusual events, such as a severe drug reaction, new and unexpected symptoms, or an adverse response to care or treatment should be charted close to the event itself. Nurses in critical areas, such as the postanesthesia room or ICU, must chart frequently throughout the shift or in the instance of the postanesthesia room, while the patient is monitored in the unit. Frequent charting should always be the rule when a patient is critical in case the record needs to be reviewed to manage a crisis.

Nurses who customarily chart at the end of the day refer to "pocket notes" or hospital worksheets to refresh their memory as to the events and findings that require formal recording. While writing their daily nurses' notes they frequently refer back to previous notes to aid them in deciding what and how much needs to be written. For example, a nurse will read previous notes to see if the amount of wound drainage is greater or less than the amount she found on the instant recording day. Thus, the nurse may record, "drainage from leg wound increased." Or the nurse may read back and record, "Patient no longer complains of pain radiating to back." By referencing back the nurse knows what needs to be highlighted and can then include the subtle changes on which nurses rely to provide subsequent care.

Occasionally a nurse will forget to document a finding (although it may have been reported) but will remember the item after leaving work. A good rule of thumb is that if the information is important and would be valuable in assisting other health care providers in caring for the patient in the shifts immediately following, the nurse should contact the nursing head of the unit and request that an addendum be added which indicates the time and event. When the amending recorder is different from the original recorder a brief explanation should be added to the record stating why the notes were updated rather than waiting until the original recorder could amend the notes in person. The original recorder should affirm the addition or correction on returning to the hospital and should date and sign it.

A cardinal rule to be applied in correcting or amending the record is that a single line should be drawn through the incorrect portion of the record—it should not be obliterated.[34] The original notation should still be legible and should remain a part of the permanent record. The amended correction should be dated and provide some explanation for the change. This is so whether the correction is because the recorder made a note in the incorrect chart or wrote a note incorrectly. Nurses should be discouraged from writing between the lines or along the margins of a record. Such a practice will always raise a credibility question in the minds of the jurors and will surely be pointed out by plaintiff's attorney.

In a recent legal article on the validity of medical records, the authors cited the following examples of problems with physician notes.[35] In one case it was found that 12 years of medical records relating to the care, treatment, and surgery of a patient had been destroyed. The woman's physician claimed not to have seen them since shortly after suit was begun. In another case involving a birth injury, it was found that the medical records introduced at trial differed from those obtained by the hospital's insurance carrier just prior to the infant's discharge. In a third case, fabrication of visual field charts was established when it was shown that the defendant ophthalmologist had provided records to a defense expert witness which did not contain the studies. The records were sent to prepare the expert to testify in the defendant's behalf. In the final case the defendant physician admitted during pretrial discovery that a note written by one of the nurses, suggesting that certain diagnostic studies had been recommended but refused by the patient, was written at his direction. It was found that the note was written 1½ months after the patient died.

Inference of Lost and Altered Records

In the leading case dealing with the inference which a jury may give to lost medical records the court held that the unavailability of the records created a strong inference of "consciousness of guilt" of negligence on the physician's part.[36] Further, the inability of the defendant to produce his original clinical records, unless explained, was evidence which the jury could weigh in their deliberations.

The physician in *Thor v. Boska* had informed the plaintiff that her breast lump was benign and no biopsy was necessary. When she consulted another physician the lump was found to be malignant with extension to axillary glands. During the pretrial discovery the physician submitted "recopied" office records, but explained that the original records could not be located and he assumed that they were thrown away. He said that the recopied records were taken verbatim from the original records. He said he recopied them when he learned that the woman was going to see another physician and he thought the physician would want to review his records, thus the recopying was for the purpose of making them more legible.

Citing *Wigmore on Evidence*, the court said that a party's suppression of evidence by spoliation is reviewable against him as an indication of his "consciousness that his case is a weak or unfounded one; and from that consciousness may be inferred the fact itself of the cause's lack of truth and merit."[37]

In a recent case, *Pisel v. Stamford Hospital*, the court held the judge properly charged the jury that they could consider the substitution of one set of records for another as a circumstance indicating the defendant's consciousness of negligence.[38] The plaintiff, a young woman, suffered severe and irreversible brain damage when her head became wedged between a bed rail and the bed frame. The evidence showed that she had been improperly monitored. Evidence was introduced during the trial that a few days following the injury the nursing director ordered the entire staff who charted the patient's care to rewrite and change the hospital records relevant to the care received the morning of the injury. The revised record contained false information and conflicted with other records and the testimony of nursing staff who were on duty at the time of the incident.

The revised records came to light after the suit was begun when a nurse informed hospital administration that she had been forced to rewrite a note on the original record. The change was done without the knowledge of the hospital administration and in violation of formal hospital policy. The defense attorneys unsuccessfully argued that, although "poor judgment" was employed in ordering the revisions, the motive was "merely one of ordering expanded notes." The court stated that an "allowable inference from the bungled attempt to cover up the staff inadequacies on the morning of January 24 was that the revision indicated a consciousness of negligence."

A spokesman for the hospital's insurance company said that the altered chart created a defense problem. "If nurses would only add to, not alter, charts when after-the-fact circumstances indicate that the charting was incomplete, we could defend them much better."[39] The jury award of $3,600,000 was upheld.

Summary

The incidence of recording errors is greater in nursing notes than physician notes because of the volume of charting that nurses do and because nurses are exposed to the patient care situation for longer periods of time. For this reason the nursing department should have a formal policy on the procedure for correcting records. There is no justification for erasure, "whiting-out," or covering the incorrect information with tape. These techniques will give a jury the impression that there was a need to hide the deleted information. This will place a substantial burden on the defense in trying to overcome the impression.

INCIDENT REPORTS

Several important points are involved in any discussion of incident reports. Such reports have gained greater prominence since risk management has become an integral part of hospital business.

The concept of risk management had been recognized by industry for at least 25 years before it was adopted by the health care system in the early 1970s. However, the "idea" of risk management has been recognized in hospitals for many years. Incident reports were used by hospitals long before the concept of risk management found its way into them. The American Hospital Association's definition of *risk management* is "the science for the identification, evaluation and treatment of the risk of financial loss."[40] The objective of a risk management program is to reduce preventable injuries and minimize the financial severity of claims. Some states have specifically enacted laws governing hospital internal risk management.[41] Risk management is only one part of a hospital's loss control program.

No risk management department can function effectively without a systematic reporting mechanism. It is essential that the definition of what constitutes an "incident" or "accident" be included in any policy statement relevant to the function of incident reports. The term "incident" is more appropriate than "accident" because it is broader in scope. In the past, few facilities bothered to define the term "incident" and as a result problems arose with respect to when such a report should be completed and by whom. The incident report should not exist just for nursing care situations.

An incident by definition covers a broader territory than an accident. The American Hospital Association has defined an *incident* as: "any happening which is not consistent with the routine operation of the hospital or the routine care of a particular patient. It may be an accident or a situation which might result in an accident."[42] The definition includes incidents involving patients, employees, or visitors although different hospital forms may be used for different groups.

Perhaps the aspect about which nurses have been most concerned with respect to incident reports is whether they will be used in litigation, either before or during a trial. The two legal rules applicable to the use of the incident report as evidence are (1) statutes dealing with *business records*, and (2) the principle of *privilege*, specifically the attorney–client privilege. In order to understand the business records exception it is necessary to understand some principles relevant to hospital medical records.

Hospital Medical Records in General

In a medical malpractice suit the patient's medical records are important because they frequently are informative and a relevant source of evidence. In some instances they may be crucial in that they form the sole basis for the plaintiff's case.[43] In common law the medical records were admissible evidence in most states. However, the procedure for admission was time-consuming and costly in that the person who wrote the specific notation was required to testify in court as to the specific note written by him. The common law approach necessitated calling numerous hospital personnel and physicians as witnesses. This procedure was followed to assure that the evidence admissible at trial was the "best" and most reliable evidence.

However, when evidence is "secondary," that is, when it is obtained from other than the one testifying or from a source, such as a medical record, it is regarded as hearsay. Even where the person is testifying about an out-of-court statement made by him, the rules of evidence regard it as hearsay evidence. The problem with hearsay evidence is its potential for being unreliable. When an attorney seeks to have an out-of-court statement, verbal or written, introduced into evidence to prove the *truth of the statement* itself, it is classified as hearsay and the attorney must identify an exception to the hearsay rule in order to have it admitted. There are of course, situations when a statement is being introduced into evidence for other than the truth of the statement. For example, an attorney may want a record admitted to show that a particular physician never treated the patient. There, the court is not dealing with the truth of the matter contained in the record and the hearsay rule does not apply.

Because of the problems associated with the requirement that the actual recorder give direct testimony, it was only a matter of time before state statutes permitted "secondary" evidence. The law carved out exceptions to hearsay evidence. One of the hearsay rule exceptions was the *business records exception*.[44] The general business records exception statutes were drafted to permit the introduction of such records, even though hearsay, because they were prepared as part of business endeavors and there was a mantle of trustworthiness associated with their preparation. The statutes refer to records "made in the ordinary course of business."

In addition to the business records exception, some states have a specific statute governing the admissibility of hospital records.[45] In states that do not have a specific statute permitting the admission of medical records, the business record statute covers their admission. Thus, the two ways of having the medical records admitted into evidence in part or as a whole, are the business records exception or a specific medical records exception. There is extensive case law dealing with hearsay exceptions.

Ordinarily the statements contained in the medical record must be from the personal knowledge of the recorder or from a compilation of personal knowledge of those who have the responsibility to transmit such medical information to the actual recorder. Thus, a nurses' aide may verbally report observations to a nurse who then records the information. However, the record should indicate that the notes were written by the nurse on behalf of the aide. In practical terms, when a medical record, or a portion thereof, is admitted into evidence, the hospital medical librarian goes to court and testifies as to the methods of preparation, and maintenance of such records. Another procedure is to have the librarian certify the records.

The Report

There are a number of concerns associated with the incident report. Most of these can be addressed in institutional guidelines. All hospital employees and physicians should be familiar with the guidelines so that each particular health care provider knows when an incident report should be completed. The hospital policy should set out the guidelines for the completion of an incident report and should include purpose, definition of an incident, situations that mandate the completion of a report, identification of the individual responsible for completing the record, processing or routing system, and general procedure for corrective action, if appropriate.

In addition to identification of the types of situations in which a report must be completed, the guidelines should contain a statement that encourages the reporting of other situations that may arise. When in doubt, a good rule of thumb is to complete a report. Another rule of thumb is that all incident reports should be completed and forwarded to the delineated individual or department within 24 hours of the incident or when the health care provider is put on notice of the incident. The specific type of incident will determine the routing process.

It may be prudent to channel all reports to the risk manager, if the facility has one, for immediate review. This would put the onus on one individual to further process the report to the appropriate department or individual and would assure timely follow-up of the incident. The number of copies of the report should be kept at a minimum to assure a willingness on the part of physicians, nurses, and other personnel to complete them. If the reports are made too readily assessible to a large number of people there is a natural tendency to "hold back" or outright disregard a policy. The practice of leaving the report at the nurse's station for a number of days or filing it under the charge nurse's desk blotter should be discouraged. The report should be completed quickly by those individuals who have a responsibility to make insertions and immediately forwarded to the risk manager or other designated individual.

In recent years the health care industry has attempted to develop a patient injury model of risk management similar in concept to the safety model of risk management of the business world. An effective hospital risk management program should detect and identify instances of patient injury that have already occurred, as well as set in motion a mechanism that identifies actual problems or potential risk circumstances. The incident report is one of the chief means of identifying patient injuries that have already occurred.

One of the major weaknesses of the use of the incident report to detect problem areas or identify potential risk situations is the mind-set that such reports only apply to nursing situations and, therefore, should only be completed by nurses. Prior to the risk management concept it was uncommon to find reports made out by other than nurses or those providing ancillary patient care assistance. Medically related incidents and situations involving other medical personnel have been traditionally excluded from the incident reporting system.[46] In order for the incident report mechanism to serve as a basis for identifying risky practice habits or situations that may lead to litigation, it must be used by all relevant hospital groups. It is essential that the incident report not be punitive. This point should be identified in the guidelines and the corrective action taken must be dissociated with a punitive attitude. This does not mean that a physician or nurse who continues to exhibit unsafe practice after corrective measures have been implemented cannot be dealt with.

The Incident Report as a Business Record

Depending on the circumstances of a case, the plaintiff or the defendant hospital may wish to have an incident report admitted into evidence at the time of trial. In addition, the plaintiff may make a demand for both the hospital policy governing the completion of incident reports and the incident report itself. It is not uncommon for plaintiff's counsel to file a pretrial motion setting out arguments as to why the document should be made available for trial preparation. If an incident report is made a part of the hospital record it will be admissible under the business record statute. For this reason, hospitals are counseled that such reports should never be made part of the medical record nor should the recorder of an incident include in the medical record the notation, "incident report completed and on file." A reference to the report in the record will incorporate the incident report into the full record. In legal terms this is known as *incorporation by reference*. However, it is noteworthy that it has been held that the mere inclusion of an incident report with other admissible records does not automatically mean that it should be admitted along with the whole medical record.[47] When asked to rule on whether or not an incident report should be admitted as part of the entire medical record, the courts will look at the surrounding circumstances. The court will consider its trustworthiness as well as the reliance placed on the report in conducting hospital business.

There is considerable case law on the issue of which records or documents are "made in the regular course of business" to justify their admission under a business record statute. Specifically dealing with incident reports, the U.S. Supreme Court in 1943 held that an accident report made out by a train engineer was not admissible as evidence at trial.[48] In that case, the nation's highest court held that the engineer's report, made out 2 days after an accident, was not made in the regular course of business because the report did not further the commercial interests of the business. The court said that the use of accident reports was for litigation and not in furthering business interests.

There has been a trend toward recognizing the appropriateness of admitting incident reports. The courts are split on exactly what constitutes the "usual business" of a hospital.

A 1955 New York case, *Williams v. Alexander*, held that documents and reports that relate to diagnosis, prognosis, or treatment come within the realm of the business of a hospital, whereas, other records, even though contained in the record do not.[49]

A federal case, *Picker X-Ray Corporation v. Frerker*, which was decided in 1969 held that hospital incident reports are part and parcel of running the hospital business.[50] That case involved the breaking of the tip of a guide wire during a radiologic catheterization. The radiologist made out one report and a supplemental report was prepared by the hospital business manager. He also distributed an interdepartmental memorandum. The radiologist's report was admitted at trial without objection. With respect to the report and document prepared by the business manager, the court, applying a Missouri business records statute, held that both documents should be admissible if made to improve treatment or hospital procedure. The case did articulate the established rule that if the sole use of the incident report was for the purpose of litigation it would be inadmissible.

The Attorney–Client Privilege Argument

The other exception to the admission of the incident report at trial is the *attorney–client privilege*. Some attorneys advise that the incident report be regarded and treated as a confidential communication, which is thereby cloaked with the *attorney–client privilege*. Such a privilege is statutory and holds that where legal advice is sought from an attorney, the communication is confidential and may not be disclosed unless waived by the client.[51]

There are two collateral issues germane to the attorney–client privilege. The first is whether an employee in preparing the incident report has sufficient authority to speak for the hospital corporation. In responding to this question, some jurisdictions hold that the corporate representative must be one who is in a decision-making capacity, that is, having authority to decide corporate policy. Presumably, in normal parlance this would exclude the staff nurse, support staff, and other allied health employees who are not regarded as part of management or administration. It is unlikely that hospitals in jurisdictions that have adopted the decision-making capacity test would rely on the attorney–client privilege to exclude incident reports from being discovered or admitted as evidence.

The more liberal test has been adopted by other jurisdictions and permits the court to take into consideration the specific facts surrounding the situation.[52] To come within the scope of the privilege, the court must find the following: the corporation has sought the advice of the attorney, the employee is one who is sufficiently identified with the corporation, and the report was completed at the direction of his superiors.

The second collateral issue germane to the attorney–client privilege, and one that raises an important legal question, is whether the privilege is lost if the report is used for purposes other than to defend a lawsuit. There is not a sufficient body of case law on this question to provide definitive direction. This is a most practical problem in view of the use of the incident report by risk management departments. Some courts have applied the "sole purpose" test, which means that the report serves the purpose of obtaining legal advice.[53] The privilege is lost where the document serves multiple uses. For example, when it is prepared for legal counsel and used to compile statistics. The more liberal test is the "dominant purpose" test which recognizes that there may be several legitimate uses for incident reports. The hospital corporation is not penalized by using the report in a particular way when it operates under a multipurpose record utilization system. If it is alleged that the multipurpose system destroys the attorney–client privilege the court, as a matter of law, would decide what the dominant purpose of the incident report is.

If a hospital decides to adopt the attorney–client privilege, and thereby exclude an incident report from discovery or admission at the time of trial, it must show that the predominant purpose of the report is to obtain legal advice. Some courts have held the privilege inapplicable unless the report has already been sent to the attorney. Generally, the courts have accepted the privilege argument if the report has been sent to the insurance carrier prior to the actual transfer of the document to the attorney. Care should be taken in the processing or routing of the report so that the confidential chain is not weakened or broken.

In responding to the fear of many hospitals that the law in their respective states will permit incident reports into evidence or will make them available during pretrial preparation, one authority suggests that they should contain only information that is or should be contained in the medical record. He cautions that the report should not contain any analysis of the cause or lay blame on any single factor. However, his position is that a complete medical record should contain objective documentation of any patient injury. Thus, he argues that an incident report that is discoverable or admitted into evidence should not make a difference.[54] His point is well taken in that a medical record without any reference to a bed fall in which an injury was sustained is highly suspect. Such an omission would not be lost on a jury. It is virtually impossible to document the care rendered after a serious incident when the details of the incident itself are vague, incomplete, or omitted.

Most attorneys are in agreement that the incident report question that asks, "How could this incident have been prevented?" is not useful and may be harmful in the event of litigation. Responses to such a question are likely to be subjective and may be written in a self-serving manner. If the report is written as factually correct as knowledge of the incident allows it will be possible to identify both risk factors and provide direction in establishing corrective measures.

In summary, each jurisdiction, either by statute, case law, or both has established what constitutes activities made in the regular course of business when the business record exception to the hearsay rule is invoked. The same is true when the attorney–client privilege is employed to shield the report from the plaintiff. When either theory is applicable, the incident report must still meet the test of trustworthiness as evidence. From the foregoing discussion, it can be seen that the frequently held belief that incident reports are inadmissible as evidence may not always be so.

Case Law

Of the following two incident report cases, one deals with the use of the report at trial as evidence and the other deals with its use in the pretrial phase.

The earliest case to raise the issue of attorney–client privilege in the context of an incident report was decided in 1968.[55]

In that case, *Barnardi v. Community Hospital Association*, the patient had suffered a footdrop, and three copies of the incident report existed. One was placed in the medical record, and the hospital administrator and the nursing director each received a copy. There was testimony at the trial that incident reports could be reviewed by legal counsel to screen for potential suits or in the face of actual suits. It was not routine policy that the attorney review all incident reports. The hospital sought to exclude the report as evidence at trial. The plaintiff sought to have the report admitted.

The court held that the report could not be excluded from evidence because it did not fit within the structure of the attorney–client privilege. There was evidence that the reports were completed during the process of seeking legal advice. Although all nurses were told to complete incident reports, there was no indication on the form that they were to be made out specifically for legal review. Also, there was no policy indicating such an exclusive use. The policy did indicate that the nurses were to complete two copies.

The court held that they were made out for "administrative" purposes and were incidentally made available to legal counsel, but only if he wished to review them. The court said that it would have applied the privilege if it was shown that the report was given to the attorney in his capacity as legal advisor for the purpose of professional advice in the face of liability.

A year before this decision, a California court, in *Sierra Vista Hospital v. Superior Court*, decided a case involving a report sent to the insurer.[56] The patient instituted a suit against a physician and the hospital, alleging that she suffered injury as a result of a dizzy spell. Shortly after the incident arose and while the woman was still a patient, the hospital administrator received information which put him on notice that the patient "would possibly file a suit." In order to obtain information to defend the hospital in the lawsuit, the administrator told the director of nursing services to gather information for use in preparing a report of the incident for the insurance company. The liability insurer supplied the hospital with printed forms on which to make a confidential report of all "incidents." Printed on top of the form were the words, "CONFIDENTIAL REPORT OF INCIDENT (NOT A PART OF MEDICAL RECORD)." These forms were in existence prior to the incident. Four days after the administrator was put on notice of the threat of suit he and the nursing director jointly prepared the report, signed it, and mailed the original and a copy to the adjuster. The administrator did not retain a copy and did not send a copy to anyone else.

During the pretrial discovery phase the administrator was asked whether any reports were prepared by him on behalf of any insurance company in the regular course of business or in preparation for litigation. He responded that such a report had been made in confidence and sent to the insurer for the purpose of preparing to defend Sierra Vista Hospital in the event of suit. He also informed the opposing lawyer that a photostatic copy was in the hands of the attorney who was defending the hospital. Subsequently the woman's attorney filed a motion which was granted, allowing inspection of the report. In subsequent litigation on the granting of the motion the court held that the communication was privileged under the attorney–client rule and was exempt from discovery. A state statute limited inspection to matters that were not privileged. The court held that the document did not lose its confidentiality status just because it went to the adjuster before reaching its final destination at the attorney's office. The court said that the attorney–client privilege must always be viewed in relationship to the particular facts of the case.

A recent case, *Kay Laboratories v. District Court*, which was decided in 1982 in Colorado, held that the court's denial of a motion to compel discovery of an incident report was improper.[57] It illustrates that the particular facts of the case are important in applying the principles of law. The facts are distinguishable from the facts in the California case. As in the California case, a state statute existed that would exempt an incident report if it came within the "work product doctrine."[58] The *work product doctrine* requires that, in order to exempt an incident report as evidence, it be submitted when the litigation process has already begun.

The patient brought suit against a hospital and the manufacturer of a chemical ice pack device. She alleged that the device leaked onto her skin causing chemical burns. A nurse completed an incident report in accordance with hospital routine. The form used was supplied by the hospital's insurance carrier and its completion was standard procedure whenever an incident occurred that could possibly result in litigation against the hospital. The procedure was that the form was to be completed in triplicate by a nurse on duty when the incident arose or was discovered. The nurse wrote the report within 6 to 8 hours of the incident which was strong evidence of the fact that the hospital had no notice of pending litigation. Although copies of the completed report were forwarded to the insurer, not all incidents reported result in suit. The insurer also did statistical analysis of the forms as part of a loss prevention plan.

When the lawyers for the manufacturer made a request of the hospital, as codefendant, to produce the report the hospital refused, saying that it was not discoverable. The manufacturer's subsequent court petition was denied when the court ruled that the document was prepared for the purpose of defending against a lawsuit and was confidential. The lawyers then appealed the decision, alleging that they were prejudiced in the preparation of their case and in fact, the document had not been prepared in anticipation of litigation. Ruling that no attorney–client relationship existed when the report was completed by the nurse, the appeals court ordered the release of the document.

In a footnote to the case, the court declined to rule on the argument that the lawyers for the manufacturer could not obtain the information contained in the report by taking a deposition of the nurse who completed the report. The attorneys for the manufacturer had sought to strengthen their argument by showing that they could not obtain equivalent information by other kinds of pretrial discovery. The court would not rule on the question because it granted their request and need not consider their argument further. However, their argument raises a good point and is one used when discovery of incident reports is requested.

A final note on the case concerns the use of the forms to analyze incidents as part of a loss prevention program. Conceivably an argument could be made that such use precludes application of the attorney–client privilege because this "secondary" use waives the privilege. Undoubtedly, use of the incident report by the risk management officer will be raised by those seeking discovery or admission at trial, who will argue that the confidential nature of the document has been violated.

These cases indicate that in some instances incident reports are available to opposing counsel in pretrial discovery or may find their way into the courtroom as evidence. For this reason, careful thought should be given before including on the form the question, "How could this incident have been prevented?" If the response is allowed into evidence it may be difficult to overcome. The information sought can be obtained by instructing nurses to complete a factual, objective report. In addition, it is customary practice to review a serious incident with those involved as soon as possible. Also, if this kind of information is helpful in identifying high-risk practices or activities, then it can be obtained at that time.

In the following case, the patient's attorney successfully argued that the trial judge's exclusion of a statement in the incident report was an error that was prejudicial to his case. The case was sent back for retrial.

In *Mercudo v. County of Milwaukee* the plaintiff was admitted after an incomplete abortion.[59] She was septic and had a temperature of 105°F. She received intravenous fluid containing penicillin and pitocin. She complained of pain when it was begun and told the nurse that the pain intensified when she later received more penicillin by bolus. Her arm began to swell and she developed a large blister which later sloughed off. Her bracelet was removed, but her arm was not restrained. She sued when she had to undergo skin grafts.

At the trial some of the contents of the accident report were admitted without objection, but the statement inquiring how the accident could have been prevented was not allowed into evidence. Her attorney wanted the response of the medical student admitted because it read as follows: "Patient (sic) arm should have been restrained so she could not thrash around while in pain." The practice in the hospital was that when an accident occurred a physician was to fill out part of the report.

The court held that the medical student's statement should have been admitted because it was made during the existence of an employee–employer relationship and the medical student was authorized to make such a statement even though it was later co-signed by a physician who was not present during the incident. The plaintiff's attorney wanted the medical student's statement entered into evidence to offset the testimony by defendant's expert that restraints were not needed. Allowance of the statement would have supported the argument that at least one medically trained person, present at the time, thought that restraints were needed and that they would have prevented the injury.

While most of the cases involving incident reports revolve around their admissibility, at least one case illustrates that the failure to complete an incident report may serve as an obstacle in defending a suit.

In *St. Paul Fire & Marine Insurance Co. v. Prothro*, a 76-year-old man recovered damages when he alleged that he developed a postoperative staphylococcal infection when the lowering device broke as he was being put into a whirlpool bath.[60] In the resulting plunge he struck his hip which had recently been pinned. The therapist covered the opened and bleeding wound with an unsterile bath towel. A nurse subsequently reported the incident, but did not fill out an incident report. The patient alleged that the nurses did not examine or treat the wound in any fashion other than applying "butterfly" tapes. When the physician inspected the wound the following day he discontinued the baths.

The issue in the case was one of causation, that is, whether the fall and lack of care were responsible for the subsequent removal of the prosthesis because of the infection. Although the patient's physician and another expert testified that they did not think the fall caused the infection there was supportive evidence indicating a connection. The patient testified that no one told him prior to the incident that he had an infection and his clinical records did not demonstrate an infection. The physician did not make any notation of the situation in the progress notes. The defendant hospital argued that the lack of a physician notation did not support the patient's allegation, since presumably if the situation was as the patient alleged some note would have been included in the record.

However, the court found that lack of notes argument was inadequate to rebut the plaintiff's testimony. The court said that the physician was dependent to some degree on records made by people in the hospital. The court went on to say that the "records were not very reliable or complete in many aspects."

If the physician or the staff had documented the situation, including appropriate follow-up care, it may have weakened the plaintiff's case. Presumably an incident report, if completed, would have included the immediate care, and in the absence of adequate medical records the hospital may have wanted it introduced into evidence to aid in the defense. It is more frequent that the defense argues to keep an incident report out of court, but there are situations where the introduction of the report may be helpful.

Contrary to a belief held by many nurses and other health care providers, incident reports may be made available, in part or in toto, to strengthen the opposing counsel's arguments. Less frequently, it may be the defense that seeks to have the report admitted. Arguably, where the medical record contains no information of an incident the plaintiff's attorney may be in a better position to argue the merits of having an incident report admitted to fill in the missing information. One authority's position is that an incident report should be admitted because it should not be at variance with content that should be included in the medical record.[61] It provides "food for thought" in dealing with the anxiety which surrounds the completion of incident reports. Suffice it to say that when either party wishes to have an incident report admitted, the respective counsel will carefully review both state law and relevant case law and set about arguing persuasively to that purpose.

Summary

If an incident report is made part of the hospital record it is likely that it will be admitted into evidence at the trial, just as the rest of the record is allowed in. When the court is asked to rule on an incident report demand, it will look to existing state statutes that particularly cover such reports. Some risk management statutes include a statement that such reports are not admissible. Two arguments are used to preclude the admission of an incident report at trial. The first is the business records exception. However, the court applies a number of "tests" to determine whether the business records exception is met. The second argument is the attorney–client privilege. This too, must pass judicial "tests."

During pretrial discovery the plaintiff's attorney will ask the nurse at her deposition if an incident report was made out. This will establish the fact that one was, in fact, made out. If one was not made out the plaintiff's attorney will elicit testimony as to the hospital policy governing such reports. The nurse will be asked in the deposition subpoena to bring all memorandums, reports, documents, and any other materials related to the incident report. However, legal counsel for the nurse will tell her not to bring them as they are business records, made in the ordinary course of business, or that such materials fit within the attorney–client privilege exception.[62]

SUMMARY

There are a significant number of nursing malpractice cases which have held that the nurse failed to verbally communicate essential patient information. Where the nurse delayed in communicating patient findings or data and the patient suffers harm because of the delay, the court may find that the nurse failed to "timely" convey the information to the physician or other health care provider. While the term, timely may be as imprecise to a nurse as "the reasonable prudent nurse" phrase, it should illustrate that the courts will find a nurse liable when certain patient observations are made without appropriate follow-up of the findings. As in all negligence cases the court will look to the surrounding facts in determining whether the timely notification occurred.

The concept of verbal communication includes information obtained from the patient or other person supplying the medical history on behalf of the patient as well as ongoing data supplied by the patient or observed by the nurse. In addition, liability may be found where the nurse was derelict in a duty to convey essential information to a transferring facility.

The medical record is always introduced as evidence at a negligence trial. Almost always, there are recordings which can both help and hurt the defendant's testimony. This is because hospital and other medical care records are not written, nor should they be, for the courtroom. However, some principles are basic, such as poor records may be viewed as evidence that improper care or inadequate care was rendered. Altered records may be viewed with suspect and missing pages may work against the defendant. Every health care facility, whether it is hospital, clinic, or physician's office should have a clear policy dealing with medical record writing protocol.

REFERENCES AND NOTES

1. Kelner, J. (Sept./Oct. 1979). Examination of hospital records. *Case and Comment, 84,* 51.
2. Garfield Park Community Hospital v. Vitacco, 327 N.E. 2nd 408 (IL, 1975).

3. Goff v. Doctor's General Hospital of San Jose, 333 P. 2nd 29 (CA, 1958).
4. Karrigan v. Nazareth Convent and Academy, 510 P. 2nd 190 (KA, 1973).
5. Kolakowski v. Voris, 395 N.E. 2nd 6 (IL, 1979).
6. Sandhofer v. Abbott-Northwestern Hospital, 283 N.W. 2nd 362 (MN, 1979).
7. Brannan v. Lankenau Hospital, 417 A. 2nd 196 (PA, 1980).
8. Hiatt v. Groce, 523 P. 2nd 320 (KA, 1974).
9. Ramsey v. Physicians Memorial Hospital, 373 A. 2nd 26 (MD, 1977).
10. Yorston v. Pennell, 397 PA. 28 (PA, 1959).
11. Pettis v. State of Louisiana, 336 S. 2nd 521 (LA, 1976); 340 S. 2nd 1108 (Dec. 1976). This case deals with indemnity cause of action against two physicians.
12. Houts, M. (Ed.). (1983). *Lawyers' guide to medical proof* (No. 15, Chapter 3000, Nurse's testimony: Proving patient's deteriorating condition). Albany, NY: Matthew Bender.
13. Krestview Nursing Home v. Synowiec, 317 S. 2nd 94 (FL, 1975).
14. Childs v. Greenville Hospital Authority, 479 S.W. 2nd 399 (TX, 1972).
15. Childs v. Weis, 440 S.W. 2nd 104 (TX, 1969).
16. Anon. (1981). *Accreditation manual for hospitals* (p. 119). Chicago: Joint Commission on Accreditation of Hospitals.
17. Collins v. Westlake Community Hospital, 312 N.E. 2nd 614 (IL, 1974).
18. Darling v. Charleston Community Memorial Hospital, 211 N.E. 2nd 253 (IL, 1965).
19. Glenn v. Kerlin, 305 S. 2nd 611 (LA, 1975).
20. Siirila v. Barrios, 248 N.W. 2nd 171 (MI, 1976).
21. Stack v. Wapner, 368 A. 2nd 292 (PA, 1976).
22. Wagner v. Kaiser Foundation Hospital, 589 P. 2nd 1106 (OR, 1979).
23. Topel v. Long Island Jewish Medical Center, 431 N.E. 2nd 293 (NY, 1981).
24. Rogers v. Kasdan, 612 S.W. 2nd 133 (KY, 1981).
25. Utter v. United Hospital Center, 236 S.E. 2nd 213 (VA, 1977).
26. Scappatura v. Baptist Hospital, 584 P. 2nd 1195 (AZ, 1978).
27. Massachusetts General Laws. Chapter 111, §70 (Acts of 1975).
28. Waltz, J. & Inbau, F. (1971). *Medical jurisprudence* (p. 140). New York: Macmillan.
29. Kelner, J. (Sept./Oct. 1979). Examination of hospital records. *Case and Comment, 84,* 51.
30. Anon. (1973). *Report of the Secretary's Commission on Medical Malpractice,* DHEW Publication no. 05-73-88, Washington, DC: U.S. Government Printing Office.
31. Babin, S. (1978). Changing notes in medical records: A proposal. *Medicolegal News, 6*(1), 4.
32. Deering's Annotated California (Penal) Code §471.5 (amended 1979).
33. Gage, S. (1981). Alteration, falsification and fabrication of records in medical malpractice actions. *Medical Trial Technique Quarterly, 27,* 476.
34. Kaunitz, K. (1981). Point of law: Medical records. *Hospital Medical Staff, 10*(6), 20.
35. Shore, S., & Coviello, R. (1979). Medico-legal documents: Admissibility and validity. *Western State University Law Review, 7*(1), 25.
36. Thor v. Boska, 113, *California Reporter,* 296 (CA, 1974).
37. Anon. (1940). 2 Wigmore. In *Evidence* (3rd ed.) (§278, p. 120). Boston: Little, Brown.
38. Pisel v. Stamford Hospital, 430 A. 2nd 1 (CT, 1980).
39. Anon. (1979). Psychiatric malpractice. *Massachusetts Nurse* (a publication of the Massachusetts Nurses Association), *48*(2), 3. Reprinted from *Nursing News* (a publication of the Connecticut Nurses Association). Anon. (1978). Psychiatric malpractice, *Nursing News, 52*(4), 1. Vose, D. (1978). Editoral. *Nursing News, 52*(4), 3.
40. Dankmyer, R., & Groves, J. (May 16, 1977). Taking steps for safety's sake. *Hospitals, Journal of the American Hospital Association, 51,* 60.
41. See, for example, Florida Statutes Annotated, §768.41 (1982).
42. Zadzilko, R. (1975). Hospital accident reports: Admissibility and privilege. *Dickinson Law Review, 79*(3), 494, footnote 4.
43. Shore, S., & Coviello, R. Medico-legal documents: Admissibility and validity. *Western State University Law Review, 7*(1), 25–37. 1979.

44. See, for example, Deering's Annotated California Evidence Code, §1270–1272 (1966).
45. Massachusetts General Laws, Chap. 233, §79.
46. Orlikoff, J., Fifer, W., & Greeley, H. (1981). *Malpractice prevention and liability control for hospitals (Parameters of the Incident Report)* (p. 36). Chicago: American Hospital Association.
47. People v. Roth, 226 N.Y.S. 2nd 421 (NY, 1962).
48. Palmer v. Hoffman, 318 U.S. 109 (1943); affirming, Hoffman v. Palmer, 129 F. 2nd 976 (1942).
49. Williams v. Alexander, 129 N.E. 2nd 417 (NY, 1955).
50. Picker X-Ray Corporation v. Frerker, 405 F. 2nd 916 (1969).
51. Zadzilko, R. (1975). Hospital accident reports: Admissibility and privilege. *Dickinson Law Review, 79*(3), 513.
52. Harper & Row Publisher, Inc. v. Decker, 423 F. 2nd 487; affirmed at 400, U.S. 955 (1970).
53. Zadzilko, R. (1975). Hospital accident reports: Admissibility and privilege. *Dickinson Law Review, 79*(3), 518.
54. Orlikoff, J., Fifer, W., & Greeley, H. (1981). *Malpractice prevention and liability control for hospitals* (p. 37). Chicago: American Hospital Association.
55. Barnardi v. Community Hospital Association, 443 P. 2nd 708 (CO, 1968).
56. Sierra Vista Hospital v. Superior Court, 56 *California Reporter, 387* (CA, 1967).
57. Kay Laboratories, Inc. v. District Court, 653 P. 2nd 721 (CO, 1982).
58. Colorado Statutes, Rules of Civil Procedure 26.
59. Mercurdo v. County of Milwaukee, 264 N.W. 2nd 258 (WI, 1978).
60. St. Paul Fire & Marine Insurance Co. v. Prothro, 590 S.W. 2nd 35 (AR, 1979).
61. Orlikoff, J., Fifer, W., and Greeley, H. (1981). Malpractice prevention and liability control for hospitals (Parameters of the Incident Report) (p. 38). Chicago: American Hospital Association.
62. Cushing, M. (Aug. 1985). Incident reports: For your eyes only? *American Journal of Nursing, 85*(8), 873.

7

CARE AND TREATMENT OF THE MENTALLY ILL

During the 1970s the courts decided a significant number of cases that dealt with mental illness. The issues covered a wide range, beginning with whether there was a "right to treatment." Two cases, one reaching the U.S. Supreme Court, decided this issue: *O'Connor v. Donaldson* and *Wyatt v. Stickney*. The courts were also called on to review and interpret state and federal laws, as well as constitutional guarantees. The courts scrutinized state commitment statutes, particularly the sections dealing with involuntary commitment. The leading cases established the rights of both minors and adults: *Addington v. Texas* and *Parham v. J. R.*

In 1976 the legal theory of a therapist's duty to warn third parties of potential danger emerged in the *Tarasoff* case. Since that time there have been a number of cases embracing that theory of recovery for damages. The most litigated concept, the right to refuse treatment, was debated in the courts for many years. Many of these cases were in litigation for 10 years.

The legal issues in these cases have been complex and a number of them worked their way to the U.S. Supreme Court. Most recently the courts have reviewed issues generated by the concept of deinstitutionalization. It remains to be seen to what extent mental health litigation will further promote change within the mental health system. Many of the cases were brought by institutionalized patients to initiate change in the system. The scrutiny by the courts has brought changes in the mental health care delivery system and has expanded the notion of accountability toward the mentally ill.

THE RIGHT TO TREATMENT ISSUE

The concept of a "right to treatment" in the context of mental illness first surfaced in the medical literature in 1960.[1] Since that time the issue of a right to treatment and humane institutional living conditions has been raised in several cases.

In 1975, the U.S. Supreme Court heard *O'Connor v. Donaldson*, in which one of the questions raised was whether an *involuntarily* committed psychiatric patient has a constitutionally guaranteed right to treatment or release. However, the court did not resolve the issue of a treatment right, but rather decided the case on other grounds.[2] Thus, although the U.S. Supreme Court has handed down rulings on specific treatment issues, it has not to date held that there is a constitutional basis for guaranteeing a right to treatment of mental illness.

Kenneth Donaldson was committed by his father to a Florida state psychiatric facility in 1957, at age 48. He was diagnosed as suffering from "paranoid schizophrenia" and at a subsequent judicial hearing was found to be mentally incompetent. At the time of his commitment Florida law allowed commitment for "care, maintenance, and treatment" purposes. During the 15 years of his commitment he refused drugs and electroshock treatment because he was a Christian Scientist. No other forms of treatment were offered to him. Throughout his confinement he unsuccessfully demanded his release.

Prior to his commitment, the patient had earned his own livelihood and it was acknowledged by the defendants in the case that he could have earned his living outside the hospital. In fact, on his eventual release he secured a responsible job in hotel administration. During his frequent and repeated attempts to gain his release from the institution, persons speaking in his behalf offered to provide him with care on release. One of the defendants told him that only his parents could bring about his release, although no such policy existed.

In the legal proceedings, brought to obtain his release, Donaldson claimed that his right of liberty, which was constitutionally protected, had been violated. The Fourteenth Amendment of the U.S. Constitution is referred to as the "due process clause" because it holds that a state may not deprive an individual of "life, liberty, or property, without due process of

law." Donaldson's confinement affected his right to liberty. He also claimed that the state hospital was not providing treatment for his supposed
mental illness. His suit did not challenge the initial commitment, but did
seek redress for the conduct of officials and psychiatrists in keeping him
confined. The court in this case and subsequent cases has not awarded
money damages, largely based on the fact that the defendants acted in good
faith.

A lower federal court in 1974 supported the "right to treatment" concept
in the *Donaldson* case and held that "a person who is involuntarily civilly
committed to a mental hospital does have a constitutional right to receive
such treatment as will give him a realistic opportunity to be cured."[3] However, the precedent-setting "right to treatment" ruling was not affirmed by
the U.S. Supreme Court in its decision in 1975. The Supreme Court did
allude to the treatment concept when it stated: "In short a State cannot
constitutionally confine *without more* a nondangerous individual who is
capable of surviving safely in freedom by himself or with the help of willing
or responsible family members or friends." The court failed to specifically
identify what it meant by the inclusion of the phrase, "without more,"
other than to say that the confinement could not be an "indefinite simple
custodial confinement." Thus, the court addressed the loss of liberty issue,
but did not, except very minimally, address the right to treatment question. "Where 'treatment' is the sole asserted ground for depriving a person
of liberty, it is plainly unacceptable to suggest that courts are powerless to
determine whether the asserted ground is present."[4] When the reason for
the commitment is to treat, a failure to treat will raise unmistakable and
serious constitutional problems.

Although the U.S. Supreme Court did not establish a right to treatment, it let stand a lower federal court ruling which held that such a
right to treatment exists. A number of federal courts have adopted the
right to treatment doctrine. The right to treatment concept, although
not as easily secured as other rights, such as a right to be free from
bodily restraint, poses, nonetheless, an issue of liberty. A legally
enforceable right such as a right to be free from bodily restraint, presents a purely legal issue. The liberty interest inherent in a right to
treatment is a less tangible interest.

The earliest case that raised the right to treatment was *Wyatt v. Stickney*,
which held that mentally ill patients "have a constitutional right to receive
such individual treatment as will give each of them a reasonable opportunity to be cured or to improve his or her mental condition".[5] The case
involved mentally ill patients confined in Alabama state-run institutions.
The plaintiffs, who were confined in three different state facilities, subsequently initiated another suit when a cut in the state cigarette tax forced
the state to fire 99 professional and paraprofessional employees. That complaint alleged that the patients would not receive adequate treatment as a
result of the employee discharges. The federal appeals court held that there
were three "fundamental conditions for adequate and effective treatment":
a "humane physical and psychological environment," qualified staff "in

numbers sufficient to administer adequate treatment," and individualized treatment plans.[6] The defendants, via a consent decree (agreement between all parties), submitted plans to correct the three deficient areas. Such plans had to be reviewed and accepted by the court in order to satisfy the agreement.

As a result of an investigation of the conditions at one of the state facilities, the court noted that it fell far short of meeting the fundamental condition of adequate and effective treatment. In a fact-finding investigation of environmental conditions, the court investigators found that one of the state facilities contained 5000 patients, one half of whom were not mentally ill but rather mentally retarded patients and geriatric patients. The facility lacked basic privacy accommodations. A number of severe health and safety problems existed, including a finding that patients had open wounds and untreated skin diseases and there was insect infestation in the kitchen and dining areas. Less than 50 cents per day per patient was spent on food, and malnutrition was a problem. The state facility for the retarded was 60 percent overcrowded. A large percentage of the patients should never have been committed and many could be discharged immediately. The court found that the seclusion and restraining policies were poor and the patients suffered at the hands of staff and fellow patients. There was testimony that several patients had died due to understaffing, lack of supervision, and brutality.[7]

The federal appeals court also held that the right to treatment must necessarily presuppose a trained and qualified staff. The court accepted a staffing plan which better met the patient's needs. Before court intervention, staffing at the facility for the retarded was one master's-prepared psychologist for every 1200 patients, a social worker for every 730 patients, and one physician for every 550 patients. At the larger facility, which housed 5000 patients, there was one physician with psychiatric training for all the patients and one social worker for every 2500 patients.

Evidence presented at the various level legal preceedings established that individualized treatment programs were nonexistent. The patient records were inadequate and incomprehensible to those staff members having prime responsibility for patient care. In addition, the records were inaccessible to the staff.

A recent federal court decision *Flakes v. Percey* held that the "Constitution guarantees to an involuntarily confined person only level of treatment minimally adequate to furnish that person reasonable opportunity to be cured or to improve his or her mental condition."[8] In essence, the court was saying that a treatment right guarantee is supported by the Constitution, albeit a minimal right. Undoubtably, the economic factor plays a significant part in designating the right as minimal, and concern about the economic impact of legal decisions will continue to be a factor.

Care and Treatment Rights of the Mentally Retarded

In 1975, Congress passed the Developmentally Disabled Assistance and Bill of Rights Act which was enacted to address some of the critical needs of the mentally retarded.[9] In May 1974, a suit was filed against Pennhurst State School in Pennsylvania on behalf of the retarded individuals who were institutionalized in the facility. Similar legal proceedings were instituted against Partlow State School in Alabama and Willowbrook State School in New York.[10] These facilities were ordered closed or ordered to eliminate existing conditions and institute reforms. The plaintiffs in Pennhurst alleged that in failing to provide the residents with minimally adequate habilitation in the least restrictive environment, the defendants violated the rights of these persons under the Fourteenth Amendment of the U.S. Constitution and state law. The complex litigation spanned over an 11-year period and was argued before the U.S. Supreme Court in 1981 and 1984 before a consent agreement was approved by the federal appeals court in 1985.[11]

The consent in the *Halderman v. Pennhurst State School* agreement was comparable to a settlement agreement and was in lieu of further litigation. Although at its conclusion there were more than 25 legal opinions published by federal courts, none of the constitutional issues or federal and state laws on which plaintiffs based the suit were decided by the U.S. Supreme Court.[12]

The impetus for the suit was to close large institutions where retarded persons were kept and to create smaller residential facilities in community settings with programs to improve "habilitative" skills. Habilitative skills referred to the education, training, and care which enables retarded persons to reach their maximum potential. One of the Pennhurst residents was Terri Lee Halderman who was brought to the facility at the age of 12 in 1966. There was testimony that while at the facility the child stopped speaking and suffered injuries. Pennhurst was founded in 1908 and is operated by the state and at the time of the initial litigation the facility was residence for approximately 1230 retarded individuals. The defendants admitted that even with improvements made in the early 1960s the facility failed to meet the professionally accepted minimum standards for the habilitation of the residents. At the time suit was brought all the parties agreed that the facility was inappropriate and inadequate for the habilitation of the mentally retarded and such individuals should be educated, trained, and cared for in community living arrangements. However, the defendants argued that this should not be accomplished by court intervention, but rather the closing and changes should be at a pace established by the state authorities.

Among its findings the court found that many of the residents had a regression of basic living skills because of the quality of the confinement. Also, the facility had no plans for improving available programs to train the residents. In addition, it found many instances of "dehumanizing practices," such as the use of physical and chemical restraints, to control the residents. Residents also suffered abuse from self-abuse, from other residents, and, in some instances, from staff.

Two lower federal courts held that the mentally retarded at the facility had a constitutional right to treatment in the "least restrictive environment." The federal trial court held that this right was based on a constitutional right to treatment. That decision was appealed by the defendants, and the higher federal appeals court, while upholding the lower court decision, said the right was grounded in the Developmentally Disabled Act. Based upon these two federal court decisions certain reforms were instituted. These included a court order to design and implement habilitation plans and transfer of residents who were able to function in a community residence. However, when the U.S. Supreme Court heard the case in 1981, it reversed the lower federal court's decision.[13] It held that the Developmentally Disabled Assistance and Bill of Rights Act did not create any substantive or legally recognized rights for retarded individuals to live in less restrictive environments. The U.S. Supreme Court held that even though Congress used the language, in the "least restrictive setting" in the 1975 Act it did not intend that such language impose an obligation on the states that they create such settings in order to be eligible for the receipt of federal funds under the act. The court said that "Congress intended to encourage, rather than mandate, the provision of better services to the developmentally disabled" because there was no clear language in the Act that the states comply with the least restrictive setting possible and Congress failed to allocate sufficient funds to renovate state hospital systems for the developmentally disabled. The later economic argument is commonly used to aid the court in interpreting legislative intent when courts are asked to interpret a law. The U.S. Supreme Court sent the case back to the lower federal court to address the claims made by the plaintiffs that a right to care in the least restrictive setting was based upon the federal constitution, or a state statute dealing with the mentally retarded and the mentally ill, or section 504 of the Rehabilitation Act of 1973. (See Chapter 12 on education law for a discussion of this congressional act.) The federal court pursuant to the Supreme Court's remand held that the state's law dealing with mental health and mental retardation granted the right to adequate habilitation in the least restrictive environment. However, the U.S. Supreme Court in 1984 rejected that decision and again remanded the case back to the lower federal court to decide the remaining federal statutory (section 504) and constitutional (Fourteenth Amendment) issues.[14] While the case was waiting to be heard for the third time before the federal Court of Appeals the plaintiffs and defendants arrived at a negotiated settlement. That in effect, stopped all future appeals of the case. In approving the agreement, the federal court held that under the equal protection clause of the Fourteenth Amendment mentally retarded individuals have a "constitutional right to receive as much education and training as is provided by the government to those whom society considers as 'not retarded'."

Under the terms of the settlement agreement the state would provide community living arrangements to residents who are capable of living in such an environment. Their capability would be determined by professionals. In addition, individual written habilitation plans would be developed and implemented in accordance with professional standards. The plans would be discussed with the resident's family or guardian and an annual review of the problem would be conducted. As part of the agreement the defendants agreed to the following: (1) protection from harm; (2) safe conditions; (3) adequate shelter and clothing; (4) medical, health-related, and dental care; (5) protection from physical and psychological abuse, neglect, or mistreatment; (6) protection from unreasonable restraint and the use of seclusion; and (7) protection from the administration of excessive or unnecessary medication.

In sum, the Pennhurst case was resolved by negotiated settlement agreement without the U.S. Supreme Court ruling on the constitutional, federal, and state law issues. However, the federal court in its 1985 decision held that the Fourteenth Amendment provided equal protection. That is, the residents were to be given the same education and training opportunities as provided nonretarded individuals. While the settlement agreement applied only to the residents who brought the suit (Pennhurst residents and those on a waiting list at the time the suit was brought), the court noted that empirical studies done while the case was in litigation demonstrated that the institutionalization of the mentally retarded could not provide minimally adequate habilitation.[15] The federal court set out a date (July 1989) at which time its supervision of the agreement would cease.

CIVIL COMMITMENT

The two most important legal aspects of civil commitment are the criteria for involuntary hospitalization and the standard of proof which must be shown before an individual can be deprived of his liberty. An individual who voluntarily admits himself to a hospital is to be contrasted with the individual who is committed against his wishes as the latter is an involuntary admission or commitment. The legal concept of *standard of proof* refers to the sufficiency of the evidence that supports the involuntary commitment.

Within recent memory the procedure for involuntary commitment failed to provide any of the safeguards which are now regarded as a fundamental right. The law regarding commitment and emergency detention of mentally ill persons varies from state to state. Each state has specific statutes and most have case law which establishes procedures for commitment proceedings.

When an individual is involuntarily committed for treatment of a mental illness the law regards such confinement as a liberty loss and a due process hearing is constitutionally mandated. In 1979 the U.S. Supreme Court handed down decisions in two separate commitment cases. *Addington*[27] established the standard of proof that had to be met before an individual could be involuntarily committed and *Parham*[31] set out the necessary procedure when the individual is a minor. (See more extensive discussion of these cases in following sections.)

The Nature of Voluntary and Involuntary Commitment Statutes

All states have involuntary commitment statutes and most have "voluntary" commitment statutes. The extent of the liberty deprivation is measured by whether the mentally ill person has been voluntarily or involuntarily committed. Involuntary commitment statutes allow the state to commit a mentally ill person to a psychiatric facility without consent from either the committed individual, his family, or a guardian. Involuntary commitment is permitted only if the mentally ill person is dangerous to self or others, or is incapable of surviving outside an institutional setting. The commitment is for an indefinite period, although there are procedural safeguards which prevent commitment for years without review and evaluation of the mentally ill person's status. If the criteria for involuntary commitment are no longer present when the review or evaluation process occurs the individual must be offered his release. An involuntary commitment raises significant constitutional liberty issues.

Voluntary commitment means that a competent adult consents to the commitment. A person who voluntarily commits himself may leave the psychiatric facility at will. Where the voluntary patient elects to leave the facility at will, most states have a statutory provision which allows the facility to detain the person for further diagnosis if there is reason to believe that the individual meets the criterion of being dangerous to himself or others. The purpose of such a statutory provision is to "convert" the voluntary commitment into an involuntary commitment in the presence of certain factors. Constitutional due process rights attach when the commitment has changed from a voluntary one to an involuntary one.[16] Due process requires a judicial hearing on the proposed commitment.

Criteria for Involuntary Hospitalization

A decade ago the criteria for commitment, as spelled out in the majority of state statutes, permitted commitment when mental illness impaired the person's ability to make a rational decision about the need for hospitalization and treatment. Prior to 1970, Massachusetts commitment law authorized involuntary confinement when there was a finding that a person was ill and that confinement was in his "best interest." As a result of *O'Connor v. Donaldson* the "best interest" test was abolished. State statutes currently frame involuntary commitment around the concept of harm or danger to self or others.

The requirement that the danger be "imminent" was created in 1975 when it was held that the "proper standard is that which requires a finding of imminent and substantial danger as evidenced by a recent overt act, attempt or threat."[17] However, the concept of dangerousness applies to an individual, but does not apply to property. A federal court in *Suzuki v. Yuen* struck down a provision in a Hawaii statute which allowed a person to be committed to a psychiatric facility against his wishes and in the absence of an emergency where the only danger was to property.[18] The statute permitted commitment of a mentally ill person who was "dangerous to property." In declaring the provision unconstitutional the court said that the statute did not strike a proper balance between protection of society from those who might harm others and preservation of the rights of the mentally ill who pose no danger to others.

The court held that while a curtailment of liberty is justified if a person is potentially harmful to himself or others, it cannot be justified when the only danger is to property. The unconstitutional provision defined "dangerous to property" as "inflicting, attempting or threatening imminently to inflict damage to *any* property in a manner which constitutes a crime, as evidenced by a recent act, attempt or threat." While the court held that such a defined harm was too broad, it did not rule out that a danger to property provision may be worked in a manner which may comply with constitutional guidelines. The court suggested that harm to property of value or significance may not be held unconstitutional.

Emergency Commitment Provisions

In addition to a general involuntary commitment admission, an individual may be involuntarily hospitalized by application of an emergency commitment or detention provision in the statute. The essential difference between an emergency detainment provision and a general involuntary commitment provision is that the emergency provision includes a time limit. A mentally ill person cannot be detained beyond the specified time limit.

The court *In the matter of Tedesco* held that a 14-day detention in a state hospital without a probable cause hearing was unreasonable and violated the patient's due process rights.[19] The individual must be released, involuntarily committed, or must voluntarily commit himself when the specified time limit has passed. In the event the individual is committed, most states either by statute or regulatory policy, require at least a yearly review of the person's status. Such a requirement safeguards against the person's status being lost in the system as frequently happened in the past.

A 1983 Tennessee statute permits the emergency detention of a person for the purposes of diagnosis, evaluation, and treatment under the following condition:

The physician must evaluate the patient and make a determination that the individual is mentally ill and because of this illness poses a likelihood of serious harm if he is not immediately detained. The phrase "likelihood of serious harm" means substantial risk of physical harm to the person himself as manifested by evidence of threats of, or attempts at, suicide or serious bodily harm; or substantial risk of physical harm to other persons as manifested by evidence of homicidal or other violent behavior or evidence that others are placed in reasonable fear of violent behavior and serious physical harm to them.[20]

The purpose of such a statute is to authorize an emergency admission to a psychiatric facility and to detain the individual for the purpose of establishing a diagnosis, and in the instance of the Tennessee statute to treat the individual. The length of time the emergency detention is operative is necessarily limited. The Tennessee statute provides that the detention cannot exceed 5 days. However, the law provides for an additional 15 days for further evaluation and treatment. When the individual is admitted to the hospital, the superintendent must immediately notify a designated judge who has the statutory authority to order the release of the individual or detainment for up to 5 days. In the event the person is ordered detained a hearing to determine the appropriateness of the hospitalization is scheduled. It is worth noting that the emergency commitment statute provides for treatment but stipulates "no treatment shall be given that will make the respondent unable to consult with counsel or to prepare to defend himself in proceedings for involuntary care and treatment."

There is some flexibility when the commitment or detainment relies on the emergency provision in a statute.

A California patient in *Doe v. Gallinot* challenged the state civil commitment statute which provided for the involuntary civil commitment of persons to mental institutions. He alleged that the standard term in the statute, "gravely disabled" which allowed a 72-hour emergency detention period, was unconstitutionally vague. The term "gravely disabled" as defined in the statute meant "a condition in which a person, as a result of a mental disorder, is unable to provide for his basic personal needs for food, clothing, or shelter." The "gravely disabled" provision was included as an alternative to an express dangerousness standard. In addition, the patient alleged that a provision allowing an additional 14 days of further treatment was unconstitutional because it was implemented without the requirement of a hearing in his behalf.[21]

The court in this case did not find that the term "gravely disabled" rendered the statute unconstitutional because of vagueness. The patient had argued that it was vague because it was subject to individual opinion with respect to what constituted an appropriate lifestyle. The plaintiff, who had a master's degree in economics, was taken into custody by a police officer after the officer observed the patient talking irrationally. The officer concluded that he should be transported to a county mental health facility. On his arrival, the patient was interviewed in the police van by a psychiatric nurse and she concluded after evaluating his mental condition that he was gravely disabled and needed hospitalization. The nurse had authority to authorize detainment for 72 hours. The nurse reported that the man was "extremely delusional, confused, and paranoid" and that he appeared potentially explosive. An hour after his admission he was placed in seclusion and a schedule of drugs were ordered and administered accordingly.

Six days later a physician sought to certify the patient in order that the commitment could be extended. The statute allowed for a 14-day extension. At that time the patient requested a judicial review and it was held 3 days later. At the time of his review, the attorney representing the patient noted that he was heavily sedated and he requested that the patient not be sedated within 72 hours of his next court appearance. However, in spite of the request, the patient received the same dosage of Thorazine (200 mg by mouth, every 4 hours) on the same schedule as preceded the first court appearance.

The court released the patient after a review of his case. The court found that neither the police officer nor the psychiatric nurse ever conducted any investigation as to whether the man had food, clothing, or shelter. In fact, when he was taken into custody he was dressed in normal street clothes, maintained an apartment in Santa Monica, and provided himself with sufficient nourishment on a daily basis.

The main issue in the case was whether the patient's due process rights were protected, particularly the adequacy of his probable cause hearing. *Probable cause* exists when it is demonstrated that reasonable grounds exist to warrant the confinement. The patient argued that due process of law required a probable cause hearing prior to certification for any confinement beyond the emergency 72 hours.

In holding the gravely disabled emergency commitment criterion valid, the court recognized that such a criterion posed considerable risk for error in implementation. Stating that a probable cause hearing was not feasible when detaining under the emergency 72-hour provision, the court held that the plaintiff must be afforded a hearing on the issue of probable cause before a neutral party in order for any detention beyond the 72 hours to be valid. Addressing the risk factor in applying the gravely disabled criterion, the court stated that the risk of error is greater when applying that criterion than when applying "dangerousness." The court went on to say that the patient's detention illustrated important procedural deficiencies in the state's civil commitment scheme. These included placing a heavy burden on the patient to contest the commitment while under the effects of tranquilizing medication and a requirement that the patient rely on the hospital staff for an explanation of his right of access to the court for review of his case.

In requiring a hearing, the court said that the probable cause determination need not be made by a judge, but could be satisfied by conducting a hearing at which a person or group of persons independent of the psychiatric facility conducted an investigation for the purpose of determining whether probable cause existed. The court allowed the state agency responsible for implementing the commitment statute to develop their plan and submit it to the court for approval.

The courts have scrutinized a number of commitment criterion statutes applicable to general commitment requirements and have declared a significant number to be unconstitutionally vague.[22] Many of the successfully challenged standards for commitment required a finding that a person was "mentally ill" and either needed or would benefit from treatment. The courts have found such laws unconstitutional because they set out a commitment standard that could not be measured and because the mental illness was not delineated. Implementation of such standards allowed commitment for a variety of behaviors which could fall anywhere within the vast range of mental illnesses.

Massachusetts requires that the person be "mentally ill" *and* that a failure to commit the person would create a likelihood of serious harm. In addition, the statute requires that no less restrictive alternative exists.[23] The department of mental health, as authorized by the statute, defines mental illness as "a substantial disorder of thought, mood, perception, orientation, or memory which grossly impairs judgment, behavior, capacity to recognize reality or ability to meet the ordinary demands of life. . . ."[24]

Under the Massachusetts statute the requirements for involuntary commitment clearly demonstrate that the commitment cannot result merely because a mentally ill person may benefit from treatment.

The mandated criterion of "dangerousness" as a necessary finding in order to involuntarily commit a mentally ill person has been challenged by psychiatrists and other health care providers who work with mentally ill persons. They argue that the necessity of a finding that the individual is "dangerous" restricts the delivery of optimal patient care, and that patients, who are unable to comprehend the severity of their mental illness or recognize the need for treatment, do not receive treatment early in the course of the illness.[25] Chodoff proposed that the following three criteria would better determine a person's need for psychiatric treatment: the presence of mental illness, the disruption of functioning with an impairment of judgment to such a degree that the patient is unable to consider his condition and make decisions about it in his own interests, and the need for care and treatment.[26]

Such a proposal inherently allows for treatment, as well as confinement. It suggests to many a conflict between the psychiatrist's philosophy to treat and the mentally ill person's right to refuse treatment. Involuntary confinement does not inherently permit treatment against the committed person's wishes. In fact, where a mentally ill person is found to be incompetent, authorization from the court or some type of internal facility review, must be obtained before the person can be treated with drugs or other treatment modalities. A finding of incompetency generally requires a separate court hearing, distinct from a hearing for probable cause on the issue of involuntary commitment.

Standard of Proof for Civil Commitment

In order for the state or other interested parties to involuntarily commit a mentally ill person, it must be shown, by a specific *standard of proof*, that the individual should be committed. In essence, the standard of proof requires that the evidence must support the commitment. This complex legal requirement can best be understood by examining the proof necessary in a criminal case. In a criminal case the government must prove "beyond a reasonable doubt" that the defendant is guilty of the alleged crime. By way of contrast, in a civil case, such as malpractice litigation, the standard is measured by a "preponderance of the evidence." Preponderance of the evidence is when there is a greater weight of evidence on one side, or "one over fifty." The law requires a standard of proof sufficient to satisfy the due process guarantees of the Fourteenth Amendment.

In the 1979 case *Addington v. Texas*, the U.S. Supreme Court identified the standard of proof which must be met before a mentally ill person can be involuntarily committed.[27] Accordingly, in order to satisfy the Fourteenth Amendment due process requirement it must be shown that the standard of proof is met. Just as it is necessary for a statute to set out the criterion for involuntary commitment (that is, dangerousness), it is equally necessary to delineate the standard of proof that must be met in order to show that the mentally ill person is, in fact dangerous. Where the applicable standard of proof is not identified in the statute, it is identified by case law. Evidence must be introduced at the probable cause commitment hearing that the criteria is met.

The legal concept of standard of proof is best understood if one views it as having three tiers or levels. The least stringent is the "preponderance of the evidence" standard. The intermediate standard of proof is "clear and convincing," and the strictest standard, which is used in criminal cases, is "beyond a reasonable doubt."

The 1979 *Addington* case held that the standard of proof which was necessary to adequately meet due process requirements was the middle tier standard, a "clear and convincing" standard. The mentally ill patient argued that the highest standard, "beyond a reasonable doubt" should be shown before he was deprived of his liberty. The defendant, the State of Texas, argued that the "preponderance of the evidence" standard should apply. At the time of the Addington decision, only one state by statute (Mississippi) permitted involuntary commitment by a mere preponderance of the evidence.

The Supreme Court said that the function of a legal process is to minimize the risk of an erroneous decision. Therefore, in order to minimize the risk of an individual being erroneously confined, the state is required to apply a standard of proof more substantial than a mere preponderance of the evidence. The court recognized that involuntary commitment to a psychiatric hospital may stigmatize the individual and have adverse social impact on his future. The court said that "Given the lack of certainty and fallibility of psychiatric diagnosis, the "beyond a reasonable doubt" standard would impose a burden on the state which would be difficult, if not impossible, to meet." Further, the court said that forced reliance on the criminal standard would force judges and juries to "reject commitment for many patients desperately in need of institutionalized psychiatric care." The court noted that 25 states had adopted the "clear and convincing" or similarly worded standard.[28]

In *Addington*, the court held that the minimum standard for commitment must be the "clear and convincing" standard, in order to provide adequate constitutional safeguards. *Addington* declined to impose, as a matter of federal constitutional law, the "reasonable doubt" standard, but nothing in the case would appear to prohibit any state from adopting the stricter standard. At the time *Addington* was argued before the U.S. Supreme Court, 14 states had, either by statute or judicial decision, adopted the "reasonable doubt" standard.[29] Since the Addington decision, at least one state, Massachusetts, has upheld the stricter criminal standard of proof in involuntary commitment cases.[30]

Commitment of Minors

In 1979, in *Parham v. J. R.*, the U.S. Supreme Court upheld the constitutionality of a Georgia statute which permits parents of a minor child to "voluntarily" commit the child to a psychiatric facility.[31] The statute had been upheld as valid in a lower court trial in 1976.[32] The Supreme Court decision has generated much comment in the legal literature.[33]

The Georgia statute permits a parent or guardian to temporarily place a minor child 12 years of age, or older, in a state hospital for observation and diagnosis. Based on a finding by the chief medical officer of the psychiatric facility that the child suffers from a mental illness that is amenable to treatment, the parent or guardian can voluntarily commit the child for an indefinite period.[34] A petition for discharge may be made by the parent or guardian. The minor may apply for release upon reaching the age of majority.

In *Parham*, two minors, J. L. and J. R., brought suit in behalf of all the "voluntarily" committed minors. J. L. died before the U.S. Supreme Court rendered its decision, but the court integrated his petition in its opinion. J. L. was committed by his mother and stepfather at the age of 6. He was discharged 2 years later, but was readmitted 10 days later. Although the staff at the hospital recommended that he be placed in a foster home, he remained institutionalized because a suitable placement could not be found.

J. R. was committed at the age of 7 by the State Department of Family and Children Services. Multiple attempts to place him in a foster home environment were unsuccessful and he was committed for an indefinite period after the hospital admissions staff determined that he would benefit from a structured setting. The plaintiffs alleged that the commitment was, in essence, involuntary and they were deprived of their liberty due process rights by being denied a hearing. They argued that the informal guidelines contained in the statute were insufficient to protect them against confinement and its associated stigmatizing effect.

The U.S. Supreme Court, in finding the statute constitutional, agreed that the minors had a constitutionally protected right, but held that the safeguards in the statute afforded them adequate protection. In weighing the interests of the parties, the court said that the parents' interest is to maintain parental authority and that the bond of affection parents have for their child, coupled with the fact that they are in the best position to determine whether their child is in need of psychiatric treatment, will persuade them to act in the minor's "best interest." The court acknowledged that parents do not always act in their child's best interest, but said that it is not the parent's exclusive decision to commit the child. The Georgia statute requires a decision by a medical officer of the admitting facility before the commitment is formalized. The Court determined that a neutral fact-finder was necessary to protect the minor's rights and a staff physician, situated in the admitting psychiatric facility, would qualify as a neutral fact-finder.

The Court said that more formal judicial-like commitment proceedings would not offer the minor greater protection and would place procedural obstacles in the path of parents seeking care for their child. The Supreme Court sent back to the lower court the question of what type of periodic review would be required during the minor's confinement. The Supreme Court decision was not unanimous and a number of significant points were raised in the dissenting opinion. There is one final note on the right of a minor to have a hearing on the commitment. While the federal Constitution does not afford a hearing, a state constitution or state law may afford the "voluntarily" committed minor such a right.

Short-Term Detention Provisions

A number of cases have considered statutory provisions permitting short-term detention without a probable cause hearing.

In *Luna v. Van Zandt* a provision in the Texas involuntary commitment statute permitted a judge to order the detention of an individual before a hearing.[35] The statute permitted the detention only after a physician determined that the individual was likely to cause injury to himself or others if not detained. However, under the law the detention could be for up to 14 days for a temporary commitment and up to 30 days for an indefinite commitment.

The court found no compelling state interest existed to justify continuing the detention beyond the initial 72-hour period because the threat of harm which was the compelling state interest justification for involuntary detention was eliminated. The court also held that the risk of erroneous deprivation of liberty was significant because the prolonged detention was based on only one physician opinion. The Texas court held the individual could not be detained for more than 72 hours without a probable cause hearing.

The similar case of *In re the Detention of Harris* posed the question of what procedural safeguards must accompany a 72-hour involuntary commitment.[36] The standard for involuntary detention was the "likelihood of serious harm." Again, applying the balancing test of compelling state interest versus the individual's interest to be heard, the Washington State court held such a commitment was a "massive curtailment" of the detainee's liberty.

The statute permitted involuntary commitment for the 72 hours if a mental health professional determined that the individual was likely to cause serious harm to himself or others. The defect in the provision was that the mental health professional's determination of dangerousness was not subject to review, thus the error risk was high. Some type of hearing was necessary to protect due process rights. In short, the court held that an impartial third party review was necessary to ensure that the diagnosis of probable dangerousness was made after sufficient investigation and that the commitment is the least restrictive alternative. However, the court said that it would not require a full-fledged probable cause hearing.

A recent federal case, *Lynch v. Baxley*, held that the use of jails for detaining individuals awaiting involuntary civil commitment proceedings violated their due process rights.[37] The court found that the state of Alabama did not have a compelling interest for the jail detention of individuals who had committed no alleged criminal act. There was evidence that jail detention could lead to a greater level of psychosis. The court ordered the state to detain such individuals in facilities that normally provide accommodations for mentally ill patients.

Summary

A *civil commitment* means that an individual is committed to a psychiatric facility against his wishes. Civil commitment is to be distinguished from *criminal commitment* because the latter means that the individual allegedly committed a criminal act. Also, commitment must be distinguished from *voluntary admission,* where an individual admits himself to a psychiatric facility or agrees to the admission which was suggested by another.

The constitutional protection for a committed individual is found in the Fourteenth Amendment to the U.S. Constitution. One has to also look to the state constitution and other laws to determine the individual's rights. A state constitution may provide greater protection than the U.S. Constitution. The Fourteenth Amendment is important because it provides "due process" rights when an individual is deprived of his freedom.

Due process rights can be substantive (dealing with the essence of the right) or procedural (dealing with how a hearing is conducted). The right to a hearing is a substantive right. Both components of the due process clause are important and enforceable rights.

All the states have enacted laws that spell out the legal requirement for commitment. All include an "emergency" section to permit a state to evaluate an individual for a short period. Many of the laws permit detention for 72 hours before a due process hearing is required for further detention. A state is not permitted to detain an individual for an indefinite period without some type of due process hearing.

The courts have been called on to closely examine commitment criteria and some criteria have been held unconstitutional because they were too vague. The courts have reviewed existing statutes in light of who is permitted to make a determination of "dangerousness." When an individual other than a physician or psychologist makes the decision the courts have required a probable cause hearing be held close to the time of commitment.

When an individual is committed, the law requires that a certain standard of proof be met—That is, that the evidence or facts of the case must support the commitment. The specific legal standard of proof varies from state to state. For example, Texas applies a "clear and convincing" standard, while Massachusetts applies the standard applied in criminal cases, "beyond a reasonable doubt." The higher the standard of proof, such as the standard applied in criminal cases, the greater will be the burden on those seeking to have an individual committed that this action is justified. Some would argue that such a heavy burden is essential before an individual's liberty is taken away.

THERAPIST'S DUTY TO WARN THIRD PARTIES OF POTENTIAL DANGER

In 1976, the *Tarasoff* case in California set a national precedent when it held that a psychotherapist and the university that employed the psychotherapist were liable when they failed to warn a potential victim of threats against her life.[38] Since that time there have been a number of similar cases calling into question the duty owed by a therapist when an individual undergoing psychiatric or psychotherapeutic care exhibits dangerous intentions toward a third party. The general rule, under the common law, is that a person owes no affirmative duty to control the conduct of another or warn the potential victim unless a "special relationship" exists. The courts have carved out an exception in cases in which the defendant stands in some special relationship to either the individual whose conduct needs to be controlled or in a relationship to the foreseeable victim of that conduct. In *Tarasoff*, the court balanced the psychiatric patient's interest in diagnosis and treatment with society's interest in the prevention of violence.

A student at the University of California who was being seen and treated by a psychotherapist who was employed by the university, confided that he intended to kill a young woman he had dated. This information was communicated to the psychotherapist 2 months prior to the murder of the woman. The treating psychotherapist wished to arrange a commitment, but was overruled by the supervising psychiatrist. On one occasion the psychologist requested that the campus police detain the patient, but the patient was released when police judged that his behavior was rational.

The patient, who was a foreign graduate student, met the victim during folk dancing classes. Although the young woman did not regard their casual dating relationship as serious, the graduate student did. When the woman informed him that she did not wish to become seriously involved, the graduate student felt rebuffed and he became despondent, neglecting both his studies and appearance. He was unable to understand why his feelings were not reciprocated. When the woman left the country for the summer the student's mental outlook improved and he regularly sought psychological assistance. He stopped seeing the psychologist on the victim's return. The psychologist alerted the campus police that the student was suffering from paranoid schizophrenia and should be committed as a dangerous person. In the early fall, armed with a pellet gun and a kitchen knife, the student went to the woman's home. When she refused to speak with him, he pursued her and shot and stabbed her, inflicting mortal wounds.

The court held that when a psychotherapist, applying professional standards, determines or should determine that his patient presents a serious danger of violence to another he incurs a duty to use reasonable care to protect the potential victim against such a danger. The psychotherapist was under a duty to take some measure to protect the woman. Although the court found no liability for the failure to take affirmative steps to bring about the student's confinement in a psychiatric facility, it did hold that the failure to warn was not reasonable care. Notifying the victim, her parents, or the police of the danger would have satisfied the reasonable care obligation.

The court stated that the special relationship, such as that which arises between a patient and his physician, or professional therapist, may support an affirmative duty for the benefit of third persons. A hospital or other health care provider must exercise reasonable care to control the behavior of a patient who potentially may endanger other persons, and a physician/therapist must also warn a patient if the patient's condition or medication renders certain conduct, such as driving a car, dangerous. The physician/therapist, because of this special relationship, must exercise reasonable care to protect others against dangers arising out of the patient's illness. For example, a physician may be liable to persons infected by his patient if he negligently fails to diagnose a contagious disease or, having diagnosed the illness, fails to warn members of the patient's family.

The defendants in *Tarasoff* argued unsuccessfully that it is impossible to accurately predict whether or not a patient will resort to violence. However, the issue of failure to predict was not involved in the case, as in fact, the therapists did predict that the patient would kill. In addressing the difficulty that a psychotherapist encounters in attempting to forecast whether a patient presents a serious danger of violence, the court said that the physician or psychotherapist's duty is to exercise reasonable care to protect third parties. Professional error in predicting violent behavior by a patient cannot negate the therapist's duty to protect others. The court stated that the risk that unnecessary warnings may be given is a reasonable price to pay for the lives of possible victims that may be saved. The therapist is not required to be perfect in making judgments, rather the therapist must "exercise a reasonable degree of skill, knowledge and care ordinarily possessed and exercised by like-professionals under similar circumstances." This standard is known as the "professional judgment" requirement. Hindsight that the therapist judged wrongly will not be sufficient to establish negligence.

In cases where the therapist is not aware of the identity of the potential victim it may not be required that the therapist conduct an independent investigation or interrogate the patient to learn the victim's identity. Noting that there is no hard and fast rule, the court said that what would constitute an obligation to ascertain the name of the potential victim would depend on the circumstances of each case. However, there may be times when routine inquiry or deduction will reveal the potential victim's identity.

Addressing the confidentiality issue, the court recognized that routine disclosures could seriously disrupt the patient's relationship with the therapist. The court said that the therapist's obligation to the patient requires that confidential information not be disclosed unless necessary to avert danger to others. In such a case, the psychotherapist's revelation of confidential information is not a breach of trust or a violation of professional ethics. The court said that "the public policy of protective privilege which favors protection of the confidential character of patient–psychotherapist communications ends where the public peril beings."

There have been a number of cases similar to *Tarasoff.* A federal case *Lipari v. Sears, Roebuck & Co.* held that the psychotherapist is required to initiate whatever precautions are reasonably necessary to protect the potential victims of the patient. The nature of the precautions that must be taken would depend on the circumstances and is not limited to a duty to warn. The Lipari court recognized the difficulty of predicting whether "a particular patient mental patient may pose a danger to himself or others. This factor alone, however, does not justify barring recovery in all situations. The standard of care for mental health professionals adequately takes into account the difficult nature of the problem facing them."[39]

However, in another case, *Case v. U.S.,* where suit was filed against the U.S. government under the Federal Tort Claims Act, no liability was found where a Veterans Administration psychiatric patient who was being treated as an outpatient, murdered a third party. The court said that there was no indication that the patient was a "clear and present danger" to himself or anyone else. The patient's condition had improved over a number of years and he was holding a job and functioning satisfactorily in the community.[40]

In an Indiana case, *Estate of Mathes v. Ireland,* the court set aside the lower court's finding and held that the issue of liability of the various named persons should be decided by a jury at a trial.[41] In 1973, a 20-year-old mentally ill person who was receiving psychiatric care abducted the plaintiff's wife from a laundromat at knifepoint. He forced her into his car, drove to a river, and forcing her from the car, he drowned her. Her husband brought suit against the patient's parents and his grandparents. He also sued two psychiatric care centers. The husband's complaint alleged that the parents and grandparents knew that the patient was violent and dangerous and that they had an obligation to supervise and control his activities. The mentally ill person lived with his mother and grandparents, but not with his father. Because there was only a familial relationship with the father, he could not be made a party to the suit.

The court said that no liability could be based on any familial relationship, but a jury may find liability if the deceased woman's husband could show that the mother and grandparents assumed "care and control" of the patient and had knowledge of the likelihood that he might cause bodily harm. However, the family had a right to reasonably rely on expert medical, psychological, or psychiatric advice. In essence, the court was saying that the family had knowledge if the therapist had put them on notice of their relative's dangerous state of mind. Conversely, if they were advised that he presented no danger, then they could reasonably rely on such advice and information. Of course, any knowledge they gained apart from the therapists, such as from their own observations of the patient's demeanor, would put them on notice independent of any therapist's advice.

Addressing the liability of the two psychiatric centers, the court in this case stated that the deceased woman's husband must show some activity demonstrating a connection between the negligence and the injury. One of the psychiatric centers diagnosed and treated the patient and the other had a contractual relationship which involved evaluating, counseling, and treating the patient prior to the killing. The complaint alleged that the staff knew or should have known that it was dangerous to release the patient without extended treatment. In order for the husband to be successful against the facilities under the respondeat superior doctrine ("let the master answer"), the husband would have to show that the staff were employees and not independent contractors, and that either or both of the two psychiatric centers had actually taken charge of the patient's care and had actual knowledge that he was extremely dangerous. Holding that the husband had a right to prove his allegations, the court sent the case back for a trial on the merits of the issues raised in the case.

Since the 1976 *Tarasoff* decision there have been a number of cases litigating the duty to warn third parties issue.

Perhaps the most notable is *Brady v. Hooper* where no liability was found against the psychiatrist who treated John Hinkley, Jr., in regard to injuries received by three men who were with President Reagan when Hinkley attempted to assassinate him.[42] The suit was dismissed because the court found that their injuries were not foreseeable because Hinkley had not made any specific threats against the President or anybody else. The plaintiffs did show that Hinckley collected books and articles on political assassinations, had guns and ammunition, and identified with the character in the movie "Taxi Driver" who assassinated people. The court held that such knowledge was too "vague, speculative, and a matter of conjecture" to reasonably predict danger toward a specific individual. Thus, the court adopted the rule that holds that threats must be specific to named victims. There are a long line of cases finding no liability.[43]

No liability was found in *Sherrill v. Wilson* where the patient did not name a particular victim.[44] The patient committed murder while on a 2-day pass from the hospital. The plaintiff unsuccessfully argued that the hospital staff was negligent in failing to take steps to have the patient returned to the hospital when he failed to come back after the 2 days had expired.

In *McIntosh v. Milano*, a jury returned a verdict for the defendant physician in a suit brought by the murdered girl's parents.[45] The physician's patient had killed his estranged girlfriend.

In response to the defendant's argument that predicting dangerousness was difficult, a Kansas court in *Durflinger v. Antiles* held that the bringing of the suit was proper.[46] The plaintiffs alleged that the physicians negligently released a patient who then killed his mother and brother. The court said that a jury would decide whether the physicians in discharging the patient exercised reasonable care in fulfilling their professional obligations. The court said it could find "no rational basis for insulating this one aspect of professional service from liability for negligence".

Some of the cases in which liability was found involved critical evidence found in the hospital record.

In *Davis v. Lhim*, a Michigan court found liability on the part of the physician for failing to warn the mother that her son posed a danger to her.[47] The court said that no duty toward the public at large existed, but when the patient makes a generalized threat towards a specific individual the psychiatrist owes a duty to warn that person. Evidence introduced at the trial contained a 2-year-old entry in the hospital record which stated that the patient "paces the floor and acts strangely and keeps threatening his mother for money."

Shortly after that case was decided, a Michigan court in *Chrite v. U.S.* held that hospital personnel were negligent in failing to warn the mother-in-law of a released patient that he posed a threat to her.[48] At the trial a note written by the patient (Henry O. Smith) and made part of the hospital record read, "Was Henry O. Smith Here Yesterday. He is wanted for murder Mother-in-Law." As in the Davis case, Chrite held that it was for the jury, as triers of fact, to decide whether the mother-in-law was a fore-seeable and readily identifiable victim. There are a long line of cases finding liability, both where the victim is identifiable and not identifiable.[49]

In a suit against the state, the court found liability in *Peterson v. State* for the negligence of its hospital staff.[50] The patient, who had been involuntarily committed for 14 days, was released, and 5 days later while under the influence of phencyclidine (PCP) he struck a person with his car. The hospital staff knew of his use of PCP because it was the prime reason for his involuntary admission. Further, he had been apprehended, while on a 1-day-pass, for driving recklessly on hospital grounds.

In *Hedlund v. Superior Court of Orange County*, the California Supreme Court held that liability could be found where a psychologist was told by the patient that he intended to harm his former girl friend.[51] The former girl friend sued on her own behalf, for her injuries, and on behalf of her young son, who was seated next her when the patient shot her, for the serious emotional injury and psychological trauma he suffered because of the event. The child who was 5 years old at the time of the shooting did not suffer any physical harm. The law makes a distinction between physical and emotional injury, imposing significant burdens on the plaintiff for recovery in emotional injury suits.

The case raised two points of law. The first was whether the 3-year professional malpractice statute of limitations should apply to the child's claim or whether the 1-year ordinary negligence statute of limitations should apply. (See Chapter 2, Establishing the Standard of Care, section on the Practical Distinction Between Negligence and Malpractice, for a discussion of the distinction between ordinary negligence and professional malpractice.) The defendant psychotherapist unsuccessfully argued that the 1-year time limit should apply because the failure to warn a third party (the son) was not a professional act. The therapist argued that only the failure to recognize "dangerousness" constituted the professional services, and that the duty to warn a third person was not within the realm of professional services. The therapist's position was that the duty to warn third parties was only ordinary negligence. However, the court held in *Tarasoff* that a duty existed to warn persons who foreseeably would be harmed by the patient's dangerous threats. Therefore, it would not fragment a cause of action by holding that the diagnosis and treatment components were professional malpractice, whereas, the duty to warn foreseeable victims was only ordinary negligence. The court held that the warning aspect of the therapist's duty is "inextricably interwoven with the diagnostic function."

The second issue raised by the defendant was that the therapist could not have known that the child would be at risk because of the failure of the therapist to warn the mother of the patient's threats to harm her. The court stated that the risk of harm to the child was foreseeable because of his close relationship to his mother. It was foreseeable that the mother would try to protect her child by throwing herself over him. The breach of the duty occurred when the therapist failed to warn the mother. The mother did not allege that the therapist owed a direct duty to the child to warn him of the threat. In short, the negligence naturally flowed from the mother to her child.

In a recent Vermont case, *Peck v. Counseling Service of Addison County*, the parents of a 29-year-old man sued a mental health facility because of the failure of one of its counselor–psychotherapists to warn them that their son had threatened to burn their barn.[52] The son had a past medical history of epilepsy with an associated brain disorder that increasingly diminished his capacity for exercising good judgment and a history of past alcohol abuse. The therapist was aware of the past medical history, as well as the patient's past history of impulsive assaultive behavior.

At the time of the events surrounding the parents' claim the son was an outpatient at the defendant's facility. On June 20, 1979, the patient who lived with his parents argued with his father. The father called him "sick and mentally ill" and told him he should be hospitalized. The son packed a suitcase and left home and went to the counseling service to speak with the therapist. He informed the therapist he had had a fight with his father and that he was angry with him. The therapist arranged for the patient to stay with his grandparents and arranged to see him the next day. He again voiced his anger with his father at that session. At a June 26 counseling session the patient told the therapist that he "wanted to get back at his father." In response to the therapist's question as to how he would get back at his father, the patient stated, "I don't know, I could burn down his barn." The patient and the therapist discussed the problem, including the consequences of burning the barn. At the therapist's request the patient made a verbal promise not to burn down his father's barn. Believing that he would keep his promise, the therapist did not disclose the patient's threats to any other staff member or to the parents. The next night the patient set fire to the barn, totally destroying it.

The state's supreme court held that the trial judge should not have dismissed the parent's suit because their claim was legitimate. The court stated that a duty to warn a third party of foreseeable harm, such as arson, to their property was as valid as a threat of physical harm to their person. The defendant unsuccessfully argued that because the man was being treated as an outpatient, it lacked control over his actions. The court, relying on case law from other jurisdictions, stated that the relationship between the therapist and the patient, not any control issue, fixes the duty owed to the patient and those who foreseeably would be harmed by his actions. Further, the court stated that the therapist did not act as a reasonably prudent counselor would have acted, and her good faith belief that the patient would keep his promise not to burn the barn was based on inadequate information and consultation. The plaintiff's psychiatric expert testified that given the patient's known history for assaultive behavior and medical problems the therapist's response to the threats was inconsistent with the standards of the mental health profession.

In addition, the evidence demonstrated that at the time of the patient's threats the therapist did not have his most recent medical history. The counseling agency did not have a cross-reference system between its therapists and the patient's treating physician. The defendant's own expert testified that a therapist cannot make a reasonable determination of a patient's propensity for carrying out a violent threat if the therapist lacks knowledge of the patient's complete medical history. Further, the agency did not have any written policy regarding formal intra-staff consultation procedures when a patient presented a threat of serious risk of harm to a third party.

The defendant argued that it could not have lawfully warned the parents because of the physician–patient privilege which did not allow the disclosure of confidential information. The defendant pointed out that although the legislature passed laws permitting disclosure of information in cases dealing with alleged child and elderly abuse and the disclosure of gunshot wounds, it did not include a therapist's duty to disclose information where the patient threatens a bodily or property harm to another. The court stated that the privilege is not "sacrosanct" and can properly be waived in the interest of public policy in appropriate circumstances.

Summary

Some courts have held liability only where the therapist had knowledge of a "readily identifiable" potential victim, while other courts have refused to impose such limits. Courts that impose liability do so because of (1) the negligent release of the patient, or (2) the therapist's failure to take reasonable precautions to protect anyone who might reasonably (foreseeably) be injured. For example, in the case where the patient on PCP injured another while recklessly driving his car (*Peterson v. State*), it was forseeable that he would injure someone. There is a mixed approach in deciding cases in which third parties are injured or killed by a patient; that is, potential victims do not have to be named if it can be shown that the patients' release was negligent.

Addressing the difficulty therapists have in predicting dangerousness, some courts have held that this uncertainty is merely one of the factors to be considered when the factual issue is whether reasonable care was exercised under the circumstances.

One state, Kentucky, recently enacted legislation which specifically identifies the duty of mental health professionals to warn intended victims of a patient's threat of violence.[53] The statute states:

> . . . no cause of action shall arise against any qualified mental health professional for failing to predict, warn of or take precautions to provide protection from a patient's violent behavior, unless the patient has communicated to the qualified mental health professional an actual threat of physical violence against a clearly identified or reasonably identifiable victim, or unless the patient has communicated to the qualified mental health professional an actual threat of some specific violent act.

Further, the act states:

> The duty to warn a clearly or reasonably identifiable victim shall be discharged by the qualified mental health professional if reasonable efforts are made to communicate the threat to the victim's residence of the threat of violence. When the patient has communicated to the qualified mental health professional an actual threat of some specific violent act and no particular victim is identifiable, the duty to warn has been discharged if reasonable efforts are made to communicate the threat to law enforcement authorities. The duty to take reasonable precaution to provide protection from violent behavior shall be satisfied if reasonable efforts are made to seek civil commitment of the patient under this chapter.

The statute also includes an immunity clause against any breach of confidence when reporting a serious threat of violence. It would be a question of fact for the jury, as triers of fact, to determine whether the mental health professional's actions were reasonable. For example, testimony by the defendant mental health professional that she got a busy signal when she attempted to telephone the intended victim to warn the person of the threat may be inadequate, especially if no alternative actions were taken.

THE RIGHT TO REFUSE TREATMENT

The right to refuse treatment concept as it applies to the use of antipsychotic medications and other invasive procedures has been a controversial issue. In the late 1970s and early 1980s a number of legal cases scrutinized and ruled on the complex issue associated with the treatment of the mentally ill. In attempting to balance the rights of the parties, the courts in rendering their opinions have sought to recognize each party's position in relationship to societal and individual needs.

The law has long upheld the right of the individual to make decisions regarding his own affairs and this right is no less significant when the individual is mentally or physically ill. Although most of the "right to refuse treatment" cases have dealt with the use of antipsychotic drugs, other issues include the use of seclusion, and other treatment modalities, such as electroshock. The cases have dealt with the rights of competent and incompetent patients.

The term *mentally incompetent* in a legal sense refers to an individual who is unable to manage his own affairs because of mental illness, physical impairment, or severely impaired intellectual capacity that so impairs his ability to reason that he is unable to make decisions necessary to function. Simply put, a person is considered mentally incompetent if he is incapable of or lacking in the capacity for choice. Where a patient is, for example, suffering from severe psychosis, is not lucid, or in a coma, the capacity to choose is lacking. *Legal incompetence* means that the person has been adjudicated incompetent in legal proceedings.

Antipsychotic Drugs

Since their introduction, antipsychotic drugs have proved valuable in treating some mental disorders and are commonly used. It is estimated that almost one-half of institutionalized patients in public and psychiatric facilities suffer from schizophrenia and some authorities consider antipsychotic drugs necessary in treatment programs for patients afflicted with schizophrenia.[54] Antipsychotic drugs do not cure schizophrenia. However, schizophrenic patients that are treated with antipsychotic medications often improve in their ability to function. Their chief benefits are to shorten hospital confinements and allow patients to function in the home or community.

Courts have increasingly become involved in treatment decisions which are intrusive in nature when the patient is incompetent. The use of antipsychotic drugs, electroshock, and psychosurgery are regarded by the courts as intrusive and invasive treatment. Psychosurgery is the removal or destruction of brain tissue in the absence of any organic disease of the brain with the primary intent of altering the behavior of the patient.

Testimony during the proceedings of a number of cases in which the use of antipsychotic drugs was in issue pointed to toxic and severe side effects of the drug in addition to its beneficial use. A number of cases have held that the involuntary administration of drugs which affect mental processes amounts to interference with Fourteenth Amendment due process rights and in some instances, First Amendment freedom of speech rights. It may also violate sections of the Civil Rights Act.[55] Because it is the patient who will suffer the consequences of treatment decisions, one court said that the patient must have the power to make the decision.[56] That court readily acknowledged that use of antipsychotic drugs yielded beneficial results, but testimony also pointed to the toxic and severe side effects which may accompany their use.[57] These include the extrapyramidal symptoms, such as blurred vision, dry mouth and throat, constipation or diarrhea, palpitations, skin rashes, low blood pressure, fainting and fatigue. *Akinesia*, which is a state of diminished spontaneity and a feeling of weakness and muscle fatigue, is not an uncommon side effect. *Akathesia*, which is another side effect, refers to an inability to be still and is manifested by a motor restlessness which may produce a shaking of the hands, arms or feet, or an irresistible desire to keep walking or tapping the feet. Akinesia and akathesia can be treated with anticholinergic drugs which may have side effects of their own. By far, the most complained of side effect, and one which may be permanent, is tardive dyskinesia. *Tardive dyskinesia* is characterized by rhythmical, repetitive, involuntary movements of the tongue, face, mouth or jaw, and is sometimes accompanied by other bizarre muscular activity. Tardive dyskinesia is associated with prolonged use and is more common in the elderly, especially women. Antipsychotic drugs, such as Prolixin, may cause agranulocytosis which may be fatal.[58]

Substituted Judgment

In handing down court rulings on treatment issue cases the courts must reach their decision by adopting a legal theory to govern their decisions. One theory is "substituted judgment." This legal doctrine is invoked by some courts in instances in which the mentally ill patient is incompetent. The substituted judgment theory originated in England and grew out of legal cases in which the courts had to resolve the question of disposition of estates of incompetent persons. In the United States the doctrine has been applied to medical treatment cases. One case, *Strunk v. Strunk* decided that the doctrine applied in a situation where authorization was sought to have an incompetent donor donate her kidney to a sibling.[59] *Substituted judgment* is a subjective test to determine the supposed wish of the incompetent. It contrasts with the "reasonable person" test which is an objective test, based on what a reasonable person or most persons would most likely do in similar circumstances.

Case Law

In reviewing the legal decisions it is important to note whether the patient voluntarily seeks admission or is involuntarily committed. Just as important is whether the mentally ill person is competent or incompetent.

> One of the first major cases, *In re Boyd* which dealt with a right to refuse antipsychotic drugs involved a 67-year-old woman who was a practicing Christian Scientist.[60] When she was admitted as an emergency patient in 1977 she had delusions of persecution and grandiosity, suffered from auditory hallucinations, and acted irrationally. Although she presented a management problem to the hospital staff she was no danger to herself or others and was found to be mentally competent. She was diagnosed as suffering from schizophrenia, or organic brain syndrome. While in a competent state she made it clear to two hospital chaplains who interviewed her that she would not accept drug treatment because of her religious beliefs and they concluded that her refusal was based on her religious conviction.

Under a District of Columbia law a person admitted for emergency psychiatric treatment is not considered legally incompetent. A separate judicial hearing is necessary to determine whether the person is mentally incompetent, in addition to suffering from a mental illness. Most states have a similar provision requiring the state to prove incompetency separate and distinct from the mental illness. In short, the law says that not all mentally ill persons are incompetent.

A court order in *Boyd* authorized the hospital to administer antipsychotic drugs. This order was given although it was known by the court that the woman had rejected, while in a competent state, the use of medications because of her religious beliefs. The order specifically stated that she "undergo whatever treatment St. Elizabeth's deems appropriate." At the time of the appeal of the court order, the emergency state no longer existed, but the woman was by now incompetent. The issue raised in the appeal procedure was whether a mentally incompetent patient, in the absence of an emergency situation, may be forced to take antipsychotic drugs. More precisely worded, the legal question became, How does the court decide whether to authorize the medication and how does an individual's incompetency affect the exercise of First Amendment religious rights? The court said that it must apply the substituted judgment approach in determining whether the now incompetent patient would opt for or against treatment. The substituted judgment theory would facilitate the courts' ability to select a course of therapy the patient herself would choose if she were capable of making a competent decision. The court found that the original legal proceedings did not give sufficient consideration to her religious views as a practicing Christian Scientist.

Another treatment question was raised in *In re the Mental Health of K. K. B.* when the superintendent of a state psychiatric hospital instituted legal proceedings to determine whether an involuntarily committed, competent patient could refuse antipsychotic drugs.[61] Oklahoma state law required that a special determination on the issue of competency be held by separate court proceedings before a person could be adjudicated incompetent. The woman in question was diagnosed with schizophrenia, but no competency hearing had been held. She refused to consent to the administration of antipsychotic drugs. The lower court ordered her to submit to treatment and authorized the hospital to take such steps as necessary to enforce treatment. The woman challenged the lower court ruling and argued that, as a legally competent person, she had a constitutional right to refuse to take powerful drugs which would affect her mental processes and might cause serious side effects.[62]

The higher court held that, based on a constitutional right to privacy (liberty), the state hospital could not force the woman to take the drugs. In the absence of an emergency, such as danger to other patients or hospital personnel, the only basis for using antipsychotic drugs would be to help the patient, and a competent patient has a right to decide whether he wished to be helped. The case dealt with consent to so-called "organic therapy" which includes electroshock, psychosurgery, and antipsychotic drugs. Such therapy can change a patient's behavior even without the patient's cooperation. The case also held that the state could not apply the parens patriae doctrine as the parens patriae relationship does not materialize until a patient is judicially declared incompetent. This doctrine gives the state the power of guardianship over an incompetent person.

One of the most significant cases of 1980, *Davis v. Hubbard*, dealt with a number of situations and findings which infringed upon the 14th Amendment rights of institutionalized psychiatric patients.[63] In addition to the right to refuse treatment issue, the case dealt with issues of seclusion and physical restraint, and medication procedures. The case set out guidelines which provide the minimal constitutional requirements which must be met. The state has to provide a level of care that will not fall below minimal constitutional guarantees. These guidelines require a physician's assessment, except in a "crisis situation," before a patient can be placed in seclusion or restraints. The order must be written and the patient's record must reflect the patient behavior which necessitated the seclusion or the restraint. The guidelines also require that the record demonstrate the alternatives to seclusion and restraint which were considered and why they were not feasible options. The nonemergency seclusion order must be limited in duration and personal hygiene opportunities must be reasonable and provided when requested by the patient. The court criticized individual and collective decision-making processes, as well as actual restraint techniques. The court found that decisions to seclude and restrain patients were actually made by attendant staff, or upon their recommendation without physician assessment. Staff shortages impacted considerably on the decision to restrain or seclude, the duration of such treatment, and the quality of care a patient received while restrained or secluded.

The court further found that there was widespread use of antipsychotic drugs in the state facility, not necessarily supported by any sound medical course of treatment. In some instances the court found that drug programs were frequently counter-therapeutic and could not be justified except for punishment purposes and for staff convenience. The court noted that many physicians, nurses, guardians, and family members failed to distinguish between manifestations of the mental illness and reactions to frustration. The court issued a guideline which stated that no medication or increases in medication may be given unless a physician has written the order or unless a crisis situation exists.

The *Davis* court, agreeing with other federal and state decisions, held that the right of an involuntarily committed but competent patient to refuse treatment, including antipsychotic medications, was based on the constitutional protection of the due process clause of the Fourteenth Amendment. However, this right is not absolute and has limitations. These limitations can be ascertained only after identifying the legitimate interests of the state and then balancing these interests against the plaintiff's interests. The court, however, did not preclude the state's use of a compulsory drug program for some patients. Obviously, constitutional protection such as a formal hearing would be required before such a program could be implemented. The state's interest translates into a duty to protect a patient from harming himself or others. It is insufficient to argue that the mentally ill person has at some time been violent. By way of illustration, the court said that prison inmates are at times violent, but the state can not drug them to prevent all possibility of their being violent while in the state's custody.[64] The court found that the majority of the patients in the facility were quite capable of rationally deciding whether it is in their best interest to take or stop taking antipsychotic drugs. The forced use of antipsychotic drugs represented a significant encroachment upon the patient's fundamental interests. A significant number of physicians testified in the case that mentally ill persons should have a right to refuse antipsychotic drugs.

Additionally, the case dealt with the impact of staffing patterns on patient care and treatment. Inadequate staffing patterns and a lack of formal continuing education were found to contribute to a number of patient care deficiencies. This case relied on the 1974 *Wyatt* case which had established that the right to treatment must necessarily presuppose a trained and qualified staff.

Supreme Court Cases

A brief scenario of the evolution of the treatment cases is important to the understanding of their ultimate decisions. In June 1982, the U.S. Supreme Court decided three cases which raised federal constitutional liberty issues. These cases were *Youngberg v. Romeo, Rennie v. Klein,* and *Mills v. Rogers. Youngberg v. Romeo* dealt with the rights of a mentally retarded institutionalized man.[65] The court issued an opinion which was to be applied in a number of subsequent treatment rights cases. The Court, however, refused to issue an opinion in *Rennie v. Klein* because it held that the *Youngberg* analysis and holding would resolve the issues presented.[66] It returned the case to the federal court for an opinion.[67] The third case to be decided was *Mills v. Rogers.*[68] Asked to decide issues similar to *Youngberg,* the *Mills* court vacated (struckdown) the lower federal court decision and returned the case to the lower court because in the interim between filing and arguing the U.S. Supreme Court case, the Massachusetts Supreme Court had decided a case on which *Mills v. Rogers* could be decided. Thus, in 1984 the federal court issued its opinion in *Rogers v. Okin,* basing much of its decision on state law.[69] Both *Youngberg* and *Rogers* set out a test for determining whether liberty rights were protected. However, a different standard or measurement was created by each decision.

As in some earlier federal cases, the U.S. Supreme Court in *Youngberg v. Romeo* looked to the liberty interests protected by the Fourteenth Amendment of the U.S. Constitution in deciding certain rights of an institutionalized mentally retarded individual. Nicholas Romeo was 33 years old and profoundly retarded. His I.Q. was between 8 and 10 and he was unable to talk or care for his basic needs. He resided with his parents until he was 26 years old, but had to be institutionalized when his father died because his mother was unable to manage his violent outbursts. He was admitted to Pennhurst, a state school and hospital in Pennsylvania, in 1974. His mother filed suit in 1976 because Romeo had been injured, both by his own behavior and from attacks by other residents on a number of occasions.

The suit alleged that the school authorities knew about the injuries, but failed to take preventive measures. She asked the court to grant her some relief, and money damages. Shortly after the suit was filed, Romeo broke his arm and was taken to the hospital wing and physically restrained. His mother added several more allegations to the suit. She objected to the use of restraints for prolonged periods on a routine basis and asked that her son be compensated for the defendant's failure to offer him appropriate "treatment or programs for his mental retardation."

The state conceded that under the Fourteenth Amendment Romeo had a right to adequate food, shelter, clothing, and medical care. The issue before the U.S. Supreme Court was whether the Constitution also provided protection for his safety, freedom of movement, and training. If such rights existed the court would then decide the test to apply in determining whether Romeo's rights were infringed.

The court first established that commitment can not deprive an individual of all substantive liberty interests. A substantive right is an "essential" right as opposed to a procedural right, such as a right to a hearing or notice that a hearing is being held.

The court held that the right to be safe and have freedom of movement were "historic liberty interests." Addressing the habilitation and training issue, the court said this same interest requires the state to provide minimally adequate or reasonable training to ensure safety and freedom from undue restraint. Romeo's attorneys had argued that additional training programs, including self-care programs, were necessary to reduce the patient's aggressive behavior. The court left unanswered the question whether Romeo had a right to habilitation to *maintain* the basic self-care skills he possessed when he entered the facility. His attorneys argued earlier that Pennhurst should provide such training as to preserve the skills he had when he entered.

Referring to the safety and freedom from bodily restraints arguments, the Supreme Court said these were not absolute liberty interests, but had to be "balanced." This is done by weighing the individual's interest in liberty against the state's justification for restraining the interest. The court held that the state had an interest in providing safety for Romeo and the other patients.

Having articulated these legal principles, the court next turned to the question, What is the proper test for determining whether a state adequately has protected the rights of the involuntarily committed mentally retarded individual? The Court rejected applying the "compelling" or "substantial" necessity test to decide whether a state could permissibly use restraints. The Court said that such a requirement would place an undue burden on the running of the facility. Instead, the Court held that the Fourteenth Amendment only required the courts, when reviewing infringement allegations, to make certain that "professional judgment" was exercised.

The court said that there was no reason to think judges or juries were better qualified than appropriate professionals in making these treatment decisions and the courts should not "second-guess the expert administrators on matters on which they are better informed." This point was emphasized when the court went further and said these decisions, if made by a professional were presumed valid. That is, the decisions had a "presumption of correctness." Thus, no liability for wrongdoing would exist unless the plaintiff could show the professionals' decision was "a substantial departure from accepted professional judgment, practice, or standards as to demonstrate that the person responsible actually did not base the decision on such a judgment."

The Supreme Court defined "professional" decision maker to mean "a person competent, whether by education, training or experience, to make the particular decision at issue. Long-term treatment decisions normally should be made by persons with degrees in medicine or nursing, or with appropriate training in areas such as psychology, physical therapy, or the care and training of the retarded."[70] Day-to-day care decisions, including those which must be made without delay, could be made by employees without formal training so long as they were subject to the supervision of qualified persons.

A recent New York court decision applied the professional judgment test. The issue in *Woe v. Cuomo* was to what extent the state has an obligation to provide care and treatment to improve the health and regain the liberty of civilly committed psychiatric patients.[71] The New York case held that accreditation by the Joint Commission on the Accreditation of Hospitals (JCAH) constitutes prima facie proof that a mental hospital's care and treatment of patients is adequate and complies with its patients' due process requirements. Finding that the accreditation criteria had a direct bearing on the likelihood that professional judgments would govern treatment decisions, the court held that such accreditation was evidence of adequate care and treatment. In allowing the fact of JCAH accreditation to demonstrate a certain level of care and treatment, the court was relying heavily on the *Youngberg* professional judgment test. However, the allowance of JCAH accreditation did not preclude other evidence to rebut the adequacy of treatment. In short, it was evidence, but its impact could be diminished if the plaintiff presented other evidence showing inadequacies in the care and treatment provided.

The second major "right to refuse treatment" case reviewed by the U.S. Supreme Court in June 1982 was *Mills v. Rogers*.[72] The origin of that case was *Rogers v. Okin* ("Rogers I") which was tried in a federal court in Massachusetts. That case went to trial in December 1977 and was decided in January 1979.[73] It ran 72 trial days and included more than 8000 pages of trial transcript. The decision in this case was appealed to a higher federal court in 1980 ("Rogers II") and ultimately the U.S. Supreme Court reviewed the case in 1982.[74] The issue before the U.S. Supreme Court was whether involuntary committed mentally ill patients have a constitutional liberty interest to be free from the forced administration of antipsychotic drugs. You will recall that the Youngberg case had decided exactly the same issue (see preceding discussion).

However, by the time the U.S. Supreme Court agreed to hear the "Rogers II" case a decision by the Massachusetts Supreme Court rendered in 1981 cast doubt on the legal significance of the "Rogers II" decision. In short, the U.S. Supreme Court, having been notified that the Massachusetts Supreme Court may have decided the same legal issue at a state level, refused to "decide" the case. The case decided by the Massachusetts Supreme Court dealt with the right of a noninstitutionalized, mentally incompetent patient to refuse antipsychotic drugs. That decision, the *Matter of Guardianship of Richard Roe III*, will be subsequently discussed in depth.[75] That decision, which was based largely on Massachusetts state laws did not follow the Youngberg analysis although it did stipulate the applicable standard of measure to be applied in deciding these kinds of cases.

In summary, the second case the U.S. Supreme Court heard in June 1982, *Mills v. Rogers*, was sent back to the federal appeals court in order that it could decide whether the *Matter of Guardianship of Richard Roe III* necessitated a revision of the holding in "Rogers II." In effect, the U.S. Supreme Court struck down the "Rogers II" holding. Following an established custom the U.S. Supreme Court refused to decide *Mills v. Rogers* because the question posed by the case may have already been resolved by the highest court in Massachusetts when it decided, *Matter of Guardianship of Richard Roe III*.[76]

In sending the *Mills v. Rogers* case back to the federal appeals court, the U.S. Supreme Court directed the appeals court to decide the question: Whether the rights and duties of the parties could be determined by looking at *state* law. Acting on that directive from the U.S. Supreme Court, the first circuit federal appeals court asked the state high court to answer nine questions concerning the standards and procedures under applicable *state* law whereby involuntarily committed patients may be medicated with antipsychotic drugs. These questions were answered in *Rogers v. Commission of the Department of Mental Health*.[77] After the state high court answered the nine questions, the case proceeded to the federal appeals court which decided the *federal* constitutional claims in *Rogers v. Okin* ("Rogers III").[78] Thus, collectively, *Guardianship of Richard Roe III*, *Rogers v. Commission of the Department of Mental Health*, and "Rogers III" answer the question raised by the 1982 U.S. Supreme Court *Mills* case. By deciding the case in 1984, the federal court placed a federal stamp on the issues, thus giving the decision more significance than if it had been merely a state supreme court decision. Although applying a different decision-making standard than the U.S. Supreme Court in *Youngberg*, the "Rogers III" decision is important. "Rogers III," applying state law, used a different standard yardstick, but was consistent with the principles laid out in *Youngberg*.

The "Rogers III" case was set in motion when in 1975 Rubie Rogers and six other plaintiffs who were psychiatric patients in a Massachusetts state hospital filed suit against the officials and staff members of the facility. They sought to stop the defendants from medicating them by force and secluding them when nonemergency situations arose. They also sought money damages, but this aspect was denied at all levels of the proceedings.

The reason the U.S. Supreme Court refused to decide the issues presented in "Rogers III" was because of the decision in *Guardianship of Richard Roe III*. The question in this latter case was whether a court-appointed guardian should have delegated authority to consent to forced medication. Roe's legal guardian was his father who was appointed because the son, as a result of his mental illness, was unable to care for himself and make decisions affecting his life. The young man was living with his family and was not in the custody of a state institution. There was no question that the guardian had legal authority to consent in an emergency situation. The guardian sought authority to authorize drug treatment at some time in the future. The son had rejected antipsychotic medications on every occasion when it was offered.

The court in the *Roe* case reaffirmed the "undisputed" right of mentally competent persons to refuse treatment. This same right must extend to incompetent individuals. The young man had the legal *right* to refuse, but was incapable of exercising that right due to his mental incompetency. The court held that the guardian did not have the right to consent and that such a decision required the "detached but passionate investigation" of a judicial determination.[79] Such a judicial determination is made by application of the *substituted judgment doctrine* which gives the court the power to decide for or against treatment, in this case, forced medication, in the same way that the incompetent individual would if he were capable of making a rational decision.

This decision is particularly significant because it set out guidelines to determine when a court order should be obtained when the question is whether an incompetent mentally ill individual should be forcibly administered antipsychotic drugs in the absence of an emergency. Additionally, it identified factors necessary to consider in applying the substituted doctrine. Factors that indicate that there should be a judicial decision include the intrusiveness of the purposed treatment; the possibility of adverse side effects, whether an emergency exists, the nature and extent of previous court involvement, and the likelihood that the guardian, in this case a parent, might have an interest that conflicts with the ward's interest. The court did not object to the physical act of injecting Haldol, but rather to the power of the drug to alter the thought processes of the mind. Antipsychotic drugs, said the court, are to be viewed in the same manner as the highly intrusive psychosurgery and electroconvulsive treatments.

The court identified the following factors as being relevant in application of the substituted judgment doctrine: the ward's expressed preferences regarding the treatment which were expressed while he was in a competent state, the religious beliefs and practices of the individual, family ties and the impact the patient's refusal or acceptance would have on the family unit, the likelihood of adverse side effects, whether a refusal will lead to a steadily deteriorating condition, and the prognosis with treatment. Applying these guidelines will ensure a degree of consistency in future judicial proceedings in which the substituted judgment doctrine is applied. The judge is to give weight to these factors and is free to consider other factors as a given case may warrant.

Following *Guardianship of Richard Roe III* the state supreme court in *Rogers v. Commissioner of the Department of Mental Health* answered the nine questions put to it.[80] In addition to answering whether involuntarily committed patients had the right to refuse treatment, it also queried the applicable standard and procedures to be followed when treating such patients with antipsychotic drugs.

Questions of Competency and Judicial Determination of Incompetence

The first three questions dealt with the right of incompetent patients and how incompetency is determined. The court first looked to state law which specifically said that no person is deemed to be incompetent solely because of admission or commitment to a psychiatric facility, whether public or private. Incompetency is not a prerequisite for commitment.

An adjudicatory hearing must be held and a determination of incompetency made before any decision to override a patient's decision can be carried out. A mentally ill person does not lose the right to make his own treatment decisions until an adjudication by a judge renders the person incompetent.

The Applicable Standard

Questions 4 and 5 dealt with the standard to be applied by the judge in deciding whether antipsychotic drugs will be given to the incompetent patient. The judge applies a "substituted judgment" test when deciding whether the patient would have consented if the patient were competent to consent. The goal of the substituted approach is to determine as accurately as possible what the desires and needs of the individual would be. It is a decision which would be made by the individual, if competent at the time of the need to decide. It would embrace all the factors that would necessarily enter into the decision-making process of the person. Several psychiatric organizations argued that the substituted judgment decision should be done by physicians and not judges. However, Massachusetts is not the only jurisdiction to use the test.[81]

A Sufficiently Compelling State Interest

Questions 6 and 7 dealt with the "police power" and the emergency exception to an individual's right. A state's police power is the power of a state to pass laws and regulations which are for the good and welfare of the state. However, only a "sufficiently compelling" state interest will override an incompetent patients' right to refuse.

The Massachusetts Department of Mental Health argued that forced medication was necessary to decrease the length of admissions and lessen the impact unmedicated patients have on the illness of other patients on the hospital unit. Further, it argued that group therapy, a necessary aspect of psychiatric care, would be difficult unless the patient was receptive.

The court noted that antipsychotic medication abuses on the part of the care provider were well documented.[82] Testimony in prior proceedings established that antipsychotic drugs had been given for staff convenience, as a substitute for treatment, and as punishment. However, the court acknowledged that psychiatric institutions must protect its staff and other patients, as well as maintain institutional security. Thus, the state must have in place, statutory and regulatory mechanisms when chemical restraints are to be used in emergency situations.

The state defined "emergency" as "an unforseen combination of circumstances or the resulting state that calls for immediate action."[83] State law addressed the "emergency" situation. The law stipulated that "only in cases of emergency such as the occurrence of, or serious threat of, extreme violence, personal injury, or attempted suicide" may a mentally ill patient be restrained.[84] The state regulations dealing with the use of seclusion and restraint state: "Restraint or seclusion of patients may be used only in emergency situations where there is the occurrence or serious threat of extreme violence, personal injury, or attempted suicide."[85]

The court also held that forced injection over the patient's objection could be done in an emergency only if no "less intrusive alternative" to drugs existed.

The Parens Patriae Doctrine

The last two questions asked whether the doctrine of parens patriae would justify forced medication in other than an emergency? Parens patriae in this context refers to the power of a state to "govern" an individual who is under some disability. In this case the court established another exception and held that the "State may, in rare circumstances, override a patient's refusal of medication under its so called Parens patriae powers". Thus, the state may force medicate to prevent the "immediate, substantial and irreversible deterioration of a serious mental illness." However, if the physicians determine that further medication is necessary to prevent deterioration, the patient must be adjudicated incompetent and a substituted judgment treatment plan prepared.

Once the state high court certified (answered) these questions the case returned to the federal appeals court. After 10 years of litigation the only issues before the federal court in "Rogers III" were the rights, under the Fourteenth Amendment due process clause, of involuntarily committed mentally ill patients to refuse antipsychotic medication. The court in *Rogers v. Okin* held that the requirements as set out in the state laws govern the use of chemical restraints and protect the patients' liberty interests.[86] In short, the federal appeals court held that the state procedures in place to protect the rights of an involuntarily committed patient with respect to forced medication measured up to those necessary to meet a federal constitution challenge. In fact, the Massachusetts standards exceeded the minimum necessary to satisfy federal constitutional scrutiny.

The third psychiatric treatment case before the U.S. Supreme Court and heard the same day as *Youngberg* and *Rogers* was *Rennie v. Klein*.[87] *Rennie*, like *Rogers*, was sent back, but for a different reason. The Supreme Court held that *Rennie* should be decided in light of its decision in *Youngberg*. You will recall that the court in *Youngberg* declined to adopt a "least intrusive means" test and instead, adopted the professional judgment test.

This subsequent *Rennie* case, decided in 1983, held that the New Jersey regulations in place satisfied the due process liberty interests of the federal Constitution.[88] To satisfy due process rights, *Rennie* adopted a two-part test to resolve the question of when forced antipsychotic medications may be given to an involuntarily committed patient. First, a professional judgment must be made that forced medication is needed to prevent the patient from endangering himself or others. Thus, there needs to be a threshold determination that there is a potential for harm. Second, professional judgment must be exercised in making the decision to administer the medication. For example, the physician must weigh the effect the drug will have on the patient. The New Jersey regulations and procedure require that the physician meet with the patient and explain "his assessment of the patient's condition; his reasons for prescribing the medication; the benefits and risks of taking the medications; and the advantages and disadvantages of alternative course of action." Additionally, the state regulations require that the physician ground his decision on one of three alternative findings: "(1) that the patient will harm himself or others without the drugs; (2) that the patient cannot improve without the drugs; or (3) that the patient can improve without the drugs, but only at a significantly slower rate."

It is instructive at this point to contrast the requirements necessary to overcome a federal constitutional challenge to forced medication under Massachusetts and New Jersey laws. New Jersey, following the mandate of the *Youngberg* decision, looked to the state procedures set in place to guide a physician when making a forced medication decision. The physician has to show that the decision complied with good and accepted medical practices. This is the standard of proof which must be met in a malpractice suit. *Rogers* required that, in the absence of an emergency, the decision to force-medicate involved a judge who will decide the question by applying the substituted judgment test. Massachusetts relies on both its case law and statutory law. New Jersey relies on its statutory law.

Forced Medication of Competent Patients

A 1984 federal court deciding Texas law in *R. A. J. v. Miller* held that, in the presence of state rules which provided a decision review right, a competent involuntarily committed patient did not have the right to refuse treatment.[89] The rules spelling out the consent mechanism also allowed for an extra review procedure if the patient was capable of appreciating the nature and consequence of his decision to refuse treatment.

Thus, the court found there was no prior case law which permitted "an absolute right on the part of the competent involuntary committed patient to refuse administration of psychotropic medications. Further, the court said, "The State is not restricted to helping the patient only if he wishes to be helped. That limitation was overcome when the patient was confined. The State may therefore make decisions about different treatments that offer some hope of improving the patient's condition and returning him to his community."

Forced Medication of Prisoners

In 1984 a federal court, in *Bee v. Greaves*, was asked to decide whether a pretrial detainee could be forcibly administered antipsychotic drugs.[90] Two constitutional provisions are important to the decision; the First Amendment (freedom of speech) and the due process clause of the Fourteenth Amendment. Suit was brought against a number of prison officials, as well as the jail physician and a psychiatrist. The jail's medical technician was not sued.

There is one fact that has significance for prison nurses although it was not a factor in the outcome of the case. The jail's psychiatrist, who ordered forced medication, testified that he ordered the drug be given by injection if the detainee refused the oral drug and that it could be repeated once more without checking with him. The order was implemented as if it were a standing order and the threat of forced injections continued over an extended period.[91]

Four days after the plaintiff was booked into jail he was referred to the mental health staff because he was hallucinating. He complained to the jail staff that he was not receiving his Thorazine and threatened suicide if not given the drug. He was placed in seclusion and evaluated. Thorazine was prescribed which was voluntarily taken at that time.

Ten days later he was evaluated and found competent to stand trial. A determination of competency was necessary because he had to understand the nature of the charges against him and assist his counsel in his defense. He was diagnosed as schizophrenic and Thorazine was again prescribed. The court ordered that the detainee be medicated with Thorazine every evening.

The detainee continued to voluntarily take oral Thorazine for the next 14 days, at which time he began to complain that he was having problems with the drug. He began to refuse the drug outright about a week later. The prison psychiatrist said the prisoner was "decompensating" as a result of the refusal and ordered that the prisoner be forcibly medicated any time he refused to take the drug orally. The medical technician testified that he gave one injection forcibly with the express purpose of "intimidating him so that he wouldn't refuse the oral medication any more." Subsequently each time the prisoner refused he was threatened with another forcible injection. In the face of this threat the prisoner agreed to take the drug orally.

The court held that the First Amendment protects the communication of ideas which must necessarily include the protection of the capacity to produce ideas. The court recognized that antipsychotic drugs have the potential to severely and possibly, permanently affect a person's ability to think and communicate. Further, the detainee has a liberty interest protection but this interest is not absolute. The court also held that the prisoner did not enjoy the full range of freedoms enjoyed by nonincarcerated persons.

The court held there was no right or duty on the part of the officials to treat a mentally ill prison detainee, but there was a right to maintain security and to prevent a violent detainee from injuring himself or others. Such was the compelling state interest. Following the professional judgment standard in *Youngberg*, the court held that a decision to administer drugs should be based on a legitimate treatment need in accordance with good and accepted medical practice.

In the presence of an emergency, forced medication would be permitted to protect jail staff and others, but the officials should consider alternative, less restrictive approaches. The court suggested the use of segregation or the use of less controversial drugs such as tranquilizers or sedatives.

Summary

Both medical treatment issues and psychiatric treatment issues have constitutional protection. Much of the case law on psychiatric treatment issues was tried in the federal courts, including a number of cases that went to the U.S. Supreme Court. Several of the cases span a long period, some as long as 10 years. The U.S. Supreme Court, as is its practice, will not decide issues that can be decided by application of state law and this is the reason why the Supreme Court would only decide one of the three cases before it in 1982.

The *Rennie* case is significant because it was decided based on the *Youngberg* analysis that the decision to force medicate incompetent involuntarily committed patients could be made by physicians in compliance with professional judgment standards. In both *Rennie* and *Rogers v. Okin* ("Rogers III") the court examined the respective state laws to determine whether these laws were adequate to satisfy the patient's due process rights when involuntary medication was an issue. In *Rogers* the court determined that the protection afforded the patient exceeded that required by the federal constitution.

Most of the decisions since *Youngberg* rely on the professional judgment standard and strictly limit reliance on the courts to resolve the decision to forcibly medicate. However, it should be noted that all decisions are subject to judicial review where there is an allegation that the physician failed to comply with professional standards. The test, according to *Youngberg*, is whether the decision was a "substantial" departure from recognized and accepted professional standards. The states have enacted laws and procedures spelling out the due process protection, and if these provide reasonable due process protection they will pass challenge. Although *Youngberg* did not adopt the least intrusive alternative standard some of the subsequent cases have adopted such a standard.

When faced with these decisions the courts have balanced the patient's due process rights with the states' interests. The law has established two exceptions to a patient's constitutional right. These are the emergency exception and the prevention of patient deterioration exception. In order to act on the emergency exception the providers must carefully document the need for emergency intervention.

One of the most important factors to be aware of is that all the forced treatment cases begin by identifying whether protections are available to the patient, what these are, and what are the limits on these rights. The courts then proceed to an analysis of the states' compelling interests. At this point, different courts set out a different standards or measurements to indicate how the practical decision is reached. Thus far, most of the courts have adopted the professional judgment standard which minimally involves the judiciary, but some of the courts have adopted a different decision-making standard, such as the substituted judgment standard.[92]

DEINSTITUTIONALIZATION

The term *deinstitutionalization* is used to describe the discharge of mentally ill patients from hospitals and returning them to the community to continue treatment and monitoring of their progress in the least restrictive setting possible. The movement became possible with the development of better drugs to treat mental illness. Deinstitutionalization has been implemented mostly in the last decade and a half. The concept of deinstitutionalization has generated both renewed hope for the plight of the mentally ill and concern for their well-being when they are released into the community. Rapidly evolving case law has contributed much in establishing the rights of nondangerous mentally ill individuals.

New law has been generated as a result of the concept. Case law, in many instances, has precluded the use of local zoning laws to keep the mentally ill from living in group homes in the community. Some of the zoning problems associated with establishing community residences for the mentally ill are mirrored in resistance to integrating the mentally retarded into society. When agencies began to implement the deinstitutionalization concept by establishing community residential and day treatment services they encountered considerable resistance. For example, towns enacted local zoning laws to keep the mentally ill from living in group homes in their communities.[93] A considerable body of law developed in response to restrictive zoning laws, and in many instances the zoning laws were struck down.

No Constitutional Right to the Least Restrictive Setting

Although many states have established programs and residences for the mentally ill and mentally retarded in the community, they are not bound to do so by the federal constitution or federal law. One of the issues raised in the 1982 *Youngberg v. Romeo* decision case was whether under the due process clause of the Fourteenth Amendment the mentally disabled had a right to "less restrictive services." The U.S. Supreme Court in *Youngberg* stated, "As a general matter, a state is under no constitutional duty to provide substantive services for those within its borders." In essence, the court held that although the state did have a duty to provide adequate food, shelter, clothing, medical care, and reasonable safety for those within its institutions, it need not provide services in community settings. In fact, many states have established community residences, but it is under no legal onus to do so unless state law *mandates* it.

In a recent case, *Mental Health Association v. Deukmejian,* a California appeals court held that there is no statutory right under either state or federal laws to provide mental health treatment in the least restrictive environment.[94] In that case suit was brought on behalf of certain, "gravely disabled persons" who were confined to two state-run hospitals to require the governor and other governmental officials to create and fund community-based mental health residential and rehabilitative programs. The commitment statute uses the phrase, "gravely disabled persons." The plaintiff's petition sought the "least restrictive" services and environment placement as alternative to the state institutions. There was testimony given by mental health officials that many persons at the two state institutions were inappropriately placed there or remained there longer than necessary because of the lack of appropriate alternative programs and services in the community. There was also testimony that less restrictive programs and services would substantially reduce the rate of rehospitalization.

They alleged that the state's involuntary civil commitment laws mandated such facilities and placement when it used the following language:

> It is the intent of the Legislature that persons with mental illness shall have rights including, but not limited to, the following: (a) The right to treatment services which promote the potential of the person to function independently. Treatment should be provided in ways that are the least restrictive of the personal liberty of the individual.[95]

The court held that the statutory language was intended to promote rather than mandate the least restrictive form of treatment. It determined that the Legislature had articulated a "preference" for treating the mentally ill in the least restrictive environment, but did not create an absolute right to it. Further, the court stated that the state is "not required to provide mental health services to its citizens. When it chooses to, it has considerable latitude in determining the nature and scope of its responsibilities." In short, the state had a duty to commit mentally ill persons in compliance with the states' commitment laws, but it need not provide "services".

In fact, the court found that the state was a pioneer in the development of community alternative to state hospitals and substantial progress had been made in the 6 years leading up to the suit. The court found that, in general, California's mental health system compared favorably with other states. It found that as a result of the deinstitutionalization movement and the civil commitment statutes, patients who were capable of community treatment had been removed to the community and the state hospitals were left by and large with the sickest "hardcore" of the mentally ill.

Summary

The period from the mid-1970s to the late 1980s has been important in revealing which direction the care and treatment of the mentally ill will follow. State institutions will never be totally eliminated, because it is recognized that some patients, because of the dangerous aspect of their mental illness, will need to be temporarily and, in some cases, permanently institutionalized. State institutions and private psychiatric facilities will always serve as a backup for deinstitutionalized patients who may have regressed because of the inherent illness or because of the failure to follow the treatment plan.

State and federal laws, as well as future case law will undoubtedly continue to afford access to employment and educational opportunities. The law has consistently recognized the stigmatizing impact of institutionalization. In recent years a great deal has been done to slowly integrate services for the mentally ill into the "mainstream" of life.

SUMMARY

In the past decade a number of important legal cases dealing with laws applicable to the mentally ill and mentally retarded have been decided by the courts. Many of the legal issues applicable to the mentally ill are similar to those affecting persons who are mentally retarded. These decisions, couched in legal language and sometimes difficult to grasp, are important to nurses caring for mentally ill individuals. Indeed, the decisions deal with the problems and dilemmas faced daily by nurses practicing in psychiatric facilities, community settings, emergency rooms, and prisons.

Nurses practicing in these settings must be familiar with their respective state laws that define the rights of competent and incompetent patients, and of voluntarily and involuntarily committed patients. Equally important are the state regulations and procedures that identify the rights of these patients. When a court is asked to examine and analyze the rights of patients, the starting point is always existing state law. When reviewing the laws one can see that the decisions of the treatment cases have been incorporated into the procedures. For example, phrases such as "least restrictive setting" will be found in the language of the regulation or procedure.

The case law of the last decade began with the *O'Connor v. Donaldson* case in which the issue was whether a right to treatment existed. That issue was not addressed by the Supreme Court because it resolved the case without deciding that particular question. The next line of cases dealt with the constitutionality of civil commitment laws. The decisions interpreted the various definitions of mental illness, including the concept of "dangerousness." Slowly, the cases established the "deterioration" exception. Commitment rights are based in the U.S. Constitution, and the courts analyzed the probable cause element and the point at which a hearing must be provided before a longer period of commitment will be permitted.

The *Tarasoff* case held that a duty to warn existed when it became known that the patient intended to harm another. Liability exists where the potential victim is identifiable, and some courts found liability for the negligent release or failure to commit where a threat existed but the potential victim could not be identified. The liability is for "foreseeable" harm.

There is extensive case law dealing with the patient's right to refuse psychiatric treatment. The three leading cases are *Youngberg, Rennie,* and "Rogers III." These three decisions resulted in the development of state law and procedure which recognized and promoted rights for the mentally ill. They established that both the patient and the care provider have rights which have to be balanced. Once the rights of the patient were set out the courts developed the exceptions. The exceptions were legally established because the patient's rights are not absolute and the state has interests it must protect. However, the state must show a compelling interest where a patient's liberty or other constitutional interest will be compromised.

The deinstitutionalization concept has given rise to its own body of law, especially in overcoming community resistance to the establishment of residences. It is not expected that there will be as rapid a growth of cases in the area of psychiatry in the coming years because many important issues have been decided and the existing decisions will serve as guidelines in enacting new laws.

REFERENCES AND NOTES

1. Birnbaum, M. (1960). The right to treatment. 46 *American Bar Association Journal, 499*. Cited in Curran, W. (Feb. 5, 1976). The holy legal war against state-hospital psychiatry. *New England Journal of Medicine, 294*(6), 318–320.
2. O'Connor v. Donaldson, 95 S. Ct. 2486, 422 U.S. 563 (1975).
3. O'Connor v. Donaldson, 493 F. 2nd 507 (5th Cir., 1974).
4. O'Connor v. Donaldson, 95 S. Ct. 2486, at 2493, footnote 10.
5. Wyatt v. Stickney, 325 F. Supp. 781 (1971).
6. Wyatt v. Anderholt 503 F. 2nd 1305 (5th Cir., 1974).
7. Ibid, at 1311, footnote 6.
8. Flakes v. Percy, 511 F. Supp. 1325 (1981).
9. 42 United States Code §6001, et seq. (1975). The Bill of Rights provision says that all persons with developmental disabilities, including retarded persons and persons with cerebral palsy, autism, cystic fibrosis, or childhood psychosis, have a right to "appropriate treatment, services, and habilitation." The law also sets out "minimum standards" for diet and dental care, as well as the use of force in state institutions receiving federal funds.
10. Anon. A relapse found at Willowbrook. *New York Times*, May 2, 1982, p. 6E.
11. Halderman v. Pennhurst State School and Hospital, 610 F. Supp. 1221 (1985).
12. See, Camper, D. (May 4, 1981). A blow to the retarded. *Newsweek*, p. 55; Dietz, J. Rights of retarded curbed. *Boston Globe*, April 21, 1981, p. 1; Anon. Rights of retarded too vague to apply, high court decides. *New York Times* April 26, 1981, p. 10E.
13. Halderman v. Pennhurst, 101 S. Ct. 1531 (1981).
14. Pennhurst State School v. Halderman, 104 S. Ct. 900 (1984).
15. Op. cit. 610 F. Supp. 1221 at 1232 (1985).
16. Tiano, L. (1980). Parham v. J. R.: 'Voluntary' commitment of minors to mental institutions. *American Journal of Law and Medicine, 6*, 125.
17. Lessard v. Schmidt, 413 F. Supp. 1318 (1976).
18. Suzuki v. Yuen, 617 F. 2nd 173 (1980).
19. In the Matter of the Petition for the Commitment of John Tedesco to a Psychiatric Hospital, 421 N.E. 2nd 726 (IN, 1981).
20. Tennessee Code Ann., §33-6-103; 33-6-104 (1983).
21. Doe v. Gallinot, 486 F. Supp. 983 (1979).
22. See, for example, Stamus v. Leonhardt, 414 F. Supp. 439 (1976); Bell v. Wayne County General Hospital, 384 F. Supp. 1085 (1974); Doremus v. Farell, 407 F. Supp. 509 (1975).
23. Massachusetts General Laws. Chap. 123, §1.

24. Massachusetts Dept. of Mental Health Regs., 104 Code of Massachusetts Regulations 3.01.

25. Rabin, P., & Folks, D. (Aug. 28, 1981). Dangerousness as the criterion for involuntary hospitalization: A time to reassess. *Journal of the American Medical Association, 246*(9), 990.

26. Chodoff, P. (1976). The case of involuntary hospitalization of the mentally ill. *American Journal of Psychiatry, 133*, 496.

27. Addington v. Texas, 99 S. Ct. 1804 (1979); see also Vitek v. Jones, 100 S. Ct. 1254 (1980).

28. Alabama, Arizona, Colorado, Connecticut, Delaware, Florida, Georgia, Illinois, Iowa, Louisiana, Maine, Maryland, Michigan, Nebraska, New Mexico, North Carolina, North Dakota, Ohio, Pennsylvania, South Carolina, South Dakota, Tennessee, Vermont, Washington, West Virginia. See Addington v. Texas, 99 S. Ct. 1804, footnotes 6, 7, and 8 for specific citations.

29. Hawaii, Idaho, Kansas, Kentucky, Massachusetts, Minnesota, Montana, New Hampshire, New Jersey, Oklahoma, Oregon, Utah, Washington, D.C., Wisconsin. See Addington v. Texas, 99 S. Ct. 1804, footnote 5 for specific citations.

30. In the Matter of Guardianship of Richard Roe, III, 421 N.E. 2nd 40 (MA, 1981).

31. Parham v. J. R., 99 S. Ct. 2493 (1979).

32. J. L. v. Parham, 412 F. Supp. 112 (1976).

33. Garvey, H. (1979–1980). Children and the idea of liberty: A comment on the civil commitment cases. *Kentucky Law Journal, 68*, 809; Harris, L. (1980). Children's waiver of Miranda rights and the Supreme Court's decisions in Parham, Bellotti, and Fare. *New Mexico Law Review, 10*, 379; Lidz, C. (1980). The rights of juveniles in "voluntary" psychiatric commitments: Some empirical observations. *Bulletin of the American Academy of Psychiatry and the law, 8*, 168; Tiano, L. (1980) Parham v. J. R.: "Voluntary" commitment of minors to mental institutions. *American Journal of Law and Medicine, 6*, 125; Watson, A. (1980). Children, families, and courts: Before the best interests of the child and Parham v. J. R., *Virginia Law Review, 66*, 653.

34. Code of Georgia Annotated, §88-503.1 (1979).

35. Luna v. Van Zandt, Southern District Court of Texas, C.A., no. B-78-13 (TX, 1982).

36. In re the Detention of Harris, 654 P. 2nd 109 (WA, 1982).

37. Lynch v. Baxley, 744 F. 2nd 1452 (1984).

38. Tarasoff v. Regents of U. of California at Berkeley, et al., 551 P. 2nd 334, (CA, 1976).

39. Lipari v. Sears, Roebuck & Co., 497 F. Supp. 185 (1980).

40. Case v. U.S., 523 F. Supp. 317 (1981).

41. Estate of Mathes v. Ireland, 419 N.E. 2nd 782 (IN, 1981). See also Edwards v. Clinton Valley Center, 360 N.W. 2nd 606 (MI, 1984), where no liability found against a public psychiatric hospital.

42. Brady v. Hooper, 570 F. Supp. 1333 (CO, 1983).

43. See Cairl v. State, 323 N.W. 2nd 20 (MN, 1982); Leedy v. Harnett, 510 F. Supp. 1125 (1981) and affirmed at 676 F. 2nd 686 (1982); Doyle v. U.S., 530 F. Supp. 1278 (1982); Matter of Estate of Votteler, 327 N.W. 2nd 759 (IA, 1982); Furr v. Spring Grove State Hospital, 454 A. 2nd 414 (MD, 1983).

44. Sherrill v. Wilson, 653 S.W. 2nd 661 (MO, 1983).

45. McIntosh v. Milano, 403 A. 2nd 500 (NJ, 1979); see also Brennan, R. (Jan. 14, 1983). Letters: Duty to warn third parties. *Journal of the American Medical Association, 249*(2), 191.

46. Durflinger v. Antiles, 673 P. 2nd 86 (KS, 1983).

47. Davis v. Lhim, 335 N.W. 2nd 481 (MI, 1983).

48. Chrite v. U.S., 564 F. Supp. 341 (1983).

49. Thompson v. Alameda, 614 P. 2nd 728 (CA, 1980); Jablonski v. U.S., 712 F. 2nd 391 (1983); Beck v. Kansas University Psychiatry Foundation, 580 F. Supp. 527 (1984);

Sharpe v. So. Carolina Dept. of Mental Health, 315 S.E. 2nd 112 (SC, 1984); Bardoni v. Kim, 390 N.W. 2nd 218 (MI, 1986).

50. Peterson v. State, 671 P. 2nd 230 (WA, 1983).
51. Hedlund v. Superior Court of Orange County, 669 P. 2nd 41 (CA, 1983).
52. Peck v. Counseling Service of Addison County, 499 A. 2nd 422 (VT, 1985). The jury found the plaintiffs comparatively negligent in causing their barn and its contents to be destroyed. The court found that the parents were aware of their son's inclination to violent behavior and they knew or should have known that the father's comments to the son would cause the son to become angry. Further, they knew that when he was angry he was capable of violent acts. The trial court found that the plaintiffs were 50 percent comparatively negligent. For further analysis of this case, see Anon. (1986). Note: Standard of care, duty, and causation in failure to warn actions against mental health professionals. *Vermont Law Review, 11*, 343.
53. Kentucky Revised Statutes Annotated, Chap. 202A, §202A.400. (Duty of qualified mental health professional to warn intended victim of patient's threat of violence.) (1986).
54. Rennie v. Klein, 462 F. Supp. 1131, at 1135-8 (1978); 653 F. 2nd 846; Rennie v. Klein, 102 S. Ct. 3506 (1982), remanded to 3rd Circuit as Rennie v. Klein, 720 F. 2nd 266 (1983).
55. Scott v. Plante, 532 F. 2nd 939 (1976). See also Winters v. Miller, 446 F. 2nd 65 (1971).
56. In re the Mental Health of K. K. B., 609 P. 2nd 747 (OK, 1980).
57. The courts use the term "psychotropic" interchangeably with "antipsychotic drug." See Rogers v. Okin, 634 F. 2nd 650, footnote 1 (Rogers II, 1980); Mills v. Rogers, 102 S. Ct. 24442 (1982); Rogers v. Commissioner of Dept. Mental Health, 458 N.E. 2nd 308 (MA, 1983).
58. In re the Mental Health of KKB., 609 P. 2nd 747, at 749, footnote 3 (OK, 1980).
59. Strunk v. Strunk, 445 S.W. 2nd 145 (KY, 1969). See also In re Weberlist, 360 N.Y.S. 2nd 783 (NY, 1974) in which the theory was used to justify nonemergency surgery for the benefit of an incompetent person.
60. In re Boyd, 403 A. 2nd 744 (DC, 1979).
61. In re the Mental Health of K. K. B., 609 P. 2nd 747 (OK, 1980).
62. Plotkin, J. (1978). Limiting the therapeutic orgy, mental patient's right to refuse treatment. *Northwestern University Law Review, 72*, 461.
63. Davis v. Hubbard, 506 F. Supp. 915 (1980).
64. Carter, J. (Sept. 1981), The use of psychotropics in the prison setting. *North Carolina Medical Journal, 42*(9), 645.
65. Youngberg v. Romeo, 102 S. Ct. 2452 (1982).
66. Rennie v. Klein, 102 S. Ct. 3506 (1982).
67. Decision is reported in Rennie v. Klein, 720 F. 2nd 266 (1983).
68. Mills v. Rogers, 102 S. Ct. 2442 (1982).
69. Rogers v. Okin, 738 F. 2nd 1 (1984), "Rogers III."
70. Youngberg v. Romeo, 102 S. Ct. 2452, 2462, footnote 30.
71. Woe v. Cuomo, 723 F. 2nd 895 (1984).
72. Mills v. Rogers, 102 S. Ct. 2442 (1982).
73. Rogers v. Okin, 478 F. Supp. 1342 (1979); "Rogers I."
74. Rogers v. Okin, 634 F. 2nd 650 (1980); "Rogers II."
75. Guardianship of Richard Roe III, 421 N.E. 2nd 40 (MA, 1981).
76. The U.S. Supreme Court will not decide cases that can be decided by applying state law, e.g., the "Roe" decision. Although *Rogers II* raised federal constitutional issues, it could be decided by applying state law. However, the findings in "Rogers I" and "Rogers II" are cited in subsequent cases, and are important when reviewing similar issues, but there were no holding (decisions) in these cases. The legal issue was finally resolved in *Rogers III*.

77. Rogers v. Commissioner of the Department of Mental Health, 458 N.E. 2nd 308 (MA, 1983).
78. Rogers v. Okin, 738 F. 2nd 1 (1984); "Rogers III."
79. Citing Superintendent of Belchertown State School v. Saikewicz, 370 N.E. 2nd 417 (MA, 1977).
80. Rogers v. Commissioner of the Department of Mental Health, 458 N.E. 2nd 308 (MA, 1983).
81. In re Boyd, 403 A. 2nd 744 (DC, 1979).
82. See Rogers v. Okin 478 F. Supp. 1342, 1375–1376, 1378 and note 49; Davis v. Hubbard, 506 F. Supp. 915, 926; Rennie v. Klein, 476 F. Supp. 1294, 1299; Halderman v. Pennhurst State School & Hospital, 446 F. Supp. 1295, 1307.
83. Guardianship of Roe, 421 N.E. 2nd 40, 54 (MA, 1981).
84. Massachusetts General Laws, Chap. 123, §21 (MA, 1984).
85. 104 Code of Massachusetts Regulations 20.08 (2) (MA, 1985).
86. Rogers v. Okin, 738 F. 2nd 1 (1984), "Rogers III." In July 1986 the U.S. District federal court, under the Civil Rights Act, awarded the team of attorneys who worked on the case over an 11-year period over one million dollars for 10,000 hours of legal work. That award is being appealed as excessive.
87. Rennie v. Klein, 102 S. Ct. 3506 (1982); remanded.
88. Rennie v. Klein, 720 F. 2nd 266 (1983). See also In re Mental Commitment of M. P., 500 N.E. 2nd 216 (IN, 1986).
89. R. A. J. v. Miller, 590 F. Supp. 1319 (1984). See also, a companion decision, R. A. J. v. Miller, 590 F. Supp. 1311 (1984) where a federal court found that the Texas Department of Mental Health and Mental Retardation failed to comply with a settlement agreement regarding patients at eight state facilities. The agreement required adequate patient treatment plans and documentation of same, adequate plans to protect the patients from harm, and adequate staff to insure minimally adequate patient care. The court ordered the defendants to submit their plan to show compliance. See also In re L. R., 497 A 2nd 753 (VT, 1985), where the Vermont Supreme Court ordered involuntary medication where it was shown that the patient's behavior changed dramatically when she refused medication.
90. Bee v. Greaves, 744 F. 2nd 1387 (1984); see also Vitek v. Jones, 100 S. Ct. 1254 (1980).
91. Bee v. Greaves, 744 F. 2nd 1387, footnote 2 (1984).
92. However, see In re the Mental Commitment of M. P., 500 N.E. 2nd 216 (IN, 1986) dissenting opinion at p. 223 where an argument was made that, under the facts of the case the professional judgment standard was an inappropriate standard when there is a need to resolve and balance "delicate constitutional rights and duties."
93. See, for example, Northern New Hampshire Mental Health Housing Inc. v. Town of Conway, 435 A. 2nd 136 (NH, 1981). See also, Deering's Annotated California (Welfare and Institutions) Code, §5115 (1970) and §5120 (1971).
94. Mental Health Association v. Deukmejian, 233 *California Reporter, 130* (CA, 1986). See also Society for Goodwill to Retarded Children v. Cuomo, 737 F. 2nd 1239 (1984); Phillips v. Thompson, 715 F. 2nd 365 (1983); Association for Retarded Citizens of North Dakota v. Olson, 561 F. Supp. 473 (1982).
95. Deering's Annotated California (Welfare and Institutions) Code, §5325.1 (1978).

8

ABORTION AND CONTRACEPTION

Conceptionally, this chapter deals with the constitutional right of privacy which serves as a basis for abortion and the attendent consent and notification issues. Many of the legal issues associated with the abortion cases parallel the contraception cases. It is worth noting that some state abortion statutes having progressed to the U.S. Supreme Court will be rewritten and reach the Supreme Court a second time. This illustrates that the abortion issue is not as well settled as one would expect in the more than a decade since the *Roe v. Wade* Supreme Court decision.

The case law has addressed such issues as the concept of viability, the rights of minors and husbands, and the funding of abortions. While access to abortion is fairly well resolved, the issue of parental notification continues to be tested in the courts.

In 1973, the United States Supreme Court handed down several precedent setting decisions on abortion. These cases established that a woman has a right to have an abortion, free from governmental interference. However, the right to have an abortion is not absolute. It is subject to limited governmental regulation in the early phase of pregnancy and increasing regulation as the pregnancy progresses. Most of the challenges to the abortion laws are directed at the first trimester period. The abortion decisions expanded the scope of earlier case law which had identified a right to privacy in the conduct of marital relations and in having access to birth control products.

> In 1965, the U.S. Supreme Court in *Griswold v. Connecticut* reversed a lower court decision which had found against a physician, employed by a planned parenthood clinic, for counseling a woman in the use of contraception.[1]

> Several years later the same court, in *Eisenstadt v. Baird*, ruled on the constitutionality of a state statute forbidding the dispensing of any contraceptive materials to unmarried persons and held that the right to be free from unwarranted government intrusion in so fundamental a decision (whether or not to have children) it applied to both married and unmarried persons.[2]

> Under the common law, an induced abortion done before "quickening," which occurred between the 16th and 18th week of pregnancy, was not an indictable offense, although an abortion after "quickening" was probably some degree of indictable offense. *Quickening* is the sensation felt by the pregnant woman of slight fluttering movements by the fetus and which gradually increase in intensity as the pregnancy progresses. Until the middle of the 19th century, English common law applied to abortions in this country. Connecticut, in 1821, was the first state to enact abortion legislation and it placed the emphasis on a woman "quick with child." By the end of the 1950s, the majority of jurisdictions banned abortions unless done to save the life of the mother. In 1967, the English Abortion Act permitted a licensed physician to perform an abortion

where two other licensed physicians agreed in a finding that continuation of the pregnancy would pose a risk to the life or mental well-being of the mother, or that the child, if born, would be at substantial risk of suffering such a physical or mental abnormality as to be seriously handicapped.[3]

EARLY DEVELOPMENT OF RIGHT TO PRIVACY

As early as 1890, legal writers held the position that the U.S. Constitution embodied a right to privacy. Shortly thereafter, the U.S. Supreme Court decided that individuals had the right to be free from invasion into their private lives.[4] The court in *Pierce v. Society of Sisters* extended the privacy concept to include family relationships.[5] By striking down a state law requiring all students to be educated in public schools, the court held that a right to privacy was inherent in such relationships.

CRIMINAL STATUTES AND ABORTION

The case that first challenged the abortion laws was *Roe v. Wade* which sought to invalidate a 1961 Texas criminal abortion statute.[6] At the time the decision was handed down, at least 36 states had statutes that imposed criminality. The Texas statute was typical of other abortion statutes which had been in effect in a number of states for many years. It made the procurement of or attempt to do an abortion a crime unless it was necessary to save the life of the mother. The suit, challenging the antiabortion statute, was brought in 1970 by a pregnant single woman in behalf of all women seeking a Texas abortion. The young woman wished to terminate her pregnancy by an abortion, performed by a competent, licensed physician, under safe clinical conditions. Because her life was not threatened by a continuation of the pregnancy, she was unable to secure an abortion in the state. She was financially unable to travel to another state to obtain a legal abortion. Her suit alleged that the state violated her rights under the Fourteenth Amendment.

The U.S. Constitution does not specifically mention a right of privacy. However, a number of legal decisions identified a concept of privacy right in the Fourteenth Amendment. This amendment holds that no state can enact laws which deprive an American citizen of "life, liberty, or property, without due process of law." Finding a fundamental guarantee of personal privacy, the judicial decisions extended the right to include activities inherent in the marriage relationship, such as procreation, contraception, and other family relationships. The *Roe* court found personal liberty (privacy right) sufficiently broad to embrace a woman's decision whether or not to terminate her pregnancy.

The Supreme Court recognized the responsibility of the state to protect and regulate the interests of different groups. The interests of a pregnant woman were balanced against those of the unborn baby. In essence, the decision attempted to distinguish two "compelling" state interests, one being, protection of maternal health and the other, protection of potential human life. Thus, the court held that, although the unborn child was not a "person," subject to constitutional protection, the state had an interest in protecting potential human life. In striking down the Texas statute, the Supreme Court said, "A state criminal abortion statute . . . that excepts from criminality only a life-saving procedure on the mother's behalf without regard to the stage of her pregnancy and other interests involved violate the Due Process Clause of the Fourteenth Amendment." The courts may not interfere with a woman's privacy right to decide to have an abortion; that is a matter between a woman and her doctor.

Conceptually, the two most important legal principles to emerge in the case were the fact that a woman's right to have an abortion was not *absolute* and the state's interest did not have the same weight throughout the 9-month pregnancy. The end of the first trimester (approximately 13 weeks) marked the parameter of the pregnant woman's health interest. The state has no compelling interest during the first trimester which would override the woman's right to privacy. The state interest increases as the pregnancy progresses. After the first trimester and up to the point of "viability" the state, in promoting its interest in the health of the mother, may regulate the abortion procedure, but only in ways that are reasonably related to maternal health. Examples of permissible state regulation include a requirement that all abortions be performed by licensed physicians and identification of the types of facility, whether hospital or clinic, at which abortions may be performed. The state interest in maintaining medical standards runs throughout a woman's pregnancy. After the point of viability, the state *may* regulate abortion, even to the point of prohibiting it, except when the abortion is necessary to preserve the life or health of the mother. While viability of the fetus allows the state to become involved in a woman's decision to abort, it does not give the fetus superior or equal status to the life of the mother.

PROCEDURAL CONSTRAINTS ON ABORTION

On the day that the *Roe* decision was handed down a companion case was also decided. The *Doe v. Bolton* case examined the procedural requirements of a Georgia criminal statute.[7] The U.S. Supreme Court struck down four of the procedural provisions. The main plaintiff in the suit was a 22-year-old indigent married woman who had been abandoned by her husband and was then living with her indigent parents, who had eight other children. The woman had three living children, the two oldest had been placed in a foster home because she was unable to care for them and her youngest had been placed for adoption. In addition, the woman had a history of emotional instability. She challenged the statute after a hospital abortion committee denied her an abortion. The statute required that a woman be a resident of the state, that two physicians confirm the primary physician's judgment; that approval from the hospital abortion committee be given, and that the abortion be done in a hospital which is accredited by the Joint Commission on Accreditation of Hospitals (JCAH). Additionally, the statute made the performance of an abortion a crime except when a licensed physician, applying "his best clinical judgment," determined that the pregnancy endangered the life or health of the woman, was a result of rape, or that the fetus would be born with a serious defect.

Addressing the physician's decision-making process in determining whether a woman's life or health interest would be affected by continuing the pregnancy, the court said, "medical judgment may be exercised in light of all the factors relevant to the well-being of the patient." Such factors may include physical, emotional, psychological, and familial findings, as well as, the woman's age. The court did not find the "best clinical judgment" provision in violation of any constitutional right. The court relied upon earlier decisions which held that a license, issued by the proper authorities, gives assurance that the holder possesses the required qualifications, and in the instance of a physician, this includes the ability to make medical judgments.

However, the court did find that the four other procedural requirements violated the U.S. Constitution. The state residency requirement violated the Privileges and Immunities clause of the Constitution. That clause provides protection for persons entering the state seeking medical services that are available in the state. The provision requiring an approval of the abortion by a hospital abortion committee placed an unreasonable burden on the woman seeking an abortion and should not be required because a primary physician would have already decided that the abortion was medically appropriate. In addition, the court found that no other surgical procedure required a special committee to clear the way for surgery. In striking down the provision requiring confirmation of the primary physician's judgment by two other physicians, the court said it could find no rational connection to the patient's need. No other circumstances required similar confirmation. Inherent in a physician's authority to practice is the fact that a physician is presumed capable of exercising acceptable clinical judgment and the provision unduly infringed on the physician's right to practice. Accepted standards of practice dictate when a physician is professionally bound to call in a consultant. If the court had upheld the provisions requiring committee approval and physician confirmation, each applicant would have had to have six physicians evaluate her abortion request. In ruling against the provision requiring abortions be performed only in JCAH facilities, the court said that it could find no link between the JCAH requirement and protection of the woman's health. No other surgical procedures were required to be done only in JCAH facilities. Extensive evidence was presented to show that facilities other than a hospital were adequate to fully meet the needs of a woman undergoing an abortion. Thus, the door was opened to doing abortions in other than hospital settings. The court recognized that a state has a right to adopt regulations applicable to abortion facilities so long as they are connected to the state interest of protecting maternal health.

As an interesting side note, seven registered nurses joined nine physicians in the plaintiff's suit. All professionals were licensed to practice in

Georgia. They alleged that the abortion statute "chilled and deterred" them from practicing their respective professions as guaranteed by the U.S. Constitution. The court held that the physicians had standing to join in the suit because they could be prosecuted under the criminal statute if they performed an abortion. However, the nurses had no standing to join in the suit. No potential for personal detriment existed for them because they were not licensed physicians. They would be reached by the abortion statute only in their capacity as accessories or as counselor-conspirators.

By way of contrast, the *Roe v. Wade* decision dealt primarily with the criminality aspect that states sought to attach to abortions, whereas *Doe v. Bolton* dealt with procedural impediments to a right to have an abortion. The *Doe* decision was based on a patient's need test.

CONCEPT OF VIABILITY

The issue of viability was considered in *Roe v. Wade* in the context of delineating the compelling state interest to protect the fetus after viability. The case defined *viability* as the point at which the fetus is "potentially able to live outside the mother's womb, albeit with artificial aid," and presumably capable of "meaningful life outside the mother's womb." In the wake of the 1973 abortion decisions, the Missouri legislature enacted legislation which it thought would be consistent with the court rulings. The plaintiffs in *Planned Parenthood of Central Missouri v. Danforth* challenged the constitutionality of a number of statutory provisions.[8] Among the challenges were three directed toward the viability issue. The viability provisions under attack included the statutory definition of viability; a prohibition against saline abortion after the first 12 weeks of pregnancy; and a requirement that the physician exercise professional care to preserve the fetus's life and health.

The statute defined viability as "that stage of fetal development when the life of the unborn child may be continued indefinitely outside the womb by natural or artificial life-supportive systems." The plaintiffs argued that the wording expanded the *Roe v. Wade* definition by failing to indicate a gestational time period or reflect the three stages of pregnancy. The mere possibility, they argued, of fleeting survival was not the medical standard of viability. The plaintiffs alleged that it was a function of the legislature to specify a specific point in the gestation period at which viability comes into being. The nation's highest court held that the Missouri viability definition did not conflict with the *Roe* definition which said that viability was a matter of medical judgment, skill, and technical ability. The high court, in *Danforth*, stated, "The time when viability is achieved may vary with each pregnancy, and the determination of whether a particular fetus is viable is, and must be, a matter for the judgment of the responsible attending physician." It is interesting to note that an earlier case had struck down a state statute that provided that a fetus would be considered potentially viable during the second half of its gestation period.[9] That court held that the definition was unreasonable, as no evidence of viability at 20 weeks had been presented.

Another statutory provision in the Missouri law prohibited saline abortions beyond the first trimester. Such abortions were categorized as, "deleterious to maternal health." The plaintiffs charged that the statute operated to preclude virtually all abortions after the first trimester. At that time, a substantial majority of all abortions performed in this country after the first trimester were accomplished by saline abortions. In order to find the prohibition valid, the court would have had to find that the restriction was reasonably related to the life and health of the mother. The court, in examining all the factors relevant to the issue, determined that the provision was unreasonable and struck it down. The court found that the alternative methods of hysterotomy and hysterectomy were, and remain today, more dangerous for the woman than the saline method. It also found that the mortality rate for normal childbirth exceeded the rate for saline abortion and that saline abortion was an accepted medical procedure in the United States. Although, today prostaglandin amnio infusion is a safe and widely used abortion agent, at the time of the decision it had been in use a short time and many physicians were unfamiliar with the method. Additionally, prostaglandin was sold only to a few medical centers in the country. Such recognition of the restrictive provision would have exposed the woman to unnecessary risk by forcing her physician to terminate her pregnancy by employing methods more dangerous to her health than the proscribed saline abortion.

The court also struck down the Missouri provision requiring a physician to exercise a standard of medical care that would preserve the fetus's life and health. The court found the provision too broad because it applied the standard to the entire pregnancy. In essence, it would require that life-support systems be instituted regardless of the phase of pregnancy. The plaintiffs argued that the provision that required the physician to use a procedure which would preserve the "fetus's life and health" would preclude abortion at any phase of pregnancy. The provision imposed a manslaughter charge against a physician for failing to utilize a standard of care equal to one that would be required to preserve the life and health of a fetus intended to be born.

In determining which abortion procedure would be best for the mother, the courts have allowed considerable physician discretion. The courts have not been receptive to statutory provisions which mandate that a physician use one method over another when the prime reason is to use the procedure least harmful to the fetus. However, where such a requirement would not interfere with either the physician's right to decide or increase the risk to the woman's health, the constitutionality of such a statute would likely be upheld. Viability remains a critical concept in determining the competing interests in abortion cases.

In 1974, Pennsylvania enacted legislation in an attempt to overcome successful constitutional attacks on statutory provisions requiring protection of a viable fetus.

The statute set out the criteria whereby a physician would be criminally liable if the physician performed an abortion on a fetus that was known or believed to be viable.[10] It required the physician to determine whether a fetus "is viable" or "may be viable," and if so, to use the abortion method which best insured a live birth. The U.S. Supreme Court ruled that the provision was unconstitutional due to its vagueness. The court said that it was unclear whether the viability determination was to be based on the physician's professional judgment, as required by *Danforth*, or some other standard, such as the judgment of an average physician. A determination of viability must be made by the attending physician in the context of the particular facts of the case. The court also held invalid the provision requiring the least harmful technique to the fetus. Evidence determined that the method most favorable to women was the saline abortion and this was almost always fatal to the fetus. The high court ruling affirmed prior case law that the mother's right to a safe abortion is superior.

DUTY OWED TO A LIVE ABORTED FETUS

A number of states have enacted legislation requiring care of an infant born alive during an abortion.[11]

A California law in effect since 1976 reads, "The rights to medical treatment of an infant prematurely born alive in the course of an abortion shall be the same as the rights of an infant of similar medical status prematurely born spontaneously."[12] The statute was enacted after complaints that some live aborted fetuses had been left unattended to die.

There have been a number of newspaper accounts of live births following planned abortions. In one case, a woman underwent a saline abortion procedure and went into labor 3 days later. The woman delivered a 2-pound, 9-ounce live infant. The parents were able to take the infant home within a month.[13] In another more complex case, a 17-year-old girl sought custody of her infant which was born alive after an abortion procedure. The infant was 19 weeks into the gestation period and weighed less than 2 pounds at birth. The state's abortion law regarded the infant as "abandoned" and awarded the state temporary custody. Hearings were held to determine the interest of the mother in keeping the infant and her ability to care for the infant.[14]

In the only reported case involving a criminal conviction for the murder of a newborn after an abortion procedure, a Texas physician was sentenced to a 15-year prison term.[15] The defendant physician argued that the infant was not born alive, but a jury agreed with witnesses who testified that the infant which was aborted by a hysterotomy was suffocated when the physician placed the placenta over her face and then immersed her in a surgical bucket filled with water. The jury conviction was upheld when the appeals court found that there was evidence of fetal development, observed signs of life, and held that the conduct of the physician justified a finding that the infant was born alive.

Summary to Preceding Content

The legal background for the abortion cases began when the courts held that individuals had the right to be free from invasion into their private lives. The test case which immediately preceded the 1973 *Roe v. Wade* decision involved the U.S. Supreme Court review of a Connecticut statute which was found to invade a right to privacy in the conduct of marital relations. *Roe v. Wade* relied on the concept of a constitutionally protected right of privacy when it was decided.

The concept of *viability* is important because the states' interest increases with viability. Viability was analyzed in depth in *Planned Parenthood of Missouri v. Danforth*. It held that viability must necessarily vary with each pregnancy and it was not feasible to legislate a specific time at which viability exists. The judgment of when viability exists must be a medical decision. A number of states have enacted statutes regulating the care that must be provided when an aborted fetus is born alive.

PARENTAL CONSENT TO AN ABORTION

Since the precedent-setting 1973 abortion ruling there have been a number of legal decisions defining the scope of *Roe v. Wade*. The cases have dealt with such diverse legal issues as state regulation of abortion clinics[16] and interpretation of municipal zoning bylaws. The bylaws issue arose when communities sought to prevent the establishment of abortion clinics.[17] Perhaps the most litigated issue in the abortion cases involved the question of parental authority to prevent an abortion procedure on a minor child.

Twice, since the original abortion decisions, the U.S. Supreme Court has dealt with a minor's decision to have an abortion. Both state statutes were challenged because they gave parents a veto power over the minor's decision to have an abortion.

The case that first tested the parental consent requirement (*Danforth*) was the same case that addressed the viability issue.[18] A section of the Missouri statute governing abortion required the written consent of a parent unless "the abortion is certified by a licensed physician as necessary in order to preserve the life of the mother." The U.S. Supreme Court held that the state lacked the constitutional authority to give a third party an absolute (and possibly arbitrary) veto over the decision of the physician and the minor patient to terminate the pregnancy.

Waiting in the wings was a Massachusetts abortion statute that was about to undergo a long course of judicial review. While the law was drafted with some imagination it ultimately allowed a third party, a judge, to have absolute veto over the minor's decision. Massachusetts, in 1974, enacted a parental consent statute which applied to minors seeking an abortion. The law was tested in various courts before it was implemented in a modified form in April 1981.[19] The statute, in its original form and subsequent modification, went before the U.S. Supreme Court twice, in 1976 and 1979.[20] The law required the consent of both parents. If one or both of the minor's parents refused to give their consent, it could be obtained by order of a judge for good cause. Drafters of the law sought to satisfy constitutional requirements by giving the pregnant minor an option to a parental veto.

However, when *Bellotti v. Baird* ("Bellotti II") came before the U.S. Supreme Court a second time in 1979, it was found to infringe on the minor's rights and was held unconstitutional for two reasons. First, the statute required parental consultation or notification in every instance and did not permit the minor to seek an independent court determination in regard to her competency (maturity) to consent or that an abortion would be in her best interests. Second, the court was permitted to withhold authorization to have an abortion from a minor even though she demonstrated that she was a "mature" minor.[21] The U.S. Supreme Court found the statute potentially more restrictive than the Missouri law because it articulated a clear veto to an abortion. A *mature minor* is a minor who is capable of making an informed decision despite the fact that she has not attained the age of majority. The mature minor rule was recognized previously in a case where an 18-year-old minor sought authorization for elective plastic surgery on her nose.[22]

Historically the courts have recognized and given great weight to parental rights. However, these rights must be balanced in order that they do not obstruct the pregnant minor's right of access to an abortion. The Supreme Court opinion did express a preference that parental consent be sought by the minor when possible. Four of the justices included guidelines in their written opinion as to how a parental consent statute could be written to survive future constitutional challenge. The suggested procedure indicated that the minor must be permitted the opportunity to go directly to the court without consulting with her parents if she did not wish to do so. If she is able to satisfy the court that she is capable of making a well-informed decision on her own, her decision must prevail. If she is unable to show that she is a mature minor, she must then be permitted to show that an abortion nevertheless would be in her best interest. The judge would be able to block her decision to abort only if he is unconvinced of her competency to make such a decision or that such a decision is not in her best interests.

After the second U.S. Supreme Court *Bellotti* decision in 1979, the Massachusetts legislature enacted a statute which was drafted according to the guidelines laid out in that decision.[23] The statutory provision provides an alternative to parental consent by allowing a pregnant minor to elect to seek judicial consent if she wishes. Judicial authorization for an abortion shall be given if the minor is found to be mature, or lacking maturity, it is in her best interest to have an abortion. In 1981, a federal court rejected a challenge to the latest parental consent provision, holding that it reflected the U.S. Supreme Court's view that the state's interest in protecting minors from immature decisions regarding abortions justified the procedural burdens which might be imposed by the statute.[24]

Although the federal court, in 1981, upheld the Massachusetts minor consent provisions in the statute, it struck down a provision requiring women of all ages to sign a consent form 24 hours before having an abortion. The court said that it imposed a burden in terms of time, money, travel, and work schedules and that such a provision served no purpose. The federal court also held unconstitutional a provision requiring the consent form to contain a description of fetal development at the time the abortion is to be performed. The form contained a detailed statement of the size and condition of a fetus during the first 20 weeks of life. The court held that the description of the fetus "presents no information whose essence most, if not all, women do not understand before receiving it." The federal court upheld a provision in the consent form which described various abortion procedures and possible complications, as well, as citing the availability of alternatives to abortion. However, 2 months later, the U.S. Supreme Court, in *H. L. v. Matheson*, when reviewing a Utah abortion consent law, struck down a similarly worded description provision, as well, as a clause requiring a 24-hour waiting period.

Shortly after the 1980 Massachusetts minor consent law went into effect, it was again tested in a state court when a judge, hearing a 14-year-old minor's petition for an abortion, declined to approve her request until she had consulted with at least one of her parents.[25] The judges decision in *Matter of Mary Moe* was immediately appealed to a higher state court which held that the judge had erred in requiring consultation with one parent because the minor consent law was designed specifically to provide a mechanism for judicial consent when a minor could not or did not want to involve her parent(s) in her abortion decision. The court said that when the judge made a finding, based on the minor's answers to questions and her courtroom demeanor, that she lacked the maturity to give an informed consent, the statute required him to move to the next level of inquiry, that is, to determine whether an abortion would be in her "best interest." When the judge determined that the minor lacked significant life experience, as well as any understanding of the responsibilities of motherhood, and the likelihood that she could be further along in the pregnancy than she suspects, his conclusion that action ought to be taken at that time was correct and he should not have made the abortion conditioned on parental consultation. The Massachusetts statute gave an unconditional judicial alternative. The court said that although the judicial alternative may have been less favored by the legislature when it enacted the statute, it was no less an available choice. "As a general proposition, not of law, but of human relations, the question whether to have an abortion is better solved with parental guidance than with judicial authorization . . . however, there are instances where the relationship between a daughter and her parents is such that this may not be so." The court said that if during the judicial proceedings it develops that the minor has not even considered talking to her parents or that the family is a loving and supporting one, the judge hearing the minor's petition may counsel her to consult with her family and offer to stay the proceedings while she does so. However, he may not insist on the parental consultation, as that is in direct conflict with the intent of the statute.

In 1983 the U.S. Supreme Court reviewed two city ordinances which raised several questions, including the minor abortion consent issue. In the wake of "Bellotti II" which laid out the guidelines which must be met in abortion consent cases involving minors the cities of Akron, Ohio, and Kansas City, Missouri enacted ordinances dealing with parental consent. Both included other provisions which will be examined later.

In *City of Akron v. Akron Center for Reproductive Health,* a physician was prohibited from doing an abortion on an unmarried minor under the age of 15 unless the physician either obtained the consent of one of her parents or a court ordered that the abortion be performed.[26] The court said that such a provision was unconstitutional in the absence of a provision authorizing the juvenile courts to inquire into the minor's maturity or emancipation. Citing *Danforth* and "Bellotti II," the court held that the Akron ordinance could not impose a "blanket determination that all minors under the age of 15 are too immature to make this decision or that an abortion never may be in the minor's best interest without parental approval." In short, the ordinance lacked a provision that would require inquiry into a minor's maturity level or emancipation status.

The City of Akron case must be distinguished from the second case, *Planned Parenthood Association of Kansas City, Missouri v. Ashcroft* at least as to the parental consent issue.[27] While the Akron ordinance was struck down the Kansas City ordinance was upheld because it met the standard set out in both *Danforth* and "Bellotti II." The Kansas City ordinance prevailed because it provided an alternative procedure whereby a minor may show that she is sufficiently mature to make the decision to abort herself, or lacking maturity, an abortion would be in her best interest. Thus, the judicial alternative standard was satisfied because: (1) a provision permitted the reviewing court to outright confer on the minor the same right to consent as a woman in her majority, or (2) to find that an abortion is in the "best interests" of the minor, or (3) deny the petition indicating the grounds. The ordinance required that the court hear evidence on "the emotional development, maturity, intellect, and understanding of the minor." Thus, the court held that the granting or denial of the abortion petition must be supported by "good cause," that is, evidence for or against the granting of the abortion request.

In the wake of these later cases there have been challenges to the process whereby a judge has determined that a minor lacked the maturity to make an informed abortion decision. In *Matter of Mary Moe*, an appeals court held that a decision by a judge at a lower court proceeding that a 16-year-old was not sufficiently mature to be capable of consenting to an abortion, was in error.[28] Based on the evidence the appeals court found the young woman mature and capable of giving an informed consent to an abortion procedure. Conversely, in *Matter of T. P.*, an Indiana court upheld the trial judge's denial of waiver of parental consent.[29] The state high court held that the trial judge's decision to deny parental waiver to a 16-year-old young woman was proper in view of the fact that she had an abortion with her parents' consent 6 months previously, but she did not want them to know of the second pregnancy. She testified that informing her parents would have an adverse effect on their relationship. She said that although birth control means had been explained to her she did not use any because she thought her parents would not approve of it.

PARENTAL NOTIFICATION

In early 1981, the U.S. Supreme Court in *H. L. v. Matheson* upheld a Utah abortion notification law. Agreeing with the lower courts, the case held that the statute "plainly served important state interests."[30] The statute requires physicians to inform parents, "if possible," that their minor daughter has requested an abortion. The case held that Utah, as well as other states, are free to set up a parent notification statutory provision if the following situations exist: (1) the minor girl is living with and dependent on her parents; (2) she is not married or emancipated; (3) she has made no assertion that she is mature enough to make the abortion decision for herself, or that her relationship with her parents might be seriously affected by notification. This last section partially acknowledges the "mature minor rule."

The Utah law was challenged by a 15-year-old girl who did not want her parents to know about her pregnancy. Her physician refused to do the procedure without notifying her parents. The minor claimed that the law interfered with her right to consult freely with her treating physician and to secure treatment in terminating the pregnancy. She ultimately had an abortion in a state other than Utah.

Specifically, the state law on abortion stated that the physician, in the exercise of his best clinical judgment, must notify, if possible, the parents or guardian of the woman upon whom the abortion is to be performed, is a minor. The court said that the statute was not unconstitutional and did not invade the minor's right to privacy. The statute did not place any restrictions upon the minor's decision to terminate her pregnancy. The court held that the parents would be in a position to provide valuable information as regards factors which the physician may want to consider in exercising his best judgment. Further, such a statute would serve to encourage an unmarried pregnant minor to seek parental advice in determining whether or not to bear the child or terminate the pregnancy. The statute also contained a provision that required that the consent form contain a description of the human fetus, as well as requiring the pregnant woman to wait 24 hours after signing the consent form before having the abortion. The U.S. Supreme Court struck down both provisions.

Two subsequent lower federal court decisions struck down other parental notification provisions. However, both reaffirmed the principle that a state's interest in protecting immature minors will permit a constitutional parental notification law. In *Indiana Planned Parenthood v. Pearson*, the court struck down an immature minor notification provision because it lacked an expeditious due process appeal procedure if in electing the alternative juvenile court procedure an adverse court decision is rendered.[31] The court held that an appeal procedure must be provided and the time frame for such an appeal must not be prolonged. In *Zbaraz v. Hartigan* a federal appeals court struck down the parental notification provision in the Illinois abortion statute.[32] The court held that a sufficient state interest existed to protect the immature minor when making an abortion decision, but the law must provide an alternative procedure to parental notification. Further, a provision requiring a 24-hour delay after parental notification was unconstitutional because it placed a direct and substantial burden on the minor.

SPOUSAL CONSENT

Although a number of states had ruled that a husband could not prevent his wife from aborting a pregnancy, it was not until the *Danforth* case that the issue came before the U.S. Supreme Court.[33] One state court held that an estranged husband could not prevent his wife from having a nontherapeutic abortion, even though the husband agreed to support and take custody of the child after its birth.[34] Another court held that, even though the natural potential father wanted to marry the pregnant woman and alleged that his own health would be affected if the pregnancy was terminated, the woman's right to abort was personal to her and no right to participate in the abortion decision rested with the natural potential father.[35]

Among the many abortion issues in *Danforth*, one questioned the statutory section requiring spousal consent to an abortion.[36] The nation's highest court held that the Missouri statute was inconsistent with the 1973 *Roe* abortion ruling. Although the decision whether to undergo or to forego an abortion may have profound effects on the future of any marriage, and the states historically had enacted legislation recognizing joint decision making by the marriage partners (adoption, artificial insemination, and disposition of jointly held property), the court ruled that the state had no constitutional authority to prohibit the wife from terminating her pregnancy, when the state itself lacked such a right. When a wife and a husband disagree on the abortion decision, only one decision can prevail. Inasmuch as it is the woman who is more directly affected by the pregnancy, the balance, the court said, must weigh in her favor.

In the most recent case, *Coleman v. Coleman,* a Maryland husband sought to stop his wife from having an abortion.[37] Following the law in *Danforth,* the state court held that a husband's consent to a wife's abortion during the first trimester is unnecessary and no state legislature can confer such a right.

SPOUSAL NOTIFICATION

The issue of spousal notification was first tried in a Utah federal court in 1981.

In *S. W. v. Wilkinson* a pregnant woman sought to strike down the provision which required a physician "if possible" to notify the husband of the intended abortion.[38] The woman was separated from her husband and was seeking a divorce. The woman testified that her husband would beat her if he knew she wanted an abortion.[39] The trial court held that the statute was constitutional because it did not prevent an abortion, but merely required that the woman's husband be told.

In another reported spousal notification decision a federal court, reviewing a 1982 Florida statute, held the law unconstitutional.[40] The law, which was tested in *Scheinberg v. Smith,* required a wife who was not separated or estranged to give her husband notice of her intent to have an abortion. The state argued that the law was designed to provide the husband with an opportunity to consult with the wife about the proposed abortion. The state also argued that it had a compelling state interest in maintaining and promoting the marital relationship and in protecting the husband's interest in the procreative potential of the marriage. Thus, the real issue before the court was whether the abortion procedure posed a substantial risk of decreasing the wife's future fertility prospects. After hearing testimony and statistics on the types of procedures used the court held that the state failed to show that the risk of infertility was increased. The testimony demonstrated that the procedures used during the first trimester were suction or vacuum aspiration and that 9 out of every 10 abortions performed in Florida were in the first trimester, using a suction or vacuum aspiration. Statistics, admitted into evidence, indicated that the rate of major complications for the suction technique were only 0.4 percent and further, not all major complications would adversely effect a woman's future child bearing potential.

Summary to Parental and Spousal Consent and Notification of Abortion

Three years after the 1973 *Roe v. Wade* decision, the U.S. Supreme Court issued the rule that parents did not have an absolute veto over a minor child's decision to have an abortion. In the *Danforth* case, the U.S. Supreme Court held that a state does have an interest in protecting immature minors and that such a state interest will sustain a requirement of a consent substitute, either parental or judicial. Statutes that also give the judge an absolute veto over the minor's decision, without hearing evidence with regard to the minor's maturity level, were also struck down. Where a minor could demonstrate that she had sufficient maturity to make an abortion decision (informed choice), the "mature minor" rule came into play. If the mature minor rule was not argued when the minor sought judicial consent rather than parental consent, the judge could alternatively make a ruling that an abortion would be in the minor's "best interests." The scenario was that after the 1976 *Danforth* case, which held that the state lacked the constitutional authority to give a third party an absolute veto over the minor and physician's decision to terminate the pregnancy, the U.S. Supreme Court issued guidelines in the 1979 "Bellotti II" decision. Since that time most of the parental consent cases have been heard in respective state and federal trial courts.

    Danforth also held that a pregnant woman's constitutional right to privacy precluded any right the husband might have to prevent the abortion, at least until the point of viability when the balance may shift. As one would expect, there were not the number of test cases surrounding the husband's right as in the parental consent cases. This is because in the spousal situation there was no right, whereas in the parental cases such a right could be recognized and the states drafted laws that had to be tested in the courts.

    Just about the time when the parental consent cases were resolving the issues, the parental notification to abortion cases were being argued in the U.S. Supreme Court. When that court reviewed a Utah parental notification statute in 1981, it held that notification laws "plainly served important state interests" and recognized the circumstances under which such a law would pass constitutional scrutiny. As in the abortion consent cases, the courts invoked inquiry into the minor's maturity or emancipation status. The courts will also review a decision by a judge that, based on the facts, the petitioning minor failed to present evidence sufficient to pass the mature minor test.

When confronted with a case involving spousal notification of the wife's intention to have an abortion, a Utah federal trial court upheld the spousal notification law, saying that it did not prevent the abortion, but merely required that the husband be told, if possible. However, another federal court in Florida held that spousal notification, at least based on the argument that the husband has an interest in preventing infertility, was unconstitutional. These two decisions demonstrate the importance of respective state laws. Some will be held to comply with constitutional guidelines and will be upheld, whereas, others will fail the constitutional scrutiny test.

CONTRACEPTIVES

Eight years before the first U.S. Supreme Court abortion decision, that same court considered the constitutionality of a Connecticut statute which prohibited the use of contraceptives by married couples.[41] The court said that the state law was an unconstitutional infringement on the right of marital privacy. The case was to be cited frequently in subsequent cases recognizing a right of privacy in medical treatment decisions. The *Quinlan* case was the first in a long line of cases which based its holding on the precept of a right to privacy. (See Chapter 9, Medical Treatment Issues: The Basis for Legal Decisions.) Sometime later, the U.S. Supreme Court held that a Massachusetts statute permitting married persons to obtain contraceptives to prevent pregnancy, but prohibited the distribution of contraceptives to single persons, violated the equal protection clause of the Fourteenth Amendment.[42]

In 1977 the U.S. Supreme Court, in *Carey v. Population Services International*, struck down a New York law which made the selling or distribution of nonprescription contraceptives to minors under the age of 16 years a crime.[43] The court held that access was a constitutionally protected right of privacy and, as such, decisions affecting procreation applied equally to minors and adults.

The case that tested parental notice prior to counseling minors was *Doe v. Irwin*.[44] That court held that parental notice was unconstitutional. The suit was brought by parents against the administrator of a publicly operated family planning clinic because the parents were opposed to their minor children receiving contraceptive information, devices, and medicines without their knowledge. The parents argued that most adolescents do not have the capacity to make birth control decisions or to understand the physical and psychological risks involved in choosing and using a contraceptive.

The court recognized three rights: the minor's right of access; the parents' right to care, nurture and have custody of their children; and the state interest in the health and welfare of all its inhabitants. The court also spent considerable time examining the day-to-day operative policies of the clinic. The minors were served without regard to whether or not they were emancipated and they were not asked if they had parental consent. The parents were not notified once the contraceptives were given, but the policy of the clinic was to require a mandatory preprescription "rap" session. If the parents made inquiry, they were encouraged to attend these sessions. Minors who attended were encouraged to discuss their sexual interests with their parents and the session leaders offered to help the minors talk with their parents. The sessions were conducted by a counselor with a master's degree in social work and students pursuing a career in medicine or social work. The minors who went to the voluntary clinic were required to have a physical examination and only if there were no medical problem was the device or medication prescribed. The decision whether the minor would receive birth control pills was made by a physician and the minor was required to have a follow-up physical if she returned after depleting her initial 3-month supply.

The parents were unsuccessful in their attempt to invoke a Fourteenth Amendment liberty right, as the court said that there was no constitutional obligation on the clinic to notify them, even though the parents may wish to know of such activities. Addressing the state interest, the court held that its interest was not compelling enough to overcome the minor's right of privacy.

Federal Regulation of Birth Control and Minors

In 1970, Congress enacted the Public Health Service Act which provides a broad range of family planning services to eligible individuals including minors.[45] In 1981, Congress passed an amendment to the act and inserted language whereby it sought to "encourage family participation" in such family planning matters. Subsequently, the Department of Health and Human Services (HHS) promulgated regulations known as the "squeal rule" which would have required federally funded family planning clinics to inform the parents of unemancipated minors under 18 years that a contraceptive device had been prescribed.

The rule was to go into effect in February 1983, but just before the implementation date two federal courts, one in Washington, D.C. and one in New York enjoined the regulations.[46] HHS appealed the injunction, but the federal appeals court held that the regulations were inconsistent with Congress's intent and purpose when it enacted the amendment. Further, the court held that the regulations exceeded the Secretary's delegated authority.[47] HHS decided not to appeal the decision and in December 1983 it withdrew the regulations.

Shortly after HHS decided to abandon the regulations at Utah law requiring parental notification when birth control devices were prescribed was struck down.[48]

In *Planned Parenthood Association of Utah v. Matheson*, the court determined that a significant percentage of sexually active minors would not cease their sexual activity if access to contraceptives was conditioned on parental notification. The law provided that any person providing contraceptives to a minor shall notify, "whenever possible" the minor's parents or guardian of such services. The court reasoned that the law would expose sexually active minors to the health risks of early pregnancy and venereal disease.

Likening this case to the parental notification required for abortion, the court held that the "state may not impose a blanket parental notification requirement on minors seeking to exercise their constitutionally protected right to decide whether to bear or to beget a child by using contraceptives." The court also found that the state law failed to include "a procedure whereby a mature minor or a minor who can demonstrate that his or her best interests are contrary to parental notification can obtain contraceptives confidentially."

Summary

Much of the law that deals with contraceptives parallels the abortion law. In 1965 when the U.S. Supreme Court reviewed a Connecticut law which prohibited the use of contraceptives by married couples, it promptly struck the law down because it infringed on marital rights. In 1972 The U.S. Supreme Court struck down a Massachusetts law which prohibited the distribution of contraceptives to single persons. It was not until 1977 that the same court ruled that laws prohibiting minor access to contraceptives were also unconstitutional. Having decided that access to contraceptives by minors was constitutionally protected the case law then proceeded to the issue of parental notification. In reviewing this issue, the U.S. Supreme Court in 1980 acknowledged the minor's access right, the parental right to care for and counsel their minor children, and the states' interest in the well-being of its citizens. The Court held that the minor's privacy rights were paramount. In 1983, HHS sought to promulgate regulations requiring all federally funded family planning clinics to notify the parents of minors that contraceptive devices had been prescribed. After two lower federal courts enjoined the implementation of the regulations HHS elected to withdraw them. Several weeks later a Utah law was struck down by another federal court when it tested the constitutionality of parental notification. In sum, the courts have consistently ruled against both state and federal laws that have required the physician or clinic to notify the parents that contraceptives were prescribed.

THE MOST RECENT SUPREME COURT DECISIONS

Since the 1973 *Roe v. Wade* decision many states have enacted abortion statutes.

In 1983, the U.S. Supreme Court heard three important cases. While all three cases involved specific abortion provisions, one, *Simopoulos v. Virginia* was brought to overturn the criminal conviction of a physician who performed an abortion on a 17-year-old student at his unlicensed clinic.[49] All three decisions, which were decided the same day, reviewed state laws that sought to spell out the type of facility in which second trimester abortions could be performed. The Simopoulos case raised the single issue of the facility, whereas *City of Akron v. Akron Center for Reproductive Health, Inc.*[50] and *Planned Parenthood Association of Kansas City, Missouri, Inc. v. Ashcroft*[51] raised the facility issue as well as a number of other issues.

In *Simopoulos*, a board-certified obstetrician-gynecologist performed a saline abortion on a young woman who was 5 months pregnant. Virginia law required that all second trimester abortions must be performed in licensed hospitals. The physician's clinic was not licensed and he had never applied for a license. After instilling the saline the young woman and her boyfriend went to a motel to deliver the fetus. The physician gave the couple an instruction sheet which counseled the patient to go to a hospital when labor began. An investigation was begun when the woman aborted the fetus 48 hours later and it was discarded in the motel. The physician was convicted for unlawfully performing an abortion during the second trimester outside of a licensed hospital.

Regulation of Second Trimester Abortions

All three cases dealt with provisions that required that second trimester abortions be performed in hospitals. However, the Virginia provision was the only one upheld, and the physician's criminal conviction was affirmed. The cities of Akron, Ohio and Kansas City, Missouri required that all second trimesters be performed in "general, acute care facilities," whereas Virginia required them to be performed only in licensed "hospitals." Virginia included licensed outpatient facilities in the hospital category. The court held that the Virginia provision was a reasonable means for furthering the states' compelling interest in protecting a woman's own health and safety. In holding the Akron, Ohio and Kansas City, Missouri provisions unconstitutional, the court said the "acute care hospital only" provision unreasonably infringed on a woman's right to have a second trimester abortion.

Twenty-Four-Hour Waiting Period

A number of states enacted abortion statutes which included a mandatory 24-hour waiting period from the time the consent form was signed to the actual abortion procedure itself. In the *City of Akron* case, the city argued that such a provision furthered its interest in insuring that the woman's decision was made after careful consideration of all the facts. However, the U.S. Supreme Court found the waiting period inflexible and without any medical justification. The court added that the mandated wait increased the cost of the abortion by making the woman return to the facility a second time and may also have increased the risks of an abortion if scheduling conflicts further delayed the surgery. However, it is worth noting that the court took notice of the recommendation by the American College of Obstetricians and Gynecologists (ACOG) that a clinic allow "sufficient time for the woman to reflect on her decision prior to making an informed decision."[52] The court reasoned that a physician should have the discretion to advise the woman to defer the abortion when he believes she will benefit from the deferment.

After this decision, a 1986 U.S Supreme Court decision, reviewing a similar provision in the Pennsylvania abortion statute, held that a mandatory 24-hour waiting period was arbitrary and infringed on the physician's discretion in the exercise of a medical judgment.[53] That suit, *Thornburgh v. American College of Obstetricians*, was brought by physicians against state officials.

In 1986 the U.S. Supreme Court in *Diamond v. Charles* held that it had no jurisdiction to hear an appeal of the federal appeals court decision holding the Illinois abortion statute unconstitutional.[54] The Pennsylvania (*Thornburgh*) and Illinois (*Charles v. Daley*) statutes contained similar provisions and will be discussed presently.

Informed Consent Counseling by a Physician Only

The *City of Akron* case also held that a provision requiring only a physician to counsel the woman when obtaining the informed consent was unconstitutional. The practice at the clinics was that the counseling was done by individuals other than the attending physician. Although in the earlier case of *Commonwealth v. Menillo* the U.S. Supreme Court stressed the importance of the physician–patient relationship, when it held that only a physician may perform abortions, the *City of Akron* court said it was not convinced that the state had a compelling reason to insist that the consent be obtained only by a physician.[55] The court said the critical state interest was not who obtained the consent, but whether the woman's consent was an informed and unpressured one.

However, the court was careful to point out that a physician may not abdicate his essential role as the individual ultimately responsible for the medical aspects of the abortion decision. The court suggested that a state may define the physician's responsibility to verify that adequate counseling had been given, as well as legislate the "reasonable minimum qualifications" for individuals who perform the counseling function.

Subject Matter of the Consent

The *City of Akron* Supreme Court decision also struck down the following provisions relevant to the specific points to be disclosed when obtaining the consent. These included the date of possible viability, developmental stage of the fetus, possible physical and emotional complications that may result from the abortion, the availability of agencies offering childbirth assistance and adoption placement service. The Supreme Court held that the provisions went beyond the permissible limits associated with the state's interest in promoting the informed consent concept because they were designed to persuade the woman to withhold consent altogether. Further, the provisions were contrary to the 1973 *Roe v. Wade* case because the Akron city ordinance adopted one theory of when life begins over other theories and used the theory to justify regulating abortions. A section of the ordinance required the physician to inform the pregnant woman that "the unborn child is a human life from the moment of conception."

The court said that the section dealing with the possible physical and emotional complications was a "parade of horribles" intended to suggest that abortions are particularly dangerous. Further, the provisions intruded into the medical judgment area and by listing the possible complications it created "obstacles" in the path of the physician on whom the woman must look to for guidance in her decision-making process.

Disposal of the Fetal Remains

Another provision in the City of Akron ordinance imposed a criminal penalty if the fetal remains were not disposed of in a "humane and sanitary manner." The U.S. Supreme Court held that such a provision was impermissibly vague and violated constitutional due process guarantees because it did not give the physician fair notice of which acts of disposal would be forbidden.

Presence of a Second Physician When Fetus Viable

One of the provisions challenged in *Planned Parenthood Association of Kansas City, Missouri v. Ashcroft* required a second physician to "take all reasonable steps in keeping with good medical practice . . . to preserve the life and health of the viable unborn child; provided that it does not pose an increased risk to the life or health of the woman." Further, it provided that the second physician "shall take control of and provide immediate medical care for a child born as a result of the abortion." Holding the provisions constitutional, the Court reasoned that the attending physician will be caring for the woman, and the aborted fetus, if born alive, would be vulnerable to immediate and grave danger if left unattended during this critical period. Although reasoning that preserving the life of a viable fetus may not often be possible, the Court said that the provision comports with the compelling state interest in preserving life.

The Pennsylvania and Illinois Laws

The Pennsylvania statute was tested in *Thornburgh v. American College of Obstetricians*.[56] The Illinois statute was tested in *Charles v. Daley*.[57] Sections of both state laws were determined to be unconstitutional in lower federal court decisions. One of the Illinois provisions found unconstitutional at the federal appeals court level included the requirement that the physician performing an abortion on a viable fetus comply with the standard of care which is required in delivering a viable fetus intended to be born. A second provision, which was also found unconstitutional, required a physician who prescribes an abortifacient method of birth control to inform the woman that he has done so.

One of the Pennsylvania provisions set out in detail the procedure to be followed by the physician in obtaining the pregnant woman's "informed consent." The woman's physician was required to present the following five explicit kinds of information at least 24 hours before she gave her consent. These five were (1) the name of the physician who would perform the abortion, (2) the "fact that there may be detrimental physical and psychological effects which are not accurately foreseeable," (3) the "particular abortion procedure to be employed," (4) the probable gestational age, and (5) the "medical risks associated with carrying her child to term." The woman must also be told that materials supplied by the state describing the fetus were available, as was a list of agencies offering alternatives to abortion. In addition, she must be informed that medical assistance benefits may be available for prenatal care, childbirth and neonatal care, and the fact that "the father is liable to assist" in the child's support, "even where he has offered to pay for the abortion." The materials describing the fetus' anatomical and physiological characteristics must be at 2-week gestational increments throughout the entire gestation period including the possibility of the unborn child's survival potential.

The court stated that the materials represented an intrusive informational source which "seem to us to be nothing less than an outright attempt to wedge the Commonwealth's message discouraging abortion into the privacy of the informed-consent dialogue between the woman and her physician." It found the 2-week fetus description interval "plainly overinclusive" which may "serve only to confuse and punish her and to heighten her anxiety." Further, the court said the financial assistance statements were "poorly disguised elements of discouragement for the abortion decision."

By mandating a discussion of unforeseeable detrimental physical and psychological effects the court said that such detail was the antithesis of informed consent and intruded on the physician's exercise of proper professional judgment. "That the Commonwealth does not, and surely would not, compel similar disclosure of every possible peril of necessary surgery or of simple vaccination reveals the anti-abortion character of the statute and its real purpose." The court also held that the statistical reporting section of the law which required the physician to identify the physician who did the abortion and list information about the woman and fetal details did not advance any legitimate state interest and "raised the specter of public exposure and harassment of women who choose to exercise their personal, private right, with their physician, to end pregnancy."

The provision requiring the use of an abortion method most likely to result in a live birth if the fetus was viable unless the procedure would result in a significantly greater risk to the mother was held invalid because the law failed to require that the woman's health be the paramount consideration. The court also invalidated the provision which required the presence of a second physician when viability was a possibility because it failed to include provisions to protect the mother who was faced with a medical emergency and the second physician's arrival was delayed.

Proponents of the laws argued that the laws protected both the rights of pregnant women seeking an abortion and the interest of the state in protecting the fetus. Proponents of the Illinois statute argued that it was chiefly concerned with a viable fetus and informing women that some birth control measures can cause abortion.

Summary

In 1983 the U.S. Supreme Court upheld the criminal conviction of a Virginia physician who performed a second trimester abortion in his unlicensed clinic. Virginia required that all abortions be performed in licensed facilities. At the same session the Supreme Court struck down a similar Kansas City, Missouri and Akron, Ohio law because both required the second trimester abortion be performed in "general, acute care facilities." The distinction was that Virginia placed the emphasis on licensed facilities and the other two limited abortions to "actue care hospital only" facilities.

The U.S. Supreme Court has clearly articulated that the two compelling state interests recognized to date are an interest in maternal health after the first trimester and the interest in protecting potential human life once the fetus is viable. These two compelling state interests are the yardsticks against which abortion laws are measured. Thus, to date, mandatory 24-hour waiting periods from the time consent is obtained to the actual abortion procedure have been held to not come within the parameters of either state interest.

The U.S. Supreme Court also held that abortion laws that require that an informed consent be obtained only by a physician are invalid because the proponents of such provisions failed to show that they met the compelling state interest test. In addition, the court has not upheld specific consent information requirements such as informing the woman of the developmental stage of the fetus or the date of possible viability because such information was designed to persuade the woman against an abortion procedure.

The most recent U.S. Supreme Court decision, *Thornburgh* found a number of provisions in a Pennsylvania law unconstitutional. The U.S. Supreme Court has agreed to hear oral arguments on the parental notification provision in an Illinois law in late 1987. The Illinois law has been the subject of considerable litigation. Illinois' parental notification law is similar to those in a number of states, many of which by court order have been enjoined from taking effect.[58] Proponents of the Illinois law argue that it meets the compelling state interests test required to pass constitutional scrutiny because the provisions attempt to protect both the rights of the woman seeking an abortion and the state interest in protecting a viable fetus.

ABORTION FUNDING

Another one of the more recent issues to arise in connection with abortion is the funding issue. Decisions on abortion funding have come from both the federal and state courts. The cases have challenged both state and federal restrictions on funding as violative of either a state's constitution or the United States Constitution. The U.S. Supreme Court has ruled on cases dealing with the refusal to fund both nontherapeutic and "medically necessary" abortions. Several state courts reviewing their own constitutional provisions have ruled that funding restrictions are unconstitutional. This is because some state constitutions provide greater guarantees than are provided by the United States Constitution.

Title XIX

In 1965 Congress created the Medicaid Act (Title XIX of the Social Security Act) which established a right of indigent persons to have "medically necessary" health care. The act was enacted for the purpose of providing federal financial assistance to states which choose to pay certain costs of medical treatment for needy persons. Participation in the joint funding program is entirely optional, however, once a state elects to participate it must comply with the requirements of the act. The majority of the states have elected to participate in the plan.

Title XIX is a cooperative program of shared financial responsibility. Nothing in the act suggests that Congress intended to require a participating state to assume the *full* costs of providing any health services indicated in its Medicaid plan. Nor is a participating state required to include in its plan any health services that Congress itself decides not to fund. When a state decides to participate in the federal assistance Medicaid program it must establish its own plan and include several federally mandated categories of health services. Once the state plan is accepted by the federal agency the federal government agrees to pay a specified percentage of the total amount expended. The state pays for the services from its own funds and is then reimbursed by the federal government. Prior to the funding restriction legislation abortions were not paid for.

Hyde Amendment

In 1976 Congress enacted legislation, commonly referred to as the Hyde Amendment, which cut off publicly funded Medicaid money for abortions. The Hyde Amendment was tacked onto an annual appropriations bill of the Department of Labor and then of the Department of Health, Education and Welfare. The original amendment restricted Medicaid funded abortions to situations in which the mother's life was endangered, but it was subsequently amended to permit federal payments for incest and promptly reported rape. Other than these three exceptions the federal government would not reimburse the state for other "medically necessary" abortions. However, it left to the individual states to decide if they wished to pay for "medically necessary" abortions.

In the wake of the Hyde Amendment a number of states enacted parallel laws to cut off state funding of abortions. Two states, New York and Illinois, enacted legislation which prohibited state Medicaid assistance payments for abortions unless a physician determined that it was "medically necessary" to save the mother's life. Although both state laws were held unconstitutional at lower federal courts, when the cases were joined and argued before the U.S. Supreme Court in *Williams v. Zbaraz* in 1980, the nation's highest court upheld the constitutionality of both state statutes.[59]

Funding Cases

In 1977 the U.S. Supreme Court held that elective or unnecessary abortions need not be paid by Medicaid.[60]

> *Maher v. Roe* held that "although the government may not place obstacles in the path of a woman's exercise of her freedom of choice, it need not remove those not of its own creation." The financial constraints a pregnant woman faces, stated the court, are a product of her indigency, not a governmental restriction on access to an abortion. Further, the court said the fact that Medicaid will not pay for elective abortions, but will pay for the expenses of childbirth, demonstrated a legitimate state interest in protecting potential life by encouraging childbirth.

Another U.S. Supreme Court decision, *Harris v. McRae*, which was decided the same day as the ruling upholding the New York and Illinois statutes, held that a woman's right to an abortion was not infringed by operation of the Hyde Amendments or the Medicaid Act.[61] The central issue in the *Harris v. McRae* case was whether the participants (states) in a Medicaid program were obligated, under Title XIX of the Social Security Act, to continue to fund those medically necessary abortions for which federal reimbursement was unavailable under the Hyde Amendment. Those who argued that the state should continue to fund abortions asserted that the participating state had an independent funding obligation under the Medicaid Act. They did not argue that they had a right to public funding of abortions or that a state had a constitutional duty to fund any medical expenses of indigent persons. They argued that when a state undertakes to provide for the medically necessary expenses of childbirth the state should not simultaneously refuse to fund the medically necessary expenses of therapeutic abortion.

The justices, in deciding the case, agreed that the 1973 *Roe v. Wade* abortion decision established that a woman's right to decide whether or not to terminate her pregnancy is a fundamental right. However, the right to decide to have an abortion did not include a constitutional right to fund the abortion from the public treasury. A woman's right of reproductive choice, continued the court, does not carry with it a constitutional entitlement to the financial resources needed to exercise the full range of such choices.

In response to the argument that a lack of funding would discriminate against the poor and, in particular, teenagers, the court said economic obstacles were not created by the government and as such, need not be removed by the government. The court also found that the "Hyde Amendment, by encouraging childbirth . . . is rationally related to the legitimate governmental objective of protecting potential life."

Approximately 200 members of Congress had urged the Supreme Court justices, in a friend of the court brief, to stay out of the question of how Congress appropriates money. Their position was that matters of money appropriations was a matter for the federal government alone. They based their argument on the separation of powers concept.

A month after the *Harris v. McRae* decision, HHS notified state Medicaid agencies that federal financing for "medically necessary" abortions would cease. The U.S. Supreme Court declined 2 months later to reconsider its decision. In mid-1981, the Senate voted to ban any federal funding for abortions for poor women except when the mother's life would be endangered if the pregnancy were carried to term. Thus, Congress forbade funding even when a woman is the victim of rape or incest.

State Constitutions and the McRae Decision

Sometimes a states' own constitution can provide greater rights than the U.S. Constitution. A state may not provide less than federal guarantees, but it may provide more guarantees. In the wake of the 1980 *Harris v. McRae* Supreme Court decision a number of state courts, reviewing their own constitutions in light of the Medicaid abortion funding issue, have rejected the McRae analysis.

A Massachusetts court, in *Moe v. Secretary of Administration and Finance,* determined that a 1979 law, which prohibited the payment of state Medicaid funds for abortions except in instances necessary to save the life of the mother, violated the due process of law provision in the state constitution.[62] The physicians consulted by the pregnant woman believed that an abortion was medically indicated, but they were unable to certify that the abortion procedure was necessary to prevent the woman's death. State law required the certification before the state would pay for the abortion out of state funds. The plaintiff also successfully argued that the decision was compatible with the Hyde Amendment because the federal legislation allowed states to decide whether or not to fund abortions.

A California case, *Committee to Defend Reproductive Rights v. Myers,* also held that a state statute providing Medi-Cal funding for childbirth, but not for abortions was invalid under the state constitution.[63] The court said that the state, having enacted a general program to provide medical services to the poor, may not selectively withhold such benefits from otherwise qualified persons. Such withholding would deprive a pregnant woman of exercising her constitutional right of procreative choice in a manner which the state does not favor or elect to support. The court went on to say that such restrictions impeded the fundamental purpose of the Medi-Cal program which is to make available needed medical care. Such restrictions, held the court, interferred with a woman's right to privacy, threatened her "interests in life, health, and personal bodily autonomy."

The New Jersey Supreme Court, in *Right to Choose v. Byrne,* held that a statute prohibiting medicaid funding for abortions "except where it is medically indicated to be necessary to preserve the mother's life" violated the state constitution.[64] The court held that protection of potential life is a legitimate state interest, but at no point in a woman's pregnancy may it outweigh the superior interest in the life and health of the mother.

However, in *Fischer v. Department of Public Welfare* a Pennsylvania court held that a statute requiring that public funds not be expended unless the life of the mother would be endangered if the fetus was carried to term did not impinge on the woman's fundamental right to an abortion.[65] The court did strike down a requirement that a rape victim report the rape within 72 hours of the rape and an incest victim report its occurrence within 72 hours of the victim's knowledge that she is pregnant in order to qualify for state funding violated the victim's constitutional guarantee of privacy. The state's interest in prosecuting and convicting those who violate the states' criminal laws are greatly outweighed by the severe invasion of the woman's privacy right.

Insurance Coverage

In 1984, a federal court enjoined the state of Rhode Island from enacting two provisions dealing with insurance coverage of abortions.[66]

In *National Education Association of Rhode Island v. Garrahy* a Rhode Island statute required all insurers doing business in the state to exclude from comprehensive health insurance policies coverage for all induced abortions, except those where the life of the mother would be endangered if the fetus was carried to term or where the pregnancy resulted from rape or incest. Coverage for the abortions excluded by the statute could be obtained only by a separate, optional rider for which an additional premium must be paid. The court held the provision invalid because it unconstitutionally burdened the right to an abortion. A second statute was also held unconstitutional. It prohibited both the state and its municipalities from providing public employees with health insurance covering abortions other than those necessary to save the mother's life. The court said that the statute must be subjected to the scrutiny mandated by *Roe v. Wade* and its progeny. The state failed, in both statutes, to show the two compelling interests recognized by the U.S. Supreme Court.

Summary

Two congressional acts, the Medicaid Act, passed in 1965 and the Hyde Amendment, passed in 1976, were integral to the first abortion funding cases. Title XIX of the Medicaid Act gave indigent persons the right to have "medically necessary" health care. The Hyde Amendment cut off publicly funded Medicaid money for all abortions except those medically necessary to save the mother's life and in cases of incest and rape. However, the Hyde Amendment left the decision whether the states would pay for other categories of abortions up to the individual states.

Two early funding cases were decided by the U.S. Supreme Court. These were *Maher v. Roe* and *Harris v. McRae* which held that neither the Medicaid program nor the Hyde Amendment compelled the government to pay for elective abortions. Further, the Court held that a government or state did not discriminate by continuing to fund programs which encouraged childbirth, but not abortion.

After these two decisions there were a number of state court suits that challenged funding statutes in light of the states' constitution. Some of the statutes were struck down while others prevailed. The most recent funding issue involves insurance coverage of elective abortions. A federal court reviewing Rhode Island law struck down a provision which required all insurers doing business in the state to exclude from coverage, without the payment of an additional premium, all abortions except those necessary to save the mother's life and pregnancy from rape and incest. The court held that such a provision unduly burdened a women's right to have an abortion.

CONTINUING THE ABORTION DEBATE

Since the 1973 abortion decision, opponents of abortion have sought to reverse the impact of the ruling. The mechanisms by which this would be done include expansion of the interpretation of the U.S. Constitution or adding an amendment to it. An argument has been made by some members of Congress that the Supreme Court exceeded its authority in a number of recent decisions, including *Roe v. Wade*. They argue that the nation's highest court is attempting to legislate from the bench.

By design the responsibility of the court is judicial, whereas the role of Congress is legislative. Article III of the U.S. Constitution created and defined the role of the Supreme Court. It lists the kinds of legal cases that the court is to decide exclusively. Among the kinds of cases the court is to decide are those in which a constitutional infringement is alleged. However, some legislators have called into question a provision which gives the Supreme Court the authority to be the final arbiter of disputes involving the Constitution. The legislators have cited, as their authority for curbing the power of the court, a section that stipulates that the Supreme Court will have jurisdiction to hear cases on appeal ". . . with such Exceptions, and under such Regulation as the Congress shall make."[67] Proponents who argue that the judicial power of the Supreme Court is limited agree that while Congress cannot tell the court how to decide a case it can take the case away from the court's jurisdiction. Conversely, those who oppose limiting the authority of the judicial branch of the government maintain that Article III was not meant to take away the Courts' jurisdiction over entire subject matters. Additionally, this latter group argues that our system of government requires a supreme arbiter of the Constitution and that role can only be filled by the Supreme Court.[68]

One of the suggested amendments to the Constitution would allow each state to set its own abortion policy. Although the amendment is based on the states' rights concept it would be framed so that Congress would have some jurisdiction over a national abortion policy. Another approach to the abortion question was the Helms-Hyde Bill which was introduced in Congress in 1981. The Bill was not enacted. The Bill defined life as beginning at conception. Conception is defined as a point when the fertilized egg begins to grow and implants itself in the uterus. Some groups propose that any legislation should define life as beginning at fertilization when a sperm cell fertilizes an egg.

A law recognizing that human life begins at conception would give the conceptus the constitutional protection of the Fourteenth Amendment, namely, due process and equal protection guarantees. In essence, "personhood" would attach at conception. The 1973 Supreme Court decision did not address the issue of "personhood." Instead, the Court applied a privacy right test. A recognition that "personhood" begins at conception would necessarily require that various homicide laws attach to abortion procedures and, it is argued by some, to birth control devices which destroy the fetus tissue after conception takes place. Unless exceptions to any similar future bill are identified, two current postrape choices, mechanical abortion and the "morning-after" pill, would be actionable crimes.

SUMMARY

Roe v. Wade established two compelling state interests: protection of the health of the pregnant woman and protection of potential life. All laws, state and federal, must be measured against these two state interests. The woman's right to an abortion can not be made secondary to either of the state's interests. A number of laws have been found unconstitutional because they placed too great a burden on the woman's right.

Roe held that the woman's right was not absolute, but any restriction on her right must be reasonably related to maternal health. However, the state's interest increases as the pregnancy progresses. The cases that immediately followed *Roe* scrutinized the procedural requirements, many of which placed obstacles in the way of a woman seeking an abortion and deterred physicians from performing abortions.

The issues of consent and notification preoccupied the court over a period of several years. The law will not permit a parent to have absolute veto over the minor's decision to have an abortion, and a husband does not have a right to veto or otherwise prevent a wife from obtaining an abortion. In 1981 the Supreme Court held that a Utah law that required parental notification, "if possible," of a minor's decision to have an abortion was permissible because it encouraged the minor to discuss the situation with her parents. The courts have also held that parental notification that a minor is on birth control is unconstitutional. In 1983 the federal government abandoned its intention to promulgate regulations that would require federally funded clinics to notify parents when such devices have been prescribed.[70]

At about that same time the Supreme Court heard three significant abortion cases. The court tested laws in Virginia, Missouri, and Ohio. The Virginia statute requiring that second trimester abortions be performed in licensed facilities was held to be a compelling state interest and was upheld. A mandatory 24-hour waiting period after consent had been obtained was held unconstitutional because it failed to promote any maternal interest. The most recent cases argued before the U.S. Supreme Court raise a number of issues dealing with the states' interest in protecting a viable fetus.

The latest abortion cases have involved the funding issue. The decisions have clearly articulated that there is no right to government payment of elective abortion procedures. Further, it is permissible for a state to promote childbirth funding over abortion funding except where the life of the pregnant woman is threatened.

It is unlikely that the issues surrounding abortion have been played out. Although many of the issues have been tested in the courts it is likely that state statutes will continue to be tested and such measures as a constitutional amendment may be raised again. Perhaps, more than any other area of the law the abortion test cases will continue to be heard by the U.S. Supreme Court as states enact laws in the hope that they will comply with constitutional requirements.

REFERENCES AND NOTES

1. Griswold v. Connecticut, 85 S. Ct. 328 (1965).
2. Eisenstadt v. Baird, 92 S. Ct. 1019 (1972).
3. Paul, E., & Schaap, P. (1980). Abortion and the Law in 1980. *New York Law School Law Review, 25*(3), 497–526.
4. Union Pacific Railway v. Botsford, 141 U.S. 250 (1891).
5. Pierce v. Society of Sisters, 268 U.S. 510 (1925).
6. Roe v. Wade, 93 S. Ct. 705 (1973).
7. Doe v. Bolton, 93 S. Ct. 739 (1973).
8. Planned Parenthood of Central Missouri v. Danforth, 96 S. Ct. 2831 (1976).
9. Hodgson v. Anderson, 378 F. Supp. 1008, affirmed at Spannaus v. Hodgson, 95 S. Ct. 819 (1975).
10. Colautti v. Franklin, 99 S. Ct. 675 (1979).
11. Massachusetts General Laws Chap. 112, § 12P (MA, 1977); West's Annotated Indiana Code, Title 35-1-58.5-7 (b) (as amended 1983); McKinney's Consolidated Laws of New York (Public Health) § 4164 (1974).
12. Deering's Annotated California (Health and Safety) Code, § 25955.9 (1976).
13. Haitch, R. Birth by abortion. *New York Times*, May 3, 1981, p. 49.
14. Crawford W. Abortion fails, mother wants to keep baby. *Chicago Tribune*, May 15, 1981, p. 3.
15. Showery v. State of Texas, 690 S.W. 2nd 689 (TX, 1985). A rehearing was denied.
16. Indiana Hospital Licensing Council v. Women's Pavilion of South Bend, Inc., 420 N.E. 2nd 1301 (IN, 1981).
17. Framingham Clinic, Inc. v. Zoning Board of Appeals of Framingham, 415 N.E. 2nd 840 (MA, 1981).
18. Planned Parenthood of Central Missouri v. Danforth, 96 S. Ct. 2831 (1976).
19. Planned Parenthood League of Massachusetts v. Bellotti, 641 F. 2nd 1006 (1981).
20. Bellotti v. Baird, 96 S. Ct. 2857 (1976); Bellotti v. Baird ("Bellotti II"), 99 S. Ct. 3035 (1979).
21. Bellotti v. Baird ("Bellotti II"), 99 S. Ct. 3035 (1979), Rehearing was denied at 100 S. Ct. 185.
22. Lacey v. Laird, 139 N.E. 2nd 25 (OH, 1956). See also *Cardwell* v. *Bechtol*, 724 S.W. 2nd 739 (TN, 1987) where the state supreme court applied the "mature minor" exception to the general common-law rule requiring parental consent to any medical treatment of minors. In that case a high school student, who was 17 years, 7 months of age, went to an osteopath who had treated her father in the past. The young woman had been under medical treatment for back pain and her parents had previously refused to consent to a myelogram. The physicians suspected that her problem was a herniated disc. The osteopath, whose practice was limited to manipulative treatments to adjust the skeletal system because he was blind, told the young woman that a disc was not her problem and he manipulated her neck, spine, and legs for subluxation of the spine and bilateral sacroiliac slip. The treatments lasted for 15 minutes. Within a few

moments after leaving the osteopaths' office she began to experience numbness and tingling in her legs. Within 2 hours she had severe pain and was unable to walk. She was diagnosed with a herniated disc when she was taken to the hospital that evening and subsequently had a laminectomy. Postoperatively she had difficulty in walking and bladder and bowel problems. In adopting the "mature minor" exception the court said it would not provide general license for treatment of minors without parental consent, as its application is dependent upon specific facts of each case. The court noted that the Tennessee legislature had carved out several exceptions to the common law rule that parental consent was necessary for individuals under 18 years, which was the age of majority, except for the purpose of the purchase of alcoholic beverages. These included emergency treatment and drug abuse or venereal disease treatment. The adoption of these exceptions indicates that "conditions in society have changed to the extent that maturity is now reached at earlier stages of growth than at the time that the common law recognized the age of majority at 21 years. The conditions and reasons that made 21 the age of majority have been eroded over time." In addition, the "Rule of Sevens" has been part of the common law for over a century. The Rule recognizes that minors achieve varying degrees of maturity and responsibility (capacity). In essence, the Rule holds that "under the age of seven, no capacity; between seven and fourteen, a rebuttable presumption of no capacity; between fourteen and twenty-one, a rebuttable presumption of capacity." A rebuttable presumption means that arguments can be presented to rebut the assumption.

23. Massachusetts General Laws Chap. 112, § 12S (Consent to abortion; persons less than 18 years of age), enacted 1974, amended 1977 and 1980.
24. Planned Parenthood League of Massachusetts v. Bellotti, 641 F. 2nd 1006 (1981).
25. In the Matter of Mary Moe, 423 N.E. 2nd 1038 (MA, 1981).
26. City of Akron v. Akron Center for Reproductive Health, 103 S. Ct. 2481 (1983). In 1986 in Akron Center for Reproductive Health v. Rosen, 633 F. Supp. 1123 (1986), suit was brought by the same Ohio birth control center challenging the constitutionality of a recently enacted legislative bill which had not taken effect. The plaintiff argued that the bill was unconstitutional on its face and should be struck down before it became law. Although the court found some parts of the parental notification abortion statute valid it found the waiver provision unconstitutional and struck the entire statute down. The court did find that states have a broader authority to regulate the abortion decisions of a minor than of adult women, thus the concept of parental notice was upheld. In an attempt to comply with the U.S. Supreme Court "Bellotti II" alternative to parental consent requirement the Ohio bill permitted a minor to file an action in juvenile court for the waiver of notification, thus getting around parental notification. After the minor filed the complaint, legal counsel would be appointed and if the court subsequently found against the minor an appeal of the decision may be taken. The fatal flaw in this part of the bill was that it specified exact time frames. "Bellotti II" had stressed the necessity of an expeditious appeal process. The appeal process in the Ohio bill would require an additional 3 weeks and the federal court found this to be unconstitutionally burdensome in view of the need to act quickly. In August 1987 an Ohio federal district court judge held a month-old parental notification statute unconstitutional.
   In August 1987 a federal appeals court in *Hodgson v. State of Minnesota* struck down that state's abortion law which required a minor to notify both parents of her abortion decision or seek judicial clearance. Hodgson v. State of Minnesota, 827 F. 2nd 1191 (1987); see lower federal court ruling at 648 F. Supp. 757 (1986). That suit was brought by two obstetricians, several birth control facilities, and six plaintiffs, ranging in ages from 15 to 17 years. The opinion contains an appendix which indicated that between August 1, 1981, and March 1, 1986, of the 3573 petitions filed, 3558 had been granted; 9 of these were denied and 6 petitions were withdrawn before the court's decision. Although the statute made provisions if the minor's parents were

divorced or one parent could not be located, the court held that the two-parent requirement did not serve any significant state interest. The court also held that the alternative judicial procedure was unconstitutional because it unduly burdened the minor. The State of Minnesota plans to appeal the federal appeals court decision. See Noble, K. Appeals court voids statute on informing parents of abortion. *New York Times*, August 28, 1987, p. 1. For an interesting case involving money damages, see Cage v. Wood, 484 S. 2nd 850 (LA, 1986) where a physician was held liable in a civil money damages suit when a minor submitted a document purporting to be her mother's written authorization for the minor's abortion. The physician was liable for a battery (unpermitted touching) for his failure to obtain a consent in compliance with the procedure set out in Louisiana law. After the minor found out she was pregnant in 1982 she gave the physician the document which in fact was written and signed by the girl's cousin. A Louisiana statute required that the statement be notarized after being written by a parent or guardian. Since the doctor testified that essentially all of his medical practice was confined to abortions he should have been aware of the legal requirements for minor consent. The minor was awarded the cost of the operation and $3,000 for pain and suffering. However, the parents claim in battery for the "deprivation of the joys of grandparenthood" was dismissed because the law does not recognize such grounds for a suit.

27. Planned Parenthood Association of Kansas City, Missouri v. Ashcroft, 103 S. Ct. 2517 (1983).
28. Matter of Mary Moe, 446 N.E. 2nd 941 (MA, 1983).
29. In re the Matter of T.P., 475 N.E. 2nd 312 (IN, 1985).
30. H. L. v. Matheson, 101 S. Ct. 1164 (1981).
31. Indiana Planned Parenthood v. Pearson, 716 F. 2nd 1127 (1983).
32. Zbaraz v. Hartigan, 763 F. 2nd 1532 (1985). See also Hartigan v. Zbaraz, 107 S. Ct. 1636 (April 7, 1987). The U.S. Supreme Court is scheduled to hear arguments in October 1987 in this case.
33. See Poe v. Gerstein, 94 S. Ct. 2247 (1976). Affirming Poe v. Gerstein, 517 F. 2nd 787 (1974).
34. Doe v. Doe, 314 N.E. 2nd 128 (MA, 1974).
35. Jones v. Smith, 278 S. 2nd 339 (FL, 1973); cert. denied at 415 U.S. 958. See also Wolfe v. Schroering, 541 F. 2nd 523 (1976); Planned Parenthood Association v. Fitzpatrick, 401 F. Supp. 554 (1975); Doe v. Zimmerman, 405 F. Supp. 534 (1975); Wynn v. Scott, 449 F. Supp. 1302 (1978), Appeal disssmissed at 99 S. Ct. 49.
36. Planned Parenthood of Central Missouri v. Danforth, 96 S. Ct. 2831 (1976).
37. Coleman v. Coleman, 471 A. 2nd 115 (MD, 1984).
38. S.W. v. Wilkinson, U.S. federal district court of Utah (central division), No. C-81-0362 (May 15, 1981).
39. Anon. Mate must be told of abortion. *Chicago Tribune*, May 16, 1981, p. 3.
40. Scheinberg v. Smith, 550 F. Supp. 1112 (1982).
41. Griswold v. Connecticut, 85 S. Ct. 1678 (1965).
42. Eisenstadt v. Baird, 92 S Ct. 1029 (1972).
43. Carey v. Population Services International, 97 S. Ct. 2010 (1977).
44. Doe v. Irwin, 615 F. 2nd 1162 (1980).
45. 42 United States Code § 300 (a), more commonly known as Title X of the Public Health Service Act. In addition, two other federal programs under the Social Security Act provide similar services. These are the Medicaid program and Aid to Families with Dependent Children (AFDC).
46. Planned Parenthood Federation of America v. Schweiker, 559 F. Supp. 658 (1983).
47. Planned Parenthood Federation of America v. Heckler, 712 F. 2nd 650 (1983).
48. Planned Parenthood Association of Utah v. Matheson, 582 F. Supp. 1001 (1983).
49. Simopoulos v. Virginia, 103 S. Ct. 2532 (1983).
50. City of Akron v. Akron Center for Reproductive Health, Inc., 103 S. Ct. 2481 (1983).

51. Planned Parenthood Association of Kansas City, Missouri, Inc. v. Ashcroft, 103 S. Ct. 2517 (1983).

52. City of Akron v. Akron Center for Reproductive Health, Inc., 103 S. Ct. 2481, (1983). See note 26.

53. Thornburgh v. American College of Obstetricians, 106 S. Ct. 2169 (1986). When the federal court of appeals for the third circuit was asked to decide the case in 1983, it held its decision over pending the 1983 U.S. Supreme Court decisions in *Ashcroft*, *City of Akron*, and *Simopoulos*, which were all decided the same day. In 1984 the federal court of appeals heard American College of Obstetricians and Gynecologists v. Thornburgh, 737 F. 2nd 283, which was appealed.

54. In Diamond v. Charles, 106 S. Ct. 1697 (1986), the U.S. Supreme Court held that Dr. Diamond, who was a pediatrician and the parent of daughter of childbearing years, did not have legal standing to appeal the lower federal appeals court decision in Charles v. Daley, 749 F. 2nd 452 (1984), which found several provisions of the Illinois law unconstitutional. The state which was involved in the lower court decision would have had standing to appeal the decision, but did not appeal. Thus, the federal appeals court decision in *Charles v. Daley* currently stands.

55. Commonwealth v. Menillo. 96 S. Ct. 171 (1975).

56. Op. cit. Thornburgh. Four of the nine justices filed dissenting opinions to the majority decision.

57. Charles v. Daley, 749 F. 2nd 452 (1984). Note that the U.S. Supreme Court refused to hear arguments on this case.

58. Noble, K. Appeals court voids statute on informing parents of abortion. *New York Times*, August 28, 1987, p. 1.

59. Williams v. Zbaraz, 100 S. Ct. 2694 (1980); 101 S. Ct. 39 (1980), rehearing denied.

60. Maher v. Roe, 97 S. Ct. 2377 (1977).

61. Harris v. McRae, 100 S. Ct. 2671 (1980); 101 S. Ct. 39, rehearing denied.

62. Moe v. Secretary of Administration and Finance, 417 N.E. 2nd 387 (MA, 1981).

63. Committee to Defend Reproductive Rights v. Myers, 625 P. 2nd 799 (CA, 1981).

64. Right to Choose v. Byrne, 450 A. 2nd 925 (NJ, 1982). See also Planned Parenthood Association v. Department of Human Resources, 663 P. 2nd 1247 (OR, 1983).

65. Fischer v. Department of Public Welfare, 482 A. 2nd 1148 (PA, 1984).

66. National Education Association of Rhode Island v. Garrahy, 779 F. 2nd 790 (1986). See also Reproductive Health Services v. Webster, 662 F. Supp. 407 (1987).

67. United States Constitution, Article III, § 2.

68. The MacNeil-Lehrer Report, "Congress and the Courts," Library no. 1516, show no. 6276 (air date, July 20, 1981).

69. Helms-Hyde Bill, Senate 158 (1981). This bill was not enacted.

70. For a discussion of recently proposed regulations affecting family planning submitted by the Department of Health and Human Services, see Pear, R. U.S. issues limits on abortion aid by family clinics. *New York Times*, August 30, 1987, p. 1. In 1970 the government's family planning program was established under Title X of the Public Health Service Act. The current law precludes using funds appropriated under the act in programs which promote abortion as a method of family planning. However, currently clinics must provide counseling on all family planning options, including abortion. The proposals would stop funding facilities that provide abortion counseling or refer clients to abortion clinics.

9

MEDICAL TREATMENT ISSUES

The Basis for Legal Decisions

The legal issues involved in the Karen Quinlan case brought the problem of complex treatment decisions to the attention of the public. Although medicine and technology had dramatically improved the quality of medical care, these advances also presented problems in some situations. While it became feasible to save the life of an accident victim who had been submerged under cold water for 30 minutes, the question was raised of whether, when, and for how long life-support technology should be continued when the prognosis became poor or hopeless. While the knowledge base was being built and experience with critical patients was being expanded the legal, moral, and ethical questions received little attention.

The questions raised by the Quinlan case were overdue and once the floodgate was opened the questions and dilemmas seemed to become increasingly more complex. Although a number of treatment dilemmas have been clarified and some specifically resolved there is continuing debate about other treatment issues. The withdrawal of treatment for severely impaired newborns is one example of an issue undergoing continuing debate.

Some of the legal decisions have been harshly criticized and for a variety of reasons. The length of time it takes for a court to hear a case and the monetary expense involved are frequently raised objections against court intervention. There is also a fundamental objection by some that the judiciary is not in a position to decide these types of issues. However, some cases must, because of their factual issues, be resolved in a judicial setting. The Chad Greene case is such an example.[1] Presumably, the courts will be less involved in treatment cases because of the guidelines established by these early cases. Also, health care facilities have developed internal mechanisms and policy guidelines to resolve questions. In addition, professional groups have adopted and published position statements. The public debate has also served to emphasize the decision-making process and has taken the nonmedical aspects of decision-making away from the exclusive realm of physicians.

Some treatment issues are of such paramount importance that even though the patient died before a court could rule on the legal issue, thus rendering the case moot, the court went forward and issued a legal opinion.[2] The basis for hearing such cases is that the issue is of substantial public interest. Factors that meet the substantial public interest test include the public or private nature of the question, the desirability of an authoritative determination for the future guidance of public officials, and the likelihood of future recurrence of the legal question.

Some of the treatment cases invoked the protection of the U.S. Constitution, while others did not. The majority of cases involved treatment or nontreatment of an incompetent adult or a minor. Most of the cases involved an issue of brain death, removal of life-support systems and drugs, or surgical procedures. There were a number of cases in which the legal issue was whether a prisoner had a legal right to refuse necessary surgery.

Prior to *Quinlan* much of the literature relevant to treatment issues dealt with euthanasia. Since 1976 there has been much written about specific treatment issues and the courts have frequently made reference to the literature in judicial rulings. The literature has played an important role in societal awareness of these complex issues. Amid the confusion and debate surrounding some of these decisions a consensus has evolved. One consensus is that the admittedly adversarial judicial setting is not an automatic forum for every treatment controversy or dilemma. The system of applying to the courts for direction in medical treatment dilemmas should probably be the exception. All the judicial decisions have emphasized the point that decisions relevant to the practice of medicine rest with physicians, but that treatment decisions interface with other critical interests, such as individual autonomy and societal mores.

There needs to be a conscious distinction made between treatment of the individual and care of that individual. This is particularly important where the individual will receive no benefit from treatment, as with a permanently comatose individual. There should be no limitations in the nursing care given to a hopelessly ill individual. Until recently little weight was given to the degree of mental and physical suffering endured by a patient, at least as it related to treatment decisions. This was particularly so with the use of life-support systems in "hopeless" conditions. Such mental and physical suffering, although somewhat alleviated with medication, has had to be endured where there is reasonable expectation and hope that the patient will benefit from the treatment. Where, however, that expectation is not present the suffering endured must be weighed heavily against continuing treatment that merely prolongs life.[3]

There has been a lack of uniformity or consensus in implementing decisions not to treat hopelessly ill individuals, although there may be consensus on what conditions or groups of individuals should not be treated when the condition is hopeless. To a large extent this has been due to a lack of guidelines. One of the more thought provoking articles on such guidelines was published in 1984.[4]

Acknowledging the patient's right to accept or refuse treatment, the authors stressed the major role physicians, because of their medical expertise, play in the decision-making process. This role includes the assumption of responsibility for recommending a particular treatment decision, including no treatment. The authors identified levels of care for hopelessly ill individuals at a given stage of their disease process. They stressed that nurses and other health-care personnel should be brought into discussions concerning the level of therapy because they are in close and frequent communication with the individual or family members.

Recognizing that any program of care must be individualized to accommodate the uniqueness of every patient the following levels of care were identified: (1) emergency resuscitation, (2) intensive care and advanced life support, (3) general medical care, and (4) general nursing care and efforts to make the patient comfortable. General medical care would include antibiotics, drugs, surgery, cancer chemotherapy, and artificial hydration and nutrition. General nursing care would include pain relief and hydration and nutrition as indicated by the patient's thirst and hunger.

Ordinarily the fourth level of care, the comfort level, is reserved for those individuals clearly in the terminal phase of an irreversible illness. The authors concluded that routine monitoring procedures as vital signs may be discontinued at this level. The same would hold true for diagnostic measures except when required to relieve an uncomfortable or painful condition. Such diagnostic tests would include blood tests and x-ray films. The authors stressed that, "Everything done for the patient at the fourth level of care should meet only the test of whether it will make the patient more comfortable and whether it will honor his or her wishes."

One of the more helpful recommendations set out by the authors was the need to aggressively treat and manage the patient's pain and suffering. Such aggressive treatment is justified even though there is the risk of respiratory depression. In caring for severely and irreversibly demented patients the authors said that the physician, in the absence of prior patient expression, should be guided by the need to provide the most humane kind of treatment. Where such an individual rejects food and water by mouth, the authors concluded that it is ethically permissible to withhold nutrition and hydration artificially administered by vein or gastric tube.

In response to the issues generated by treatment decisions, President Carter created a commission to study and take testimony relevant to the ethical, medical and legal aspects of such decisions. The commission published their findings and recommendations in early 1983. A similar study was conducted by the Canadian government. The group, known as the Law Reform Commission of Canada, issued their report in November 1983.[5] The report dealt with euthanasia, aiding suicide, and cessation of medical treatment. Most of their report dealt with the cessation of medical treatment because the other issues did not generate as much discussion. In defining euthanasia as the intentional killing of a person for compassionate motives the commissioners recommended that such acts be covered by the criminal code. They also recommended retaining as a crime any action that would aid in suicide, including furnishing the individual with a lethal medication which the patient would then administer to himself.

With respect to stopping medical treatment the commissioners said the legal presumption in favor of life, while always recognized, should not be regarded as "absolute." One unique aspect of the Canadian Report was its emphasis on the "quality of life" factor. The U.S. courts have been reluctant to adopt a quality of life test in reaching judicial decisions. The commissioners said that Canadian law would require that the value of human life should be considered from a "quantitative" prospective, as well as from a "qualitative" viewpoint.[6] It is noteworthy that the quality of life as a factor has been recommended by a number of authors writing on the subject of treatment decision making, but the failure of the U.S. courts to embrace the concept in legal decisions has prevented its inclusion in formal guidelines. This is somewhat ironic in that the legal doctrine of informed consent is based on the patient's freedom to choose or refuse treatment, and such decisions always bring into play individual choices of the quality of life in view of the risks associated with treatment or nontreatment. Recent decisions dealing with the withdrawal of nutritional devises deal head-on with the quality of life factor, and thus it is only a matter of time before it is adopted into other treatment issues.

DETERMINING MENTAL INCOMPETENCY

The issue of whether a person is competent to make a treatment decision has been discussed at great length in the amputation cases and for that reason this category of cases will be discussed in relationship to the material on incompetent patients. The issue of competency, of course, is involved in every decision to treat, or not treat, a particular condition.

Whenever a petition is initiated with a court seeking to have a guardian appointed for the alleged incompetent, the crucial question is whether the individual lacks the mental capacity to the extent that the individual is unable to make a treatment decision. It must be shown by evidence that the impairment is to the point of legal incompetence. If it is shown that the individual is competent the court will refuse to hear the case and of course, will not appoint a guardian. There is a legal presumption that a person is competent unless a judicial proceeding has found otherwise. The burden is on the court or the individual seeking the guardianship appointment to prove the proposed ward is incompetent. The question of competency is not an either or question. Frequently the question is one of degree. The courts consider the issue of guardianship to be serious because of its effect of stripping the ward of certain liberties, including the right to make his own decisions.

From a practical point of view, the competency issue becomes a factor when the physician first discusses or sees a need to discuss with the patient the necessity of performing an invasive procedure. Traditionally if the patient was incompetent the surgeon sought permission from the family. However, few if any hospitals had guidelines in place to assure consistency in the decision-making process. Recently the courts have looked with favor on use of the family in deciding treatment decisions where the patient is incompetent. However, the courts suggest that formal guidelines be established which recognize the rights of the parties involved. Many of the legal cases involved patients who had no family or family who had not maintained ties with the patient. Recent decisions suggest that even patients without families need not go to court so long as there are policies to protect the patient. Presumably, this attitude will become more universal.

Test for Competency

Two early Washington state cases serve to illustrate the competency issue.

> The first case, *Peterson v. Eritsland,* which involved a contractual agreement (contract for child support) held that the test in deciding whether mental competency existed was whether the person in question, at the time of executing the contract, possessed sufficient mind or reason to enable him to understand the nature, the terms, and the effect of the transaction.[7]

> The second case, *Grannum v. Berard,* held that it was a well settled law that sanity and competency is presumed until there is satisfactory proof to the contrary.[8] The competency issue arose when the patient alleged (unsuccessfully) that the surgical consent form he signed was invalid because he was under the influence of drugs when he gave it. The patient failed to meet the judicial standard of proof showing that he was incapable of exercising a sufficient mental faculty to make an intelligent choice. The court said that the mental capacity necessary to consent to a surgical operation is a question of fact to be determined from the circumstances of each individual case.

Two Holdings

In two New Jersey cases, each reaching different results, the court provided tangible guidelines for determining whether or not competency existed. Both cases involved a request to permit amputation.

> In *Matter of Schiller,* the court said that in terms of mental capacity to consent, the test may be stated as: "Does the patient have sufficient mind to reasonably understand the condition, the nature and effect of the proposed treatment, attendant risks in pursuing the treatment, and not pursuing the treatment?"[9] The initial hearings were conducted in the hospital because the surgeon said the man's condition had suddenly deteriorated and immediate surgery was necessary. At the proceedings the following facts came to light.

On admission to the hospital the man was covered with his own excrement and his foot was overtly gangrenous with purulent drainage. Three of his toes were black, his lower leg and ankle was red and swollen, and his entire involved leg was flexed against his abdomen. The condition had developed over a period of several months. The fact that it was a diabetic gangrene was significant because the use of antibiotics would slow, but would not stop the infection process. The healing process would not be as good as in nondiabetic gangrene conditions, such as frostbite or a traumatic injury. In those conditions the infection can frequently be "walled off" and spontaneous amputation can occur without the danger of systemic infection which can occur with diabetic gangrene.

When the physician first discussed the need to amputate to prevent the spread of infection the patient said that he wanted to think about it. In the presence of increasing spread of the infection the surgeon had a staff psychiatrist examine the patient and render an opinion as to his mental capacity. The psychiatrist found that the man had organic brain damage and that he did not have the mental capacity to knowingly consent or refuse to consent. The patient did not ask any questions. Although he said he wanted to live he always responded that he did not want the operation.

The surgeon reviewed his records during the proceedings and informed the court that a few days delay would not be life-threatening. The court appointed an attorney to represent the man and an independent psychiatrist. Another hearing was scheduled, but because of the infection the man was not present in the courtroom. At that hearing testimony was heard from both psychiatrists. Both agreed that the man was incapable of understanding his present condition and the fact that the amputation was a life-saving technique. The court-appointed psychiatrist testified that the man evidenced the five tests for organic brain damage. He was disoriented as to time and place and did not understand who was talking to him. As a result of the organic brain damage he was unable to read and could not do the simplest addition requests. In response to questions he answered instantaneously and these responses were not based on any judgment or insight. The patient was found to be incompetent and the court appointed a family member as special guardian with authority to consent.

In the second New Jersey case, *Matter of Quackenbush*, the court held that the patient was competent to decide whether he wanted the amputation or not. The evidence showed he was capable of appreciating the nature and consequences of his treatment decision.[10] The patient, a 72-year-old man who did not have any relatives, originally signed the consent, but later the same day withdrew it. The operation involved bilateral above the knee amputations. He presented an extreme picture; his left leg was black from the knee down and was partially mummified with the foot dangling. The tibia and tendons of his right leg were exposed and draining fluid. From the midcalf down the leg was also mummified and black. His leg was septic and he had "wet" gangrene. The physician's sworn affidavit indicated the likelihood that one foot would fall off and the man would probably die within 3 weeks unless he had the operation.

The hospital psychiatrist saw the patient and concluded that he was suffering from organic brain syndrome with psychotic elements. However, he thought that the syndrome was acute and was a result of the septicemia. If so, it was subject to change. The psychiatrist based the syndrome diagnosis on the patient's findings which included disorientation to place (unaware he was in a hospital) and person. He was visually hallucinating. Although agreeing that his mental state may have been secondary to the septicemia, the psychiatrist concluded that the patient fully appreciated the magnitude of the illness and the consequences of his refusal. Although the man would lose his train of thought and his discussions would wander the court held, under the circumstances, that these findings did not constitute mental incompetency. Further, he fluctuated in his mental lucidity which is not an uncommon finding. The man said that he hoped for a miracle, but realized that there was little likelihood of its occurrence. The fact that he was not in pain was important. He had previously stated that if pain occurred he would likely change his mind in favor of surgery. Finding that the events and conditions documented by the hospital psychiatrist were of a temporary and curative nature the court would not declare the man incompetent. In short, the court held that it had not been proved that he could not make his own decision. His rights outweighed the States' right to preserve life.

Some Observations

It is important to remember that although the decision to amputate may seem obvious from a medical perspective, such a perspective must not outweigh the individual's wishes not to have it done, even if necessary to save his life. The tradition of medicine is to cure, when able. In the face of extreme physical findings or certain death it is understandable that nurses and physicians have difficulty with a patient's decision to forego amputation. Because the focus of nursing and medicine is to do what is best for the patient it is difficult to merely stand by while a limb wastes away. It is particularly difficult for nurses who must care for the limb on a daily basis.

Another observation is that the courts and the physicians, including the psychiatrists, underwent an educational process in these early competency determination cases. Both learned the right questions to ask in order to obtain the most complete information. It is clear from reading the *Quackenbush* case that the medical facts surrounding the need to amputate, as well as the psychiatric's observations and findings, and the individual's personal wishes were necessary to reach a decision. The judicial process served to provide an in-depth analysis.

Quackenbush pointed out that incompetency may be transitory and secondary to the immediate disease process. Presumably as the man's condition was medically managed, especially management of the infection process, he presented with less mental impairment symptoms. This last point should be of extreme interest to nurses who observe a patient over continuous period of time. Fluctuations in mental lucidity do not necessarily indicate mental incapacity to make a rational decision. A patient may not be lucid when the surgeon visits, but may be lucid during the administration of daily care. Accurate nursing records are particularly important when the patient's mental competency is at issue. Nursing notes, as well as direct dialogue with the surgeon or psychiatrist serve to guide all parties on how best to proceed.

Incompetence May Be a Matter of Degree

In 1978, the Mary Northern case attracted national attention.[11] The case is particularly interesting because the court found that her incompetence was limited to her denial of or inability to realize her extreme situation. The opinion stressed that this was not a "right to die" case, rather it was a judicial proceeding limited to the issue of competency to consent to treatment. If found incompetent the court would then set in motion the mechanism whereby "competent consent" could be obtained.

It is clear in reading the *Northern* opinion that the court went to great lengths to obtain information. In addition to hearing testimony on the psychologic impact of surgery on the woman, the court heard evidence on the prognosis with and without surgery, survival statistics, and the nature of the emergency. In every so-called treatment case a judicial inquiry is made as to the level of pain and the impact of delay in withholding treatment. Where the court petition indicates that the nature of the situation is an emergency, as in the need for immediate electroshock treatment or transfusions in a hemorrhaging postpartum patient, judicial authority can be rendered immediately. It is not uncommon for judicial proceedings to be conducted at the bedside as was done in the *Matter of Schiller* amputation case. As both the courts and the medical community develop guidelines, the process, where judicial inquiry is warranted, will be expedited.

Mary Northern was 72 years old when she was brought into a Tennessee hospital. She had no family and no one to care for her. She was found when a fire occurred in her home. Shortly thereafter protective services measures were instituted. The proceedings to have her declared a ward of the state and to obtain consent for amputation of both her feet extended over a period of several months. She suffered from "wet" gangrene of both feet, probably secondary to frostbite which was complicated by thermal burning of the feet.

Psychiatrists filed affidavits which stated that she was generally lucid and sane, but was functioning on a psychotic level with respect to ideas concerning her gangrenous feet and was utilizing a psychotic mechanism of denial. The court found that she was intelligent, communicative, and articulate. However, when she appeared before the judge he found that her comprehension of the seriousness of her situation was "blocked, blinded or dimmed to the extent that she is incapable of recognizing facts which would be obvious to a person of normal perception." In the presence of the judge she looked at her feet and refused to recognize the obvious fact that the flesh was dead, black, shriveled, rotting and malodorous. She told a psychiatrist that her feet were black because of soot or dirt. She believed that her feet would heal without surgery and she rejected the surgeon's assessment that the infection process represented a real life threat. She was unwilling to discuss how she would care for herself if she returned to independent living.

She did not express a wish to die and did express a strong desire to live. However, she expressed a strong desire to keep her dead feet and when asked if she would prefer to die rather than lose her feet, her answer was "possibly." The courts always look for a presumption by way of a statement or attitude expressed by the proposed ward while in a competent state to ascertain the patient's wishes. No such presumption existed in the *Northern* case. The court cited an earlier case which involved a woman who based her refusal to consent on delusional reasons.[12] However, that court refused to order diagnostic tests and surgery because the woman had previously refused the same treatment while in a competent state.

Mary Northern's chances of survival without amputation were from 5 to 10 percent and only 50 percent with surgery. The court held her "delusion" rendered her incapable of making a rational decision as to whether to undergo surgery to save her life or to forego surgery and forfeit her life. Ultimately the court authorized the Commissioner of Human Services to act on Mary Northern's behalf in consenting to amputation when her surgeons certified in writing that her condition had progressed to the critical stage where immediate surgery was needed to save her life. However, she died as a result of a blood clot which originated in her gangrenous feet. The surgery had not been scheduled because of intervening complications.

One last aside in the *Northern* case was her attorney's argument that the phrasing of the statute under which the case was brought was too vague for interpretation. However, the court held that the phrase, "capacity to consent" interpreted in the context of the statute meant, "mental ability to make a rational decision, which includes the ability to perceive, appreciate all relevant facts and to reach a rational judgment upon such facts."

About the same time the Tennessee court was faced with the question of the degree of impairment sufficient to constitute legal mental incompetence a Massachusetts court was faced with a similar question.[13]

In the case of *Lane v. Candura*, the patient's family did not agree with the woman's decision not to have surgery. The woman was a 77-year-old widow who had diabetic gangrene in her lower leg and foot. The surgeon recommended that the leg be amputated without delay. She vacillated and finally resolved not to have the operation.

Her daughter, one of four children, petitioned the court to be appointed temporary guardian in order to give the consent. A psychiatrist testified that the woman was unable to make a rational choice. When the court allowed the daughter to act as temporary guardian the attorney representing the patient appealed and the decision was set aside. The appeals court found the following facts which set the case apart from the *Northern* case. One such distinction was that Mary Northern elected both to live and reject the surgery.

The Massachusetts woman stated that she was lonely and depressed since her husband died 2 years previously. Her diabetes was discovered 4 years earlier when she had to have a toe amputated because of infection. A year later she had to have a portion of her foot amputated because of gangrene. At that time she also had an arterial bypass to prevent further diabetic complications. After that surgery she was discharged to a rehabilitation facility where she stayed for 5 months. She was readmitted to a hospital when the gangrene returned. Just prior to surgery she withdrew her prior consent for amputation and was discharged to her daughter's home. She was readmitted, gave her consent, and retracted it almost immediately. She discussed her reasons with some staff. She said that she did not want to be a burden to her children, did not wish to live as an invalid or be sent to a nursing home. She did not believe that the amputation would take care of her problem and was unafraid of death. The failure of her previous surgery added to her depression.

Testifying before the judge, she expressed a desire to get well, but was resigned to death and was adamantly opposed to the operation. There was testimony that she was lucid on some matters and confused on others, that her train of thought sometimes wandered, and that she was hostile to certain doctors. A second psychiatrist found her to be competent. The appeals court held that the woman had made a knowing choice with full appreciation of the consequences. The court went on to say, "The most that is shown is that the decision involves strong, emotional factors, that she does not choose to discuss the decision with certain persons, and that occasionally her resolve against giving consent weakens." The court also noted that the issue of irrationality did not surface until she changed her mind. In short, her competence was not questioned so long as she agreed to the operation.

Summary

Two of the mental incompetency cases involved situations where the patient did not have family. A third case permitted a family member to consent after the patient's incompetency had been adjudicated. The last case held that vacillation does not, in and of itself, demonstrate incompetency. From the facts of the four cases it would seem clear that all required judicial intervention. Although the courts may differ in the language used to define capacity to consent, each required that the patient be unable to make a reasoned judgment, under the particular set of facts, before incompetency will be found.

BRAIN DEATH

Traditionally the law has had a need to define death as an event that occurs at an identifiable instant. An example is where two individuals have died simultaneously and the instant of death of both must be ascertained to determine inheritance.[14] From a medical perspective,

death is seen as a gradual process at a cellular level, with tissues varying in their ability to withstand oxygen deprivation.

The common law definition of death is irreversible cessation of
cardiac and respiratory function. Prior to transplants there was no need
to define death in terms other than the common law definition. The first
kidney transplant was done in the late 1950s and this procedure set in
motion the need to define death in other terms. The donor for the first
kidney transplant was the twin brother of the recipient. In the early
years of kidney transplants the donors were blood-related or cadaver
donors whose tissue studies were compatible with the recipient. Subsequently, nonrelated individuals with healthy organs became a prime
source of organs. Most of the donors are fairly young people who have
been severely traumatized in accidents. It became necessary to establish criteria whereby such individuals could be terminated from life-
support systems and their organs, with the consent of next of kin, transplanted into individuals with compatible tissue study findings. Once
the concept of brain death was translated into criteria for defining its
existence, it naturally evolved to include situations other than the
transplant cases. However, it was not until a decade after the first transplant that criteria for determining "irreversible coma" was published
by the medical community.

The Harvard Criteria

The first criteria were developed by the Ad Hoc Committee of the Harvard Medical School to Examine the Definition of Brain Death.[15] Although the committee did not define death, it did take the position that
a patient in a state of irreversible coma may be considered dead and,
thus, their criteria came to be equated with brain death. The criteria
published in 1968 were established for two reasons: (1) response to
advancements in resuscitative and supportive measures which resulted
in increased efforts to save severely injured persons, and (2) establishment of uniform or standard criteria to be used when "harvesting"
organs for transplantation from patients in an irreversible coma.

The Ad Hoc Committee identified four characteristics of irreversible coma which were as follows: (1) unreceptivity and unresponsitivity
to externally applied stimuli (painful stimuli), (2) no spontaneous movements and absence of spontaneous breathing, (3) lack of reflexes (both
superficial and deep tendon reflexes), and (4) flat or isoelectric electroencephalogram.[16] The electroencephalogram (EEG) requirement
was a confirmatory measure and was to be repeated in 24 hours. Applying the Harvard criteria, electrocerebral silence and absent spinal reflexes were required in order for a determination of irreversible coma to
be made. It was recognized at that time that primary hypothermia,

some metabolic and endocrine diseases, and drugs would produce false findings, seemingly confirmatory of irreversible brain death and so a caveat was affixed to these conditions. The caveat remains in effect and will be discussed presently.

Shortly after publication of the criteria, various medical experts criticized them for their rigidity. Other groups published their own criteria. The fact that different criteria were proposed and the Ad Hoc Committee did not define the term "brain death" lead to a lack of uniformity in implementing the brain death concept. Other terms, such as "cerebral death," "neocortical death," and "apallic syndrome" were used to indicate brain death. Irrespective of these problems, the idea of translating the concept of brain death into measurable criteria was an important step. In retrospect, the criteria were too rigid. For example, cases have been reported where spinal cord reflexes persisted as long as 2 weeks after a finding of electrocerebral silence.

Another group, from Minnesota, established criteria that were less rigid than the Harvard Criteria.[17] This group from the University of Minnesota did not require a mandatory EEG. They also took the position that spinal reflexes may exist in death. They placed greater emphasis on absent brain stem reflexes.[18] Absent brain stem reflexes included dilated and fixed pupils, absent corneal reflexes, absent ciliospinal reflexes, absent gag reflex, absent oculovestibular reflex, and absent tonic neck reflex. When the respirator was removed there would be no spontaneous respirations.

A number of European countries, including Sweden, published criteria which included angiography to assess cerebral blood flow. None of the criteria published by the U.S. groups made angiography a requirement. In addition to the groups that established their own criteria, a number of surgeons who were involved in heart transplant surgery established and published their own criteria. Barnard of Cape Town, Cooley of Houston, and Shumway of Palo Alto are examples of surgeons who established their own criteria.

Lack of Anatomic Definition

In addition to the lack of uniformity in brain death criteria, there was a lack of consensus as to the anatomic definition of brain death. *Brain death*, that is, death of the whole brain must be distinguished from clinical findings diagnostic of cerebral death. *Cerebral death* means that both cerebral hemispheres are in a state of irreversible total dysfunction.

Persistent vegetative state and neocortical death is the same as cerebral death. Karen Ann Quinlan remained in a persistent vegetative state. Her brain stem functioned, permitting spontaneous breathing and primitive motor responses. However, the perceptive, cognitive part of her brain was dead. The higher functions, such as speech, voluntary movement, emotional reaction, and memory were absent. When Karen was first examined she exhibited electroencephalographic activity, normal intracranial blood circulation, and a number of reflexes.[19]

By way of contrast, the death of the entire brain includes both cerebral hemispheres, the cerebellum, and the brain stem. When there is complete loss of function of the whole brain cardiac arrest will occur in about 1 week.[20] A requirement of whole brain death would be impractical for the purpose of organ donation or for removal of life-support systems.

The problems that can result from failing to uniformly define the term "brain death," are illustrated by a wrongful death case which was tried in Virginia in 1972.[21]

The brother of Bruce Tucker in *Tucker v. Lower* brought a wrongful death action against five physicians who were directly or indirectly involved in removal of the brain-injured decedent's respirator. The decedent, who was 54 years old, was brought unconscious to the emergency room and his identity was not known. Examination showed that he had a subdural hematoma, and he subsequently had a craniotomy and a tracheostomy. His condition deteriorated postoperatively and 19 hours after his admission he was examined by a neurologist to determine brain activity. A single EEG showed flat lines with occasional artifact and there was no evidence of cortical activity. His vital signs were within normal limits and a respirator controlled his breathing. Seven hours after the surgery, arrangements were made to harvest his heart and kidneys. Attempts to locate family members to obtain permission to use the organs were unsuccessful. The surgeon was told to call the medical examiner after Tucker had been pronounced dead. The medical examiner, on notification of the death, "consented" to the use of the organs. In fact, family members had been searching for Tucker. A card with a brother's name was on the victim when he arrived at the emergency room, but was not discovered by the hospital. His heart was transplanted by one of the defendants. His kidneys were also removed at this time. The transplantations occurred within 24 hours of his injury.

The issue in the case was the interpretation of the word "death" as used in the Virginia wrongful death statute. The jury was instructed by the judge that they could accept the common law definition of death or an alternative definition, "neurological death," in their deliberations. The jury applied the alternative medical definition and held in favor of the defendant physicians. If the jury had been instructed to apply the common law definition of death, undoubtedly it would have found in favor of Bruce Tucker's brother. However, the court itself refused to adopt the alternative definition of death. The defendant physicians had requested that such a judicial decision be handed down. The court took the position that such an undertaking rested with the state legislature and not the courts. Virginia enacted a brain death statute the following year.[22]

Brain Death and Criminal Homicide

In 1974, Dr. Shumway, who was a pioneer in heart transplant surgery in California, transplanted the heart of Samuel Moore, a victim of a shooting.[23] The defendant, who had been caught after the shooting, unsuccessfully argued that the death resulted from the surgery and not the gunshot to the victim's head. The victim was declared brain dead whereupon his ventilator was disconnected. The court held that, "A person may be pronounced dead if, based on the usual and customary standards of medical practice, it has been determined that the person has suffered an irreversible cessation of brain function."

Three years later, the Massachusetts Supreme Court in a criminal case held that the defendant was not deprived of a possible defense to his act of murder.[24] A 34-year-old man was struck on the back of the head with a baseball bat by the defendant. He had cranial surgery and was placed on a ventilator. He had some degree of brain stem function. Two days later his EEG was isolectric and he could not breathe when the ventilator was removed. By this time all brain stem function had ceased and within 48 hours he had no reflex action or response to painful stimuli. With the consent of the family his respirator was removed 2 days later and his heart ceased to beat. An autopsy revealed a decomposed brain without structure, a finding that is consistent with brain death.

Although the hospital had developed brain death criteria less rigid than the Harvard Criteria, the physicians used the Harvard Criteria as a basis for pronouncing the victim brain dead. The internal criteria were based on brain death studies which came after the 1968 Harvard Criteria. The jury found that the victim's death occurred before he was disconnected from the respirator.

In 1975, a New York court was asked to rule on the meaning of the word, "death" as used in the state Uniform Anatomical Gift Statute.[25] The term was not defined in the statute, which was enacted to encourage anatomic gifts by donors or their next of kin. The situation that triggered the judicial request arose when a 27-year-old man was admitted to a city hospital suffering from a gunshot wound to his temporal area. He was totally unresponsive with no spontaneous respirations or movement. After intensive treatment he was determined to be neurologically dead. His parents consented to the removal of his kidneys. However, the kidneys were not removed because of a lack of a legal definition of death. In addition, policy of the medical examiner prohibited organ removal from homicide victims. Within 48 hours of his admission to the city facility he had a cardiac arrest, but the homicide victim policy precluded donations.

The next day Daniel Sulsona, aged 21, was admitted to the same hospital suffering from a gunshot wound to the parietal region of his head. He too, was declared medically dead and his mother authorized removal of his kidneys. The hospital then petitioned the court to have him legally declared dead. Four hours after the court petition was filed he also suffered an arrest and met the common law definition of death. The surgeons, acting on advice of attorneys, immediately transplanted the kidneys into recipients.

Because these types of cases occur on a daily basis in many New York hospitals the court agreed to issue a ruling. It heard testimony from medically recognized experts. There was unanimous agreement that kidneys obtained from cadavers at that time had a higher incidence of post-transplant renal failure, whereas those transplanted from brain dead patients had an optimal chance of acceptance by the recipient. There was testimony that the lack of a definition of brain death was a source of undue stress for family members who wanted to donate organs. Hospital administrators did not know how to proceed in implementing the Gift Statute. Physicians were also reluctant to expose themselves to potential civil or criminal liability. All parties to the court proceeding were in agreement that there was a uniformly accepted medical standard of death which defined death in terms other than spontaneous cessation of cardiac and respiratory functions, and that the alternative definition was established according to generally accepted medical standards. Further, the court found that it was the intent of the state legislature, in enacting the Uniform Gift Act, to devise a systematic procedure to effectuate the public policy of encouraging organ donations. The court urged the state legislature to take affirmative action to provide a statewide remedy for the problem. In short, the court was urging the legislature to enact a statute that would at least recognize the concept of brain death.

In 1979, in the case of *Lovato v. District Court,* the Colorado Supreme Court recognized the concept of brain death when it ordered that the life support measures be removed from a 17-month-old child who had been allegedly beaten by his mother.[26] The state has since enacted legislation adopting the brain death standard. The child "died" minutes after the physicians disconnected the ventilator. The mother sought to persuade the court that the common law definition should be applied. However, the child while on advanced life-support systems showed no response to pain or other stimuli and there was a total absence of activity in his brain. This case is an example of the court, by judicial opinion, adopting the concept of brain death.

When confronted with a brain death question, an Illinois court looked to the wording in the state's existing Uniform Anatomical Gift Act which defined death for the purposes of the act as meaning irreversible cessation of total brain function, according to usual and customary standards of medical practice. The court noted that the legislature's definition was in harmony with the consensus of the medical community which defined legal death in the same terms. In that case, *In Re Haymer,* the parents and special guardian opposed removal of a ventilator from a 7-month-old infant.[27] Three physicians, including a pediatric neurosurgeon, confirmed that total, complete, and irreversible brain death existed. The court authorized the removal of the machine after finding that the child had been legally dead for 8 days prior to the initiation of the proceeding by the hospital. The infant died while the case was being appealed. The higher court upheld the trial court's decision.

Statutory Recognition of the Concept

In 1970, Kansas became the first state to enact legislation that recognized the concept of brain death.[28] The statute is wordy, but does set out the common law definition in addition to the brain death concept. The statute used an over-broad standard, "absence of spontaneous brain function" but failed to define the term. Later state statutes attempted to eliminate this omission. A number of states enacted identical or similar statutes. They included Alaska, Maryland, Virginia, New Mexico, and Oregon.

Two years after the Kansas statute was enacted, Capron and Kass proposed that brain death is "irreversible cessation of spontaneous brain function." Alexander Capron was to be appointed the Executive Director of the President's Commission For the Study of Ethical Problems in Medicine and Biomedical and Behavioral Research. A number of states, including Iowa, Louisiana, Michigan, Montana, and West Virginia based their brain death statutes on the Capron-Kass proposal.

In 1975 the American Bar Association adopted the following simple definition, "For all legal purposes, a human body with irreversible cessation of *total* brain function, according to usual and customary standards of medical practice, shall be considered dead." It was the basis for statutes in California, Georgia, Idaho, Illinois, Tennessee, and Oklahoma. The American Medical Association did not endorse the act of establishing the standard of brain death by legislation until 1979. The American Bar Association standard indicated that brain death included the total brain and not just cerebral death.

In 1980 the Uniform Law Commissioners developed a proposal in an effort to bring about uniformity in a brain death definition. The Law Commissioners are a confederation of state commissioners whose function is to draft legislation addressing problems common to all states. The group proposed a Uniform Determination of Death Act (UDDA) which states:

> An individual who has sustained either (1) irreversible cessation of circulatory and respiratory functions, or (2) irreversible cessation of all functions of the entire brain, including the brain stem, is dead. A determination of death must be made in accordance with accepted medical standards.[29]

The UDDA was endorsed by the following groups: American Bar Association, American Medical Association, American Academy of Neurology, and the American Electroencephalographic Society. Some states that had statutes on brain death, revised them to reflect the UDDA. These included Idaho, West Virginia, and Maryland. Others, such as Arizona, Indiana, Mississippi, Nevada, and Vermont legislatively adopted the model definition and enacted statutes for brain death for the first time.

The first state to adopt the UDDA by judicial decision was Washington.[30]

> In *In re the Welfare of William Bowman*, a 5-year-old boy had been physically abused and within 2 weeks of his admission to the hospital his neurologic findings were total absence of blood flow to the brain, no superficial or deep tendon reflexes, no response to painful stimuli, and no electrocerebral activity. Although the court determined that the child was brain dead it allowed the child's court-appointed guardian to appeal the court's decision that the child should be removed from the respirator to the state supreme court. During this interim period of 7 days all of the child's bodily functions ceased and he was declared dead under the traditional heart-lung death standard.
>
> The Washington State Supreme Court said that it viewed defining death as a matter of law because the law has an independent interest in defining death. It acknowledged the essential role medicine had in the brain death concept, that of setting out the medical criteria which must be met before the standard of brain death is diagnosed. The court distinguished the standard (definition) from the means whereby it was to be met (medical criteria).

There are, of course critics of the UDDA. Although it is redundant, the words, "entire brain" and "including the brain stem" was included to eliminate any confusion that neocortical or cerebral death would constitute brain death. There are those who would prefer that the brain death concept embrace destruction of the cerebrum because they argue that it is the cortex, not the brain stem, that gives the attributes of self-awareness and perception, and that gives man his human qualities. There are some commentators who would not regard patients whose brain stem continues to function as possible organ donors.[31] Their position is that there is insufficient scientific data on cerebral death. Future advances in diagnostic technology and research in clinical cases may eliminate resistance to the cerebral death concept.

In July 1981, the President's Commission for the Study of Ethical Problems in Medicine and Biomedical and Behavioral Sciences issued its report on brain death.[32] In its report, the commission recommended that the UDDA model be adopted in every jurisdiction. The commission picked up where the UDDA model left off. The commission developed criteria or guidelines for implementing the UDDA model definition and stipulated them as "advisory" in nature. The Commission added that the criteria would help medical practitioners and hospital committees who were developing their own internal policies and protocols.

The Criteria

The criteria reflect the general consensus of cardiologists, neurologists, neurosurgeons, philosophers, and attorneys. In its introduction to the criteria, the commission stated that it would be undesirable for any guidelines to be mandated by legislation or regulations, or to be inflexibly established in case law. The criteria, which were widely circulated, sought to encourage local, state and national institutions and professional organizations to examine and publish their own practices. The criteria began by stating that the common law definition of death and the brain death criteria are independent of each other and each stands alone as a determination of death.

The meaning of "cessation" and "irreversibility" as set out in the UDDA model definition were spelled out. *Cessation* refers to both cerebral and brain stem functions. Cessation of cerebral functions means deep coma (unreceptivity and unresponsibility) and may require confirmatory studies. Such confirmatory studies would include angiography and electroencephalography if circumstances warrant such confirmation tests. A determination of the cessation of brain stem functions requires "reliable testing." The criteria indicate that brain stem reflexes should be tested, but it does not go so far as to identify specific tests. It does, however, stress the importance of apnea testing and sets out one accepted method.

In evaluating the *irreversible* component, it is essential that the cause of the coma be identified and a determination made that it is not reversible. It is, of course, not always possible to identify the cause of coma with any degree of medical certainty. Although the criteria state that the length of the observation period is a matter of clinical judgment it does set out some figures. For example, where the cause of the coma is a result of anoxia an observation period of 24 hours is recommended. This time period may be reduced if angiography shows cerebral blood flow cessation or an EEG shows electrocerebral silence.

It is worth noting that the commission's advisory criteria did not attempt to mandate certain tests. The commission recognized that more sophisticated diagnostic tests will make some current tests obsolete for the purpose of diagnosing brain death. An example of new technology that may have future impact in diagnosing the physiologic effect of injury to the brain is computer analysis of evoked potentials (EPs).

The criteria set out four instances in which a false brain death finding may occur. These are drug and metabolic intoxication, hypothermia, increased resistance in infants and young children, and shock. While not identifying what category of physician should be employed to make a brain death diagnosis, the commission recommended a "competent and judicious physician, experienced in clinical examination and the relevant procedures." Although the criteria are silent on documentation, accepted medical practice standards would require complete clinical assessment records.

For the physician, the problem of defining brain death translates into a question of the accuracy of the criteria used to describe a dead brain. The President's Commission proposed the authority approach to validate the existence of brain death. The authority or consensual approach is based on clinical expertise and judgment. For example, the combined medical organizations of the United States might declare that an identified group of criteria will constitute brain death. Establishing criteria via this approach gives some assurance that they will be uniformly implemented.

It is not just the large urban medical centers that will need medical staff competent in diagnosing brain death. The rural facilities will be faced with the same problem. With the search methods for organ transplants becoming more organized and society accepting the need for noncadaver organs, even rural medical facilities will be pressed to identify potential donors who meet the brain death standard. One of the problems that urban hospitals may face which rural ones probably will not see are the indigent or "street people" who enter the emergency room in a coma. One problem when diagnosing and treating this group is that an exact history is frequently impossible to obtain. Evaluating a persistent coma may require the use of confirmatory tests, even invasive ones, to more accurately evaluate blood flow.

It is unlikely that the courts will become more involved in the brain death standard, as a number of judicial opinions have been handed down and there appears to be a momentum for states to adopt a brain death definition by statute. Whether or not a state statutorily adopts the UDDA, the criteria developed and published by the President's Commission will serve as advisory criteria. They are broad enough to be workable in the context of current technology, yet provide some degree of uniformity. The idea of uniformity is important to society as well as to the medical community who will be involved in various phases of care of the brain dead patient. Society needs the reassurance to maintain trust in health care providers, both as consumers and individuals making donation decisions. Colleagues need to know that ethical and professional tenets are being upheld.

Summary

The brain death concept became important with the advent of transplantation because of the need to identify potential donors and to obtain and transplant the organ without undue delay. Many of the early problems resulted from the lack of consensus of what constituted brain death. Some states approached the problem by enacting laws defining death. Other states dealt with the problem by judicial decision. Some states resorted to both mechanisms. Some courts in their decisions encouraged the legislature to enact brain death statutes. Conversely, there were those who did not want any legislation or court involvement, preferring to leave the brain death issues to the medical profession. However, this last option created instability and uncertainty in dealing with both brain dead and non-brain-dead patients.

The Harvard Criteria were important because they represented an early effort to both define brain death and formulate criteria for diagnosing its existence. The extensive work done by the President's Commission on brain death criteria focuses attention on the need for each facility to formulate its own guidelines to aid the staff in diagnosing and implementing policy. The Commission's advisory criteria encourage facilities to formulate committees to develop its own protocols to meet the needs of a specific patient population.

Some states have not adopted a statutory definition of brain death. This, of course, does not mean that a facility is prevented from establishing its own internal guidelines. A significant number of states do not have a legal definition and the hospitals in such jurisdictions operate on protocols which have been developed by a specific committee or ad hoc group within the hospital setting. The internal criteria must comport with existing standards of accepted medical practice.

LIFESAVING AND LIFE-PROLONGING TREATMENT DECISIONS

Occasionally a legal decision attracts national interest and the Karen Ann Quinlan case in 1976 did just that. It also generated a great deal of worldwide interest. Ordinarily such interest subsides with the passage of time, but this has not been so in the medical treatment cases. Undoubtedly one of the factors that continues to make the treatment issues so compelling is the fact that society can identify with the issue readily. The Quinlan case brought into sharp focus the need to decide these types of cases with some sort of structured deliberation. *Quinlan* served to focus attention on a dilemma generated in part by scientific and technological advancements.

It was just a matter of time before the courts would become actively involved in treatment decisions. This is because the scientific advances unexpectantly, although not altogether unforeseeably, began to be applied in situations involving hopelessly ill patients. The courts were forced to deal with these cases when they came to them for resolution. A number of writers have criticized judicial intervention, and the medical and legal literature contains sharp criticism of individual holdings and the role the court itself played in some treatment decisions. Most authorities agree that the role of the courts should be limited. The courts have begun to arrive at a consensus concerning when and to what extent they should be involved.

The judicial approach has been criticized for a number of reasons. First, it lacks the expertise to make these kinds of decisions. Second, the judicial process is, by its nature, slow and thus not a proper vehicle for many treatment decisions. Third, it can be expensive. Fourth, it intrudes into an area of decision making that has traditionally been done by physicians and sometimes by the family. However, it is doubtful that the judiciary will ever be entirely excluded from the treatment decision dilemmas. This is because traditionally the courts have been the means whereby conflicting interests and rights have been resolved. Although the courts in different jurisdictions have not formulated a uniform approach to treatment decisions, the decisions have served to identify principles applicable to treatment cases.

The courts, in relying on previous judicial decisions and having the unique mechanism (the appeal process) of being able to review lower court proceedings, are in a position to provide "consistency over time."[33] *Quinlan* set in motion an overdue examination of some fundamental societal beliefs as they impact on complex medical treatment decisions. The courts have provided significant direction, albeit not in the form of step-by-step guidelines. They have, in a number of cases, encouraged resolution by the legislative process. The amount and depth of the materials written on the subject of treatment decisions has added dimension to the topic. Areas of agreement have emerged from both legal rulings and the literature.

Quinlan

The facts of the case are well known.[34]

> Karen Ann Quinlan lapsed into an irreversible coma in 1975, possibly from the combined effect of tranquilizers and alcohol. After several months her parents requested that her respirator be disconnected. They anticipated and had been advised that withdrawal of the ventilator would accelerate her death. Karen's physicians refused to remove the ventilator, saying that such an act would "not conform to medical practices, standards and traditions." Her father, Joseph Quinlan, filed a court petition requesting that he be appointed her guardian in order that he could authorize the removal. He was appointed guardian of her property, but not of her person. The case eventually was heard in the state Supreme Court.
>
> That court granted the relief requested by finding that the constitutional right of privacy was broad enough to encompass a patient's decision to decline medical treatment under certain circumstances. The Constitution

does not explicitly identify a right to privacy, but the U.S. Supreme Court in prior decisions recognized such a right and held that certain areas of privacy are guaranteed under the Constitution. The New Jersey court said that neither the right to religious belief or protection against cruel and unusual punishment applied to Karen's plight. In the presence of Karen's persistent vegetative state, her father as guardian was permitted to exercise her right to terminate treatment.

The court acknowledged that the ventilator served only a maintenance function and was not curative. It also stated that the state had an interest in the "preservation and sanctity of human life and defense of the right of the physician to administer medical treatment according to his best judgment." However, it stated that these two state interests were diminished in the presence of a significant degree of bodily invasion. In essence, the court recognized that Karen's right to be free from intrusion outweighed the state interest.

Karen required intensive round-the-clock nursing care, antibiotics, respiratory maintenance, a catheter, and a feeding tube. The court said, "We have no doubt, in these unhappy circumstances, that if Karen were herself miraculously lucid for an interval (not altering the existing prognosis of the condition to which she would soon return) and perceptive of her irreversible condition, she could effectively decide upon discontinuance of the life-support apparatus, even if it meant the prospect of natural death." The court observed "that physicians distinguish between curing the ill and comforting and easing the dying, that they refuse to treat the curable as if they were dying or ought to die, and that they have sometimes refused to treat the hopeless and dying as if they were curable."[35]

The court declined to give any weight to the testimony of her mother and friends concerning any supposed choice Karen might have uttered, as such testimony lacked sufficient evidentiary weight. A subsequent New York case stated that such statements would have to be more than a casual statement uttered at a social function.[36] The court did not give absolute authority to Karen's father to exercise her right to refuse. It stipulated that "should physicians attending the patient. . . conclude that there was no reasonable possibility of the patient's emerging from her comatose condition to a cognitive, sapient state and that the life-support apparatus should be discontinued, physicians, upon concurrence of the guardian and family of the patient, should consult with a hospital ethics committee or a like body and if the consultative body agrees with physicians' prognosis, the life-support system can be withdrawn without any civil or criminal liability. . . . The court appeared to be saying that the collaboration was for the purpose of confirming the medical findings and that the function and role of the committee was not advisory.

One final point regarding *Quinlan* should be made. The court was disinclined to grant immunity to the physicians for their decisions and actions. However, some courts have granted immunity to both physicians and hospitals against civil or criminal liability.[37] Nevertheless, the *Quinlan* court recognized that undue concern might inhibit physicians in their medical judgment when treating dying patients.

The court viewed the ethics committee approach as providing a safeguard for the patients and their medical caretakers because such a committee structure would involve multidisciplinary members in the decision-making process and would undoubtedly screen out "less than worthy motivations of family or physician." The court stated that once the treatment decision was made by that body it would be inappropriate to go to court to confirm the decision. It regarded such a measure as a "gratuitous encroachment upon the medical profession's field of competence," as well as an impossibly cumbersome burden. Thus, the New Jersey model was based on an ethics committee concept.[38] In the wake of the *Quinlan* decision, New Jersey developed guidelines to aid health care facilities in the development and implementation of procedures concerning the care of comatose, noncognitive patients.[39]

Saikewicz

Just about the time that Karen Quinlan was being weaned from her respirator, events in a Massachusetts state facility raised many of the same issues.[40]

In *Superintendent of Belchertown State School v. Saikewicz*, the Massachusetts courts articulated many of the legal principles cited in *Quinlan*, but rejected the ethics committee decision-making approach to such treatment problems. The Massachusetts decision was widely criticized because it carved out a more definitive role by the courts than *Quinlan*. The medical issue in *Saikewicz*, as in *Quinlan*, involved life-prolonging treatment as opposed to lifesaving treatment. A number of groups, including a mental health legal advisory committee and state association for retarded persons, submitted friend of the court briefs. The court declined to formulate a comprehensive list of guidelines that would be applicable to emergency medical situations involving incompetent persons. The court viewed that as the role of the legislature.

At the time of diagnosis, Joseph Saikewicz was 67 years old and had resided in a state facility since he was 14. He was profoundly retarded and incapable of consenting to treatment. Family members did not wish to be a part of the decision. In April 1976, it was discovered that he had acute myeloblastic monocytic leukemia and his physicians recommended against treatment because even with aggressive chemotherapy his life would be extended for only a short time. Additionally, there was concern that because of his profoundly retarded state he would not understand or cooperate with the treatment. There was also concern that he might suffer emotional harm because of the nature of the treatment. The facility petitioned the court for the appointment of a guardian who could make the necessary decisions. The judge appointed a special guardian whose duty it was to investigate the case and report back to the court. After investigating the situation the special guardian recommended that treatment not be given because of the pain and fear that would be experienced. These factors weighed against the limited benefit associated with treatment. The judge, relying on the testimony of Saikewicz's attending physicians who also recommended against chemotherapy, ordered that treatment not be given. The man died 5 months later.

Because of the importance of the decision the judge requested that the state high court rule on the case. The high court asserted four state interests: preservation of human life, protection of third parties, maintenance of the ethical integrity of the medical profession, and the prevention of suicide. Two of the articulated state interests, suicide prevention and the protection of third parties, were not applicable to Saikewicz's situation. The two remaining interests were weighed against his rights.

Addressing the preservation of life interest, the court said that prolonging a life must be reconciled with the interest the person has to reject the traumatic cost of that prolongation. The therapy available to Saikewicz would not be curative. Addressing the maintenance of the ethical integrity of the medical profession, the court said that the force and impact of this interest was lessened by the prevailing medical ethical standard which does not demand that all efforts toward life prolongation be made in all circumstances. The medical community clearly recognized and accepted a patient's right to refuse necessary treatment in appropriate circumstances. The court upheld the lower court decision and said, "It is not necessary to deny a right of self-determination to a patient in order to recognize the interests of doctors, hospitals, and medical personnel in attendance on the patient."

Deciding for an Incompetent Person

Once it was determined that Saikewicz had as much right as a competent person to decline treatment, the question became: What legal standards would govern the decision-making process? The court first considered the decision-making process that a competent person would embark upon. The process would necessarily involve such factors as, age, prognosis (with and without treatment), the pain or discomfort associated with chemotherapy, and other factors. Applying the legal doctrine of "substituted judgment," the court then sought to reach a decision that would factor-in Saikewicz's position. The *substituted judgment* doctrine facilitates a treatment decision that would be made by the incompetent person, if that person were competent, and takes into consideration all the known factors that would necessarily enter into the decision-making process of that individual. Although similar to the "reasonable man" standard, the substituted judgment test is more subjective and takes into account with as much accuracy as is possible the wants and needs of the individual involved.

The Saikewicz court also addressed the "gratuitous encroachment" on the domain of medical expertise argument raised in *Quinlan*. The Saikewicz court said that the awesome question of whether potentially life-prolonging treatment should be withheld from a person incapable of making his own decision, requires "the process of detached but passionate investigation and decision that forms the ideal on which the judicial branch of government was created." The Saikewicz court viewed the ideal as the responsibility of the court, not to be entrusted to any other group purporting to represent the "morality and conscience of our society."

Spring Reaffirms *Saikewicz*

More than a year passed from the time of Joseph Saikewicz's death to the court opinion. When the long-awaited opinion was issued it was heralded by some and criticized by others. It completely rejected the *Quinlan* approach and was interpreted by some as requiring *all* treatment decisions involving life-prolonging or life-saving treatment of incompetent individuals to go to the courts. It was not until the *Spring* case that *Saikewicz* was placed in a more reasonable light. The case, *In the Matter of Spring* did not generate the controversy that the earlier Massachusetts case had, but it was criticized for placing an unreasonable burden on the family and dragging on for an unreasonable length of time.[41] *Spring* was entirely consistent with the Saikewicz opinion.

Earl Spring, a Massachusetts resident, was mentally competent until he got a systemic infection after injuring his foot in a hunting accident. Within 4 months he was diagnosed as having end-stage renal disease and was placed on hemodialysis. When he was first placed on dialysis he consented to the treatments, but his mental state deteriorated and he was subsequently diagnosed as having chronic organic brain syndrome. At the time his wife of 55 years and his adult son petitioned the court, it had already been determined that both the renal disease and senility were permanent and irreversible. Because of his age he was not a candidate for transplant.

A lower court authorized the son, who had been appointed guardian, to consent to stopping the dialysis treatments. However, the state supreme court, in keeping with *Saikewicz*, said that once the case came before the court it was the responsibility of the court to decide the legal question. It should not delegate it to some private person or group and it disapproved of a shift of the ultimate responsibility away from the court.

The *Spring* court held that the legal standard of substituted judgment was applicable to the *Spring* facts. The only state interest involved was the preservation of life issue. The court ultimately ruled that the state interest was insufficient to compel *Spring* to undergo the invasive treatment.

The holding was particularly helpful in responding to some of the questions raised by the medical and legal community in the wake of *Saikewicz*. The court stated that *Saikewicz* was not intended to set a standard that prior judicial approval was necessary before life-prolonging treatment could be withheld from an incompetent patient. The court listed some circumstances that may be used as a guide in deciding whether judicial approval is necessary. These include "the extent of impairment of the patient's mental faculties; whether the patient is in the custody of a state institution, the prognosis without the proposed treatment; the prognosis with the proposed treatment; the complexity, risk and novelty of the proposed treatment; its possible side effects; the patient's level of understanding and probable reaction; the urgency of the decision; the consent of the patient, spouse, or guardian; the good faith of those who participate in the decision; the clarity of professional opinion as to what is good medical practice; the interests of third persons; and the administrative requirements of any institution involved." The court declined to cite what combination of circumstances would make prior court approval necessary or desirable. Further, it acknowledged that the development of both medical advances and opinion made the establishment of legal criteria unreliable.

The high court stated that it in no way disapproved of the practice by hospitals of using a committee to review medical decisions. It emphasized that such decisions must be made responsibly and, as with any medical decisions, are subject to judicial scrutiny if bad faith on the part of the decision-makers is alleged.

Shortly after these two decisions, several situations arose that involved treatment decisions and prisoners. One case involved a 24-year-old prisoner who was on hemodialysis.[42] The court held that the state's interest in upholding orderly prison administration outweighed the prisoner's right. The prisoner's refusal of the hemodialysis treatments was not based on any religious objection and he did not express a wish to die. In fact, the court found that his protest was based on his request to be transferred to a minimum security prison and he was refusing the treatments for this reason. Another prisoner who was a diabetic refused his insulin as a manipulation tactic.[43] In a similar case the court ordered necessary x-ray films and blood tests where a prisoner refused them after swallowing razor blades.[44]

New York Cases

A New York case became the third model decision after the New Jersey and Massachusetts decisions.

Like the Massachusetts case, the "Brother Fox" case generated considerable controversy.[45] There was also a companion case which was equally criticized. The two cases were consolidated and heard by the state high court. By the time the cases were heard both patients had died, but the court elected to address the issues because of their public importance.

Brother Fox

In *Eichner v. Dillon*, Brother Joseph Fox was a retired member of a Catholic teaching order. At the age of 83 he underwent a hernia repair during which he had a cardiac arrest. As a result there was significant oxygen deprivation and he was placed on a respirator. He remained in a vegetative state and his prognosis was hopeless. The religious director and president of the school where Brother Fox resided asked the physicians to remove the respirator, but they refused, stating that once such intervention had begun it should not be withdrawn. The hospital directed him to seek a court order and as a result the court appointed the director, Father Eichner, as guardian. The district attorney opposed Father Eichner's court petition to remove the respirator.

At the court hearing there was evidence that Brother Fox on a number of occasions had made it known that he did not want extraordinary measures in the event he suffered a fate similar to Karen Quinlan. He first expressed his opinion after the Quinlan case came into prominence. At that time discussions at the school revolved around Catholic moral principles and the use of extraordinary means in hopeless cases. His last expression of opinion occurred several months before he was hospitalized.

The Storar Case

In the case of *Matter of John Storar*, the patient was profoundly retarded and at the time of the court petition he was 52 years old.[46] He had been a resident of a state facility since the age of 5 and his mother visited her only child almost daily. In July 1979 he was diagnosed as having cancer of the bladder. His mother was appointed guardian and consented to radiation therapy which brought about a remission. However, 7 months later he had another bout of hematuria and his cancer was diagnosed as terminal. When the physicians sought the mother's permission to administer blood transfusions she, at first, refused. A month later she requested they be discontinued. The transfusions were needed every 8 to 15 days. The facility brought a petition to continue the transfusions. The physicians feared that the son would hemorrhage to death and the continued bleeding deprived him of sufficient oxygen levels.

By this time the cancer had spread to his lungs and it was determined that he would live between 3 and 6 months. At times he resisted the transfusions and had to be restrained and sedated before the treatment. He needed regular doses of narcotics to alleviate the pain from the cancer.

In deciding these two cases, the court declined to recognize a constitutional argument as was the case in *Quinlan* and *Saikewicz*. The New York court held that the right to refuse treatment was based on the common law right of every person of adult years and sound mind to determine what should be done with his body. The court did say that such a right may have to concede to a greater state interest. In *Eichner*, the court held that before it could grant the relief sought by Father Eichner it must be shown by "clear and convincing evidence" that Brother Fox had left instructions to terminate life-support measures. Because Brother Fox had articulated his preference on several occasions, that standard was met. The court observed that the statements made by him were "not casual remarks made at some social gathering," and that he was not so young as to be unaware of the consequence of his remarks. This observation was in response to the New Jersey court in *Quinlan* finding that remarks made by Karen to her mother after the death of an elderly family friend that she would not want to linger on, would not serve as evidence of a knowing statement. The New York court imposed this standard of proof to emphasize the critical nature of the decision and to preclude evidence that is "loose."

The chief criticism of the *Eichner* opinion was that it recognized no alternative means to provide judicial relief if one has not articulated a preference. Another criticism was that this was the type of case that should not have gone to court.[47] The New York ruling placed in limbo the recognized medical practice of withdrawing extraordinary treatment measures, including ventilators and aggressive drug therapy, from hopelessly ill incompetent adult patients. While the court said that those responsible for the care of these patients could apply to the courts before the contemplated activity was carried out, such a procedure was optional. Thus, the court did not preclude withdrawal, but said that prior court approval could be sought when the legal consequences were in question. The responsible parties "need not act at their peril." Both the Massachusetts and New York courts refused to confer civil or criminal immunity on the physicians. Such a refusal is in line with the role of the judiciary. Physicians should be supported and encouraged to make medical decisions that conform to recognized and accepted medical practice standards. Physicians should not make it a practice to look to the courts solely to reduce their potential for civil or criminal liability. Such an approach would severely compromise the rights of patients and, in addition, would set a precedent that these types of cases are best dealt with in a judicial setting. The courts should be used for the unusual case or in cases where there is potential for civil or criminal liability.

The *Storar* decision has been subject to considerable criticism, including a dissenting opinion written by one of the New York justices.[48] That court declined to apply the substituted judgment test. It rejected the "proxy" decision-making approach and would not allow John Storar's mother to refuse the transfusions on his behalf. The court acknowledged the right of a parent to consent to medical treatment on behalf of an infant. In New York this is accomplished by statute. However, no such recognized right exists to refuse *lifesaving* treatment on behalf of the minor, no matter how well intentioned. The court likened John Storar's situation to the case of a child who may bleed to death because of the parents' refusal to consent to a blood transfusion because of their religious belief. Although understanding and respecting the mother's despair, the court said, "a court should not in the circumstances of this case allow an incompetent patient to bleed to death because some, even someone as close as a parent or sibling, feels that this is best for one with an incurable disease."

In writing one of two dissenting opinions, Judge Jones said that the question before the court was whether, and under what circumstances, a surrogate or proxy decision could be made where the decision related to the withholding or withdrawal of extraordinary life-support medical measures in situations similar to that presented by John Storar. He recognized that "few areas of judicial activity present such awesome questions or demand greater judicial wisdom and restraint" than these types of decisions. In a footnote, the judge noted that the practice of turning off machines to allow the patient to die is a fairly common practice in hospitals, and he cited the American Medical Association policy statement that states that the decision to stop life-prolonging extraordinary measures where there is evidence that biologic death is imminent is the decision of the patient or his immediate family. Judge Jones took the position that medical care providers should resort to judicial authorization in cases like these only in extraordinary circumstances and the judicial approach should not be normal practice.

Recognizing that the discontinuance of transfusions would "eventually" lead to John Storar's death sooner than death by cancer, the judge concluded that Mrs. Storar should be permitted to authorize the discontinuation of the transfusions. He applied a "best interests" test, that is, because the son was incapable of making a "reasoned choice" and his mother knew and loved him more than any other individual, she was in a position to make the crucial decision of what was in his best interests.

> In the wake of the *Eichner* and *Storar* cases, two New York trial court judges ordered hospitals to remove the life-support systems from two patients. In one case the patient was brain dead, but the hospital had refused the family's request that the respirator be turned off.[49] The other case involved an 88-year-old woman who was comatose after suffering massive brain damage as a result of strokes.[50] That court ruled that the woman had a common law right to refuse treatment, and that the family could enforce her right if they could show by "clear and convincing evidence" that she was fatally ill and when competent had requested that treatment should be stopped if she became irreversibly ill.

Summary

The three judicial models on the withholding or withdrawal of medical care and treatment are *Quinlan, Saikewicz,* and *Eichner* and *Storar.* Of the three models, *Quinlan* generated the least amount of criticism. *Quinlan* went the route of the ethics committee. In *Saikewicz* and *Spring,* the court adopted a substituted judgment test as the standard of proof in deciding such cases. *Spring,* of all the models, was the only one to articulate some judicial guidelines in deciding which cases should go to court. Although these guidelines were broad, they did serve to help during the initial decision-making process at the bedside. In the past, such decisions were not arrived at with any degree of analytical precision. The court in *Spring* also said that *Saikewicz* was never intended to set the standard that all life-prolonging cases must go to court. In an uncommon break with judicial tradition, the justice who authored the Saikewicz opinion discussed it publicly.[51] He faulted physicians, and in particular, attorneys who advised the physicians and hospitals, for creating problems by misinterpreting the ruling.

Although most of the hospitals who had their own in-house legal counsel or utilized outside counsel with experience in treatment cases, continued to remove respirators without going to court, a significant number of cases did crowd the courts. *Spring* and the coverage the topic received in the literature helped to place restraint on this approach.

Eichner did little to clear the air. The standard of proof adopted by the New York court was "clear and convincing." This contrasted with the substituted judgment and best interest" standards adopted by the earlier decisions. The standard adopted in *Eichner* was difficult to prove because it required "formal" articulation of a preference while the patient was competent. However, both Massachusetts and New York were helpful by ruling that not every case warranted judicial intervention. The *Storar* decision went wrong when it likened the patient's situation to cases where an infant needs blood and the parents refuse because of their beliefs. The *Storar* decision was criticized because it involved applying inappropriate case law. Much of the problem with *Saikewicz* was the interpretation given to it.

Some observations can be made about the lessons of these cases. An important one is that where a spouse or family disagrees with a patient's prior articulated decision, the case should be resolved in court. This would also be true where adult family members disagree among themselves. Although not all third party interests mandate judicial intervention, such a factor should be discussed thoroughly before a decision is implemented.

RESPIRATORY SUPPORT CASES

There have been other state court decisions, but none established the precedent of the New Jersey, Massachusetts, and New York opinions. Some of these indicated that the decision was confined to the case before the court and that other treatment issues would have to be resolved on a case-by-case basis. That is not to say that these courts required judicial intervention in all instances, only that they were reluctant to establish precedent. Many said that such cases should be guided by legislation rather than the courts. When the physicians in *Quinlan* refused to remove Karen's ventilator they opened the door to the courts. Ironically, the practice of removing patients from ventilators had existed for some time prior to *Quinlan*. The problem was that such decisions had not been made ad hoc.

In 1980, the state of Delaware did not have enabling legislation to permit the next of kin to serve as proxy in decisions to terminate life-support systems.

Thus, in *Severns v. Wilmington Medical Center*, the husband of a 55-year-old woman who had been in an irreversible coma after an automobile accident, went to court to be appointed her guardian with authority to have her ventilator removed.[52] He also sought authority to have other supportive treatment stopped. The woman had been an active member of the Euthanasia Council of Delaware and had said that she did not want to be kept alive as a "vegetable." She had not left any written instructions, but had made verbal statements that she wanted to make a living will.

Her attending physician indicated that he would continue the use of the respirator and medications as needed unless there was an order from the court to permit stopping them. Further, he indicated that he would not write a "no code blue" order unless the court determined that it was permissible to write such an order. The medical center did not have an ethics committee or like body whereby it would approve or disapprove of the discontinuance of the systems. In his complaint the husband asked that the court order the removal and restrain the authorities from bringing a criminal action against any parties involved in the decision or act. He also requested immunity for any physician for civil liability, including any allegation of unprofessional conduct.

Noting that other courts had granted such relief in the absence of legislation, the Delaware Court held that it had the authority to grant the requests. The court based its authority on the wife's constitutional right. However, the court required a full hearing on the facts before it would rule on the husband's requests.

In a Ohio proceeding that same year, a trial court in *Leach v. Akron General Medical Center* permitted the removal of a respirator from a 70-year-old woman who had amyotrophic lateral sclerosis (ALS).[53] The woman had been on the ventilator for 5 months. The husband had unsuccessfully requested 29 physicians to remove the ventilator. She died shortly after the ventilator was disconnected.

The case set out the procedural requirements for removal. These included certification by two physicians (one a neurologist) that the patient is in a permanent vegetative state, prior notice to the county coroner and prosecutor that the examination would be conducted, and a 48-hour delay after the examination in order to notify the coroner and prosecutor. A representative from the coroner's and prosecutor's office may be present when the support is withdrawn.

Two cases heard in California in 1979 allowed parents to have their children taken off ventilators. Neither patient met any brain death standard. The first case involved a 3-year-old child and the second case involved an 18-year-old young man who was in a coma for 5 months following an automobile accident.[54,55] Both petitions were based on the state constitution which recognized a right to privacy.

Because of cases in the Los Angeles area and intense public concern surrounding the issues, several local groups took positions on the issue.[56] The California Board of Medical Quality Assurance said that as long as the prevailing standards of medical care were followed physicians should not fear disciplinary action by the Board for withdrawal of life support systems. The then-district attorney covering the Los Angeles area publicly stated that as long as good medical practices were followed his office would not initiate criminal prosecution. He stated that the families should be consulted and concur with the decision. He also advocated the use of necessary consultations to confirm the diagnosis and prognosis, and cautioned that detailed records should be kept.

In 1981 the Los Angeles County Medical and Bar Associations developed guidelines for the discontinuance of life-support systems under specified circumstances.[57] The guidelines set out five broad principles that govern decision making and three sets of circumstances whereby decisions to discontinue the use of cardiopulmonary life-support systems can be made without prior court authorization (see Appendix C in the back of the book.) Two of the principles are particularly noteworthy. First, family members of adult patients should always be consulted, although they have no legal standing under present California law to make such decisions on behalf of the patient.[58] Second, a physician is not required to continue the use of cardiopulmonary life support systems solely because such support was initiated at an earlier time. The three specific sets of circumstances in which life support can be withdrawn without prior court approval include brain death, natural death, and irreversible coma. The California Uniform Determination of Death Act deals with brain death and a natural death, however the irreversible coma situation is not specifically recognized in any present California statute.[59]

Criteria for the discontinuance of life-support measures in the presence of irreversible coma require that the medical record indicate the following: (1) confirmation of the diagnosis by a physician qualified by training or experience to establish such a diagnosis; (2) no indication that the patient expressed a wish to be maintained on life support systems; (3) concurrence by the family or guardian.

In a case that was widely reported in the news media, a California appeals court held that the individual's wishes were "paramount to the interests of the patient's hospital and doctors." In *Bartling v. Superior Court*, a 70-year-old patient who suffered from a malignant lung tumor, abdominal aneurysm, arteriosclerosis, and emphysema with chronic respiratory failure requested that his respirator be removed.[60] He was mentally competent and efforts to wean him from his ventilator were unsuccessful. His medical record indicated that he had tried to disconnect the tubes himself. While competent he had signed a "living will" and all his family were in agreement that his respirator be disconnected.

The trial court had refused to permit the withdrawal. It held that although his illnesses were serious they were not terminal and he was not comatose. It took the position that Mr. Bartling had the potential for being restored to a "cognitive, sapient life." However, the appeals court said it was incorrect for the lower court to hold that the disconnection of life support equipment was limited to comatose, terminally ill patients. Also addressing the physicians argument that disconnecting the machine would aid in the patient's suicide, the court said that such an act would not cause death by unnatural means, but would merely hasten his inevitable death by natural causes.

An earlier Florida case decided in 1978 also dealt with an elderly man who was competent, on a ventilator, and wanted it discontinued. The *Satz v. Perlmutter* case dealt with a 73-year-old man with advanced ALS.[61] He had no minor children and his family agreed with his decision. His condition was terminal and his situation wretched. Both the trial court and the state high court acknowledged that no state interests existed which would vitiate his consent. The *Satz* case was the first case to specifically address the suicide issue. The court found that the man wanted to live, but not in misery. No action on his part had placed him in his miserable state. The court held that it saw no difference in his wish to die a natural death and a situation where a terminal cancer patient declines surgery or chemotherapy. The court stated that although disconnection of a ventilator requires an affirmative act the principle upon which the wish was based was the same.

However, the *Satz* court failed to provide any reassurance for families, physicians, or hospitals in the manner in which they should be guided in their future conduct. The Florida Supreme Court, in adopting the lower trial court decision, said that it did so only based on the particular facts of the case. Thus, future Florida cases would be decided on a case by case basis. The court did take a firm position that such matters are better dealt with on a legislative level. Thus, in 1981 Florida enacted a brain death statute.[62]

In 1984 the Florida Supreme Court was asked to certify the question of whether a court order was necessary if a patient had executed a living or "mercy" will before support measures could be withdrawn. The facts involved in *John F. Kennedy Memorial Hospital v. Bludworth* were that in 1975 the patient had executed a living will.[63] In April 1981 his wife requested that all support measures be withdrawn because he was irreversibly comatose and in a vegetative state. The hospital filed a petition seeking court direction because it was uncertain of its liability. Although the court expedited a hearing the man died before it could be convened.

Rejecting the opinions of two lower courts that heard the case, the Supreme Court held that "the right of a patient, who is in an irreversibly comatose and essentially vegetative state, to refuse extraordinary life-sustaining measures, may be exercised either by his or her close family members or by a guardian of the person of the patient appointed by the court." The Supreme Court said that it was "too burdensome" to require prior court approval in such cases where the patient is irreversibly brain damaged, comatose, and unable to personally express his wishes. "If there are close family members such as the patient's spouse, adult children, or parents who are willing to exercise the patient's right to refuse treatment. . . there is no requirement that a guardian be judicially appointed." Both the family and the guardian must have the primary physician certify that the patient is in a "permanent vegetative state and that there is no reasonable prospect that the patient will regain cognitive brain function and that his existence is sustained only through the use of extraordinary life-sustaining measures." Two other physicians must concur with the primary physician.

Further, the court said that guardians, consenting family members, physicians, the hospital, and its administration would be relieved of potential civil and criminal liability so long as they acted in good faith. Liability would attach if it was shown that their actions were not in good faith, but rather were intended to harm the patient.

In 1984, a Connecticut court ruled that a 42-year-old woman who had multiple sclerosis for 24 years and who was in a vegetative state could have her ventilator removed.[64] In *Foody v. Manchester Memorial Hospital* the young woman's month-long court battle finally ended when she died an hour after she was removed from the respirator. She became paralyzed from the neck down with only her brain stem functioning after suffering a respiratory arrest 3 months previously.

In a West Virginia petition brought in 1981, a trial judge said that he had been prepared to rule in favor of a 76-year-old woman's request that her life-support systems be removed so she could die.[65] The woman, who was mentally competent, developed a severe infection six weeks after hepatic surgery for cirrhosis of the liver. She previously told the judge that she wanted to die, but died before a judicial decision was reached.

In a similar New York case, the hospital initiated suit after the patient who was mentally competent had been examined by two psychiatrists and had signed the necessary hospital forms.[66] He was in a terminal stage of diabetes, had bilateral amputations, and was blind. He asked that his hemodialysis treatments be stopped and while the legal proceedings were underway he had a respiratory arrest and remained in a vegetative state until his death. The court held two bedside judicial hearings and said that the man had a right to die a natural death.

In 1985, in *Tune v. Walter Reed Army Medical Hospital,* a federal court was asked to rule on the rights of patients in a federal hospital to have life support systems removed in the "face of mortal illness."[67] A woman who was competent throughout the judicial proceedings was admitted to the government hospital for sudden onset of respiratory problems which was believed to be caused by pneumonia. She was placed on a ventilator 2 days after admission. However, subsequent cytologic examination of fluid in the pericardial sac revealed the presence of a malignant adenocarcinoma. She quickly developed adult respiratory distress syndrome (ARDS) and deteriorated. The court petition for the removal of the ventilator was filed 6 days after her admission to the hospital. She told the court appointed guardian ad litem she had "no reservations at all" about removing the ventilator and wrote, "I would like to get off the life support system under which I am now having to live." Her physicians who were sympathetic to her wishes told her it was the policy of the Department of the Army not to remove artificial life support once it was begun. The physicians were unaware of the full extent of her illness initially and testified, that had they known the circumstances they would not have ordered the ventilator originally. The court held that the well-established rule of general law "that it is the patient, not the physician, who ultimately decides if treatment—any treatment—is to be given at all" is as binding upon the government as it is upon the medical profession at large. ". . . such a patient who enters treatment in ignorance, with or without the physicians' connivance, has the right to insist that the treatment be halted once he is fully informed of the consequences and does not wish to incur them." Further, the court concluded that any state interests "are insufficient to outweigh plaintiff's interest in dying as she chooses."

In June 1987 the New Jersey Supreme Court decided three termination of treatment cases and one of these was *In the Matter of Kathleen Farrell* which held that a competent, terminally ill patient who was kept on a ventilator in her home could be allowed to have the machine removed.[68] Her case was tried in June 1986 and she died while still connected to the ventilator right after the trial. Factually, *Farrell* was distinguished from *Quinlan* and *Matter of Conroy* because Mrs. Farrell was competent and receiving home ventilator care. (See Chapter 10 for a discussion of *Conroy* and the two other 1987 New Jersey decisions.)

Mrs. Farrell was a 37-year-old mother of two teenage sons with terminal ALS and was maintained on a ventilator in her home. When she was first placed on it in the hospital she refused to allow the insertion of a nasogastric tube and left DNR instructions to the staff. At the time of the trial she could not eat any solid foods. She was paralyzed and needed around-the-clock nursing care. After an experimental program which was "their last hope," Mrs. Farrell told her husband that she wanted to be disconnected from the machine. Some of the trial was held at her home in order to permit her to testify. She told the court that she was "tired of suffering" and a court-ordered examination by a psychologist determined that she was mentally competent. The case is important because it set out the procedures to be followed when a patient living at home wishes to terminate life support measures.

The court said, "As in *Quinlan* and *Conroy*, we do not today determine whether life-sustaining medical treatment should be withdrawn from any of the patients in these cases, but rather define who may make such a decision and how it may be made." The procedures applicable when competent patients who wish to terminate life-sustaining medical treatment live at home are as follows: (1) two nonattending physicians must examine the patient to confirm that he or she is competent; (2) two nonattending physicians must ascertain that the patient is fully informed about his or her prognosis, the medical alternatives available, the risks involved, and the likely outcome in the withdrawal of life-sustaining treatment; and (3) it is determined that the patient made his or her choice voluntarily and without coercion. The court noted that many people wish to die at home in familiar surroundings and that home care of the terminally ill is increasing. It said the right to exercise this choice does not vary depending on whether the patient is in a medical institution or at home. The court said that the procedures which must be done before the withdrawal of treatment in the home could occur were designed to protect the patient. It said that in a hospital setting the patient is observed by more people and the issues of competency treatment alternatives and noncoercion are more easily resolved. Only "unusual circumstances, such as a conflict among the physicians, or the family members, or between the physicians and the family or other health care professionals, would necessitate judicial intervention."

The court found that the states's interest in protecting innocent third parties (her two teenage sons) did not outweigh her decision to stop treatment. Addressing the issue that many competent patients are physically unable to separate themselves from life-support equipment and need to rely on others to do it for them the court held that no civil or criminal liability will be incurred by any person who, in "good faith" relies on the court adopted procedures when terminating such home life-supporting equipment.

Summary

Most of the withdrawal or withholding of treatment cases have involved incompetent patients. The majority have based the right to stop treatment on constitutional grounds. The legal principle brought into focus by these cases is that a competent adult has a right to make a reasoned choice about the management of his medical care. This is so, even if the reasoned choice results in an accelerated death. In the instance of incompetent patients the courts have evolved legal theories to permit them to enjoy the same rights as competent patients. The right to make a reasoned choice is not an absolute right and may be outweighed by a greater state interest.

There is a consensus emerging from the various judicial opinions, as well as from the vast amount of literature on the subject of lifesaving and life-prolonging treatment issues. Many of the major treatment decisions have taken the opportunity to encourage the legislature to address the issues. Some of the decisions have provided direction in the form of legal guidelines or suggestions. Some, of course, are impractical or impose undue burden upon the right to refuse treatment. There appears to be some hesitation in complying with the request of a competent patient to stop treatment, especially in instances where the patient is alert.

In conclusion, first, the fact that a patient has been placed on a ventilator should never preclude its removal when a medical determination is made that the patient is hopelessly ill or in an irreversible state. Second, where the patient is alert, medication should be given to control the fear and anxiety of stopping the machines. If the patient is being sustained only by medications the termination is generally physically comfortable. Third, a facility should prepare its staff to meet the needs of the family when the treatments are stopped. This is especially important if the family wishes to be at the bedside while the patient is actually dying. The last point is that the events leading up to any decision to terminate life-support systems should be clearly reflected in the patient's record and all staff members should be aware of the institutional policy. The policies should be developed by all interested parties and any disagreement resolved. The policies should be reviewed frequently to reflect scientific advancements and societal interests.

THE THREAT OF CIVIL LIABILITY

In the wake of the treatment decisions, some families brought suit against the hospital and physicians for refusing to terminate ventilators. In the first such case, *Estate of Leach v. Shapiro* the court held that where the patient had expressly told the defendants that she did not wish to be placed on life-support systems and where the placement was not to treat a life-threatening emergency, the next of kin had a right to sue for wrongfully placing and maintaining the patient on the life-support systems.[69] The suit alleged that the hospital and the neurologist failed to get the family's consent before connecting the 70-year-old woman who was suffering from ALS to a ventilator and later refusing to disconnect it when requested by the family. The family was unable to get any local physician to disconnect the machine and finally got an out-of-town physician who had to wait for hospital privileges to be granted before he could disconnect the ventilator. Mrs. Leach died 26 minutes later.

The hospital settled with the family.[70] After 2 days of the trial against the physician the judge rendered a verdict in favor of the doctor saying that the evidence on informed consent was lacking. He also questioned whether state law allowed a physician to disconnect the ventilator where the physician found such an act conflicted with his own moral beliefs.[71]

In another case in which the hospital delayed for 3 days the removal of a ventilator from a brain dead 20-year-old young man who shot himself, a court held that the parents had no grounds to sue for the delay.[72] A jury in *Strachan v. John F. Kennedy Memorial Hospital* had awarded the family $140,000, but an appeals court set aside the verdict because it had not been shown that the hospital should have had consent forms available for all the parties to sign before withdrawing the ventilator. The delay was caused because the hospital had to consult with its attorneys. The court said that the family had not shown that it suffered any harm recognized under state law. The family alleged that they suffered emotional distress watching their child after they had requested the removal of the machine.

In the most recent case a New Jersey court in *McVey v. Englewood Hospital Association* held in favor of the hospital, its administrator, and the physicians where a deceased patient's daughters alleged they failed to honor her wishes to terminate life-support measures.[73] The patient was taken to the hospital after suffering a stroke at the age of 91 years and the neurologist informed the family on the day she was admitted that brain stem activity was minimal and that death would ensue if she was removed from the ventilator. The daughters demanded that the mother be removed from the machine saying that she had orally expressed the wish that she not be kept on a machine if she should suffer this kind of fate. The hospital refused to remove her from the machine in the absence of a court order. However, as soon as the daughters obtained the court order the woman was removed and died 4 days later. The court held that there was no actionable breach of a legal duty by the hospital or physicians to the patient of her family in the absence of a written directive. No duty existed on the part of the defendants to determine the "existence, veracity, and effect" of the patient's orally expressed wishes with respect to extraordinary treatment measures to preserve life.

A California court in *Bartling v. Glendale Adventist Medical Center* held that the hospital in which William Bartling died after 7 months of treatment could not be sued for money damages.[74] The family alleged that the hospital deliberately disregarded the constitutional rights of the decendent by maintaining him on a ventilator in spite of a living will made out by the patient 6 weeks after being admitted to the hospital. He formally released the hospital and its physicians from any civil liability. Both the patient and family members signed the release papers. In addition to the violation of constitutional rights the family alleged that the defendants actions were extreme, malicious, and outrageous, and violated the patient's constitutional right of privacy.

The court found that the hospital acted sincerely as a pro-life-oriented hospital in declining to respect the patient's wishes, especially because California law was not clear with regard to treatment rights in 1984. In addition, the hospital had been unsuccessful in getting him transferred to another hospital because they were unable to find another hospital willing to accept him because of the cost of caring for him and the fear of criminal and civil liability. The court found that "no common or comprehensive legal standard was in place to guide the medical community at the time . . . which clearly should have compelled Glendale Adventist to 'pull the plug' on Mr. Bartling's ventilator. . . . What the Bartlings insist was a reckless disregard of Mr. Bartling's rights, Glendale Adventist saw as a responsible regard for the preservation of life." The court said that this commitment was sincere and rooted in their belief that their actions reflected the prevailing medical and legal standards.

In *Iafelice v. Luchs,* a suit for money damages was brought on behalf of an infant and her parents for injuries due to premature birth.[75] The child, who was 4-weeks premature and weighed 2 pounds and 14.5 ounces, went on a ventilator because of severe respiratory distress and was transferred to a tertiary center for specialized perinatal care. The parents consented to treatments including an exchange transfusion and insertion of a replogle (feeding) tube in the stomach to prevent air or fluid distention. The child developed hyperbilirubinemia, hyaline membrane disease, and lung congestion. The child responded well and began to breath on her own. At the age of 4 weeks a diagnosis of intraventricular hemorrhage with secondary hydrocephalus was made and a shunt was done after consulting with the parents. After discussing the shunt surgery and being advised of the seriousness of the situation and the fact that the child would die without the shunt the father signed the consent form. After discharge from the hospital, the infant had to be institutionalized with severe neurological deficits.

The parents based their suit on a claim that the physicians failed to inform them that they could have opted for not doing the shunt surgery and other lifesaving procedures. They testified that if they knew they had the right to withhold their consent, even if they had to go to court to get authorization they would have done so. All parties agreed that the infant was treated in compliance with the highest standards of medical care and probably would not have survived if cared for in other intensive care units.

There was medical testimony that there was no way to determine the extent of damage the child's hemorrhage would cause. There was a reasonable medical probability that the shunt surgery would result in minimal brain damage and the medical literature reflected that surgically managed hydrocephalus results are better in the treated groups. The court found that the measures undertaken for the infant were designed to save her life. Further, the court concluded that there was no legal duty upon the defendants to inform the parents of an alternative to withhold treatment and to let the infant die because such was not a legally sanctioned alternative.

Summary

To date there have been only a handful of cases in which the plaintiffs sought money damages because the hospital or physicians kept the patient alive against either the patient's wishes or the families' wishes. None of the courts have held in favor of the families. Several of the cases discussed the fact that the hospital and physicians could not have known how the law would view the removal of ventilators and feeding devices due to the fact that technology had surpassed ethical thinking in the treatment of hopelessly ill patients and legal guidelines were nonexistent.

THE PRESIDENT'S COMMISSION

In 1974, a National Commission for the Protection of Human Subjects of Biomedical and Behavioral Research was created. Its charter, which expired in 1978, was to advise the then Department of Health, Education and Welfare on rules to govern research. On its expiration, in 1978 Congress created another commission whose scope was considerably broader. This latter commission was the President's Commission for the Study of Ethical Problems in Medicine and Biomedical and Behavioral Research (hereinafter called The Commission; see 42 U.S. Code § 300v). Its mandate extended beyond research to include health care. By the time its charter expired in December 1982 it had conducted a number of nationwide public hearings on various health care topics. The Commission also contracted with private groups to conduct studies. One study was on informed consent practices and another reported on a national survey of hospital ethics committees.

Among the individuals who testified at the Commission hearings were physicians, nurses, patients and family members, philosophers, theologians, and lawyers. A survey of the 12 hearings on treatment decisions are included in one of the President's Commission Reports.[76] The Commission began its work by examining the existing definitions of death. It ultimately recommended the adoption of the UDDA.[77] The Commission next considered an issue which perhaps generated the greatest amount of public interest, that of refusing lifesaving and life-prolonging treatment and care. The Commission expanded its study of consent for participation in research projects to other more routine medical procedures. It ultimately published a three-volume report on health care decisions.[78] The Commission's study of access to health care was reported in three volumes.[79] The remaining topics dealt with compensation for research injuries, genetic engineering, and "whistleblowing" in biomedical research.

The Commission's Report, *Deciding to Forego Life-Sustaining Treatment*, is 255 pages long and includes a nine-part appendix. The appendix contains model statutes for natural death and health care consent legislation, as well as a model child protection act. The appendices also included a report of the findings of a national survey on ethics committees and published guidelines for establishing a hospital ethics committee. Without specifically recommending the establishment of an ethics committee, the Commission concluded that access to such a group would be in the interests of both the providers and recipients of health care. In a survey initiated by the Commission it was found that only 1 percent of hospitals have ethics committees. The Commission offered no definitive explanation for such a finding, but did raise several factors that might account for the low figure. The Commission queried whether there were internal hospital forces that might hamper their formation and function. It also raised the question whether they were simply neither needed nor useful. The report traced the beginnings of hospital ethics committees and set out a model bill identifying the salient criteria necessary in establishing such committees.

The addition of the Commission's findings and reports to the health care literature is timely and of considerable value. Both the findings and reports have been frequently cited in recent treatment decision cases. Perhaps the Commission's greatest value and contribution lies in the process of gathering data and information. The national hearings served to structure input from a variety of experts who are faced with treatment dilemmas. The sharing of their experiences and the input of patients and their families served as an excellent resource and provided the necessary consensus of national thinking.

ETHICS COMMITTEES

The idea of an "ethics committee" was raised during the 1960s in Seattle when it was concluded that some sort of mechanism must be established to determine who would be eligible for the then-new treatment, hemodialysis, for renal failure. Shortly before the Karen Quinlan case attracted national attention, Dr. Karen Teel, a Texas pediatrician, published a frequently cited law review article in which she argued the merits of multidisciplinary hospital ethics committees.[80] Dr. Teel counseled that such committees would be helpful in the review of individual circumstances and would provide assistance and advice to safeguard both patients and their careproviders. A survey done by the president's commission during the period when national hearings concerning treatment decisions were conducted indicated that only 17 of the 400 hospitals surveyed had "ethics committees."[81] There were no committees in hospitals with fewer than 200 beds, and larger hospitals, especially teaching hospitals were most likely to have such committees.

There were two important study conclusions: (1) the use of ethics committees had not been widely adopted, with only 1 percent of the hospitals having such committees, and these bodies only reviewed a single case per year; (2) the composition and function of the committees were dominated by physicians and other health professionals. The majority did not allow patients to attend or to request meetings. However, some permitted family members to attend the meetings.

It is worth noting that although the Quinlan decision used the term, "ethics committee" in its application, such committees were really "prognosis committees." The existence of prognosis committees was first described in the medical literature in 1976.[82] By way of distinction, a prognosis committee deals with medical considerations, whereas an "ethics committee" reviews multiple factors. Although "ethics committees" are not found in every hospital setting, there is evidence that such committees can serve a valuable service.[83]

Ethics Cases

In a few reported decisions the courts have incorporated the concept of ethics committees into the legal opinion.

In *Matter of the Guardianship of Hamlin*, the court-appointed guardian refused to consent to termination of treatment for a mentally retarded 42-year-old patient who had extensive brain damage after an arrest.[84] When he was examined by several physicians all agreed that the man had virtually no prospect of recovery. The appeals court said that the lower trial court had complied with all the procedural guidelines established by the court and court approval was not required if the treating physicians and the prognosis committee were unanimous that life-sustaining efforts, including CPR and the use of a ventilator, should be withdrawn.

In 1984, the Minnesota Supreme Court reviewed a trial court's termination of treatment decision.[85] In *Matter of the Conservatorship of Torres*, 2 weeks after a 57-year-old man was hospitalized for a fall he was found with a Posey restraint around his neck. During a subsequent hearing two neurologists testified that the man had no chance of regaining consciousness and both recommended removal of the respirator. Three biomedical ethics committees supported their recommendation. The Minnesota Supreme Court, noting the language of the *Saikewicz* court which stated that an ethics committee could be of "great assistance" in these kinds of decisions, agreed with the ethics committees recommendation.

In another 1984 decision, the Georgia Supreme Court in *In re L.H.R.* held that in a case of a severely brain damaged 15-day-old infant who suffered a "medical catastrophe" neither court approval or prior judicial approval were required for removal of life-support systems.[86] The infant was in a chronic and vegetative state and 90 percent of her brain tissue had been destroyed. The neurologist and parents agreed that life-support systems should be removed. The hospital's infant care review committee which was made up of two pediatricians, a registered nurse, a social worker, the hospital administrator, and a parent of a handicapped child agreed with the decision to terminate treatment. The court stated that although it did not require the use of such committees it did not foreclose the use of such committees if the hospital or staff elected to use such a committee.

SUMMARY

The threshhold question in withdrawal or withholding of medical treatment cases involving an alleged mentally incompetent patient is always whether the person is, in fact, incompetent to decide the issue on his own behalf. Surprisingly, the courts first addressed patient autonomy rights as early as the beginning of this century. The case law developed slowly and many of the early cases dealt with amputations.

With the advent of major organ transplants, namely, the kidney, a need to define death in terms other than cardiopulmonary cessation was needed. Hence, the concept of brain death was introduced. The first criteria were introduced in 1968 when the Harvard Criteria was published. Because of the advances in medical science and technology, it became obvious that the brain stem death requirement was too impractical a prerequisite to govern when a patient was brain dead and his organs could be harvested. A number of states adopted laws defining brain death. Those states that did not have a definition looked to what the prevailing medical practice was in a "brain death" situation. Both approaches served as a basis for the removal of respirators and for the limitation or withdrawal of other life-support measures.

In 1976, the precedent-setting Quinlan case focused attention on the process whereby respirators and supportive measures could be discontinued. That court and subsequent courts expanded on the concept of patient autonomy and its limitation. The courts based their opinions on either a common law right or a constitutional right of privacy. However, the right was held not to be absolute and the courts ruled that it must yield to state or societal interests. In the wake of Quinlan a number of decision-making models were adopted. Massachusetts and New York followed in the case's immediate wake, both adopting a different standard or test in deciding how to give an incompetent patient the same right as a competent patient.

The Quinlan case, decided in New Jersey, adopted an ethics-prognosis committee approach. Massachusetts courts adopted a substituted judgment approach, and New York courts a clear and convincing evidenciary standard. The courts spoke in terms of lifesaving and life-prolonging treatments. It was not until the withdrawal of food and fluid cases in 1983 that the term "life-sustaining" appeared in legal opinions.

There have only been a few cases in which the family sued the hospital or doctors for not stopping medical treatment earlier. To date, all of these have been unsuccessful. The courts will look to the "good faith" element on the part of the hospital and physician before imposing liability.

In response to the withdrawal of treatment cases, a number of state medical societies took formal positions and developed guidelines to cover such situations. In 1978, a President's Commission was created to

study specific medical care and treatment problems and after conducting many nationwide hearings it published its findings and conclusions.
The Commission recommended the adoption of a uniform brain death
statute and while, not recommending it, it suggested that the creation
and utilization of hospital ethics committees would be beneficial. Presumably, the Commission held back on recommending it because a
commissioned study indicated that it may be too early to determine
their effectiveness. One of its studies indicated that the use of hospital
ethics committees has not been significant. It is interesting to note that
several recent cases have taken specific notice of the role of such
committees.

A recent Congressional study reported that severely or terminally ill
patients are often left out of the decision-making process when decisions
are made regarding whether they should be kept alive on ventilators or
have feeding tubes inserted or when other treatment choices are made.[87]
The study made recommendations which included the establishing of
national standards governing the writing of advance directives, such as
"living wills." The report noted that as of January 1987, 38 states and the
District of Columbia had enacted laws setting out the requirements for
the recognition of living wills as legally enforceable directives in the event
a person becomes incompetent and is terminally ill. To date, there is
almost no case law testing the concept of living wills. However, in
Saunders v. State of New York a 70-year-old woman with progressive
emphysema and lung cancer petitioned a New York court to declare the
living will she prepared in another state as valid in the state of New
York.[88] Because of her illness she moved to New York to live with her
daughter. Although the living will was valid where it was made, the New
York court said that it could not recognize it as a living will because the
state had not passed any law recognizing the validity of living wills. The
court said if it recognized living wills it would be tantamount to usurping
the function of the legislature whose role it was to enact such a law.
However, the court held that the document was in the nature of an
informed consent and as executed by the woman was a "clear and
convincing demonstration that while competent she clearly and explicitly expressed an informed, rational, and knowing decision to decline
certain medical treatment by artificial means while in a terminal condition and it should be given great weight by hospital authorities and
treating physicians."

The use of "advance directives" are a useful tool, because in addition to explicitly setting out an individual's wishes they may incorporate such things as power of attorney or the identification of a surrogate
decision maker in case of incompetency. A power of attorney gives legal
authority to another to carry out explicit activities in circumstances as
set out in the document. Because of the enormous number of treatment
cases since the Quinlan decision in 1976, hospitals and health care pro-

viders are more likely to carry out a patient's directive than they were even a few years ago. The cases have served to solidify a national consensus against using medical technology in all cases.

REFERENCES AND NOTES

1. Custody of a Minor, 393 N.E. 2nd 836 (MA, 1979).
2. See, for example, Superintendent of Belchertown State School v. Saikewicz 370 N.E. 2nd 417 (MA, 1977); and in the Matter of Clair C. Conroy, 486 A. 2nd 1209 (NJ, 1985).
3. Schain, R. (Oct. 6, 1983). Correspondence: "Allowing the debilitated to die." *New England Journal of Medicine, 309*(14), 862.
4. Wanzer, S., et al. (Apr. 12, 1984). The physician's responsibility toward hopelessly ill patients. *New England Journal of Medicine, 310*(15), 955.
5. Law Reform Commission of Canada (Nov. 1983). Report on Euthanasia, Aiding Suicide, and Cessation of Treatment (no. 20). Ottawa, Canada. The Law Reform Commission of Canada is an official national body charged with periodically recommending the substantive reform of federal law throughout Canada. In 1976 the commission was established as a special group to work on the "protection of life project."
6. Curran, W. (Feb. 2, 1984). Law-medicine notes: "Quality of life and treatment decisions: The Canadian Law Reform Report. *New England Journal of Medicine, 310*(5), 297.
7. Peterson v. Eritsland, 419 P. 2nd 332 (WA, 1966).
8. Grannum v. Berard, 422 P. 2nd 812 (WA, 1967).
9. Matter of Schiller, 372 A. 2nd 360 (NJ, 1977).
10. Matter of Quackenbush, 383 A. 2nd 785 (NJ, 1978).
11. State Department of Human Services v. Mary Northern, 563 S.W. 2nd 197 (TN, 1978).
12. In Re Yetter, 62 Pa. D. & C. 2nd 619 (PA, 1973), C.P. Northampton County.
13. Lane v. Candura, 376 N.E. 2nd 1232 (MA, 1980).
14. Thomas v. Anderson, 215 P. 2nd 478 (CA, 1950).
15. Becher, H., Adams, R., Barger, A.C., Curran, W., & Denny-Brown, D. (Aug. 5, 1968). Ad Hoc Committee of the Harvard Medical School to Examine the Definition of Brain Death. A definition of irreversible coma. *Journal of the American Medical Association, 205*(6), 337–340.
16. Ibid., note 2, at pp. 337–338.
17. Mohandas, A., & Chow, S. N. (1971). Brain death—a clinical and pathological study. *Journal of Neurosurgery, 35,* 211.
18. Goodman, M., & Aung, M. (May/June 1978). Cerebral death: Theological, judicial, and medical aspects. *Heart & Lung, 7*(3), 477.
19. Korein, J. (1978). Preface to brain death: Inter-related medical and social issues. *Annuals of the New York Academy of Sciences, 315,* 1–10.
20. Walton, D. (1980). *Brain death.* West Lafayette, IN: Purdue University Press (p. 80).
21. Tucker v. Lower, Law & Equity Court, Richmond, VA, C.A. no. 2831, May 23, 1972.
22. Virginia Code, Chap. 19, § 32-364, 3.1 (1974).
23. People v. Lyons, an unreported case, Oakland, CA. (May 21, 1974); See also Editorial (Nov. 1973). "How did Samuel Moore die?, *New Scientist,* 487. See also State v. Shaffer, 574 P. 2nd 205 (KA, 1978), a case dealing with a similar gunshot homicide which occurred in 1970 and resulted in Kansas being the first state to enact a brain death statute.
24. Commonwealth v. Golston, 366 N.E. 2nd 744 (MA, 1977). See also People of the State of New York v. Eulo, 472 N.E. 2nd 286 (NY, 1984). Thus, New York became the 38th state to legally recognize brain death.

25. New York City Health and Hospitals Corporation v. Sulsona, 367 N.Y.S. 2nd 686 (NY, 1975).
26. Lovato v. District Court, 601 P. 2nd 1072 (CO, 1979).
27. In re Haymer, 450 N.E. 2nd 940 (IL, 1983).
28. Kansas Statutes Annotated, § 77-202 (1970).
29. National Conference of Commissioners on Uniform State Laws, Uniform Determination of Death Act (UDDA), 1980.
30. In re the Welfare of William Matthew Bowman, 617 P. 2nd 731 (WA, 1980).
31. Walton, D. (1980). *Brain death*. West Lafayette, Indiana: Purdue University Press (pp. 78–79).
32. Anon. (1979). Guidelines for the determination of death, Report of the medical consultants on the diagnosis of death to the President's Commission on the Study of Ethical Problems in Medicine and Biomedical and Behavioral Research. *Journal of the American Medical Association, 242*, 2184–2186.
33. Beyer, H. (Sept. 1982). Correspondence. *Law, Medicine & Health Care, 10*(4), 185.
34. In the Matter of Karen Quinlan, 355 A. 2nd 647 (NJ, 1976).
35. Ibid. p. 667.
36. Eichner v. Dillon, 438 N.Y.S. 2nd 266; 429 N.E. 2nd 64 (NY, 1981). But, see 1985 decision of In the Matter of Conroy, 486 A. 2nd 1209 (NJ, 1985) in which the N.J. Supreme Court receded from *Quinlan* and held that even oral directives to family members or health care providers are to be considered as relevant evidence.
37. See, for example, In re Moschella, *N.Y.L.J.*, May 22, 1984, at 12 (NY Sup. Ct., Queens Cty., Special Term, Part 6).
38. Forty-six days after the landmark decision, Karen Quinlan was weaned off the ventilator and was able to breath independently. She was transferred from the hospital to a nursing home where she remained until her death in 1985. During this period she received antibiotics and was fed a high-caloric liquid through a feeding tube.
39. Anon. (Jan. 27, 1977). *Guidelines for health care facilities to implement procedures concerning the care of comatose non-cognitive patients*. Department of Health, State of New Jersey.
40. Superintendent of Belchertown State School v. Saikewicz, 370 N.E. 2nd 417 (MA, 1977).
41. In the Matter of Spring, 405 N.E. 2nd 115 (MA, 1980).
42. Commissioner of Correction v. Myers, 399 N.E. 2nd 452 (MA, 1979); the prisoner subsequently consented to a kidney transplant.
43. Commissioner of Correction v. Ferguson, 421 N.E. 2nd 444 (MA, 1981).
44. Unreported decision, Commissioner of Correction v. R.C., Suffolk County Superior Court, C.A. No. 39780, (MA, 1980).
45. Eichner v. Dillon, 438 N.Y.S. 2nd 266 (NY, 1981).
46. In the Matter of John Storar, 438 N.Y.S. 2nd 266; 420 N.E. 2nd 64 (NY, 1981).
47. See, in particular, Paris, J. (Oct. 9, 1980). Sounding Board: Court intervention and the diminution of patients' rights: The case of Brother Joseph Fox. *New England Journal of Medicine, 303*(15), especially footnotes 5 and 6.
48. In the Matter of John Storar, 438 N.Y.S. 2nd 266, pp. 276–281 (NY, 1981).
49. Malcolm, A. Medicine, law and the American way of death. *New York Times*, Dec. 30, 1984, p. E7.
50. In re Moschella, N.Y. Sup. Court, Queens Cty., May 22, 1984.
51. Liacos, P. (1979). Dilemmas of dying. *Medicolegal News, 7*(3), 4.
52. Severns v. Wilmington Medical Center, 421 A. 2nd 1334 (DE, 1980).
53. Leach v. Akron General Medical Center, Ohio Court of Common Pleas, Summit Cty., No. C80-10-20 (Dec. 18, 1980).
54. In the Matter of Benjamin C., L.A. Juvenile Court, California, no. J914419 (Feb. 16, 1979).

55. In the Matter of Vincent Martin Young, California Superior Court, Orange County, no. A100863 (Sept. 11, 1979).

56. Rothenberg, L. S. (Apr. 1981). A matter of life and death, *Los Angeles Lawyer, 4*(2), 6.

57. Anon. (Apr. 1981). Agreement reached on life support guidelines. *County Bar Update,* a publication of the Los Angeles County Bar Association, *1*(4), 4.

58. Aponte v. U.S., 582 F. Supp. 65 (1984). The wife of an incompetent patient who had his who had his left testicle removed recovered $1000 in damages after the Veterans Administration failed to obtain her informed consent. The husband recovered $9000.

59. Deering's Annotated California Health and Safety Code, §7181 (1974). See also, §7185 and sequelae for Natural Death Act (1976).

60. Bartling v. Superior Court of the State of California for the County of Los Angeles, 209 *California Reporter, 220* (CA, 1984).

61. Satz v. Perlmutter, 362 S. 2nd 160 (FL, 1978); this decision was upheld by the Florida Supreme Court in 379 S. 2nd 359 (FL, 1980).

62. Florida Statutes Anotated § 382.085 (1981).

63. John F. Kennedy Memorial Hospital v. Bludworth, 452 S. 2nd 921 (FL, 1984); overruling 432 S. 2nd 611 (FL, 1983).

64. Foody v. Manchester Memorial Hospital, 482 A. 2nd 713 (CT, 1984).

65. Anon. A dying woman gets wish. *Boston Globe,* Sept. 1, 1981, p. 3.

66. Gaylin, W. Still, a person owns himself. *New York Times,* December 7, 1982, p. A31. But see Anon. Dying man denied wish to disconnect device. *New York Times,* March 4, 1984, p. 22. This article tells of a 75-year-old patient who was suffering from a severe chronic cardiopulmonary disease and had consented to being attached to a respirator. He later wished to be disconnected, but doctors said they could not honor his request because of his initial request to be connected to the life-support system. There was testimony that he would die within minutes if the respirator was disconnected. A trial judged denied the man's request to have the respirator turned off.

67. Tune v. Walter Reed Army Medical Hospital, 602 F. Supp. 1452 (March 1985). See case footnote 2, p. 1453, which says that the federal hospital was not subject to the provisions of the District of Columbia Natural Death Act, D.C. Code §6-2421, which would permit Mrs. Tune to have the machine removed by signing a declaration in the presence of disinterested witnesses. Since the Tune case was decided, the Department of the Army has changed its policy and will permit the removal of life-support measures in situations similar to Mrs. Tune's.

68. In the Matter of Kathleen Farrell, slip opinion no. A-76, N.J. Supreme Court argued November 5, 1986, and decided June 24, 1987, 529 A. 2nd 404 (NJ, 1987). See footnote 2, pp. 4, 5 for a list of state natural death statutes.

69. Estate of Leach v. Shapiro, 469 N.E. 2nd 1047 (OH, 1984).

70. Anon. (Dec. 1985). The latest word. *Hastings Center Report, 15,* 52.

71. Anon. Akron doctor goes on trial in "right to die" case. *New York Times,* Sept. 18, 1985, p. A17. See also Anon. Judge clears doctor who refused death plea. *New York Times,* Sept. 19, 1985, p. A24.

72. Strachan v. John F. Kennedy Memorial Hospital, 507 A. 2nd 718 (NJ, 1986). This case had an interesting dissenting opinion which would have recognized the right to sue.

73. McVey v. Englewood Hospital Association, 524 A. 2nd 450 (NJ, 1987).

74. Bartling v. Glendale Adventist Medical Center, 229 *California Reporter, 360* (CA, 1986).

75. Iafelice v. Luchs, 501 A. 2nd 1040 (NJ, 1985).

76. President's Commission for the Study of Ethical Problems in Medicine and Biomedical and Behavioral Research (1983). *Deciding to forego life-sustaining treatment* (No. 83-600503), Appendix A, The commission's process, p. 259. The Reports are available from the U.S. Government Printing Office, Washington, DC.

77. President's Commission (1983). *Deciding to forego life-sustaining treatment,* p. 9.

78. President's Commission (1982). *Making health care decisions. Report* (Vol. 1); *Appen-*

dices (empirical studies of informed consent) (Vol. 2); *Appendices (foundations of informed consent).* (Vol. 3).

79. President's Commission (1983). *Securing access to health care. Report* (Vol. 1); *Appendices (socio-cultural and philosophical studies)* (Vol. 2); *Appendices* (Vol. 3).

80. Teel, K. (1975). The physician's dilemma—A doctor's view: What the law should be. *Baylor Law Review, 27,* 1 p126.

81. President's Commission (1983). *Deciding to forego life-sustaining treatment,* Appendix F (Hospital Ethics Committees: Proposed Statute and National Survey), p. 439.

82. Pontoppidan, H., Abbott, W., Brewster, D., Buckley, M., & Cassem, N. (Aug. 12, 1976). Optimum care for hopelessly ill patients—a report of the Clinical Care Committee of the Massachusetts General Hospital. *New England Journal of Medicine, 295*(7), 362.

83. See Cranford, R., & Doudera, E. (Feb. 1984). The emergence of institutional ethics committees. *Law, Medicine and Health Care, 12*(1), 13. Also see Cushing, M., Hall, D., Houy, M., & Covner Weiss, E. (Mar./Apr. 1985). The role of hospital ethics committees in decisions to terminate treatment. *Boston Bar Journal, 29*(2), 22.

84. In the Matter of the Guardianship of Hamlin, 689 P. 2nd 1372 (WA, 1984).

85. In the Matter of the Conservatorship of Torres, 357 N.W. 2nd 332 (MN, 1984).

86. In re L.H.R., 321 S.E. 2nd 716 (GA, 1984); a rehearing was denied.

87. Anon. Planning treatment of terminally ill is urged. *New York Times,* Aug. 2, 1987, p. 27.

88. Saunders v. State, 492 N.Y.S. 2nd 510 (NY, 1985).

10

MEDICAL TREATMENT ISSUES

Specific Problems

Once the courts articulated the broad legal principles that formed the basis for the treatment issues cases they were forced to turn their attention to some of the more novel treatment issues. These included the rights of parents to refuse blood transfusions and the right of a minor to have a blood transfusion. The rights of unborn but viable fetuses were tested in 1981 in the Georgia Supreme Court. The earliest "no code" or *do not resuscitate* (DNR) cases involved an elderly woman who was "hopelessly ill" and a young infant with an uncorrectable cardiac birth defect.

In 1983 two novel treatment issues were decided by the courts. One case questioned the appropriateness of removing routinely used nutritional devices from an elderly nursing home patient. Two other cases, one in California and one in New York, dealt with the issue of whether a patient could refuse to be fed. These cases were considered unique because they did not involve technology, but rather an activity considered basic for life.

Although there were cases that dealt with treating minors it was not until 1978, when Massachusetts courts ruled that a young child should have chemotherapy over the objections of his parents, that national attention was focused on parental rights. Two other treatment issues involving minors are important. These are organ donation, especially from mentally incompetent minors to siblings, and sterilization of mentally incompetent or intellectually impaired minors.

BLOOD TRANSFUSION CASES

A significant number of cases deal with the treatment issue of blood transfusion refusals. The problem arises when an individual refuses to have a blood transfusion because of his religious belief. The courts have also had to resolve legal questions involved in cases where a pregnant woman refuses to be transfused and when parents refuse a transfusion for their minor child. Most often the cases involve Jehovah's Witnesses who will not accept whole blood, blood cells, or plasma. They base their refusal on specific Bible passages.

In a large number of these cases there is advance opportunity to plan an alternative to whole blood use, such as blood expanders in the event that the patient hemorrhages. When care of a patient whose religious beliefs preclude whole blood products takes place prior to a surgical procedure or birth there is generally an opportunity to discuss any limitations placed on care or treatment by the patient. When the patient is in shock, intubated, or otherwise compromised it is difficult if not impossible to determine exactly what his beliefs and wishes are and whether the patient will consent to receiving any blood protein.

In one of the earliest blood cases suit was brought after the fact of a transfusion.[1]

The issue before the court in *In re Brook's Estate* was, "Could the patient (incompetent and weakened by her condition) without minor children, be judicially compelled to accept treatment of a nature which, although it may save her life, is forbidden by her religious convictions, and refused, knowing, that death may result from the refusal?" The plaintiff sought to show that the appointment of a conservator for the purpose of giving consent to the whole blood violated her basic constitutional rights.

The patient and her husband, as well as their two adult children were Jehovah's Witnesses. The woman had been under treatment for 2 years for a peptic ulcer and had informed the physician that she did not want to receive any blood products. The physician assured her that she would not be persuaded to accept blood after both she and her husband signed a document releasing the hospital and the physician from all civil liability which may result from their failure to transfuse. However, a blood transfusion was given after her physician and state agency lawyers successfully petitioned the court for appointment of a guardian who had authority to consent to the transfusion.

In the suit brought by the family, the court said that it would not countenance state action that sought to decide the best course of action for an individual where that individual had previously refused treatment because of a religious conviction. The court said that, "Even though, the refusal, based upon certain belief, may be considered unwise, foolish or ridiculous, if the refusal offers no overriding danger to society, the court will not permit interference."

However, in another case decided 7 years later, the court ordered a blood transfusion for a 22-year-old unmarried woman who was injured in an automobile accident.[2]

In *John F. Kennedy Memorial Hospital v. Heston*, a young woman's parents refused transfusions which the surgeons said were necessary during an operation. The woman was unable to consent because she was in shock and the parents' refusal was based on religious grounds. After successful surgery the woman affirmed her parents' decision. The case went to the state supreme court which upheld the decision to permit the transfusion. The court found that a "compelling state interest in the preservation of life" existed. Preventing suicide is considered a state interest. The court went on to say that the physician's right to administer medical treatment according to his best judgment should prevail over the patient's religious claim. It is worth noting that the refusal did not come from the young woman, but rather through her parents.

A federal court in *Application of the President and Directors of Georgetown College* also upheld the giving of a transfusion in an emergency situation.[3]

The U.S. Supreme Court refused to review the decision. The husband of a 25-year-old woman brought her to the hospital for emergency care. The woman, who had a 7-month-old child, had lost two-thirds of her blood from a ruptured ulcer. Both the husband and wife were Jehovah's Witnesses and both refused to consent to a series of transfusions deemed necessary to save the woman's life. When the physicians approached the husband he stated that if the court ordered the transfusion, the responsibility would not be his. The wife subsequently told a judge that a transfusion would be "against my will" and would not be her responsibility. When death, without the blood, appeared imminent the hospital petitioned the court and their petition was denied. Two days later they sought a review. After speaking with the surgeons the judge visited the couple and a short time later the order for the necessary lifesaving transfusions was signed.

The fact that the woman said that she did not want to die and regarded the need to refuse as an unwanted side effect of a religious scruple was an important fact. In finding for the hospital, the court held that when the woman elected to come to the hospital for medical care she placed the hospital and the physicians in a position that required them to treat her in accordance with medical standards. Their only option was to let her die. With the woman's life in the balance the judge "opted to act on the side of life." The fact that the couple had a young child was important as the courts are reluctant to "orphan" a child.

In *In re Caine* a juvenile court ordered a 35-year-old father of three minor children to have necessary blood transfusions.[4]

The man had been admitted because of bleeding ulcers and would not survive surgical repair without transfusions. The hospital attorney brought a care and protection petition on behalf of the children in juvenile court. The court held that the welfare of the father and children were "inseparable." The court invoked the state's right to protect its citizens and said that its interests outweighed the father's religious rights. The court, in ordering the transfusions, if they became necessary, said they were not "overly intrusive."

The Balancing Test

When constitutional issues are involved, one of the tests the court will apply is a *balancing test*, that is, balancing or weighing one right against another. The prevailing law holds that the patient's valid and knowing choice in deciding the events of his life is the governing criterion when balanced against the preservation of life argument.

In a 1972 case a patient hemorrhaged after a tree fell on him.[5] Both the man and his wife in *In the Matter of Osborne* refused a transfusion on religious grounds. The court found that the man was competent and not under the influence of drugs. He had expressed a desire to live, but without a blood transfusion. He told the court that he would be accountable to God and even if the court forced the decision on him he would lose everlasting life. Thus, the court refused to appoint a guardian to override the man's refusal.

Minors

The courts early on were confronted with the question of parental rights when parents refused to consent to blood transfusions for their minor children.

The court in an early Massachusetts case, *Prince v. Massachusetts*, which involved parental rights and a child's educational process, held that "neither rights of religion or rights of parenthood are beyond limitation."[6]

In a 1952 Illinois case, a court ordered that an 8-day-old infant suffering from erythroblastosis fetalis should receive a blood transfusion.[7]

In *Wallace v. Labrenz*, there was medical testimony that the infant would suffer mental impairment or death without the transfusion. The parents believed that if they allowed the infant to receive the blood, their future spiritual life and that of the infant would be lost.

The court petition was brought under the state's child neglect statute. Ruling against the parents, the court recognized that both the right to practice one's religion and the right of parents to decide the direction of care and training of their children are rights that are accorded the highest possible respect. However, neither right is limitless. The cases involving lifesaving blood transfusions for minors have consistently held that the transfusion should be given.

Blood and the Pregnant Woman

In addition to the compelling interest argument, the state has carved out another exception, that is, the third party interests argument.

In *Raleigh Fitkin-Paul Morgan Memorial Hospital v. Anderson*, it was held that it was unnecessary to determine whether the mother ("quick with child") could be compelled to accept a transfusion to save her own life because the issue was so inextricably interwoven with that of the child that it became impossible to distinguish between them.[8] Where a blood transfusion is necessary to save the life of the pregnant woman, the courts have ordered it. Of course, such cases must be decided in light of the 1973 *Rowe v. Wade* abortion decision.

Akin to the issue of transfusing a pregnant woman is the issue of in vitro exchange transfusion for the sole benefit of the fetus. Recent scientific and medical advances have made it possible to transfuse the baby while it is still in the womb. The degree of bodily invasion would be a factor in deciding such a case. *Quinlan*, in setting out the distinctions between the blood cases and removal of life-support measures, said that transfusion is a "minimal bodily invasion." However, where a case can be made that a transfusion presents a substantial risk to the mother it is unlikely that the court will order it. The law has long recognized that it cannot order a treatment that poses substantial danger, especially a life threat, to the mother. Another factor in the fetal exchange transfusion (Rh factor) would be the benefit received by the fetus by prenatal transfusion.

Negligence and Blood Refusal

There are two recent cases where the need to give blood to a patient who refused it on religious grounds was because of negligence of the physician. In the first case, *Randolph v. City of New York*, the husband of a Jehovah's Witness sued when his wife's urinary bladder was lacerated during an emergency hysterectomy following a cesarean section.[9] The laceration caused a massive hemorrhage. The wife had refused blood under any circumstances. Within 15 minutes of the accident, the patient had lost 40 percent of her blood supply. In spite of the administration of a crystalloid solution by the anesthesiologist the woman had lost 80 percent at the end of 45 minutes. After receiving authority from the hospital attorney, whole blood was given 1 hour after the initial laceration. However, the patient had a cardiac arrest one-half hour later.

The obstetrician settled with the husband before the trial. The defendant anesthesiologist said that the death occurred because of the obstetrician's negligence. The husband argued that the anesthesiologist should not have waited for the hospital attorney's authorization. The jury found against the anesthesiologist, but their verdict against him was overruled on appeal. The court said that the husband's argument that the anesthesiologist had a duty to give the blood in spite of the woman's refusal—because she had minor children—lacked persuasion because the husband could give the children parental support. In addition, the court held that by the time the hospital attorney authorized the transfusion, the woman's condition was irreversible because she had already lost 80 percent of her blood.

However, in *Shorter v. Drury*, a surgeon was not released from liability for the wrongful death of a Jehovah's Witness when he negligently lacerated her uterus during a D and C.[10] Both the husband and wife signed forms refusing any blood transfusions and releasing the hospital and physician from any responsibility. The woman refused any blood even when she knew she was bleeding profusely. The court said that while the signed release did not relieve the surgeon of his negligence in performing the surgery it did show that the husband and wife fully accepted any risk which might flow from their refusal to accept the blood. The jury held the plaintiff 75 percent negligent and the surgeon 25 percent negligent. The plaintiff was apportioned that extent of negligence because he "assumed the risk" of what the refusal might bode. However, there were four dissenting opinions in the case which would not have found the plaintiff assumed the risk. The dissenters said they would have looked to why the necessity for the blood arose.

Summary

It can be seen from these cases that even when constitutional rights and issues are raised, the courts do not view such rights as absolute. The courts frequently apply a balancing test. As early as 1940, in *Cantwell v.*

Connecticut, the U.S. Supreme Court identified two distinct concepts in the right to practice one's religious beliefs as guaranteed by the First Amendment of the U.S. Constitution. "The freedom to believe and the freedom to act. . . . The first is absolute but, in the nature of things, the second cannot be. Conduct remains subject to regulations for the protection of society."[11] The courts have recognized such state interests as the protection of third parties, preventing suicide, and preserving life.

The courts have uniformly permitted blood transfusions if the recipient is a minor. This is because the child is unable or has not adopted the religion of the parents. In the face of a strong religious belief that eternal life would be lost if a blood product were given, the courts are unlikely to order the transfusion in the case of an adult recipient. Recent advances, such as Rh factor in utero exchange transfusions, have added another dimension to the transfusion cases. When the court finds that the benefit to the fetus significantly outweighs the risk to the mother it will opt for transfusion.

Some of the more specific treatment issues cases, such as the blood transfusion cases, actually preceded the seemingly more dramatic withdrawal of life-support systems cases. These cases were, of course, a basis for the more profound respirator cases, but as a whole they did not generate the public concern or extensive literature that the latter did. Perhaps this is because the refusal of blood was based on a constitutional religious right, and thus was more personal in nature.

The courts were quick to make a distinction between an adult's refusal to receive blood from those cases involving minors. As in the ventilator cases the courts identified compelling state's interests that had to be balanced with the individual's wishes. The rights of a viable unborn child was first decided by the U.S. Supreme Court in 1964 in the *Raleigh Fitkin-Paul Morgan Memorial Hospital* case. That court articulated the third party interest concept.

COMPELLING TREATMENT FOR THE PREGNANT WOMAN

There are procedures other than blood transfusion and Rh blood exchange procedures that can conflict with a pregnant woman's religious beliefs on privacy rights.

In 1981 the Georgia Supreme Court was asked to rule on an order of a lower court. The lower court in *Jefferson v. Griffin Spaulding County Hospital*, had granted custody of an unborn child to a state agency and ordered the mother to undergo a cesarean section if the physicians deemed it necessary to save the infant's life.[12] The high court upheld the decision. The woman who was in the thirty-ninth week of pregnancy had been receiving prenatal care at the defendant hospital for several weeks. Her physician informed her that she had a complete placenta previa and it was unlikely that the condition would reverse itself. A vaginal delivery would almost certainly result in a dead baby. The mother was also at substantial risk if she delivered vaginally. The woman and her husband refused to consent to a cesarean section or blood transfusion. The refusal was based entirely on their religious beliefs.

The hospital sought a court order seeking authority to perform a section if she came to the hospital and the physicians considered it necessary to save the infant's life. The hospital argued that both the infant and mother would be saved if the surgery was done before labor began. The infant was viable and capable of sustaining life independent of the mother. In taking measures to protect the unborn child the court relied on the 1973 *Roe v. Wade* U.S. Supreme Court abortion decision which held that a viable unborn child has a right to be protected under the Constitution.

The original court order gave the hospital authority to administer all medical procedures deemed necessary to preserve the life of the unborn child, but such authority would only operate if the woman voluntarily sought admission to the hospital. The court refused to order the woman to submit to surgery before the onset of labor. In an unusual move the next day, the state agency for human resources returned to court and was granted temporary custody of the unborn child. The state's custody right would terminate after the infant was safely delivered. Because the birth could occur at any moment, the court ordered the woman to proceed immediately to the hospital for a sonogram. If the test indicated that the life-threatening condition persisted, the woman was to submit to a cesarean section and related procedures considered essential to save the infant's life.

The court held that, "Because the life of defendant and of the unborn are, at the moment, inseparable, the Court deems it appropriate to infringe upon the wishes of the mother to the extent it is necessary to give the child an opportunity to live." The opinion continued on to say that the intrusion into the life of the woman was outweighed by the duty of the state to protect a living, unborn human being from meeting his or her death before being given the opportunity to live.

A year later, a Chicago juvenile court judge ordered a 20-year-old woman, who refused to sign an operative consent form, to undergo a cesarean section to preserve the life of a viable fetus.[13] The mother, who arrived at the hospital in labor, refused surgery, citing her religious beliefs as the reason. She had previously delivered her three other children by cesarean section.

In 1983, a Massachusetts court dealt with another novel question. In *Taft v. Taft*, a husband sought a court order to compel his wife, who was a recent "born-again Christian," to have a "purse string" operation for an incompetent cervix.[14] The wife was in her fourth month of pregnancy and the couple had four children. Three of the children were born after the wife underwent a similar cervical procedure to hold those pregnancies. Another pregnancy terminated in the seventh month without the benefit of the purse string procedure. That fetus died. Both husband and wife wanted this fifth child.

A lower court ordered the wife to submit to the procedure, but the higher court held that she could not be ordered to submit to the operation. The woman testified that she believed that no harm would come to her baby and that God would protect them both. The court found that her beliefs were sincere. At the time of the lower court proceeding neither party was represented by legal counsel and the court record was sparse. The judge had appointed a special guardian for the unborn child and after ordering the surgery he appointed counsel for all the parties.

The woman's obstetrician wrote a letter to the husband stating that the surgery was necessary for the delivery of a full-term infant. On appeal the court held that the wife had presented a case showing that her religious beliefs and right of privacy would be violated, and the state had failed (on the record) to establish a state interest sufficient to compel such a procedure. It is important to note that in this case the fetus was not viable as in the transfusion cases. The court recognized that in some situations there may be justification for ordering such surgery.

Summary

In the novel 1981 *Jefferson* case, the Georgia Supreme Court ruled that a pregnant woman in her third trimester could be compelled to undergo surgery in the event it was necessary to save her viable fetus's life. Since that case, the courts have been petitioned to address a number of issues involving fetal rights. The threshold question when such petitions are brought is the viability of the fetus. Such inquiry recognizes the balancing of the pregnant woman's rights and the interest of the state in protecting viable fetuses as articulated in the 1973 *Roe v. Wade* U.S. Supreme Court decision.

In the past year the court cases have been asked to establish the rights of a fetus where the mother disregarded medical advice, thus putting the fetus at risk (physical damage or death), and where a pregnant woman became comatose.[15] In Santa Clara, California, Marie Odette Henderson was declared brain dead several months before her 26 weeks' gestated infant daughter was born; and in Augusta, Georgia, a pregnant brain dead woman was kept on a ventilator for 4 weeks until the delivery of her infant son. In the California case, the child is deemed healthy a year after its birth and the Georgia infant, born with multiple defects, died. In the latter case, the judge ruled against the woman's husband who wanted the life-support systems discontinued.

In another similar case in New Britain, Connecticut, a judge denied the request of the mother of a 24-year-old comatose pregnant woman to permit an abortion.[16] The woman's doctors testified that there was a 90 percent chance that the comatose woman would bear a healthy baby. At the time of the petition, the woman was 4½-months pregnant. The petition was instituted because the physicians differed in their opinion whether the abortion should be performed.

These lines of cases are indicative of the expanding kinds of legal issues which can surround fetal rights. In addition to the impact of AIDS on fetuses there is also the issue of fetal experimentation. It is expected that the judiciary will become increasingly active in the area of fetal rights.

DO NOT RESUSCITATE ORDERS

By the late 1950s, medicine had developed a technique whereby a sudden cardiac arrest could be successfully managed in some cases. The basic resuscitation technique began to be used outside the acute care setting by both laypeople and emergency medical technicians. However, it was in the hospital setting where its use on all patients, regardless of prognosis, was a problem. The situation appeared to be one where scientific advancement and skill had moved forward without the benefit of moral reasoning. It took the medical community some time before its all-out use began to be questioned. Ironically, the fear of suit because of potential injuries resulted in some hospitals not adopting the cardiopulmonary resuscitation procedure (CPR) as quickly as the large teaching hospitals.[17] Thus, just when these smaller facilities began to teach hospital staff the technique, the large teaching hospitals began to write "no code" orders.

In the beginning many physicians were giving the order verbally, but refused to write the order in the patient's medical record, and the "no code" order took on a subrosa aspect. As a result of not writing the order, nurses were placed in a difficult position because of their continual presence at the bedside. Nurses were the providers who had to initiate, or not initiate, the order when a patient arrested. This do nothing or negative order was new to both medicine and nursing and neither discipline seemed comfortable with it initially. A considerable amount of anxiety was experienced by nurses because of the legal implications of not coding a patient in the absence of a formal medical directive.

Acknowledging the Problem

In May 1973, the American Heart Association and the National Academy of Sciences–National Research Council sponsored a national conference which resulted in the development of standards and guidelines for CPR. The *Standards* were published and subsequently updated in 1979 and again in 1986 to reflect the state of the art in medical practice.[18] The *Standards* were important for a number of reasons, not the least of which is that they dealt with the medicolegal aspects and included recommendations. The 1974 *Standards* defined the purpose of CPR as the "prevention of sudden, unexpected death" and stated that it was "not indicated in certain situations, such as in cases of terminal irreversible illness where death is not unexpected." Included in the *Standards* was the forceful statement, "Resuscitation in these circumstances may represent a positive violation of an individual's right to die with dignity." It included a recommendation that the hospital progress notes should reflect the basis for not coding a patient. The 1974 *Standards* stated that it was "appropriate" to indicate the medical directive on the order sheet. The 1979 *Standards* stated that such an order should be "expressed clearly on the physician's order sheet for the benefit of nursing and other personnel who may be called on to initiate or participate in CPR."

The 1974 criteria should have relieved much of the anxiety that surrounded the question of whether a "no code" order was appropriate and could be justified in a legal sense. However, the practice of "verbal" no codes continued in far too many acute care facilities. Shortly after the *Quinlan* decision was handed down the *New England Journal of Medicine* published an article dealing with orders not to resuscitate. The article was the first major article to appear in medical literature and reflected the internal guidelines developed by a major teaching hospital in Boston.[19] The article identified the process of decision making in arriving at a "no code" treatment decision. It dealt mainly with the identification of categories of special concern and outlined concepts on which internal policies could be based.

Absence of Litigation

The fear that a failure to initiate the resuscitation procedure in all cases would result in suits by family members was not founded in fact or based on reason. Essentially all of the judicial decisions involving cardiac resuscitation concerned a failure to timely diagnose a cardiac arrest or improper technique when carrying out the resuscitation procedure.[20]

There is a notable absence of case law dealing with situations in which legal proceedings were instituted because the physician wrote a "no code" order. However, two such situations have been reported. In 1981 a Minnesota court struck down a *do not resuscitate* DNR order when it was found that the guardian of the young woman did not comprehend the irreversible nature of such an order.[21]

> Further, in *Hoyt v. St. Mary's Rehabilitation Center* there was no evidence, on which the guardian could rely, that the 41-year-old brain-damaged woman had ever expressed an opinion on how she would want to be managed if she arrested. The woman resided in a nursing home and had been mentally competent until she suffered trauma to her brain during an operation 5 years prior to the court hearing.

In 1982, a New York grand jury was called to investigate the deaths of two elderly patients who were not resuscitated during an arrest.[22] The hospital did not have any written policy or guidelines dealing with DNR orders.[23] As a direct result of the criminal investigation, the New York Medical Society in September 1982 approved guidelines for hospitals and physicians in deciding whether such an order is appropriate.[24] (Appendix D in the back of the book). The New York guidelines are modeled after the DNR Guidelines developed by the Minnesota Medical Association in January 1981 (Appendix E in the back of the book). The New York guidelines add two significant points to the Minnesota model. The New York guidelines state that, "A verbal or telephone order for DNR cannot be justified as a sound medical or legal practice." In the New York Medical Association's preamble statement, hospital medical staff and governing bodies are encouraged to develop internal policies within the parameters of their corporate bylaws.

The Alabama Medical Association also published DNR guidelines which were modeled exactly after the Minnesota guidelines (Appendix F in the back of the book). In May 1981, the Texas Medical Association adopted a resolution encouraging physicians to develop general guidelines pertaining to "no cardiopulmonary resuscitation (CPR)" decisions (Appendix G in the back of the book). The association did not adopt specific guidelines as did Minnesota and the other states because of a feeling that such guidelines may be too "rigid." However, the general guidelines provide clear direction for the development of internal policy.

The Minnesota and New York situations dealing with "no code" orders need to be put in proper perspective. The Minnesota case dealt with a woman, now incompetent, who had never given a directive or expressed a preference to aid either the guardian or court in making a decision. This, coupled with the fact that the consent given by the guardian was not informed, placed the court in a position where it had little choice but to rescind the DNR order.

The New York grand jury hearing illustrates the increased exposure of risk when a facility elects not to adopt a uniform procedure. Institutional policies will serve to demonstrate that a consensus exists among various disciplines and level decision makers. If the policies give evidence of prevailing medical and hospital practice it is unlikely that problems of this nature will proceed to the level it did in New York.

Judicial Review of DNR Orders

To date, there have only been a few judicial decisions dealing with the legality of a DNR order. It is unlikely that there will be a significant number of cases because the DNR order does not present the complex dilemma that the withdrawal or withholding of treatment and supportive measures present. The first litigation in the country to raise the question of the legal status of the DNR order occurred in Massachusetts in 1978.[25] The case, *Matter of Shirley Dinnerstein* was brought to the court in the immediate wake of the Saikewicz case. It was intended to be a test case to determine the legal status of DNR orders which some believed to be in doubt after *Saikewicz.*

Aside from the large metropolitan teaching hospitals most facilities did not have formal DNR policies or guidelines. The Saikewicz ruling did not pose a problem for those acute care facilities that had policies in existence. This is because they had worked with legal counsel to develop policies prior to *Saikewicz* and did not give the weight to *Saikewicz* that some of the hospitals that lacked policies gave to it. For those hospitals and staff that had no policies the period between *Saikewicz* and *Dinnerstein* was troubled with indecision. A number of hospitals issued directives to their medical and nursing staff that forbade DNR orders unless the patient consented to it. If the patient was incompetent and had not previously consented to a DNR order the directive required court authority before such an order could be written. Thus, even though a patient was in the death process of a terminal disease a DNR order was not written.

Although the Dinnerstein decision was decided at an intermediary court level it has been cited by many jurisdictions. The case held that, under the facts of the case the law did not prohibit the writing of a DNR order and prior judicial approval was unnecessary. In essence, the court looked to prevailing medical standards which reflected a medical consensus. The lesson is clear and that is that if the profession or literature is silent on the criteria or standards to be applied, then the courts must search for and adopt the appropriate standard.

In *Dinnerstein* the family and physicians were in agreement that a no code order was appropriate. Shirley Dinnerstein was a 67-year-old woman who was diagnosed in 1975 as having Alzheimer's disease. She had to be cared for in a nursing home because of deteriorating motor and sensory functions. In February 1978 she suffered a massive stroke and was admitted to an acute care hospital. In addition to her primary disease she had labile hypertension, arteriosclerosis with resultant coronary artery disease, and severe osteoporosis. Her life expectancy was no more than a year and because of her complicated condition it was anticipated that she could suffer a cardiac or respiratory arrest at any time.

The court found that the CPR procedure would be highly invasive and would offer no cure for the underlying disease process. In consultation with the family the physicians agreed with their wishes to write the order. In the face of her irreversible terminal illness the court held that prior court review was unnecessary. The court said that to attempt to resuscitate dying patients in most cases, without the exercise of medical judgment, would be characterized as a pointless, even cruel, prolongation of the act of dying.

The case placed the onus on the medical profession to keep within the highest traditions of medicine in deciding whether to write a DNR order.

The court said that such decisions would be subject to review only where it was alleged that the physician failed to exercise competent medical judgment. While the decision did not suggest what course of action should be taken by the physician in the event of family disagreement it is clear that the facility would need to develop guidelines to address such a disagreement.

Another DNR case, *Custody of a Minor*, involved an infant who was a ward of the state.[26] The case, referred to as the "Baby Billy" case in the media, involved an infant who was born with congenital heart defects. Surgery done when he was 3 days old was unsuccessful and the surgeons believed that he would die before his first birthday. When he was 5 months old he was admitted to a hospital with pneumonia, a bacterial infection, and meningitis. His immediate prognosis was poor. Because he was a ward of the state the hospital asked the Department of Social Services to authorize a DNR order. As a matter of policy the Department refused and the hospital petitioned the court which approved the order.

The infant survived the life threat and shortly thereafter it was found that his life expectancy had substantially improved because he had developed collateral circulation which maintained his oxygen levels at 80 percent. However, the infant's ultimate prognosis was hopeless. At a subsequent hearing the physicians testified that given the change in the infant's condition he should be resuscitated if he should arrest. The judge of the juvenile court ruled that the DNR order should remain in effect. That order was appealed.

The higher court held that the judgment to continue the DNR order was supported by the evidence and findings. The judge's decision was based on the fact that the order would involve a "substantial" degree of bodily invasion and would do nothing but prolong the child's "agony and suffering." The court rejected the argument that the case involved a "right-to-life" issue. It determined that the case dealt with the question of the "manner of dying." Citing *Dinnerstein*, the court stated the question was, what "measures are appropriate to ease the imminent passing of an irreversibly, terminally ill patient in light of the patient's history and condition."

The fact that the infant was a ward of the state is significant. He lacked parents who ordinarily would consent to such an order. The court said that absent a loving family with whom physicians may consult regarding the entry of a DNR order, the question is best resolved by requiring a judicial determination.

One final point should be made. The hospital and Department of Social Services argued that the highest standard of proof should be met in any decision to uphold a DNR order—That is, the criminal standard, "beyond a reasonable doubt." The court rejected that argument, saying that such a high standard would require judges when reviewing medical judgments to reach a level of moral certainty. Further, the court said that imposing such an evidentiary burden would ultimately cause unnecessary pain and loss of dignity. The court said, "We refuse to lay down a rule requiring a physician to testify that he or she has personal knowledge, to a moral certainty, that the ward's future is hopeless." It said that it was sufficient to rely on the expert testimony of the child's physician that it was unlikely that the child would survive beyond a year and that the child was "irreversibly terminally ill."

Summary

Of all the treatment dilemmas the DNR order is the easiest to resolve. The problem is confined to the manner in which a DNR order is communicated. In the past physicians would not write the order, principally because they believed that a "negative" order exposed them to liability. Thus, nurses were placed in the position of having to implement a verbal order without any documentation in the medical record about the patient's medical condition or prognosis which would justify their failure to affirmatively respond to an arrest.

There was little case law concerning DNR orders although there were a number of cases on the failure to diagnose a cardiac arrest.[27] The standards for CPR and emergency cardiac care, first published in 1974, did not alleviate the anxiety surrounding the DNR order, although they should have. This was probably due to the fact that many physicians were unaware of its existence. Publication of an article in an international medical journal in 1976 served to bring the DNR issue out in the open. Subsequently a number of state medical associations proposed guidelines for DNR orders.[28] In the fall of 1983 the Veterans Administration (VA) adopted a DNR policy.[29] The VA had resisted adopting protocols for some time.

A number of interesting CPR articles have recently begun to appear in the medical literature.[30] One such article reported the survival rates after CPR in a hospital setting. The findings will undoubtedly prove helpful when discussing the technique with a patient or family member. Another article dealt with a prospective survey of the use of CPR in residential facilities for the elderly.[31] The residents of an Illinois residential home were canvassed as to their wishes regarding resuscitation in the event they arrested in the facility or in a hospital. As a result the facility has formalized in writing the resident's wishes should such an event occur.

In another study conducted at a Boston teaching hospital the researchers concluded that many physicians, although they believe in the concept of informed consent, did not openly discuss the nature of CPR with their patients.[32] The DNR order was one of the issues dealt with by the President's Commission for the Study of Ethical Problems in Medicine and Biomedical and Behavioral Research. The commission recommended in one of its reports that "health care institutions should have explicit policies and procedures governing orders not to resuscitate, and accrediting bodies should require such policies."[33] The commission concluded that DNR policies should be in written form and delineate who has the authority to write such an order.

In June 1987, the Joint Commission on Accreditation of Hospitals (JCAH) which is the principal agency accrediting U.S. hospitals said it would require hospitals to develop formal policies on withholding resuscitation.[34] The policies are effective as of January 1988 and apply to all of the hospitals that the Joint Commission accredits. The policies define the roles of nurses, physicians, patients, and family members in deciding when a patient will have a DNR order placed in the medical record and plan of care.

REMOVAL OF FEEDING DEVICES

The issue of discontinuation of Karen Quinlan's feeding tube which was her main source of nourishment was not a predominant one in the case. The Quinlan court, however, did not decide the issue and her parents later took the position that such an act would be tantamount to killing her. The question was one which sooner, rather than later, was bound to reach the courts. Since the first case was cited in the news media in 1982, courts in New Hampshire, Massachusetts, New Jersey, New York, California, and Maine have dealt with the legal issue.[35]

Criminal Indictment for Removal of Feeding Tube

The California Natural Death Act permits adults to execute a directive for withholding or withdrawing life-sustaining treatment if their illness is terminal.

However, in *Barber v. Superior Court of the State of California*, Clarence Herbert had not signed such a directive in August 1981 when he entered a California hospital to have his colostomy closed.[36] He suffered a cardiac arrest in the recovery room and was placed on life-support equipment. He had suffered severe brain damage, but was not brain dead. After the physicians informed the family that his prognosis for recovery was poor, the family requested that he be removed from the machines. This was done, but he continued to breathe. Two days after the ventilator was withdrawn the physicians ordered the removal of his intravenous tubes. They had consulted with the family who consented to the action. He died 6 days later from dehydration and pneumonia.

A year after these events the Los Angeles district attorney filed a criminal charge against the surgeon and the attending physician for murder and conspiracy to commit murder. A magistrate issued findings in favor of the physicians, but authorities appealed that decision and the murder indictment was reinstated. That court based its decision on the Death Act which "does not allow anyone to shorten anothers life unless the latter's condition is 'irreversible' ". The murder indictment was ultimately set aside by a California appellate court in 1983, but a civil suit against the hospital and the physicians was allowed to proceed.[37]

The appellate court said, "we view the use of an intravenous administration of nourishment and fluid, under the circumstances, as being the same as the use of the respirator or other form of life-support equipment." Further, the court said that once life-sustaining treatment becomes futile there is no duty to continue its use. The court emphasized that a determination that it would be futile must be made by qualified medical personnel. The court concluded that it was unnecessary to seek authorization from the courts to remove life-sustaining treatment. The facts of each case will determine whether the efforts at treatment are "futile."

The criminal indictment in the California case did not come about because of the removal of the respirator. The patient did not die, as expected, from that act. It should be noted that the nurses were asked to remove the respirator 2 days after the recovery room arrest.[38] While it would be premature to remove life-support systems within hours of a resultant coma following an arrest, there should be no need to keep a patient on machines for an extended time where the condition has been diagnosed as "irreversible." The staff should see in the medical record the process whereby the patient was evaluated. The amount of time between the unfortunate event and the withdrawal of treatment and devices should be reasonable. This requires medical consultation, frequent evaluation of progress or deterioration, and a consensus among the medical evaluators.

Thus far, the courts have not indicated a specific time frame as to the removal of life-support devices. It is unlikely that any time frame will be dictated by the courts. However, in a recent Washington state decision, two judges, in a dissenting opinion, said that the time between a 69-year-old woman's out-of-hospital cardiac arrest and the removal of her respiratory support was "shockingly short."

In fact, in *Matter of Colyer*, a judicial hearing was not sought until 17 days after her coma ensued.[39] Since the California case the moral aspect of stopping intravenous fluids and tube feedings has surfaced in professional literature.[40]

The Nursing Home Dilemma

Until recently feeding devices such as Levine and gastrostomy tube feedings were not regarded as "extraordinary" means of sustaining life.[41] Such devices are commonly used for nursing home patients, especially those who have suffered a severe stroke whereby the swallowing mechanism is totally lost or severely impaired. It may also be used in elderly individuals who have severe organic brain syndrome.

In a newspaper account of the plight of a New York man it was reported that the 85-year-old retired engineer who resided in a nursing home, began to fast in December 1983.[42] The man, who was mentally competent, suffered from heart disease, hardening of the arteries, and arthritis which confined him to a wheelchair. After a month the nursing home reported the fast to the city health department and it brought a petition before the court.

After hearing testimony and reviewing medical reports, a trial judge ruled that the man could not be "force fed." The court based its decision on the man's constitutional right of privacy under the First Amendment and on a state public health law which permitted patients to refuse medically necessary treatment.

In 1985, 9 years after the historic Quinlan decision, the New Jersey Supreme Court issued a lengthy and equally historic opinion.[43]

In *Matter of Conroy*, the New Jersey court expanded on many principles articulated in the earlier case and its progeny. The case is historic because it was the first state supreme court case to deal with the troublesome issue of when, if ever, and under what standards may the feeding device of an elderly patient who resides in a nursing home be permanently withdrawn. It is apparent that the well-reasoned decision is the beneficiary of almost 10 years of extensive scrutiny by the courts, as well as in-depth analysis by countless writers.

Claire Conroy was an 84-year-old mentally incompetent woman whose nutrition was derived almost exclusively from nasogastric feedings. She had been incompetent since 1979 and her nephew, who brought the court petition, was her legally appointed guardian. The woman suffered from severe organic brain syndrome, diabetes, arteriosclerotic heart disease, and necrotic ulcers of her foot and leg. The nephew had earlier refused to consent to an amputation because he felt it was not in her best interest. The court noted that the nephew had no financial gain in his aunt's death. In his petition, he sought authorization to consent to removal of the Levine tube.

The trial court allowed his petition, but stayed the order until the appropriate appeals could be taken. She died 13 days later. The appeal went forward because of its importance. The appeals court expressed concern that removal "would establish a dangerous precedent" and reversed the trial judge's order. The appeals court said that it rejected the extension of the Quinlan decision to active euthanasia.

In striking down the appeals court decision, the state supreme court held that the right to reject treatment by both competent and incompetent patients does not depend upon the quality or value of a person's life, and that "no distinction is to be made between withholding and withdrawing life-sustaining treatment." The court said that the decision-making procedure for vegetative patients suggested in the Quinlan opinion is not appropriate to nursing home patients who are similarly situated in Claire Conroy's petition. The court noted that significant differences in patients, health care providers, and the institutional structure of nursing homes and hospitals. Thus, the Conroy decision and guidelines are limited to the nursing home setting. Also of note is the fact that the court bypassed the ethics/prognosis committee approach and instead adopted the ombudsman approach. The states' ombudsman program came into being when New Jersey created it to investigate patient abuse complaints in nursing homes.

The court set out the required procedure to be followed in determining whether withholding or withdrawing life-sustaining treatment from an incompetent nursing home resident is justified. A person who believes the withdrawal or withholding action would effectuate an incompetent's wish or "best interests" should notify the office of the ombudsman of the intended action. Such notification can be done by the patient's guardian or by another interested party, such as a family member, attending physician or the facility. An individual who believes such an action is an abuse of the patient should also report the fact to the office. The court suggested that the ombudsman should treat every notification as a "possible abuse" and thus, under state law would be required to investigate the situation and report within 24 hours to the appropriate state regulatory agency.

The attending physician and nurse should provide evidence regarding the resident's condition. Two independent physicians and the attending physician would confirm the patient's condition and prognosis. Once the medical condition and prognosis are confirmed the guardian may terminate the life-sustaining measure. The attending physician must concur with the guardian's decision to terminate the treatment.

Once the court established the procedure it turned its attention to the standard or test to be applied in deciding whether the treatment should be stopped. It established three standards, one of which would permit incompetent nursing home residents who suffer from "serious and permanent mental and physical impairment" and who will "probably die within approximately one year" to have life-sustaining treatment withheld or withdrawn.

The first standard, a "subjective" standard, applies when it is clear that the resident would have refused the treatment. Evidence such as a living will, an "oral directive" to a family member or a health care provider, or a power of attorney will meet the subjective test.

The second and third standards are objective in nature. Under the "limited objective" test the court looks for some "trustworthy evidence" that the resident would have refused the treatment. This standard would be applicable where the resident did not express any wish. In addition, the court must be convinced that the burden of living outweighs the benefits to the patient. For example, the burden of pain outweighs the emotional enjoyment of life.

The third standard, a "pure objective" test, would be applicable where there is an absence of any reliable evidence of the patient's wishes. Under this stringent standard it would have to be shown that the patient's life is unbearable. The court expressed this as, the net burden of the patient's life with treatment should clearly outweigh the benefits the patient would derive from life. This would encompass pain so severe that keeping the patient alive by life-sustaining treatment would be "inhumane." The New Jersey Supreme Court held that the evidence in the Conroy case failed to meet any of the three standards. However, its clear and detailed language makes the case an important precedent.

The language of the Conroy decision makes it clear that the court was aware of the unique situation many nursing home residents are in. That is, frequently there are no relatives to protect their interests, they are visited by a physician only on a monthly basis or less, and there are other factors that make these individuals "a particularly vulnerable population."

The language of *Conroy* make it clear that these types of decisions cannot be made on an ad hoc basis.

In Minnesota the Department of Health investigated a situation where an 89-year-old nursing home resident died in 1984 after not being given water or food for a period of 6 days.[44] Although the investigator concluded that the care was "thoughtful, comprehensive, and appropriate," he found that there was no physician's order for withholding the oral feeding. The nursing staff stated that they deprived the woman of water at the request of her daughter. The department of health directed the hospital to develop more explicit supportive care guidelines and to include patients in discussion about their care.

In the spring of 1984 a Massachusetts intermediary court was asked to render a decision on the authority of a guardian ad litem to consent to the administration of antipsychotic drugs and surgical procedures necessary to provide adequate nutrition.[45]

In *Matter of Hier*, a 92-year-old woman had suffered for many years from severe mental illness and her physical problems included a hiatal hernia which prevented adequate nutrition by mouth. After pulling her gastrostomy tube out many times the site had closed, necessitating new surgery. She resisted any attempts to replace the tube and the administrator of the nursing home and a nurse filed the court petition.

The trial court authorized the administration of the antipsychotic drugs, but would not authorize the surgery. On appeal, the decision was upheld. The court rejected the guardian ad litem's argument that a distinction should be made between the right to choose for or against medical treatment, and the right to choose not to have procedures necessary to maintain adequate nutrition forcibly administered. The court reviewed the literature and found much support against such a position. Although the woman was mentally incompetent and her verbal refusal and behavior could not be given a legal effect, it was considered by the court in its decision.

When the Massachusetts court applied the "substituted judgment" test to the Saikewicz case in 1977 it provided a legal means whereby treatment decisions could be made for incompetent patients. Recall that the New York law seemingly provides no mechanism if the patient is incompetent and has not expressed a view against treatment. The Massachusetts court said that it found no inconsistency in deciding for antipsychotic drugs and against surgery for nutritional support. It viewed the administration of Thorazine, even if by injection, as relatively nonintrusive. The patient had not experienced side effects and the drug had relieved the torment of her mental illness. Conversely, the surgery was burdensome and there was no guarantee that she would not pull the tube out as she had done frequently in the past. A month after the appellate decision the case was taken back to the trial court and based on new medical evidence the court authorized the gastrostomy operation.

The pivotal factor in *Conroy* was the fact that she would probably die within 1 year even with treatment. A year after *Conroy* two other feeding tube cases were decided by lower New Jersey courts.

In the case of *In re Visbeck* the court ordered the insertion of a feeding tube in a 90-year-old incompetent hospitalized patient when it found that the woman had expressed no preference against any life-prolonging treatment.[46] The court found that the surgical procedure was simple and there would be minimal discomfort associated with the procedure. The court said that the "real risk of making bad decisions if we allow quality of life factors to be considered should not lead us to exclude those factors . . . . If we require treatment decisions to be made without any reference to quality of life factors, we will be creating other kinds of risks of bad decision making."

In the event that her son who was appointed her guardian wished to remove the feeding tube he would be required to obtain the agreement of a hospital prognosis committee if his mother was still hospitalized or to obtain the agreement of the ombudsman for the elderly, the attending physician, and outside physicians if she resided in a nursing home. Such protections were in accord with those which had evolved in the state in the aftermath of *Quinlan*.

Two months later the second New Jersey intermediary court feeding tube case was decided.

In that case, *In re Clark*, the hospital sought direction as to whether a 45-year-old man who was not in a vegetative state should have a "life-saving" enterostomy because he was unable to sustain proper nutrition via oral intake.[47] In accordance with the New Jersey Supreme Court guidelines outlined in the *Quinlan* and *Conroy* decisions the *Clark* court required the concurrence of the guardian, family and physicians. Seven of Clark's twelve siblings testified. All, but one of the testifying siblings said they would refuse to consent to the enterostomy, mainly because of Clark's perceived quality of life and negative potential for any neurological recovery. There was also disagreement among the physicians. Thus, lacking concurrence as required by *Quinlan* and *Conroy* it became necessary to resort to the court. The court appointed a guardian for the purpose of consenting to the surgery. The court held that such surgery was in the "best interest" of the man. It looked to the *Quinlan* and *Conroy* standards in deciding the outcome, mainly looking to the three Conroy standards, namely, the subjective, limited-objective, and pure objective test. The later two are really, "best interest" tests. Because there was no reliable evidence as to whether Clark would have accepted or rejected the surgery the subjective and limited-objective tests were inapplicable. Applying the pure objective test the court looked to a "determination of whether certain treatment should be provided or withheld . . . by strictly weighing the burdens of life with the treatment versus the benefits of that life to the patient". Based upon evidence from the physicians and nurses, as well as from the family that the patient was not suffering present pain, and was deriving some benefits from life, the court found that it was in Clark's "best interest" to have the surgery and "that the net burdens of Clark's life with the enterostomy do not markedly outweigh the benefits that he derives from life. Administering this type of treatment is not inhumane in this case, since it would not cause or prolong suffering for Clark."

Clark, unlike Quinlan and Conroy was not in a coma or vegetative state. While the *Quinlan* court would not give legal weight to Karen Quinlan's expressed wishes made before she went into a coma (the court found them unreliable) the *Conroy* and *Clark* courts would have given weight to the statements of Conroy and Clark. However, there was no evidence that either made any such statements.

Two other nutritional devices cases decided in 1986 and 1987 were as precedent setting as *Conroy*. These cases were the Massachusetts *Brophy* case and the New Jersey *Jobes* case.

In *Brophy v. New England Sinai Hospital*, the Massachusetts Supreme Court held that the gastrostomy tube of a patient in a persistent vegetative state could be removed.[48] After the state supreme court ruled on the case the attorney who had been appointed by the court for Paul Brophy tried to get Justices of the U.S. Supreme Court to stop the order to remove the tube pending a review by the full bench of the U.S. Supreme Court but the request was refused. (This route was also followed in the *Jobes* case.) Brophy was then moved from the defendant hospital to another Massachusetts hospital where the tube was removed and he died of pneumonia 8 days later.

Paul Brophy was a 47-year-old fireman who was also an emergency medical technician. In March 1983 he had a ruptured basilar artery aneurysm which was operated on 2 weeks later. He never regained consciousness from the surgery. Eight months later he had a gastrostomy tube inserted. He was not terminally ill or in danger of imminent death. Brophy's wife who was a nurse was appointed his legal guardian and sought court authorization to remove the tube in February 1985. All the family members approved of the request. However, the hospital refused to remove the tube and thus became a defendant.

There was ample evidence that before becoming incompetent Brophy had expressed his wishes against life-prolonging treatment if he was ever placed in a condition similar to the one he ultimately faced. In the wake of the Karen Quinlan publicity he stated to his wife, "I don't ever want to be on a life-support system. No way do I want to live like that; that is not living." Between the time he suffered the ruptured aneurysm and his surgery he told one of his daughters that he would rather be dead than be unable to sit up and kiss his children.

Applying the substituted judgment test as articulated almost 10 years previously by that same court in *Saikewicz*, the *Brophy* court overruled a trial judge's decision refusing to authorize removal of the tube. The substituted judgment test or standard requires the court to determine with as much accuracy as possible the desires and needs of the incompetent person. Once the court found that Brophy would have decided for either removal or clamping of the tube, knowing that death would result it considered whether any state interest should override Brophy's wishes. On this issue the court reviewed its own holdings, as well as other state treatment decisions. Addressing the "quality of life" argument the *Brophy* court said, ". . . we make no judgment based on our own view of the value of Brophy's life, since we do not approve of an analysis of state interests which focuses on Brophy's quality of life." The court found that although the presence of the tube was not highly invasive or an intrusive procedure, allowing Brophy to remain in his present state was intrusive. The court reaffirmed its position that removal of the tube feedings would not be the "death producing agent set in motion with the intent of causing his own death." Thus, the court disposed of the state's interest in preventing suicide.

The last issue which the court dealt with was the refusal of the hospital to remove the tube. On that issue the court held that the hospital and its medical staff "should not be compelled to withhold food and water to (sic) a patient, contrary to its moral and ethical principles, when such principles are recognized and accepted within a significant segment of the medical profession and the hospital community." The court took notice of the American Medical Association statement on "withholding or withdrawing life-prolonging medical treatment issued in 1986 (Appendix H at the back of the book)[49] and the 1985 resolution passed by the Massachusetts Medical Society which stated that recognizing the autonomy rights of vegetative individuals by carrying out their wishes to refuse treatment did not constitute unethical medical behavior (Appendix I at the back of the book).[50] No law existed in the state requiring the hospital to take any active measures to stop hydration and nutrition upon request of the guardian. The court noted that there is substantial disagreement in the medical community over the appropriate medical action in situations similar to Brophy's. In addition, the hospital was willing to help in arranging a transfer of the patient to a facility which would not object to affirmatively removing or clamping the tube. The court held that "A patient's right to refuse medical treatment does not warrant such an unnecessary intrusion upon the hospital's ethical integrity. . . ."

Two additional points about the *Brophy* decision are worth noting. First, referring to language in the President's Commission Report the court said that the distinction between extraordinary and ordinary treatment may obscure the real issues in a termination of care or treatment case because applying such distinctions "can lead to inconsistent results, which makes the terms of questionable value in the formulation of public policy in this area."[51] Second, the court when discussing the right of the hospital to refuse to actively participate in the withdrawal of the feeding device said that its ruling did not violate the integrity of the medical profession. The need to recognize that legal concept was articulated in the *Saikewicz* opinion.

Of all the feeding device cases to date, the one that attracted the most national attention was the Elizabeth Bouvia case in California. Her case was different because she was a young woman who was competent and alert and not faced with the immediate certainty of death. However she was severely incapacitated with cerebral palsy and quadriplegia. She also suffers a great deal of pain from degenerative and crippling arthritis. In 1983 when she was 26 years old she was admitted to a hospital and began a food fast several weeks later. She admitted that she wanted to die. When petitioned, the court issued an order to the hospital that it continue to force-feed the young woman. However, in 1986 in *Bouvia v. Superior Court* the court held that she had a constitutional right to refuse feeding by nasogastric tube even if the act would hasten her death.[52] When the court reviewed her petition in 1986 it said "Here Elizabeth Bouvia's decision to forego medical treatment or life-support through a mechanical means belongs to her. It is not a medical decision for her physicians to make. Neither is it a legal question whose soundness is to be resolved by lawyers or judges. It is not a conditional right subject to approval by ethics committees or courts of law. It is a moral and philosophical decision that, being a competent adult, is her's alone." Further, the court said, "We do not believe it is the policy of this State that all and every life must be preserved against the will of the sufferer." The court said it found no evidence that Bouvia's refusal to accept the feeding tube was suicide.

Shortly after the appeals court ruled in her favor the patient filed a petition with the courts when physicians at the hospital informed her that they would be decreasing her narcotic medication (morphine) because it was too addictive.[53] She had been receiving a morphine drip to control the pain from her severe arthritis. She appealed to the courts on the narcotic issue and a judge ordered a temporary injunction against the physicians' stopping her morphine. However, at a later hearing the injunction was lifted. Bouvia's physicians argued that the court should not be permitted to intervene in medical judgment and treatment decisions.

Another withdrawal of a feeding device case, *In the matter of Nancy Ellen Jobes* was decided by the New Jersey Supreme Court in 1987.[54] That court held that the patient who is in an irreversible vegetative condition has a right to refuse life-sustaining medical treatment and this right may be exercised by the patient's family or close friend. If the patient has "close and caring" family members who are willing to make the decision they are the best qualified decision makers to make substituted judgments for incompetent family members. Family members close enough to make a substituted judgment would be a spouse, parents, adult children, or siblings. The court said that it would not ordinarily countenance health care professionals deferring to a patient's relative who lacks a close degree of kinship, but if the health care provider determines that another functions as the patient's nuclear family, then that person can be regarded as a close and caring family member.

If there are no close family members to make the decision then a guardian should be appointed. Where a health care professional becomes uncertain about whether family members are protecting a patient's interests then, guardianship proceedings should be begun. So long as the health care provider acts in good faith that person will not incur any criminal or civil liability where guardianship proceedings are instituted due to uncertainty of family motives.

In 1980 Nancy Ellen Jobes, who was 4½-months pregnant, was involved in an automobile accident which killed her fetus. During an operation to remove the dead fetus she suffered severe and irreversible damage. She was transferred to a nursing home 4 months later and in 1985 after having trouble with other feeding devices she had a jejunostomy (j-tube) inserted. She was severely brain damaged and in a vegetative state. In May 1985 her husband and her parents asked the nursing home to withdraw the j-tube, however, they refused on moral grounds. Before her injury Mrs. Jobes did not express in any legally reliable manner how she would have wished to deal with the j-tube.

Thus, the issues before the high court were to determine who decides for the incompetent patient, the standard or test that the surrogate decision maker must use, and who must be consulted and concur in the decision. The New Jersey court specifically pointed out that it was not the court who was to decide whether to remove the j-tube, but rather to establish for those who will make the decision the criteria and procedure to follow. In short, the *Jobes* court was asked to determine who decides for the incompetent patient, what standard the surrogate decision maker must use, and who must be consulted and concur in the decision.

In the absence of a clear directive the substituted judgment test will ensure that the surrogate decision maker effectuates as much as possible the wishes of the patient. The surrogate decision maker considers the patient's personal value system for guidance. For example, the patient's likely attitude toward the impact of the choice on loved ones. As in *Quinlan* the court said the family members were the proper parties to make a substituted medical judgment on Mrs. Jobes's behalf.

> Family members are best qualified to make substituted judgments for incompetent patients not only because of their peculiar grasp of the patient's approach to life, but also because of their special bonds with him or her. Our common human experience informs us that family members are generally most concerned with the welfare of the patient.

Thus, the court held that the patient's right to stop the treatment may be exercised by the patient's family or close friend. If there are no close family members and the incompetent person is not elderly, a guardian must be appointed. The court said the process of surrogate decision making should be substantially the same regardless of where the patient is located. The surrogate decision maker must obtain statements from at least two independent physicians experienced in neurology that the patient is in a persistent vegetative state and that there is no reasonable possibility that the patient will ever recover to a cognitive, sapient state. If an attending physician exists, then the physician must likewise submit such a statement. These independent neurological confirmations will substitute for the concurrence of the prognosis committee for patients who are not in a hospital setting. Further, the court said if there is a dispute among the family members physicians, or guardian, any interested party can seek judicial assistance to insure that the patient is protected.

Conroy, Brophy, and the three New Jersey Supreme Court feeding cases decided in June 1987 will serve as guides for other jurisdictions. There are other removal of feeding devices cases which are worth noting because of their factual distinctions.

In *Workmen's Circle Home v. Fink* the daughters of a 79-year-old incompetent woman with an inoperable brain tumor petitioned the court for an order permitting them to withhold their consent to a gastrostomy.[55] The woman had orally told her daughters that she did not want any life-support procedures done for her if there was no hope for recovery. The court allowed the petition to withhold consent to the gastrostomy, but would not permit the daughters to withhold consent to administer antibiotics or IV therapy.

In *Corbett v. D'Alessandro* A Flordia court held that a 75-year-old woman who had been in a vegetative state for over 3 years could have her nasogastric tube removed.[56] It is noteworthy that the court permitted the removal even though the legislature had passed a right to decline life prolonging bill in 1984 which specifically stated that measures to comfort the dying included, "sustenance . . . deemed necessary to provide comfort, care or to alleviate pain."[57] In holding that the tube could be removed the Florida court relied on another provision of the act which said it was not intended to impair any existing rights. Relying on the privacy right under both the U.S. Constitution and the state constitution the court held that while the statute did not authorize the removal of the tube, neither could it prevent its removal because to do so would violate Mrs. Corbett's privacy rights.

In *In re Requena* a New Jersey court upheld the right of a competent patient with ALS to refuse artificial feedings.[58] The woman who was 55 years old had been in the hospital for 15 months and her swallowing problems were increasing. When she informed the hospital of her decision the hospital asked her to leave because it had a strong institutional policy against participating in the withholding of foods or fluids. When the woman refused to leave, the hospital petitioned the court. The court held that the hospital must comply with the patient's informed decision exercising her right to a peaceful death. An alternative suggested by the hospital that she be transferred to a hospital 17 miles away was not appropriate because the woman expressed confidence in being with familiar nursing staff and in familiar surroundings. The court held that although the hospital's policy was valid and enforceable it could only be enforced in instances where it did not conflict with the patient's rights. Some courts appear to be suggesting that when a hospital has institutional policies against stopping feeding devices, it informs the patient in advance of such policies.

In *Rasmussen v. Fleming* an Arizona court held that although an incompetent nursing home patient had never expressed an opinion about life prolonging procedures, she had a constitutional right to have her feeding tube removed.[59] The court applied a "best interest" standard. The woman had lived in the nursing home for 6 years and in addition to extensive cerebral damage from several strokes she had a degenerative muscular condition and organic brain syndrome.

In a New York petition, *Delio on Behalf of Delio v. Westchester County*, the wife of a 33-year-old patient in a vegetative state after an arrest during rectal surgery was not permitted to remove his feeding tube.[60] However, that decision was not upheld on appeal.[61] The lower court although sympathetic to the family's plight said that there was no "clear and convincing" evidence that the man would have wanted the tube removed. Also, the physicians who examined him were unable to conclude that he was "terminally ill." The lower court indicated it's reluctance to decide these kinds of cases when it said that intervention by the legislature would be a preferable way of approaching them.

Force-Feeding of Prisoners

In 1984 a New Hampshire high court held that a prisoner who had received a 30-year sentence should be force fed against his wishes.[62] The 36-year-old prisoner had lost 80 pounds during a 3-month fast. The prisoner said he wanted to "die with dignity," rather than spend the rest of his life in jail. The court held that where the prisoner was not dying from an illness, but rather was attempting to set the "death-producing" agent in motion to cause his own death, the state's interest in maintaining an orderly and effective criminal justice system and its interest in preserving life would prevail. The prisoner had no right to starve himself under either the federal or state constitutions.

Summary

The withdrawal and withholding of life-sustaining treatment, in the form of gastric feedings, from irreversibly ill patients is the latest treatment issue to be brought to the courts. The moral and legal issues surrounding the withdrawal of feeding tubes were initially so strong that they resulted in a criminal indictment for two California physicians. The courts recognize that the cases have tremendous significance for many patients in nursing homes where many are incompetent, "hopelessly" ill, and without family. Of all the treatment decisions, perhaps, this area requires the strictest guidelines for decision making because of the potential for abuse.

To date there are three precedent-setting withdrawal-of-feeding-devices cases, *Conroy*, *Brophy*, and *Jobes* (and the two companion cases decided with *Jobes*). All were decided by the state's highest court and the U.S. States Supreme Court refused to review two of the cases, *Brophy* and *Jobes*. In *Conroy* the court set out three standards or tests necessary to justify the withdrawal of her feeding tube; ironically, *Conroy* did not fall within any of the criteria but she had died by the time the case was decided. The court limited its decision to elderly nursing home patients. As a result, New Jersey set up a state ombudsman office for the institutionalized elderly to intervene in cases where the incompetent nursing home resident has no family or guardian. *Conroy* set up a life expectancy criterion. While *Quinlan* would not accept an "oral directive" the *Conroy* court would have. The court in *Quinlan* said that the testimony of Karen's prior statements about life-prolonging treatment was unreliable, given her young years and the "casualness" of the remarks.

Brophy held that it was in the man's best interest to have the feeding device removed. The court, applying the substituted judgment test was able to determine that *Brophy* would have refused the device. Its removal would not be suicide. The *Jobes* court said that the decision is one to be made by a "loving" family in compliance with the protection criteria set out by the court to establish a medical confirmation of irreversibility and hopelessness. In the absence of family, a close friend with firm ties to the incompetent will suffice. Where neither exist, the ombudsman will protect the incompetent's rights. In *Farrell*, the New Jersey court held that patients who are cared for in a home setting have the same rights as those in hospitals and nursing homes.

In the immediate wake of the *Conroy* decision, the New Jersey Legislature created a Commission on Legal and Ethical Problems in the Delivery of Health Care to study the issues created by the evolution of medical technology.[63] The commission's first report to the governor, legislature, and the public is scheduled in late 1988 and 3 years thereafter. New York has a similar commission which was started in late 1984.[64] Several prominent physicians in the beginning of the removal-of-feeding-devices debate wrote that removal of hydration and nutrition from "hopelessly ill" elderly patients may be in their best interests.[65] One cannot help but be aware in reading the feeding device cases, especially the *Jobes* and companion decisions, that the courts paid keen attention to the vast amount of literature published by medical, legal, and ethical writers beginning with the debate surrounding *Conroy*. The court was also aware of public attitudes about the role of surrogate decision making and the perceived role of the judiciary in these types of decisions.[66] In addition to the many articles published on the hydration issue, the President's Commission concluded that, "no particular treatments—including such "ordinary" hospital interventions as parenteral nutrition or hydration, antibiotics, and transfusions—are universally warranted and thus obligatory for a patient to accept."[67]

TREATMENT DECISIONS INVOLVING MINORS

Under the common law parents have the right to consent to medical or surgical treatment for their minor children. Thus, physicians seek parental consent when faced with such surgical procedures as the removal of tonsils, appendectomy, and setting fractured bones. However, the rights of the parents are different when they elect to forego a life-saving treatment in favor of one not supported by existing medical standards or elect no treatment when medical opinion supports treatment.

A recent Pennsylvania court found the parents of a 2-year-old boy guilty of involuntary manslaughter.[68] The parents, who belonged to a fundamentalist religious sect, refused to seek medical attention or treatment for the child, stating that they believed in prayer and faith as the source of healing. The child died and an autopsy showed that a 5-pound abdominal mass was a Wilms's tumor. There was medical testimony at the trial that the child's chances for survival were 95 percent if the tumor was localized to the kidney and detected early. In addition, there was evidence that both parents had received regular dental treatment, both before and during the child's illness.

In a similar case in Colorado, a father was convicted of felony child abuse when he failed to seek medical attention for his 5-week-old daughter.[69] The parents, who belonged to a fundamentalist Christian sect, took their child to the home of another sect member who was a practical nurse. The infant died in her home a day after the parents brought her there for care. In related nursing board proceedings it was found that she was not engaged in the practice of nursing and thus they could not take action against her. The Colorado nursing practice statute authorized the nursing board to discipline for conduct unrelated to professional acts only in instances where the nurse was convicted of a felony, or had a drug or alcohol problem.

A similar case occurred in California when the state accused the parents of a 17-month-old child of involuntary manslaughter.[70] The boy died of acute bacterial meningitis after the parents took him to the home of another Christian Scientist where all three prayed over the child.

In a widely reported Tennessee case the court declared a 12-year-old girl neglected when her parents refused to seek treatment.[71] The young girl was suffering from Ewing's sarcoma and received chemotherapy after the state took temporary custody of her. The girl's father who was a fundamentalist minister believed that the girl's faith would heal her, although her leg had swollen to twice its size and doctors said she would die within a year if untreated.

Limitations on the Right of Parents to Refuse Treatment

In 1978 the plight of 2-year-old Chad Green came to the attention of the national media. There was tremendous debate in the media about the parents right to choose the treatment modality for the child who suffered from the most common type of leukemia among children, acute lymphocytic leukemia. The Greens sought to treat Chad's leukemia with a natural and metabolic regimen. Although the public debate generated much sympathy for the parents' right to choose the type of treatment, the child's rights did not get the same attention, at least initially. At the time of Chad's death in September 1979 he was being treated at a clinic in Mexico and was receiving laetrile, a diet high in vegetables and low in meat, high doses of vitamins, and enzyme enemas. The parents objected to the traditional chemotherapy treatment and finally ceased giving the chemotherapy pills 3 months before Chad died. Physicians at the clinic regarded chemotherapy as part of the treatment regimen and had prescribed it along with the metabolic treatments.

The child's leukemia was diagnosed when he was 22 months old. Left untreated the disease is fatal. Subsequent medical testimony established that the only known medically effective treatment was chemotherapy which consisted of an aggressive 3-year treatment regimen given in three distinct phases. The treatments consisted of antileukemia drugs given orally, intravenously, and by spinal injection. The first two phases consisted of a 4-week and 6-week period and the third phase was a maintenance period which continued to the end of the 3-year period.

The parents moved from Nebraska to Boston partly because the Nebraska physician recommended cranial radiation which they did not want. The father had been born in the Boston area. On return to Massachusetts the parents took Chad to a specialist at Massachusetts General Hospital. The physician in charge acceded to the parents' request to include a diet of distilled water, vegetarian foods, and high doses of vitamins. However, he explained that alone, the diet regimen was not appropriate treatment.

After a month of treatment at the hospital the child was in remission and the third phase was begun in November 1977. The third phase consisted of monthly vincristine injections and oral drugs. At this time the parents requested the physician to stop the injections and he reluctantly agreed to substitute another drug which could be given orally. When asked by the parents what would happen if the chemotherapy was terminated, the physician informed them that the chance for relapse was 100 percent. The parents stopped the daily 6-mercaptopurine pills, but continued the monthly visits.

In January the physician noted some deterioration and was reassured that the 6-mercaptopurine pills were still being given. However, in February 1978 when Chad presented with an enlarged liver and hemorrhage spots on his arms, and leukemic cells were found in his blood, his mother stated that the oral medication had not been given for over 3 months. The parents refused to continue therapy in spite of pleadings by the physician.

The First Legal Proceeding

The hospital obtained a court order under a parental neglect statute and the chemotherapy was restated, resulting in a quick remission. Subsequently, a court found the child to be in need of "care and protection" within the meaning of a state statute.[72] During these legal proceedings the parents failed to offer evidence that any alternative treatment would be consistent with "good and accepted medical practice." The court order required the parents to continue chemotherapy treatment under the supervision of any Massachusetts certified pediatric hematologist selected by them. The Greens retained physical custody of Chad.

The drugs were administered to the child in his home by a visiting nurse. If the child had remained in remission for 1½ years, his chances of being completely cured would be in a range of 80 percent. With the interruption his chances of cure dropped to approximately 50 percent. The court had acted quickly in ordering the resumption of chemotherapy because time was of the essence in that the leukemia cells double in number every 4 days.

The court recognized the strong precedent of parental rights, but subscribed to the established rule that parental rights are not grounded in any "absolute property right." In effect the court said that the concept of family autonomy may be limited and subject to the interests of the state, and the "best interests" of the child when parental decisions jeopardize the life of the child. By contrast, the majority of decisions involving elective, non-life-threatening treatment have held in favor of the parents right to decide against treatment if they so choose.

The Second Legal Proceeding

In January 1979 the parents sought a redetermination of the need for care and protection.[73] For the first time, they testified that they now accepted the need for the chemotherapy treatment. They sought full custody of Chad and authority to supplement chemotherapy with the metabolic therapy. Up to this point the Department of Public Welfare had custody of Chad only to the extent of supervising the child's medical treatment. At these proceedings the Greens presented experts, none of whom were licensed to practice in Massachusetts or had expertise in treating leukemia. All agreed under the judge's examination that laetrile and metabolic therapy had no observable effect in curing Chad's type of leukemia. The state presented testimony of physicians who were experts in treating childhood leukemia or doing research in leukemia. At this time Chad was in his second remission.

Evidence presented at these proceedings showed that Chad had not suffered significant side effects and his drug doses were modified to minimize side effects. Although the family had been informed that cyanide was an end-product of laetrile, they began the metabolic treatment in September 1978 and it continued up to the second legal proceeding. The court found that the daily ingestion of laetrile had produced a low-grade chronic cyanide poisoning. Chad had hypervitaminosis A which was deemed the likely source of his impaired liver function. There was testimony that high doses of vitamin C had a potential for kidney toxicity.

In view of these findings the court ordered the Greens to cease these aspects of metabolic therapy because of their potential for harm. Because of Chad's somewhat depressed immunologic system the enzyme enemas posed a risk of breakdown of the cells in the colon and subsequent bacterial infection. The court concluded that the judgment of the parents had been consistently poor and no matter how well intentioned, had seriously threatened the well-being of the child. The court upheld the previous order requiring the chemotherapy. By the time the court decision was issued the parents had left the state and remained out of it until Chad's death. They were not prosecuted for violating the court order in taking the child from Massachusetts.

The Chad Green case is not an isolated instance. In 1977 a Milwaukee court returned a 7-year-old girl to the custody of her parents after they agreed to seek leukemia treatment at a recognized facility.[74] Originally the parents began conventional therapy, but discontinued it because they lost faith in it. In 1979, Florida parents took their young daughter to West Germany for metabolic therapy after having her treated with chemotherapy for 2 years in the United States.[75] Her physician discovered recurrent leukemia cells in her brain, and the court found that she had not been on laetrile for several months prior to the legal proceedings. After the court found there was no probable cause to rule against the parents they took her to Germany. In 1981 a California couple fled a hospital with their 2-year-old leukemia-striken child and took her to the same clinic where Chad Green was treated.[76] The Los Angeles authorities agreed to allow the treatment because the child would be receiving chemotherapy in conjunction with the metabolic treatments.

These cases appear to be distinguished from *Chad Green* in that it was not shown that the metabolic therapy was harming any of the children. In addition, all of the children were receiving chemotherapy in addition to the metabolic therapy.

A case that is frequently compared with the Chad Green case is *Matter of Hofbauer*, decided by the New York courts in 1979.[77] The issue in the case was whether the parents of an 8-year-old child suffering from Hodgkin's disease were neglectful in failing to follow the diagnosing physician's recommendation regarding radiation and chemotherapy. The condition had been diagnosed when the boy was 7. After making numerous inquiries the parents rejected the recommended treatment and took the boy to Jamaica where he received metabolic therapy, including laetrile injections for a period of 1 month. On their return a child neglect proceeding was initiated and the child was temporarily removed from the custody of the parents. A month later he was returned to the custody of his parents and all parties agreed that the child would be medically managed by a New York physician who was a proponent of metabolic therapy. It was ordered that another physician would be consulted on a regular basis and the child's medical reports would be submitted to the court periodically.

At a subsequent hearing, medical evidence submitted by both parties relevant to medical treatment was in sharp conflict. One medical group testified that radiation and chemotherapy was the accepted method of treatment and metabolic therapy was ineffective. There was evidence that the disease had progressed. Physicians testifying on behalf of the parents supported metabolic therapy and were of the opinion that the child was responding favorably to that mode of therapy. They also testified that they would not rule out the adjunct use of traditional therapy if his condition appeared to be deteriorating beyond control. The boy's father testified that he would permit conventional treatment if the primary physician recommended it. All the physicians testified to the potentially dangerous side effects of radiation and chemotherapy.

Finding in favor of the parents, the court held that a parent may rely upon the recommendation and competency of the attending physician if that physician is licensed in the state. The court held that a state license provides some assurance that the physician is capable of exercising acceptable clinical judgment. The court found that the parents sought medical assistance and embarked on a course of care that was recommended by their physician and that had not been totally rejected by all responsible medical authorities. The New York court noted that the state medical licensing board had not taken any disciplinary action against the New York physician who was treating the boy with metabolite therapy. The distinction between the New York and Massachusetts cases is that, in Massachusetts, there was no expert testimony from recognized authorities that metabolite therapy was an accepted and recognized medical practice.

Summary

It is important that the nurse who is an advocate for both the child and the parents be aware of potential conflicting interests. The courts have been reluctant to deprive the parents of their right to make treatment choices for their children and, generally, will not do so if the treatment involves an elective routine procedure. However, when the election involves a lifesaving course of treatment the courts will weigh the child's rights against those of the parents.

The test for the child is that which is "best" for the child. As in any legal proceeding the court will hear testimony from relevant experts and decide what is the "best interests of the child." It should be evident from the evidence presented during the Chad Green case that the courts bypass the emotional aspect of these difficult cases and rely heavily on medical testimony.

ORGAN DONATION BY MINORS

With the advent of kidney transplantation a new treatment issue was raised. Because kidney transplantation between blood relatives decreased the risk of organ rejection, parents and siblings became a prime source of kidneys. Little problem beyond the issue of consent was involved when the donor was a parent or adult sibling. However, when the source of a healthy kidney was a minor sibling different consent issues were raised. A minor is under a legal disability because of the age factor and special factors must be considered to obtain a valid consent. The early cases involved court authorization for organ donation from a retarded sibling, but soon parents began requesting the courts to authorize an organ donation from a mentally competent child to another sibling. The various state jurisdictions have reached different judicial decisions.

Donation by a Retarded Sibling

The earliest case arose in Kentucky in 1969.[78] In *Strunk v. Strunk,* the mother of a 27-year-old institutionalized son petitioned the court for authorization to permit him to donate one of his kidneys to a 28-year-old sibling who was on hemodialysis for chronic glomerulous nephritis. The latter son frequently visited his retarded brother at the facility. The mental age of the institutionalized brother was approximately 6 years. He was the only tissue compatible source.

The court authorized the operation on the retarded brother because it found that he would derive a personal benefit from the fact that his brother's life might be saved. The retarded brother, who was emotionally dependent upon the ill brother, would derive more benefit by donating his kidney, and would be severely jeopardized by the loss of his brother. The death of his brother would deprive him of intimate communication and loving concern which the court deemed necessary to the stability and optimal functioning of the retarded brother.

A decade later, in *Little v. Little,* after a full judicial hearing during which the donor's interests were protected, a Texas court allowed a 14-year-old Down's syndrome sibling to donate her kidney to a younger brother.[79] Although the court found that no physical benefit would be conferred on the sister it said that she would receive substantial psychologic benefit and should not be denied such benefits as are conferred on competent donors when they donate to family members.

In 1972, *Hart v. Brown,* a Connecticut case, dealt with identical 7-year-old twins.[80] The court again applied the psychologic benefit test and allowed the donation.

Not all the courts followed the early decisions.

In 1973 a Louisiana court in *In re Richardson* would not allow a sibling to donate as it found that it was not in the mentally retarded donor's best interest to donate his kidney.[81] The retarded minor brother had a mental age of 3 or 4 years and his tissue studies showed him to be more compatible than his elder siblings. The court found that there was only a 5 percent chance of rejection with the retarded brother's organ compared with a 20 to 30 percent chance if other sibling organs were used. In spite of these findings the court determined that the retarded brother would derive no benefit as it was not shown that his ill adult sister had any significant relationship with him.

In *In re Guardianship of Richard Pescinski*, a Wisconsin court would not allow an adult schizophrenic who had few lucid moments and whose decision-making reasoning was impaired, to donate his kidney to his adult sister.[82] The brother was committed to a state facility and the court failed to find that any interests of the brother would be served by donating his kidney.

Summary

In surgical procedures which confer a physical benefit on the donee, but not on the donor, the courts will permit a minor to donate an organ if it finds that a psychological benefit will be conferred upon the donating minor. Thus, the courts offset the risks of surgery and living with only one kidney by weighing the positive psychologic benefit. The courts will also give significant weight to the mental capacity of the donor to understand the implications of the donation. A "mature minor," that is, one under the age of majority, but able to fully understand the implications of his consent, or lack of consent, is viewed by a number of courts as freely able to consent. For example, in *Masden v. Harrison* a Massachusetts court permitted a willing 19-year-old twin to donate his kidney to his twin.[83] At that time the age of majority in Massachusetts was 21 years.

The courts have expressed concern about the motivational conflict of interest that may exist between the parent and donor child, whether or not the child is retarded. The rule is that where the donor is a minor the court will appoint an independent person to investigate and evaluate the donor's willingness to donate his organ.

STERILIZATION OF MINORS

Another area of controversy is the sterilization of minors and mentally incompetent adults.

In 1978 the U.S. Supreme Court in *Stump v. Sparkman* held that a judge who had authorized the sterilization of a "somewhat retarded" 15-year-old girl was immune from civil liability when the woman brought suit a number of years later.[84] The woman married and only discovered that she was surgically sterile when she and her husband could not conceive. She had been told that the surgery was an appendectomy. The woman alleged that her constitutional due process rights had been abridged because she had never received notice or had a hearing on her mother's petition for sterilization. The Supreme Court held that even though the judge exceeded his authority and acted erroneously in personally managing the petition, no statute existed that specifically prohibited his action and thus judicial immunity protected his act.

Three years before the U.S. Supreme Court decision an Indiana court refused to permit sterilization unless it was necessary to save a minor's life.[85]

In *A. L. v. G. R. H.*, the parents sought court authorization to consent to a vasectomy for their 15-year-old son who was intellectually impaired as a result of brain damage from an accident. His parents feared that he might become sexually active with girls he met in his special education classes. Noting that sterilization transcends the ordinary medical treatment concept because it involves irreversible consequences the court said, "the common law does not invest parents with such power over their children even though they sincerely believe the childs' adulthood would benefit therefrom." Finding no life preserving factor or statutory authority, the court refused the parents' petition.

Judicial Versus Statutory Authority

In New York state there are two trial level decisions that have held two different holdings. In the first case, *Matter of Sallmaier*, the court relied on the common law authority of the state to act as guardian for incompetent individuals.[86] The mother of a 23-year-old retarded woman was permitted to consent to have the daughter sterilized. In the second case *Application of A. D.* the court refused to intervene under essentially the same set of facts.[87] The court said it was reluctant to authorize the procedure in the absence of a statute permitting sterilization of incompetents.

The California courts have been reluctant to authorize sterilizations, stating, "such awesome power may not be inferred from the general principles of common law, but rather must derive from specific legislative authorization.[88] California does not have a statute permitting sterilization and thus, in *Guardianship of Tulley*, the parents of a 20-year-old girl with a mental age of 3 years could not authorize sterilization. Both the state and U.S. Supreme Court refused to review the decision. A Wisconsin petition brought by the guardian of another profoundly retarded woman was similarly dismissed.[89]

In the early 1980s a series of cases held that, even in the absence of express legislation, authorization could be granted.[90] A Washington court in *In re Hayes* ruled that it had inherent authority to consider a sterilization petition.[91] That court imposed an evidentiary standard that is less than the high "beyond a reasonable doubt" standard required in criminal cases, but higher than the "based upon a preponderance of the evidence" standard required in civil suits. The standard imposed by the Washington court is, "clear, cogent and convincing." That standard applied in analyzing the following questions: whether the ability to procreate existed, whether any less drastic contraceptive measure existed, whether the incompetent individual is likely to engage in sexual activity, and whether the individual is incapable of caring for a child. The court established a procedure whereby a guardian would be appointed to assist the retarded individual at the legal proceedings and the court would have access to independent professional consultants.

About the same time a New Hampshire court in *In re Penny* also established procedures to be followed in sterilization petitions.[92] That state had an enabling statute and the petition was brought on behalf of a 14-year-old child with Down's syndrome. The state's highest court established guidelines similar to those adopted in a New Jersey case. The New Jersey court in *Matter of Grady* set out the following guidelines: an independent guardian to protect the interests of the retarded individual, independent medical and psychologic examinations for the court, and a judicial determination that the retarded individual is incapable of making a decision about sterilization and unlikely to be able to so do in the future.[93] In deciding whether the sterilization is in the "best interests" of the individual the judge must consider the possibility of pregnancy and childbirth, the individuals inability to benefit from other contraceptive methods, and the motivations of those proposing the sterilization. An Alaska court, in *Matter of C. D. M.*, also adopted procedural guidelines similar to those of New Jersey and New Hampshire.[94]

Colorado courts will authorize sterilization if the court finds that it is "medically essential."[95] A finding of medically essential is met if the court finds sterilization is necessary to preserve the life or physical or mental health of the mentally retarded person. In one of the most recent decisions *Motes v. Hall County Department of Family and Children Services*, which dealt with the sterilization of retarded individuals, the Georgia Supreme Court struck down a state statute that adopted the legal standard, "by a legal preponderance of all the evidence."[96] The statute required the judge to apply that evidentiary standard in finding that the retarded individual is unable to provide care and support for any child because of irreversible retardation or brain damage. In holding the statute unconstitutional the court said that "procreation is a fundamental right" and the higher "clear and convincing" standard should be applied in sterilization cases.

Summary

In the absence of the state statute permitting sterilization of retarded individuals the courts have been reluctant to grant such a petition. The courts have leaned heavily toward the right of everyone to procreate. If a court is relying on a state statute the evidentiary standard must be embodied in it or the court will impose a standard. None of the courts have adopted the lowest evidentiary standard, undoubtably because of the fundamental right to procreate and the irreversible nature of sterilization.

Just as individuals who are mentally ill are considered mentally competent unless adjudicated incompetent, the retarded individual is competent unless there has been a legal determination of incompetency. It is important to note that there are many causes of retardation other than genetic and this factor would be important in an adjudicatory hearing. When the issue of consent to a hysterectomy, radiation ablation, or vasectomy for a mentally retarded individual arises the consent must come from an enabling statute or a judicial hearing.

SUMMARY

There is a significant body of law dealing with the right to refuse blood transfusions. Where there are no compelling state interests the courts have been uniform in granting patient autonomy. However, where there are minor children who will be orphaned in the event the parent dies the courts have been reluctant to permit the adult to refuse the blood. The courts have generally refused to uphold a right of the parent(s) to refuse a transfusion for their minor child. The courts have also required a pregnant woman to have blood where the fetus is viable because the fetus and the mother's life are inextricably bound.

In 1981 the Georgia Supreme Court addressed the novel question of whether a near-term pregnant woman could be compelled to submit to surgery that her physicians said was necessary to save the fetus's life. That court brought a juvenile court into its decision because of the need to protect the rights of the unborn child. The court ordered the woman to submit to any tests and procedures to save the fetus's life.

The failure of physicians to formally write a no code order was a problem for nurses. While many of the teaching hospitals adopted a policy requiring that such orders be written, far too many nonteaching facilities, including nursing homes, were resistent to putting orders in writing. The first case to specifically address the legality of the no code order was the 1978 Dinnerstein case. There was some confusion in the wake of a prior decision about whether no code orders could ever be written without a court order. The Dinnerstein court, as anticipated, looked to the medical aspects of the procedure and framed its ruling around this important aspect. Ironically, it was the first time that many physicians learned that a recognized medical group was on record that such orders should be in writing. Perhaps this was because many nurses presumed that every physician was as knowledgeable about the cardiopulmonary resuscitation procedure as nurses were. In fact, this was not the case. To date, almost all of the no code cases involve a failure to diagnose it or to correctly carry out the CPR technique.

The most recent treatment issue is the withdrawal of feeding devices. The *Jobes* and companion decisions decided together in 1987 went beyond the *Brophy* decision decided by the Massachusetts high court in 1986. In that they set out the procedure for withdrawing the feeding tube in hospitals, nursing homes, and homes. The Jobes family was represented by the same attorney who represented the Quinlan family 10 years previously. A review of *Conroy, Brophy,* and *Jobes* indicates that the court analyzed this latest treatment problem with deliberation and care. All the courts were quick to say that feeding devices are to be viewed as life-support systems not unlike ventilators. Initially, because feeding devices were so firmly associated with life itself the courts went to great length in dispelling this concept. In addition, the courts were careful to spell out the patient protection measures for individuals in both acute and nonacute facilities.

In a January 1985 Gallup Poll of over 1500 adults in 300 U.S. communities, 81 percent favored the removal of all life-support measures, including food and fluids, from both competent and incompetent terminally ill patients if that is what they wanted or would want. The poll was taken in the immediate wake of the New Jersey Supreme Court case involving withdrawal of a feeding device.[97]

Treatment issues involving minors have been litigated for many years. The issues include situations in which a minor may request surgery, but the parent will not consent to it or where the parent(s) outright refuse surgery. As a general rule of law the courts will not find in favor of the minor, against the parents' wishes, unless the surgery is lifesaving in nature. For example, the courts will not find in favor of the minor in a case involving elective plastic repair for cosmetic reasons. In cases in which the physician believes that surgery or a particular form of treatment is essential to life and the parents disagree with the treatment modality, the courts are likely to rule on the side of providing the treatment. There is also a growing body of law dealing with organ donation requests by minors and the courts have been split on these decisions.

REFERENCES AND NOTES

1. In re Brook's Estate, 205 N.E. 2nd 435 (IL, 1965).
2. John F. Kennedy Memorial Hospital v. Heston, 279 A. 2nd 670 (NJ, 1971).
3. Application of the President and Directors of Georgetown College, 331 F. 2nd 1000 (1964).
4. In re Caine, Juvenile Court, Boston Division, C.A. No. 83164-N (MA, 1983).
5. In the Matter of Osborne, 294 A. 2nd 372 (Washington, DC, 1972). For cases where the court petition was brought after receipt of blood to prevent its reoccurrence see: Wons v. Public Health Trust of Dade County, 500 S. 2nd 679 (FL, 1987), where a court decided that a 38-year-old mother of two teenage children who was a Jehovah's Witness should receive a transfusion because she had lost over 90 percent of her available blood cells. At that hearing her husband and brother testified that they would care for the children if she died. After she recovered she appealed the decision saying she might be in a similar situation and did not want any blood. The appeals court upheld her right to refuse when it found no evidence of abandonment of her minor children would occur where her husband and family agreed to care for them. See also, In re Brown, 478 S. 2nd 1033 (MS, 1985), where after blood was given against the wishes of a woman who was shot she appealed because she would face further surgery and transfusions. Because she was a potential witness in the criminal case as a result of the shooting the district attorney had obtained a court order to transfuse her. The appeals court held the woman's right to the free exercise of her religious beliefs and her right to privacy outweighed the state's interest.
6. Prince v. Massachusetts, 64 S. Ct. 438 (1944).
7. Wallace v. Labrenz, 104 N.E. 2nd 769 (IL, 1952).
8. Raleigh Fitkin-Paul Morgan Memorial Hospital v. Anderson, 201 A. 2nd 537 (NJ, 1964); The U.S. Supreme Court refused to review the decision in 84 S. Ct. 1894 (1964). See also, In the Matter of the Application of Jamaica Hospital, 491 N.Y.S. 2nd 989 (NY, 1985) where the court ordered a transfusion for a Jehovah's Witness who was 18-weeks pregnant and in danger of dying because of bleeding from esophageal varices. A physician testified that the fetus was in mortal danger. The court appointed the physician as special guardian of the unborn child and ordered him to do all that in his medical judgment was necessary to save the fetus' life, including administering a blood transfusion.
9. Randolph v. City of New York, 501 N.Y.S. 2nd 837 (NY, 1986).
10. Shorter v. Drury, 695 P. 2nd 116 (WA, 1985).
11. Cantwell v. Connecticut, 60 S. Ct. 900 (1940).
12. Jefferson v. Griffin Spalding County Hospital (In the Interest of John or Mary Doe, a Thirty-Nine-Week-Old Unborn Child), 274 S.E. 2nd 457 (GA, 1981). See also, Brigham & Women's Hospital v. Britto, Massachusetts, Suffolk Superior Court (Boston), Civil Action No. 84532 (July 1986), where the hospital using the court's Emergency Judicial Response System petitioned the court in the middle of the night for a ruling with respect to a 32-week-old fetus' rights where the mother refused treatment and tests in the presence of 20–50 percent placenta abruptio condition. The condition had been confirmed by ultrasound the evening before. The hospital's chief resident in obstetrics testified that if the placenta abruptio remained untreated and worsened, which it could at any time, the fetus would die and the mother would risk going into cardiovascular collapse. The side effects of the proposed treatment were minimal, short term, and not a significant danger to the mother's health. The mother who was single wanted to leave the hospital. The court authorized the hospital to compel the patient to receive the medically necessary treatment. It held that the states' compelling interest in preserving the viability of the fetus justified the interference with the woman's constitution right of privacy. See also, Rhoden, N. (1986). The judge in the delivery room: The emergence of court-ordered cesareans. *California Law Review, 74,* 1951.

13. Anon. Judge orders caesarian. *Lawrence Eagle Tribune* (Lawrence, MA). Feb. 5, 1982, p. 2.
14. Taft v. Taft, 446 N.E. 2nd 395 (MA, 1983).
15. Anon. (Jan. 2, 1987). Courts face questions on legal status of fetus (The Year In Review). *American Medical News.* p. 23.
16. Madden, R., Comatose woman's fetus is focus of dispute. *New York Times.* March 8, 1987, p. 39. Author has no further information of the disposition of this case, and cites it as indicative of an emerging legal issue in defining the extent of fetal rights.
17. The risks of injury associated with the technique include fractured ribs, injury to the oral pharyngeal structures, cardiac contusions, pneumothorax, and rupture of the liver. See Nagel, E., et al. (1981). Complication of CPR. *Critical Care Medicine, 9,* 424.
18. American Heart Association and National Academy of Sciences–National Research Council. (1974). Standards for cardiopulmonary resuscitation (CPR) and emergency cardiac care (ECC). *Journal of the American Medical Association, 227*(7) 883–886, See also Anon. (1980). *Journal of the American Medical Association, 244*(5), 453–509. Anon. (1986). *Journal of the American Medical Association, 255*(21), 2841–3044.
19. Rabkin, M., Gillerman, G., & Rice, N. (Aug. 12, 1976). Orders not to resuscitate. *New England Journal of Medicine, 295*(7), 364.
20. A number of these suits have arisen in an operating room or recovery room setting. See for example, Czubinsky v. Doctors Hospital, 188 *California Reporter, 685* (CA, 1983).
21. Hoyt v. St. Mary's Rehabilitation Center (District Ct., Hennepin Co., MN, no. 774555, January 2, 1981); State of Minnesota v. Jane Douglass Hoyt, 304 N.W. 2nd 884 (MN, 1981).
22. Margolick, D. Hospital is investigated on life-support policy. *New York Times,* June 20, 1982, p. 34.
23. Anon. Life, death and accountability. *New York Times,* March 25, 1984, p. E6. The New York state special grand jury did not issue any indictments, but criticized the system the hospital employed for communicating DNR orders to the staff. See also Sullivan, R., Law on emergency life-saving care is proposed. *New York Times,* April 20, 1986, p. 38.
24. Sullivan, R. Medical unit issues standards on resuscitation of the dying. *New York Times,* September 19, 1982, p. 1.
25. Matter of Shirley Dinnerstein, 380 N.E. 2nd 134 (MA, 1978).
26. Custody of a Minor, 434 N.E. 2nd 601 (MA, 1982). See also In the Matter of the Welfare of Steinhaus (Minn. Cty., Juvenile Division, Redwood, CO, Sept. 11, 1986).
27. See Lowry v. Henry May Newhall Memorial Hospital, 229 *California Reporter, 620* (CA, 1986).
28. Op. cit., Rabkin, M., Gillerman, G., & Rice, N.
29. Lesparre, M. (1983). VA hospitals adopt right-to-die policy. *Hospital Medical Staff, 12*(11), 12.
30. Bedell, S. (Sept. 8, 1983). Survival after cardiopulmonary resuscitation in the hospital. *New England Journal of Medicine, 309*(10), 569.
31. Wagner, A. (Apr. 26, 1984). Cardiopulmonary resuscitation in the aged. *New England Journal of Medicine, 310*(17), 1129.
32. Bedell, S. (Apr. 26, 1984). Choices about cardiopulmonary resuscitation in the hospital. *New England Journal of Medicine, 310*(17), 1089.
33. President's Commission for the Study of Ethical Problems in Medicine and Biomedical and Behavioral Research. (Mar. 1983). *Deciding to forego life-sustaining treatment (A report on the ethical, medical, and legal issues in treatment decisions).* Washington, D.C.: U.S. Government Printing Office.
34. Anon. Hospitals must define policies on resuscitation, *New York Times,* June 7, 1987, p. 30E.
35. For selected readings, see Steinbock, B. (Oct. 1983). The removal of Mr. Herbert's

feeding tube. *Hastings Center Report, 13*(5), 13. Also see Lynn, J., & Childress, J. (Oct. 1983). Must patients always be given food and water? *Hastings Center Report, 13*(5), 17; Callahan, D. (Oct. 1983). On feeding the dying. *Hastings Center Report, 13*(5), 22; and Annas, G. (Dec. 1983). Nonfeeding: Lawful killing in CA, Homicide in NJ. *Hastings Center Report, 13*(6), 19.

36. Barber v. Superior Court of the State of California for the County of Los Angeles, 195 *California Reporter* 484 (October 12, 1983).

37. Anon. (Oct. 1985). The latest word column. *Hastings Center Report, 15*(5), 51.

38. Kirsch, J. (Nov. 1982). A death at Kaiser Hospital. *California Magazine, 5,* 79.

39. In the Matter of Colyer, 660 P. 2nd 738 (WA, 1983). The dissenting judges based their dissent on the critical issue of the bounds of reasonable medical certainty or probabilities and whether the woman would have recovered brain functions. They relied on medical testimony in cases in other jurisdictions which placed a 4- to 6-month comatose period as a prognosis criteria for recovery to a cognitive state.

40. Micetich, K., Steinecker, P. & Thomasma, D. (May 1983). Are intravenous fluids morally required for a dying patient? *Archives of Internal Medicine, 143,* 975; Curren, W. (Oct. 10, 1985). Defining appropriate medical care: Providing nutrients and hydration for the dying. *New England Journal of Medicine, 313*(15), 940.

41. For a stimulating discussion about the problems with the use of the terms, "ordinary" and "extraordinary," see Green, W. (Dec. 1984). Setting boundaries for artificial feeding. *Hastings Center Report, 14*(6), 8.

42. Margolick, D. Judge says ailing man, 85, may fast to death. *New York Times,* Feb. 3, 1984, p. 1.

43. In the Matter of Conroy, 486 A. 2nd 1209 (NJ, 1985).

44. Anon. (Oct. 1985). The Latest Word column: Another case of withholding nutrition. *Hastings Center Report, 15*(5), 51.

45. In the Matter of Hier, 464 N.E. 2nd 959 (MA, 1984).

46. In re Visbeck, 510 A. 2nd 125 (NJ, 1986).

47. In re Clark, 510 A. 2nd 136 (NJ, 1986).

48. Brophy v. New England Sinai Hospital, 497 N.E. 2nd 626 (MA, 1986).

49. Anon. (March 15, 1986). Opinion of the American Medical Association Council on Ethical and Judicial Affairs, Withholding or Withdrawing Life-Prolonging Medical Treatment. See also, Anon. (July 25, 1986). Letters to the editor: Withholding or withdrawing treatment. *Journal of American Medical Association, 256*(4), 469–471.

50. Anon. (July 17, 1985). Massachusetts Medical Society resolution recognizing the autonomy rights of terminally ill and/or vegetative individuals. See also Mancusi, P. Medical group backs right-to-die policy. *Boston Globe,* July 18, 1985, p. 23.

51. President's Commission for the Study of Ethical Problems in Medicine and Biomedical and Behavioral Research. (1983). Deciding to Forego Life-Sustaining Treatment—A report on the ethical, medical, and legal issues in treatment decisions, at p. 83; and Brophy v. New England Sinai Hospital, 497 N.E. 2nd 626, at 637. See also Green, W. (Dec. 1984). Setting boundaries for artificial feeding. *Hastings Center Report, 14*(6), 8, citing concern of members attending a conference in Philadelphia March 23–24, 1984, sponsored by The Society for Health and Human Values that a "clear-cut distinction between ordinary and extraordinary treatment is neither possible nor necessary," footnote 1.

52. Bouvia v. Superior Court (Glenchur), 225 *California Reporter, 297* (CA, 1986).

53. Chambers, M. After winning right to starve a new fight, *New York Times,* April 20, 1986, p. 26, where a judge ordered continuation of Bouvia's morphine drip. See also, Anon. Quadriplegic loses plea to retain morphine. *New York Times,* April 23, 1986, p. A10.

54. In the Matter of Nancy Ellen Jobes, 529 A. 2nd 434 (NJ, 1987). Mrs. Jobes husband and her parents settled their malpractice action for her injuries for $900,000. Although Mrs. Jobes was in a nursing home she did not fall within the ombudsman procedures set out in *Conroy* because Jobes was only 31 years old. The court also noted that since

Quinlan about 85 percent of New Jersey's acute-care hospitals have established prognosis committees that check the attending doctor's prognosis when decisions for the withdrawal of life-support systems or treatment of a vegetative patient is being considered. In a footnote the court suggested that nursing homes should consider affiliating with such committees of nearby hospitals, or as suggested in the *Peter* case, decided that same day, the Department of Health might consider the feasibility of developing regional prognosis committees for nursing homes. Mrs. Jobes was transferred to Morristown Memorial and her j-tube was removed. She died August 7, 1987. In the Matter of Hilda M. Peter, 529 A. 2nd 419 (NJ, 1987). A 65-year-old-nursing home patient, in a persistent vegetative state and not expected to die in the near future and fed by a nasogastric tube, had left clear and convincing evidence (a power of attorney which authorized her friend with whom she lived for 2 years before her stroke to make all decisions) with respect to her health if she became incompetent. Her friend, Mr. Johanning, was appointed her guardian and asked the court to remove the feeding tube after the ombudsman decided her life expectancy would permit her to survive many years. The life expectancy test was articulated in *Conroy*. The Supreme Court held that the choice of an elderly nursing home patient in a condition similar to Mrs. Peter who has left reliable evidence of her medical preference to withhold medical treatment must be respected regardless of his or her life-expectancy. The ultimate decision is not for the court, but that of the patient, competent or incompetent, and the patient's family or guardian and physician. The court said it would have been better if Mrs. Peter had specifically provided Mr. Johanning, in her power of attorney, the authorty to terminate life-sustaining treatment. Judicial review of such authority is unnecessary unless a conflict arises among the surrogate decision maker, the family, the physician, and the ombudsman. See also Anon. When sophisticated medicine does more harm than good. *New York Times*, March 30, 1986, p. 8E for a brief discussion of the role of the New Jersey ombudsman in the *Peter* case.

55. Workmen's Circle Home v. Fink, 514 N.Y.S. 2nd 893 (NY, 1987).
56. Corbett v. D'Alessandro, 487 S. 2nd 368 (FL, 1986).
57. Florida Statutes Annotated, § 765.03 (1984). In the wake of the *Corbett* case legislation was introduced to amend § 765.03 of the Life-Prolonging Procedure Act to redefine the term "life-prolonging procedure" by inserting: "The provision of sustenance through artificial means, including intravenous feeding and tube feeding shall be considered a 'life-prolonging procedure' that may be withdrawn or withheld when such provision would serve only to prolong the process of dying." Oral feeding would not be considered a "life-prolonging" procedure. Florida House of Representatives, House Bill 670 (1986).
58. In re Requena, 517 A. 2nd 869 (NJ, 1986).
59. Rasmussen v. Fleming, Arizona Court of Appeals, no. 2 CA-Civ. 5622, slip opinion (1986). This case and the Bouvia case were the earliest cases to take notice of the AMA opinion statement, issued March 15, 1986, withholding or withdrawing life prolonging medical treatment (see Appendix H).
60. Delio on Behalf of Delio v. Westchester County, 510 N.Y.S. 2nd 415 (NY, 1986).
61. Verhovek, S. "Right to die" inquiries rise after rulings. *New York Times*, June 26, 1987, p. B1.; Feron, J. Comatose man's family seeks removal of his feeding tube. *New York Times*, April 19, 1987, p. 35.
62. In re Caulk, 480 A. 2nd 93 (NH, 1984).
63. New Jersey Statutes Annotated § 52:9Y-2 (November 12, 1985).
64. Severo, R. Cuomo appoints 23 to study issues in medical technology. *New York Times*, December 23, 1984, p. 22. See also Sullivan, R. Cuomo asks panel for brain death proposal. *New York Times*, March 17, 1985, p. 44.
65. Wanzer, S., Adelstein, S., Cranford, R., Federman, D., & Hook, E. (Apr. 12, 1984). The physician's responsibility toward hopelessly ill patients. *New England Journal of Medicine 310*(15), 955. In response to letters responding to the article, the authors stated that "identification of the hopelessly ill patient does not relegate that patient to less

rigorous standards for decision making." See Correspondence (Aug. 2, 1984). *New England Journal of Medicine, 311*(5), 335. See also Neu, S., & Kjellstrand, C. (Jan. 2, 1986). Stopping long-term dialysis: An empirical study of withdrawal of life-supporting treatment. *New England Journal of Medicine 312*(1), 14.

66. Op. cit., In the Matter of Jobes, p. 26, footnote 11.

67. President's Commission. (1983). Deciding to forego life-sustaining treatment, p. 90.

68. Anon. Faith healers could face seven year prison term. *Lawrence Eagle-Tribune* (Lawrence, MA), March 17, 1983, p. 3.

69. Cox, J. Study due on role of nurse. *Denver Post*, September 23, 1982, p. 5B.

70. Anon. Three are accused of failing to get aid for a baby. *New York Times*, June 24, 1984, p. 16. For an interesting medical discussion regarding faith healing and Christian Science, see a series of articles in the December 29, 1983, issue of *New England Journal of Medicine, 309*(26): Relman, A. Christian science and the care of children (p. 1639); Swan, R. Faith healing, Christian Science, and the medical care of children (p. 1639); Talbot, N. The position of the Christian church (p. 1641).

71. Anon. Parents ask court to stop treatment. *Boston Globe*, September 29, 1983, p. 14.

72. Custody of a Minor, 379 N.E. 2nd 1053 (MA, 1978). By statute, the parents had the right to have a judicial hearing on the care and protection order every 6 months.

73. Custody of a Minor, 393 N.E. 2nd 836 (MA, 1979).

74. Anon. Girl with leukemia returned to parents. *Boston Globe*, August 28, 1977, p. 20.

75. Anon. Parents take girl to Germany for leukemia therapy. *Boston Globe*, February 18, 1979, p. 53.

76. Anon. Father feared U.S. hospital care. *Boston Globe*, July 19, 1981, p. 39.

77. Matter of Hofbauer, 393 N.E. 2nd 1009 (NY, 1979).

78. Strunk v. Strunk, 445 S.W. 2nd 125 (KY, 1969). See also Matter of Doe, 481 N.Y.S. 2nd 932 (NY, 1984). This case concerned a bone marrow transplant from a retarded brother to his sibling.

79. Little v. Little, 576 S.W. 2nd 493 (TX, 1979).

80. Hart v. Brown, 289 A. 2nd 386 (CT, 1972).

81. In re Richardson, 284 S. 2nd 185 (LA, 1973).

82. In re Guardianship of Richard Pescinski, 226 N.W. 2nd 180 (WI, 1975).

83. Masden v. Harrison, Equity Court, no. 68651 (MA, 1957).

84. Stump v. Sparkman 435 U.S. 349 (1978).

85. A. L. v. G. R. H., 325 N.E. 2nd 501 (IN, 1975).

86. In the Matter of Sallmaier, 387 N.Y.S. 2nd 989 (NY, 1976).

87. Application of A.D., 394 N.Y.S. 2nd 139 (NY, 1977).

88. Guardianship of Tulley, 146 *California Reporter, 266* (CA, 1978).

89. Bernstein, A. (1983). Sterilization of incompetents: The quest for legal authority. *Hospitals* 56(3), 13. This article cited Matter of the Guardianship of Eberhardy, 294 N.W. 2nd 540 (WI, 1980).

90. Rosenberg, N. (1980). Sterilization of mentally retarded adolescents. *Clearinghouse Review, 14*(5), 428.

91. In re Hayes, 608 P. 2nd 635 (WA, 1980).

92. In re Penny N., 414 A. 2nd 541 (NH, 1980).

93. In the Matter of Grady, 426 A. 2nd 467 (NJ, 1981).

94. In the matter of C. D. M., 627 P. 2nd 607 (AK, 1981).

95. In the Matter of A. W., 637 P. 2nd 366 (CO, 1981).

96. Motes v. Hall County Department of Family and Children Services, 306 S.E. 2nd 260 (GA, 1983).

97. The Hastings Center has recently developed guidelines on the use of life-sustaining treatment and the care of the dying which were prepared by a committee of doctors, nurses, lawyers, and ethicists. See Postell, C. (1987). Treatment to sustain life, *Trial*, 23(12), 88.

IMPACT OF THE LAW ON NURSING PRACTICE

The law impacts on nursing in significant ways. Conceptually all the cases in this book can be viewed as a formal process whereby disputes between the parties are resolved or redressed. The chapter on the care and treatment of the mentally ill dealt almost exclusively with the establishment and recognition of rights, whereas the negligence cases dealt with financial redress. This chapter considers the wide range of disputes that confront the nurse in three areas: the employer–employee relationship, discrimination in education, and disciplinary proceedings before a licensing board.

EMPLOYMENT STATUS

The case law in the area of employee–employer relationship is fairly extensive. Generally the law will allow considerable latitude in disciplining personnel in a setting such as a health care field. It is important to distinguish employment termination rights which are protected by a collective bargaining agreement from a situation in which no such agreement or contract exists. The employment termination cases presented in this chapter deal with cases outside of a collective bargaining agreement.[1] Under the proper circumstances federal laws may apply, such as the Equal Employment Opportunities Act which forbids discrimination in hiring or termination based on age, race, color, religion, sex, or national origin. In addition to protection offered by federal legislation some state statutes forbid a dismissal based on an employee's race, sex or religion. Although the courts have traditionally upheld the right of an employer to dismiss an employee for no reason the long-recognized legal doctrine that an employer can fire an employee at will is changing. Recently a California jury ordered IBM to pay $300,000 in damages to a 12-year employee.[2] The woman who held a managerial position had been told to cease dating a sales manager from a competing firm or be transferred to a lesser position at IBM. The woman elected to quit and sued on grounds that her constitutional privacy rights had been invaded and that their ultimatum constituted a wrongful discharge.

The legal issues that are germane to the employer–employee relationship include unjust dismissal, violation of safety regulations in the work setting, justification for refusing to carry out orders that violate the law or are against public policy, and denial of employment benefits.

Employment That Is Terminable at Will and Unjust Dismissal

The majority of persons working in the private sector have essentially no contractual protection from unjust job dismissal. Although in recent years there has been some erosion of the rule that an employer may "terminate at will" an employee, the rule prevails in many situations. In the absence of a state law or a contractual agreement, an employer may dismiss an employee without notice and without cause. Contractual agreements exist when there is a collective bargaining relationship, but are uncommon otherwise except where the employee is in a top managerial position, such as a nursing director. Fortunately, a number of employers have established some form of internal grievance procedure which has the effect of forcing the employer to give notice and to examine the facts surrounding a complaint or discharge. Recently some legal commentators have advocated legislation that would preclude disciplinary actions and job loss except for just cause.[3] In addition to evolving case law numerous legal commentators have advocated the recognition of an employee's right to retain employment absent "just cause" for termination.[4]

The firm rule that an "employment at will" agreement could be terminated at any time for any reason or for no reason at all was applicable in a case where a long-term salesman for U.S. Steel was terminated because he called to the attention of his superiors the fact that tubes he was selling constituted a danger to users. The discharge was upheld even though the tubes were ultimately withdrawn from the market. However, some of the more recent line of cases have not upheld a discharge if it violated a strong public policy. Examples of discharges that violate the public policy principle include refusing to commit perjury, filing a worker's compensation claim, serving on a jury, refusing to engage in illegal activity, and refusal by a woman to "be nice" to her foreman.[5] These cases represent a change from the long-standing rule that no cause or "even for cause morally wrong" would justify a discharge. It is noteworthy that not all courts have recognized the "public policy" exception to employee termination.

The old rule was also upheld by a recent Georgia court when it upheld the dismissal of a suit brought by a husband and wife against a nursing home.

> Applying prior case law, the court in *Andress v. Augusta Nursing Facilities* said, "where a plaintiff's employment is terminable at will, the employer with or without cause and regardless of its motives, may discharge the employee without liability.[6] The husband was an administrator and the wife was a dietician. Both were fired by the president of the nursing home when the husband discovered that the facility conspired to cause the husband's signature to be forged on a 1977 report filed by the facility. The report was part of a scheme to obtain additional Medicaid monies from both state and federal governments which the nursing home was not entitled to receive. With respect to the discharge, the court held that in the absence of a contract and where the employment relationship is terminable at will, it was legally irrelevant that the motivation for the firing was improper. It would not award damages for the termination, however, the plaintiff's request for money damages for the forgery was allowed because the husband had been exposed to a criminal investigation with the potential for prosecution.

> In *Hinrichs v. Tranquilaire Hospital*, an Alabama court also upheld the terminable at will principle in a case that involved record changes.[7] The plaintiff had been employed by a psychiatric facility and the employment agreement was oral. She alleged that during the course of her employment she was ordered to falsify certain medical records. When she informed her supervisor that she intended to stop this practice the supervisor transferred and eventually terminated her. Arguing against the employee's position that public policy should preclude the discharge, the court said that the

employer's justification may be for "a good reason, a wrong reason, or no reason." The court said that it based its opinion on recognized Alabama case law and that the public policy concept was a vague expression which did not justify the creation of a new tort theory.

The case is particularly interesting because three of the judges wrote a strong dissenting opinion in which they said that denying the plaintiff a remedy would permit grave violations of public policy without substantial legal sanction. Their dissent reflects the change adopted by some courts. They said that the need for accuracy and integrity in medical records is critical to patient life and health decisions, and is essential to the awarding of grants from public funds. Also, in affording the employee redress for a wrong in these circumstances, it would place the employee in a far better position to withstand oppression at the hands of the employer. By providing a remedy to such a discharged employee, there is less likelihood that such improper and public policy violations would ever occur.

The Alabama court made a distinction between a *right to employment* and the right of an employee not to be obliged to the employer in ways bearing no legitimate connection to the employment. No right to employment exists. The dissenting judges held that termination of an agreement at will was wrongful and tortious in nature when both the motivation and practical effect is contrary to public policy. Responding to the facility's claim that the "against public policy" theory is too nebulous, the dissenting judges said they would limit such claims to those acts cognizable as a crime or to conduct so morally reprehensible as to be commonly recognized as offensive to the public good.

A New Jersey court in *O'Sullivan v. Mallon* applied the public policy concept in ruling that the discharge of an x-ray technician who was an at-will employee was not justified.[8] The technician had been ordered to catheterize a patient although she informed her superiors that she had never been taught the skill and additionally, that such an activity would violate the state nurse practice act. When she was fired she brought suit and the court held that the termination was not permissible because the grounds for the dismissal were for an illegal act and public policy mandates against such acts.

Where a nurse's evidence is strong the courts will find in favor of the nurse if the discharge is against public policy.[9] In December 1980, an occupational safety nurse who worked at the Cooper River plant of E. I. du Pont de Nemours in South Carolina informed company officials that she believed complaints from employees about skin rashes and eye irritation were attributable to chemicals to which the employees were exposed. In accordance with policy the nurse reported her findings and informed the facility's medical director. She documented the complaints in the plant's employee medical records. In May 1981 the nurse was fired. She alleged that her firing was done in an outrageous manner and was "publicly offensive." In her suit she sought money damages for intentional infliction for emotional distress. To recover on that claim she had to prove that the manner of firing was outrageous and shocking to the senses. In 1984 a federal jury awarded the nurse $1 million. That verdict was set aside and a federal judge categorized the firing as an "ordinary industrial firing" which was not extreme or abusive. A federal appeals court in *Meierer v. E. I. du Pont de Nemours and Company* granted a new trial and a second jury also found in favor of the nurse. The defendants set a further appeal in motion, but in May 1987 the nurse settled out of court for an undisclosed amount.[10]

Discharge for Cause

In a suit for unfair labor practice against a nursing home a court held that the firing of a licensed practical nurse was legitimate and was not a pretext for the nurse's past union activities.[11]

The nurse in *Edgewood Nursing Center v. N.L.R.B.* made a medication error in 1973 and followed then-existing hospital policy in reporting the incident. The patient was not harmed by the mistake and the nurse was spoken to regarding the incident. Three months later a patient died as the result of a medication error by another nurse. That nurse resigned after she was given the option of being discharged or resigning. Shortly thereafter the facility instituted a new policy which stipulated the manner of investigating future errors and included a warning that serious medication errors would result in discharge and a second medication error would result in immediate discharge. There was some testimony at the nurse's hearing as to whether the nurses had been informed of the policy, however, the administrator testified that the new policy went into effect within 6 months of the patient's death and that the staff was aware of the new policy.

Two and a half years after the new policy went into effect the nurse in question committed her second medication error. She administered a double dose of a bedtime sedative in addition to the correct dose of a tranquilizing drug. In fact, the higher dose had been ordered for a patient on another floor. The patient suffered no ill effects and the nurse reported the error immediately. When she informed the physician of the error she failed to indicate that the patient also had received the ordered tranquilizer. The physician testified that he was not aware that his patient had received the incorrect double-dose in addition to the "correct" ordered dose. The physician told the nurse not to worry about the overdose as he did not believe it would harm the patient. The next morning when the incident was being investigated the total picture came to light and one of the physicians attending the patient recommended that the nurse be fired because he considered the combination of the drugs to be potentially dangerous. The nursing director also recommended discharge. After an investigation and a review of the recommendations, the administrator discharged the nurse. She was not given a hearing or the alternative of resigning.

Although the initial National Labor Relations Board (NLRB) hearing determined that the nurse was discharged because of her prior union activity, the federal court held that the facility's concern was for the health and welfare of its patients and that the evidence did not support the nurse's contention that the firing was in retaliation for her union activities.[12]

Due Process Rights on Termination

A Florida case, *Nelson v. Mustian*, considered the extent substantive and procedural due process rights applied when a nurse manager alleged that the hospital dress code was arbitrary and capricious.[13] The nurse, a "valued" employee who had consistently received superior evaluations, stated that she would not comply with a pending policy which limited the number of rings a nurse may wear on duty to three. The policy, which was developed with input from all interested parties, was subsequently passed. The nurse, who was a supervisor, continued to exceed the ring limit even though on several occasions she was told she would be sent home if she continued to ignore the rule. Ultimately she was sent off duty and the next day the assistant director of nursing completed a "notice of corrective action" form indicating that the suspension, without pay, was for failure to adhere to the dress code, insubordination, and failure to support administrative decisions. Various hospital administrators tried to get the supervisor to comply with the policy, but she refused and stated that she would resign. However, she sought and was allowed to proceed with the facility's four-level grievance procedure. The stated objective of the grievance procedure was to effect a resolution at the lowest management level.

The grievance committee, which was the last level of the grievance process, recommended that she be reinstated with the proviso that she comply with the code and forfeit the pay lost during the 5-week suspension. The grievance hearing dealt exclusively with the issue of suspension without pay. The defendant, who was the chief executive officer, wrote to the nurse inquiring about her return date. In correspondance, the supervisor failed to indicate whether she would return to work, but repeatedly requested a hearing on the issue of the ring policy. Ultimately the defendant wrote to her, stating that since the grievance committee recommendations were not acceptable to her she would be terminated. Plaintiff appealed her termination to the hospital board which upheld the grievance committee recommendations.

The nurse then initiated suit alleging that she was denied *procedural* due process (right to a hearing on the policy itself) and denial of *substantive* due process rights because such a rule was arbitrary and capricious. The court held that the nurse had abandoned her position at the facility. Her initial suspension, based on her refusal to comply with policy, was conditional and she could have returned to work by simply removing the excessive rings. The court also said that her managerial position required that she obey, as well as enforce the rule. The court viewed her resistence to the policy as an "ideological struggle" and held that her asserted right to wear the rings did not raise to the level of a fundamental freedom, thus the hospital need only show that the rule was rationally related to a permissible objective. In order to establish that the rule offended the tenets of substantive due process, the nurse had the burden to show that the ring restriction was wholly arbitrary.

Addressing the procedural due process issue, the court held that the nurse had a property interest in her employment sufficient to permit her to invoke procedural due process protections. The handbook stipulated that an employee who had worked at the facility for less than 6 months could be dismissed without notice, but a permanent employee may be dismissed only for cause. Finding that procedural due process protections were owed, the court went on to say that the plaintiff had been afforded more due process than her situation required.

Hazardous Working Conditions

Although a majority of nurses work in a hospital setting they may be unaware of the increased risk to their own health and safety. This is so even in spite of the fact that they take appropriate measures to protect their patients from environmental harm.

> In a suit against a large New York teaching hospital the court found that the common practice of requiring nurses to immobilize patients while X-ray films were taken violated an existing city health code.[14] The city code provided that "fertile women and individuals under 18 years of age shall not hold patients under any conditions." Although other hospital employees fell within the category of occupationally exposed, nurses were not included in the category. Thus, radiologists, radiology technicians, anesthesiologists, and others who used radioactive materials in diagnosing and treating fell within the broad group considered to be occupationally exposed.
>
> While the suit dealt with nurses working in a pediatric intensive care unit, it also has implication for nurses working in emergency rooms, adult intensive care units, or any area when it is expected that a nurse will help immobilize the patient or position a limb during the actual x-ray examination. The violation was first picked up by an inspector during a site visit and the facility was cited and fined when the violation was found during a subsequent visit. The hospital challenged the regulation in court. The hospital argued that it needed the expertise of the pediatric nurses because of the complex life support equipment attached to the infants. Ninety-nine percent of the pediatric nurses were female. The hospital failed to show why male orderlies or physicians could not be used to restrain the infants. In upholding the legitimacy of the code the court said it was designed to protect future generations from deformities due to the effect of ionizing radiation. The issue of low-level exposure to radiation is particularly troublesome for nurses because of their unmonitored exposure to it.
>
> The case illustrates the need for nurses to be aware of city or state regulations that may apply to their work situations. In the absence of such regulatory protection it is incumbent on nurses working in potentially harm-producing situations to initiate steps to reduce or eliminate the hazard.

Civil Service and Nurses

Nurses who work for governmental agencies, such as the state or municipal government, are protected by civil service laws. Individuals who work for the federal government are protected by the federal civil service laws. It is a well-established rule that in the absence of contractual agreements or unlawful reasons, such as discrimination, private sector employees are terminable at the will of their employers. The civil service system came into existence to promote job tenure. However, the objective of the laws was to confer a benefit on the governmental agency and not to provide a benefit to public employees. The impetus for the laws was to create a stable pool of public employees who would, if their job was protected, provide continuous meritorious service to the government agency. Prior to civil service in most states there was a high rate of turnover and the government lost both time and money in training new employees.[15] One element of the civil service system was the protection of public employees from termination except for "just cause." A private facility such as a hospital may provide as much substantive and procedural due process rights as a governmental agency, but it is not required to do so.

In *State Employees Association v. Department of Mental Health* a Michigan nurse sought and was granted a preliminary injunction enjoining a state agency from dismissing her from her job.[16] A court-ordered injunction is a legal device to stop a party from doing a particular act. For example, a person can be enjoined from selling their house if there is a lien or legal claim against the property owner. The nurse was in charge of a unit in a state institution and a 17-year-old patient drowned in a bathtub after suffering an epileptic seizure. After an investigation, the plaintiff, the head nurse of the children's unit, who was not on duty at the time of the drowning, and the child care worker who had taken the child to the bath and shower room were dismissed for patient neglect. The three were fired the same day the investigator's report was submitted. Each filed grievances and within days filed suit for an injunction to prevent their dismissals until completion of the grievance procedure.

In order to successfully argue an injunction the plaintiff must prove to the court that she will suffer "irreparable harm" if it is not granted. Examples of irreparable harm include loss of insurance benefits, in the presence of a showing that there is serious immediate or ongoing need for medical treatment, or foreclosure of a mortgage. Although, the plaintiff was the sole support of herself and her son she failed to present sufficient evidence to the court that she would be irreparably harmed by the dismissal. The nurse failed to present any evidence that she would be unable to meet other financial obligations, could not obtain other nursing employment, or be eligible for unemployment benefits.

When the court granted the nurse her petition and enjoined the hospital "until further order of the court" from dismissing her, the defendant hospital appealed the court's decision. While the case was waiting to be heard on appeal the hospital changed the dismissal to a 6-month suspension. At the fourth level of the grievance procedure the dismissal was reversed and she was ordered reinstated with full back pay and benefits by the committee. However, the dismissal was not reversed until almost a year after the child's drowning.

The state high court held that while there is no ban on the courts to grant an injunction in cases involving civil servants, the court should restrict its involvement where civil service procedures are followed and constitutional requirements are being met. The court should stop the dismissal discharge of a civil servant only in extraordinary circumstances. For to do otherwise would undermine the civil service procedures in discharge cases. The role of the courts in such cases should be reserved for providing review or last resort measures where there is an allegation that the civil service procedures were not complied with.

In another civil service case, *Stoker v. Tarentino*, the highest court in New York held that where insufficient evidence was presented at a civil service hearing to support the allegation of patient neglect the nurse's employment record should be expunged of the incident.[17] The neglect charge against the nurse was for allegedly leaving a wheelchair patient by herself in the bathroom. The plaintiff had assisted another nurse in moving the patient from the bed to a wheelchair and then to the bathroom. There was evidence that the plaintiff left the bathroom for about 1 minute and the nurse admitted that she did not stay with the patient while she was on the commode.

The assistant director of health services testified at the hearing that in her opinion the failure to remain with the patient constituted neglect especially in view of the fact that it took two people to get her out of bed and into the wheelchair. All the nurses who testified said that there was no order, written or verbal, requiring a nurse to remain with the particular patient in the bathroom and nothing in the health department policies and procedures concerning commode procedures for wheelchair patients mandated that a nurse remain with the patient. In fact, wheelchair patients were routinely left alone in the bathroom. Whether a nurse remained with a patient in the bathroom was a matter of nursing judgment. After the hearing the disciplinary action was annulled and the nurse instituted the suit to have her employment records cleared.

Dismissal for Asserting a Protected Right

A nurse has a right to refuse to participate in professional activities that contravene the nurse's religious beliefs. A religious belief that a non-therapeutic abortion is wrong is perhaps one of the main reasons for refusing to participate in that surgical procedure. However, the right to refuse may be contingent on the fact that such refusal will not place the patient in jeopardy. For example, where there is no other nurse to participate in the surgery and delay would increase the risk to the woman, a nurse may not refuse to assist in the necessary procedure. Of course, the hospital or clinic has a responsibility to make reasonable attempts to secure the services of another nurse when time and other factors permit.

A recent Montana case, *Swanson v. St. John's Lutheran Hospital*, held that the hospital wrongfully dismissed a nurse-anesthetist who had refused to participate in a sterilization procedure.[18] Two state statutes were pertinent to the ruling. One statute, known as the "conscience" statute, stated that a medical person could refuse to participate in sterilization procedures "because of religious beliefs or moral convictions." State law also required the employer to furnish to a discharged employee a "full, succinct and complete reason of discharge" if the employee demanded such a letter. Many states have a similar statute requiring some type of service letter which is supposed to provide the discharged employee with a true reason for the discharge. Although the service letter set forth that she "untimely refused to perform customary and needed services" it made no reference to deficiencies in "team work" or other employment deficiencies.

Although the nurse had previously participated in sterilization procedures she informed the hospital a day in advance that she would not participate in abortion or sterilization procedures in the future. She was asked to reconsider and was discharged when she persisted in refusing. Ruling in favor of the nurse, the high court held that her past participation in such operations did not preclude her present refusal and her right to refuse under the conscience statute was not outweighed by the hospital's needs.

The lower court had determined that she was an "employee of questionable value" because the hospital alleged that she made excessive demands upon the administrator in requesting a pay raise, had caused disharmony when she abrasively handled a situation involving a unit of blood, had caused disharmony when she refused to proceed with a tonsillectomy, and had caused considerable difficulty because of excessive demands and a failure to recognize authority. In addition, she was accused of refusing to stay with recovering patients and maintaining outdated drugs.

When the high court reviewed these allegations it held that none of them should have been presented at the lower court proceeding because they had not been included in the service letter. Further, none of the allegations were supported by evidence. The nurse received favorable evaluations indicating that she performed as a team member and the blood incident resulted when she objected when the hospital laboratory sent packed cells instead of the whole blood which had been ordered by the physician. The court said that she was not to be blamed for alerting the hospital to a disregard of the physician's orders. The court also found that the refusal to proceed with the tonsillectomy was because the patient had an elevated temperature. No evidence was submitted by the hospital on any of the other allegations. Although the nurse asked to be reinstated the court held that it had no authority to reinstate her because the term of her contract was for a 1-year period and that period had lapsed. However, the court did rule that she was entitled to money damages.

A New Jersey trial court held that a hospital did not discriminate against a nurse who refused to care for patients who had undergone an abortion.[19] State law prohibited any disciplinary action against medical personnel who declared a religious objection to abortions. The nurse, who worked on a obstetric and gynecologic unit, was transferred to a medical and surgical unit. Two other nurses who worked on the unit and who also voiced their objection against abortions were allowed to remain on the unit. The hospital did not transfer the two nurses because both had longer tenure at the hospital and their presence was compatible with necessary staffing levels. Ruling in favor of the hospital, the court held that the nurse did not have an absolute right to work in the obstetric unit and thus her rights were not violated.

Summary

The employment termination cases have begun to swing in favor of the employee after a long history of favoring the employer. For many years there was an absolute "hands-off" attitude which was based upon the principle that an employer has the right to decide who will be employed in the facility. Recent decisions have looked to the public policy issue which is, in effect, a balancing test. If the employer fires an individual for reporting or refusing to do a criminal act, the courts will not leave the employee without a remedy.

Once a private employer gives the employee a right to a hearing it must be conducted fairly. There is, of course, no mandate that a private employer provide a hearing as there is in the public sector. The courts will look to the language in employment manuals to determine what the rights are when there is a dispute.

There is no absolute right to employment, thus when a nurse is moved from one area of a hospital to another, there is no guarantee she will be employed in the job she has requested.

The courts have recently begun to rule in favor of plaintiffs who allege that their discharge was in response to their reporting alleged wrongful acts of superiors. In these kinds of cases there are substantial legal hurdles to overcome, but under the proper circumstances the nurse will have the opportunity of judicial review.

DENIAL OF UNEMPLOYMENT BENEFITS

Under existing unemployment insurance laws an employee who is discharged for misconduct is disqualified from receiving benefits. This is known as discharge "for cause." It is not uncommon for a discharged employee to appeal the discharge on grounds that no misconduct existed or that the discharge was for other reasons.

In a recent Pennsylvania case, *Slayton v. Commonwealth of Pennsylvania Unemployment Compensation Review Board*, a licensed practical nurse who was denied benefits alleged that the hearing board capriciously disregarded her version of the events when it ruled against her.[20] The nurse discovered that $20 had been taken from her purse while she was working the night shift with two other hospital employees. Hostility developed between the three when her colleagues thought they or one of them was being accused of the theft. In an effort to resolve the situation the director met with them. The practical nurse refused to apologize to her co-workers as requested by the Director and voluntarily terminated her employment by leaving work. Applicable state law required that in a voluntary quit case the ex-employee has to prove eligibility for benefits by showing that the termination occurred through no fault of the employee. The nurse claimed that she was discharged for not apologizing whereas the director testified that she only requested an apology and that it was not an order.

The compensation review board held that the referee and hearing board, in the proper exercise of their discretion, found the director's version of the events more credible. The review board said that even though it may have reached a different conclusion than the hearing board, it could not set aside the decision unless the practical nurse showed that the decision was capricious. Although the director's request that an apology be made may have been unreasonable under the circumstances, there was sufficient evidence presented before the board that it was a request and not a condition for continued employment. The Compensation Review Board held that a conditional order would have resulted in a finding that the nurse was discharged through no fault of her own.

Applying statutory law, a California court in *Davis v. California Unemployment Insurance Appeals Board* held that a nurse was ineligible to collect unemployment benefits where it was shown that her discharge was for misconduct in carrying out a professional activity.[21] The California Unemployment Insurance Code provided that "An individual is disqualified for unemployment compensation benefits if the director finds . . . that he has been discharged for misconduct connected with his most recent work."[22] An earlier case had ruled that misconduct is "conduct evincing such wilful or wanton disregard of an employer's interest as is found in deliberate violations or disregard of standards of behavior which the employer has the right to expect of his employee. . . ."

Davis was an employee at a California hospital from 1960 to October 1972 and was discharged for failing to comply with hospital policy when administering prescribed narcotics for postoperative pain. The patient's surgeon had ordered 100 mg for pain and Davis administered 50 mg without seeking permission to change the order from either the surgeon or the on-call physician. The procedure for medication modification was included in a hospital procedure book and all new employees were informed of the policy during orientation. In addition, the procedure was communicated to the nursing staff in frequent floor bulletins. At a hearing Davis, stated that she did not administer the full dose because the patient exhibited drowsiness. She testified that she consulted with the charge nurse who concurred that the decreased dose would be appropriate. Testimony at the hearing supported Davis's judgment in administering the reduced dose. The patient's surgeon also testified that he had no objection to a nurse making a judgment that a patient should have less medication and that "many nurses do this. . . ." However, the legal issue was one of misconduct; not questionable judgment. More precisely, the key issue was whether Davis's action, in failing to obtain the permission of the surgeon, was a deliberate, intentional and willful violation of hospital policy.

Evidence presented at the hearing before the compensation board established that Davis had a predisposition toward not giving narcotics for pain. She testified that she did not wish to give "excessive" pain-controlling drugs and there was testimony that several patients had complained that they did not receive requested narcotics. Four months prior to her discharge she had signed a performance evaluation which specifically identified narcotic withholding as a weakness. Weighing the evidence, the higher court determined that the findings and judgment of the lower court was proper when it held that Davis's action fell within the realm of misconduct.

INTERFERENCE WITH EMPLOYMENT RIGHTS AND ADVANTAGEOUS RELATIONSHIPS

Most nurses do not have a formal contractural agreement with their employer. In a contractural agreement such things as salary and length of the contract will be spelled out, as well as other items of mutual concern to the parties. A written contract provides protection in ways in which an employment "at will" does not. If either party to the written contract breaches it, then the injured party may sue on that contract.

An employment relationship that lacks a formal written contract is an *employment at will*. Although an employment relationship may be at the will of both parties there is case law in which nurses have successfully sued either their employer or a third party for interfering with a legally recognized right. When the suit is brought against the employer it is for interference with a right to earn a living. When the suit is brought against a third party it is referred to as tortious interference with prospective advantage or advantageous relationship. With respect to a suit against a third party the nurse must present evidence sufficient to establish "malice." Malice can be established when the interference was spiteful or motivated by a desire to do harm to the nurse-employee.

In an early Massachusetts case, *Owens v. Williams*, suit was brought when a nurse was barred from a hospital with the effect of depriving her of her means of livelihood.[23] Several years prior to the events that resulted in the suit, the plaintiff, a private duty nurse, requested that the defendant's patient cease ringing her call bell as the nurse's patient was becoming annoyed at the constant ringing. The nurse informed the staff nurses that defendant's patient required attention that was not emergency in nature. The following day the defendant physician demanded that the nurse apologize to his patient which the nurse did. The nurse testified that the physician said at that time, "I will get you off the registry if it is the last thing I do."

Five years later while the nurse was working in the same hospital, another incident occurred that gave rise to the suit. One of the defendant's patients became excited when the plaintiff asked the floor nurses to remind patients that visiting hours were over. The defendant's patient was in the same semiprivate room as the plaintiff's patient. Two days later the hospital superintendent removed the nurse from her case and said that the defendant wanted to talk to her on the telephone. The nurse testified that he criticized her for making derogatory remarks about his medical skill in front of the patient and for asking the visitors to leave. The nurse alleged that the physician said: "I have told the supervisor that you are never to work in this hospital again and if you come back I won't send another patient. It is either you or me." She told him that he had no right to interfere with her.

Ruling in favor of the nurse, the court held that there was no privilege to justify the measures taken by the defendant physician. The evidence developed during the trial indicated that in 1940 the defendant admitted 540 patients of the total 3000 hospital admissions and his alleged threat, which the jury elected to believe, carried great weight with the hospital authorities.

In a more recent case, an Alabama nurse sought damages because of lost time and earnings when a hospital refused to allow her to continue to practice as a private duty nurse.[24] The nurse in *Byars v. Baptist Medical Center* had worked almost exclusively at the hospital for a number of years. While on duty in the summer of 1968 she slipped in a corridor and was permanently injured. She brought suit against the hospital, alleging that it was negligent or careless in not maintaining the hallway in a safe condition. She was awarded $20,000. Immediately after the trial she informed the nurse's registry that she was able to work at the defendant's hospital now that the trial was completed. She was informed by them that the hospital refused to allow her return.

In her complaint she alleged that the hospital "willfully, maliciously and wrongfully" interfered with her "employment, trade or calling as a registered nurse" and further, that the hospital's refusal was predicated on her injury suit. During the injury trial her physician said that she suffered a 25 percent permanent partial back injury. The hospital, at the later trial, said that it based their rejection on her permanent disability as well as her "obesity and female problems." Hospital officials stated that she would be incapable of caring for acutely ill patients. At the trial the nurse had two witnesses testify in her behalf indicating that her disability did not interfere with their nursing care needs. The hospital administrator who observed the nurse during the injury trial had informed the nursing director that it was not in the best interests of patients to have her return to nursing work. The court held that if the hospital had refused to allow her to return because of the outcome of the injury suit, then she could correctly bring a suit for wrongful interference with her right to earn a livelihood. However, if the refusal by the hospital was based on a valid assessment of the nurse's physical ability to perform her nursing duties, then she did not have a legal recourse. While noting the distinction between an employment currently in existence from an employment opportunity, the Alabama court recognized no difference, as in either case an individual is prevented from enjoying the benefits of the property right to earn a livelihood.

In reaching its decision the court cited a similar case which held that:

"One of the rights incident to many, if not all, contracts is to be protected from malicious interference. A contract between master and servant is one of these contracts, although the contract of employment be at will, and the master be free from liability in discharging the servant; yet if the discharge was wrongfully or maliciously procured by a third party, such third party is liable to the servant and the motive with which the discharge was procured may . . . determine the liability, as well as go to the amount of damages."[25]

A federal judge overruled a lower court decision and held that a former director of nursing had grounds to bring a civil rights action against a city hospital.[26] In *Rookard v. Health and Hospitals Corporation* the plaintiff claimed that the corporation violated her First Amendment right to free speech when it first demoted her and then fired her because she disclosed illegal and wasteful practices at the municipal hospital. In that case it was shown that the nurse began her employment at the hospital as its nursing director in 1980 where she supervised a staff of approximately 1000 nurses. The nurse was hired by the hospital's acting executive director who shortly thereafter asked that she sign permits authorizing unlicensed nurses from nursing employment agencies to work at the hospital. She refused believing that such permits could only be issued to nurses directly employed by the city hospital. Thereafter, the executive director ostracized her.

The nurse subsequently noted a number of irregularities in the nursing department, such as abuse of the hospital's "sign-in" procedure, the use in specialized areas of nurses who lacked proper credentials, the use of foreign nurses who failed to have proper documentation of their immigration status, and an inability to properly account for monies paid to outside nursing agencies.[27]

The director reported these irregularities to the acting executive director, but he ignored her. However, she herself took steps to eliminate the problems and improve the efficiency of the nursing service and thus earned the enmity of some nurses. She began to receive threatening calls and letters. Six months after the plaintiff began her job the acting executive director resigned and he was succeeded by a permanent director. Two months later the plaintiff told the new director she intended to inform the corporation's inspector general of the threats against her and of some of the problems she had discovered. The executive director told her that was all right and she reported the problems. She was promised an investigation by the inspector general's office. The next month the executive director informed the nursing director that he intended to relieve her as director of nursing and transfer her to the corporation's headquarters to serve as assistant to the director of nursing at the corporate office. He told her that she had been "battered enough" at the city hospital and that she would be reinstated as nursing director when matters "cooled down." The plaintiff objected to the transfer, but assumed her new position. She was to continue to work at her previous salary which exceeded that of her new nursing superior. She was assigned a windowless cloak room for an office.

Several months later the inspector general's office issued its report. It stated that the nursing registry had overcharged the city hospital by one-half million dollars between September 1977 and May 1981. The hospital had repeatedly paid the registry for full working shifts when the nurses had only worked parttime shifts. Although the plaintiff took measures to reduce the hospital's use of the registry nurses when she first took over her position the hospital increased them again during the plaintiff's 4-month leave for illness. The report also found that the acting executive director's plan to use unlicensed agency nurses was a clear violation of state rules and regulations.

Two months after the report was issued the plaintiff was informed by the vice president for corporate affairs that she would have to find a new position because of budget cuts. She offered to employ the plaintiff as an entry-level nurse. This offer was refused. Ten days later the plaintiff received notice of her discharge.

In order for the plaintiff to be successful in her suit against the city corporation she would have to show that the constitutional wrong complained of resulted from official corporate policy. In short, she had to show that the corporation had a policy of punishing "whistle-blowers" and that policy caused the plaintiff's transfer and discharge. Further she had to establish that the officials' actions in firing her could be regarded as the municipality's own actions. The court held that both the executive director and the vice president of corporate affairs who actually fired her had authority to make corporate policy. It was shown that their authority over personnel decisions was final.

In addition to proving that the corporation had a policy to punish "whistle-blowers" the plaintiff had to prove that her speech was constitutionally protected and her speaking out on the practices at the hospital was a "substantial factor" in the discharge. The court stated that the First Amendment protects a government employee from discharge for speech upon matters of public concern. However, this free speech guarantee could be outweighed by the state's interest in efficiency in providing public services. The court found that the plaintiff's speech was clearly constitutionally protected. The test to be applied is whether the employee's ability to perform her duties was impaired by speaking out. Other tests included whether the free speech disrupted working relationships requiring personal loyalty and confidence, or otherwise impeded the regular operation of the employing agency. The court found that the matters discussed by the nurse were her concern and concerned the public good.

The court further found that there had been no expressed discontent with the plaintiff's work, thus the defendants could not successfully argue that her discharge was "for cause." The court stated that in light of the plaintiff's long and distinguished career as a nursing administrator and previous successful service as director at a different city hospital her treatment can only be explained as retaliation.

DISCRIMINATION IN EMPLOYMENT RIGHTS

Most of the case law in the area of employment discrimination in nursing involves male nurses. Historically the nursing profession has been comprised mostly of women, and to a large extent that is still true.

Whereas female nurses face no practice-setting limitations, such is not the case for male nurses. There appears to be no universal agreement, even among some nurses, that men should be able to practice in any setting. A review of the testimony offered by nurses in the recent *Backus v. Baptist Medical Center* case illustrates this. It is conceivable that the nursing profession will be the only profession to place or have placed upon it limitations with regard to career choices or mobility. It should be recognized that this limitation most frequently takes the form of artificial practice barriers and in some instances, as in *Backus*, these are created by judicial rulings.

Some of the nurse employment discrimination cases have been brought under Title VII of the 1964 Civil Rights Act. Title VII makes it an unlawful employment practice for an employer to engage in certain enumerated forms of discrimination on the basis of sex. When an individual believes that employment discrimination exists a complaint is filed with the Equal Employment Opportunity Commission (EEOC) which is a federal agency.

If a state agency provides the same or similar protection as the federal agency then a complaint may be filed with that agency. Additionally, many state constitutions have an employment discrimination clause which may be invoked. Under EEOC, an employer is defined as a "person engaged in an industry affecting commerce who has 25 or more employees."

A 1972 federal case, *Sibley Memorial Hospital v. Wilson*, involved a male nurse who worked as a private duty nurse in a private hospital in the District of Columbia.[28] He alleged that on two occasions the supervisor of nurses at the hospital rejected him because he was male. The procedure at the hospital was that when a patient requested a private duty nurse the hospital nursing office telephoned the Professional Nurse's Official Registry which matched the request with the registered nurses available that day. The nurse would then obtain the patient's name, situation, and hospital room number. The registry had a payment policy to insure that no nurses were victimized by "invidious" discrimination. The policy was that when the nurse arrived at the patient's room, if the patient, for any reason, found the nurse unacceptable, the patient was obliged to pay the nurse for a full day's work.

The male nurse alleged that during the period between 1936 and 1970 every patient he attended at the defendant hospital was male, despite the fact that female nurses routinely served both male and female patients. The basis for his suit was that on two occasions in 1968 and 1969 the supervisors at the hospital rejected him because he was male and the requesting patients were female. The nursing supervisors prevented his reporting to the patient's room. He filed a complaint with the District of Columbia Council on Human Relations, as well as with the EEOC which found "reasonable cause" to believe that the defendant hospital violated Title VII. The hospital argued that no direct employment relationship was ever contemplated, since they were not an employer as to the nurse under the Civil Rights Act.

The case was sent back to the trial level to resolve material factual issues. The most important holding of the case was the court's finding that the objective of Congress in enacting Title VII was "to achieve equality of employment opportunities" and that "one of Congress' main goals was to provide equal access to the job market for both men and women." The court recognized that a labor organization, employment agency, or employer may have significant control over access to the job market. Specifically addressing the hospital's argument that it was not an "employer" as to the private duty nurse, the court held that the spirit and language of the act recognized an employer–employee relationship under the facts which were sufficient to create a nexus and come within the reach of Title VII.

A second important sex discrimination case appears to have laid the legal groundwork for the *Backus* case. In *Fesel v. Masonic Home of Delaware*, a third-year nursing student of the University of Delaware responded to a newspaper ad for a position as a nurse's aide at a residential retirement home.[29] There were 22 female and 8 male residents. He was advised by the nursing service director that the home did not employ male aides. He then had a female friend call and she was asked to fill out an application. He continued to seek employment as an aide and was subsequently hired by a Pennsylvania hospital a short time later. The nursing student also sued another nursing home that had run similar ads, but reached a money settlement agreement in lieu of trying the case.

Initially, he had to establish grounds for sex discrimination. He did so by showing that he applied, was qualified, was refused, and that the facility continued to advertise the job. Once he established a case, the burden shifted to the retirement home to articulate a legitimate, nondiscriminatory reason, or a statutory defense for rejecting him. The facility raised the bona fide occupational qualification (BFOQ) defense. This defense holds that sex is a bona fide occupational qualification for the job. The facility demonstrated that the duties of an aide include dressing residents, giving baths, changing bed pads, catheterizing, and assisting with toilet use. In order to meet the BFOQ exception the court required that, first, the facility must show that a factual basis existed for believing that women would object to intimate touching by a man, and second, by showing that the schedules of the employees could not be adjusted to avoid the privacy violation.

The first criteria was met when officials at the home submitted testimony in which other personnel offered their opinions supporting the privacy concept and when some of the patients testified that they would object to such intimate touching. Addressing the second criteria, the facility demonstrated that rescheduling could not avoid violating patient's privacy. Their evidence indicated that scheduling around the nurse would require a female nurse to either do the intimate care or to remain with the male nurse while such intimate care was being administered.

The court in dicta said, "customer preference" will not justify a job qualification based on sex, but an invasion of privacy will. Dicta is not the recognized rule or principle legal finding in the case, but rather a judge's opinion. In essence the court said that while attitudes associated with customer preference may overlap with personal privacy interests, it is only the latter that are protected by law. The employer may recognize such interests in conducting the business. The court articulated the argument that the purpose of the sex provisions of the Civil Rights Act is to eliminate discrimination in employment, but is not intended to force a change in accepted mores or personal sensitivities of society.

The recent *Backus* case has generated the most interest.[30] It contrasts with prior sex discrimination cases in that it is not limited to routine care of female patients, but involves the exclusion of a male nurse from a practice speciality. Backus became certified as a registered nurse in May 1978. In April he put in a request to work in the obstetrics and gynecologic department and was refused. He began to work in the intensive care unit (ICU) nursery after appealing to the hospital's executive director, who upheld the refusal. Nine months later he requested to work in the obstetrics department and was again refused. He filed a discrimination suit 5 months later.

The hospital had a policy in effect which stipulated that whenever a patient's genital area was examined by a person of the opposite sex, a third person must accompany the examiner to act as a chaperone. In order to justify the policy or practice the hospital was required to demonstrate that the challenged policy was reasonably necessary to the normal operation of its business or enterprise. The stated purpose of the policy was to protect the hospital against a charge of sexual abuse. Thus, any male nurse would have had to have a second nurse accompany him when he carried out cervical checks, uterine massages, and perineal pad assessments and changes.

However, the policy standing alone would not have precluded Backus from practice in an obstetric setting. The hospital had to show that scheduling accommodations could not be made. The hospital addressed the scheduling criteria by presenting two arguments. First, it argued that it subscribed to a concept of continuity of care which meant that a nurse, selected randomly, was assigned to follow a patient through the entire birth process. Thus, the need to have a nurse chaperone Backus when certain care was provided would take a female nurse away from her assigned patient. Second, if Backus were permitted to work in this area the chaperone policy would necessitate duplicative staffing which would cause unmanageable staffing rotation problems.

The hospital offered substantial evidence to show that a factual basis existed which supported their position that women would object to any male nurse. A woman who had delivered twice at the hospital testified that she would not accept a male nurse. A female physician testified that one-half of her patients would object, as would their husbands, and that she herself would object to a male nurse. A male physician testified that a majority of his patients would object and that one of his patients who was cared for by Backus had objected to his presence. In addition, a number of female nurses, including one who taught the LaMaze technique to over 2000 women, testified that patients would object. Many of these nurses also testified that they would object to a male nurse in labor and delivery.

It is necessary when invoking the BFOQ exception that the defendant demonstrate that all or most men would be ineligible to practice in a labor and delivery room setting. The defendant successfully argued that the intimate touching required by patient needs precluded all male nurses from working labor and delivery. A male nurse is precluded because of the very fact that he is male, not because of some trait equated with his maleness or lack of competence. In *Backus* the court spent considerable time dealing with the issue that Backus was an intruder by virtue of the fact that he was not selected by the woman. In that manner the distinction was made between the male nurse and the male physician who was selected.

The hospital also argued that it would lose patients to other hospitals, thus suffering an economic loss if it permitted male nurses to care for female patients. Undoubtedly none of these arguments would prevail if Backus sought a position that was limited to teaching LaMaze technique because there would be no exposure of the woman's genitals and the woman's husband or other coach would be present. The holding has been publicly criticized.[31] It should be noted that Backus did not provide multiple witnesses who would support his position or rebut the testimony of the nurses and physicians who spoke against the presence of a male nurse in the department.

In a federal case, *Buckley v. Hospital Corporation of America* a nurse brought a suit alleging age discrimination.[32] The suit was brought under the Age Discrimination in Employment Act.[33] The suit was initially dismissed, but an appeals court held that the plaintiff should be permitted to have her suit tried on its merits before a jury.

The nurse who was 62 years old at the time she resigned was hired by the defendants as a charge nurse on the night shift in 1968 and was promoted to the position of day shift supervisor in 1978. In 1978 a new administrator was appointed and at one of the early meetings he conducted with the hospital staff he expressed surprise at the longevity of personnel and stated he wished to attract younger doctors and nurses. He stated he thought the hospital needed "new blood." Subsequent to these series of meetings with the staff, the plaintiff discussed her concerns about plans to hire a former patient who had a history of drug abuse with a hospital physician. The administrator and the plaintiff's supervisor were away from the hospital at that time, but met with her later and told her she had acted improperly and that she would be terminated if she ever went outside the "chain of command" again. The nursing supervisor inquired about the plaintiff's retirement plans on several occasions after this admonishment and the plaintiff found out that other nurses had been asked to report to her nursing supervisor whether the plaintiff said anything against administration.

In September 1980 an incident occurred which prompted the nurse's resignation. The plaintiff who had been working in the emergency room went to the pharmacy to get a vial of tetanus toxoid and was given the wrong medication. She stated that she was unable to read the label immediately because of frost on the vial, but took the vial back and obtained the correct medication. The defendants said that they had two witnesses who said the plaintiff threw the vial down and shouted in a loud voice when she returned to the pharmacy. The plaintiff denied this and after the incident gave her version to the administrator. During the investigation of this incident the administrator did not interview three witnesses who later testified favorably on behalf of the plaintiff although the names of the employees were made known to him. The nurse denied that she shouted, used profane language, or threw the vial down. However, he told her she was under stress and due to her advanced age, she had lost her temper. He told her to take a week off while he considered what he would do about the situation. She testified that her nursing supervisor a short time later asked her if she thought it was time to retire and enjoy life with her family.

On her return the administrator told her she would have to step down from her position as supervisor and take a staff nursing position. Her immediate superior would be one of the nurses who told the administrator that the plaintiff shouted and used profane language during the pharmacy incident and who, in the past, had asked other employers to report anything they heard about the plaintiff's conduct. The plaintiff told the administrator she would not step down from her supervisor's job and work in the staff position. She said that it would be "demoralizing and humiliating." No other position was offered. When the plaintiff wrote to the administrator pointing out why she could not take the staff position he terminated her employment. Following her departure her duties were divided among 12 other employees, ten of whom were over 40, while only two were under 40. Subsequently, a 45-year-old assistant director of nursing was hired and she absorbed some of the plaintiff's former duties. In May 1983 the nurse under which the plaintiff would have had to work as a staff nurse became clinical coordinator, absorbing other duties in the plaintiff's old job. The court noted that the two nurses who absorbed the bulk of the plaintiff's duties were more than 15 years her junior.

Defendants contended that the plaintiff resigned from her position, however, the court held that she was "constructively" discharged. The defendants contended that the offer of another position at the same pay and benefits precluded a constructive discharge allegation. A constructive discharge exists where the employer deliberately makes an employee's working condition so intolerable that the employee is forced into an involuntary resignation. The court stated that it was a fact for a jury, as triers of fact, to determine whether a reasonable person would find the working conditions under which the plaintiff would have to work so intolerable that she would be forced to resign.

Discussing the issue of age discrimination the court applied the following evidentiary test: (1) the plaintiff must prove that she was a member of the protected group, (2) that she was discharged, (3) that she was replaced with a person outside the protected group, and (4) that she was qualified to do the job. The plaintiff could also prove her case by presenting evidence showing that the hospital had intended to discriminate against her when she was discharged. A third way of proving her case would be to establish statistical proof showing a pattern of discrimination. The court held that the plaintiff's testimony, if believed by a jury, was sufficient for a reasonable jury to conclude the defendant acted in a discriminatory manner.

Summary

In nursing, the employment rights issue is most frequently raised by male nurses when they are prevented from working on a particular unit, and in some cases, in a particular facility which has female patients. Suits are begun by filing a complaint with the EEOC, a federal agency. The Civil Rights Act is the legal basis for the discrimination suit. There is an exception to discrimination, based on the sex provision in the act, and that is that sex must be a bona fide occupational qualification for the job. There are, of course, tests that must be met before this defense is available to the employer.

DISCRIMINATION IN EDUCATION

In 1973, section 504 of the Rehabilitation Act of 1973 was enacted.[34] The regulations essential to the implementation of the Act were promulgated in June 1977. The basic principle of Section 504 is equal opportunity. The act was modeled on Title VI of the Civil Rights Act which was passed in 1964. Section 504 is aimed at discrimination on the basis of disability and section 601 of the 1964 Civil Rights Act bases discrimination on race, color, and national origin. In Section 504 Congress mandated that: "No otherwise qualified handicapped individual in the United States . . . shall, solely by reason of his handicap, be excluded from participation in, be denied the benefits of, or be subjected to discrimination under any program or activity receiving federal financial assistance."

While all school nurses were familiar with the Rehabilitation Act, it was not until *Davis v. Southeastern Community College* in the mid-1970s that nurses gained an appreciation for its impact on nursing education.[35] The regulations embodied many important concepts, but two in particular had direct application to the *Davis* case. The concept of *due process* in the evaluation of the handicapped individual requires that determinations about the abilities of that individual be made on an individual basis. The concept of *accommodation*, much akin to "affirmative action," was necessary to overcome the historical exclusion of handicapped individuals in many facets of life experiences. Such accommodations necessarily included the removal of architectural barriers, modifications in curriculums, and auxilliary assistance when feasible. The most common auxilliary assistance were readers for the blind and interpreters for the deaf. A third concept, *integration* or "mainstreaming" provides the opportunity for handicapped individuals to learn, work, and live with nonhandicapped individuals and was implicit in *Davis*.

Section 504 and its regulations apply to any private or public entity which receives financial assistance from Health and Human Services

(HHS) [formerly Department of Health, Education and Welfare (HEW)].[36] The financial assistance includes funds and federal services and may be by grant, loan or any other arrangement. Thus, every state, county, and local government program, as well as every private entity that receives financial assistance directly or indirectly from HHS falls within the Act.

The Balance Between Patient Safety and Educational Rights

The *Davis* case was the first in which the U.S. Supreme Court was called upon to interpret the language of section 504.[37] A number of "friend of the court" briefs on behalf of both sides were filed with the court. It is important to note that the case is limited to the realm of higher education and its findings would have limited effect on other levels of education.

> Francis Davis, a licensed practical nurse (LPN) sought admission to a state-funded community college in pursuit of an associate degree in nursing. At that time she had irreversible bilateral, sensorineural hearing loss and had not worked as a nurse for several years prior to applying to the college. As part of the application process she was interviewed by a faculty member and acknowledged a hearing problem when it became apparent during the interview. She was asked to consult an audiologist who advised a hearing aid to augment her lip-reading skills. Although the hearing aid permitted her to detect gross sounds she essentially was dependent on the technique of lip-reading for effective communication. Even with the hearing aid she could not discriminate among sounds sufficiently to hear normal spoken speech.

> The college then consulted with the North Carolina Board of Nursing and was advised that Davis not be admitted because such a practitioner would be unsafe. Additionally, the board held the view that she would be unable to participate in the clinical component of the educational program and that necessary program modifications would place substantial limitations on the educational process itself. When the college refused her admission Davis sought and received a review of the decision. The full faculty reviewed the situation and voted to deny her admission. Davis filed suit in a federal court alleging that her due process rights had been violated as well as her rights under Section 504.[38]

> The trial court placed great weight on the issue of patient safety. The court noted that: "In many situations such as an operation room, intensive care unit, or post-natal care unit, all doctors and nurses wear surgical masks which would make lip reading impossible. Additionally, in many situations a registered nurse would be required to instantly follow the physician's instructions concerning procurement of various types of instruments and drugs where the physician would be unable to get the nurse's attention by other than vocal means."

> Davis did not testify, nor was evidence introduced with regard to the ability, or lack of ability of other practicing hearing impaired nurses. How-

ever, at least one friend of the court brief filed at the Supreme Court level discussed examples of hearing-impaired nurses who have successfully practiced as registered nurses. The trial court did take note of the fact that her abilities and responsibilities as a registered nurse would differ from that of her role as an LPN. There was little testimony with regard to Davis's own past nursing performance.

Addressing the alleged Section 504 violation the trial court held that Davis was not an "otherwise qualified handicapped individual" as mandated by the Congressional Act. It dismissed the violation of constitutional due process claims. When Davis appealed the decision the higher court took into consideration regulations that were promulgated just prior to the appeal process and held that the college should have considered her application without regard to her impairment.[39] It should have limited its inquiry to her academic and technical qualities although it need not discount her impairment.

The regulations stated that a "qualified handicapped person" is "with respect to post-secondary and vocational education services one who meets the academic and technical standards requisite to admission or participation in the school's education program or activity. . . ." The appeals court ordered the college to reevaluate her with emphasis on her academic and technical capabilities. Second, it ordered the college to consider the accommodations that could be made to enable her to participate in the program. The court did not order the college to admit Davis, but to evaluate her on criteria not limited to her impairment. Perhaps the most significant suggestion was that the College "affirmatively" modify its program to accommodate the disabilities of applicants.

Subsequently the college appealed to the U.S. Supreme Court which in an unanimous decision upheld the original trial court ruling in their favor. The Supreme Court held that an "otherwise qualified person" is one who is able to meet all of the program's requirements in spite of his handicap. The act imposed no requirement on an educational facility to lower its standards or undertake affirmative action that would dispense with the need for effective oral communication. It held that it was unlikely that Davis would benefit from any affirmative action the college might have undertaken such as providing her with individual supervision whenever direct patient care was rendered or dispensing with some required courses. The court would not "compel" a facility to undertake such action. There was no discrimination on the part of the facility in not making the necessary major program adjustments. It found the physical admission requirements imposed by the college to be reasonable. Davis had persuasively argued that it was not necessary for the college to prepare her to undertake all of the tasks required of a registered nurse. The court noted that a registered nurse may choose to practice in industry or a physician's office where lip-reading alone may suffice. However, not withstanding different career choices basic admission criteria may operate to exclude a handicapped individual.

The court left unanswered the question of whether state licensing requirements might serve to identify "legitimate and necessary" physical standards. One final observation in light of the *Davis* opinion is that in the American Nurses' Association Suggested Legislation for Nursing Practice

Acts, the concept of issuing a "limited" license is raised.[40] The question of such a license is timely and it is not unlikely that state laws pertaining to the licensing of nurses will recognize the concept. In the absence of such a law or regulation, individual state boards, applying their discretionary authority, may issue a limited license.

Failure to Admit

In contrast to *Davis*, a young woman in Los Angeles who sought to enter a state-run collegiate nursing program was granted an injunction after the school denied her admission.[41]

In *Kling v. County of Los Angeles*, the nursing program received federal financial assistance. Mary Kling, a 25-year-old woman with a history of Crohn's disease, applied for admission in February 1979 and was admitted in April. She proceeded to be fitted for uniforms and to purchase textbooks. During this time she was examined by the school physician and subsequently was informed that she could not enroll. She was denied admission because the school contended that she would be unable to meet its requirements and would miss an excessive number of classes. The authorities assumed that because she had the disease, her health was not sufficiently sound and stable to successfully complete the program. Kling's physician testified that it was unlikely that she would miss excessive time, as she was well controlled and that even if she required hospitalization it could be scheduled to minimize interference with her course work. He said that her illness would not prevent her from completing the full program.

The court in ordering the school to admit her for the 1981 semester held that the school was not required to make the extensive modifications in its program as would have been required in the *Davis* case. Relying on the holding in *Davis*, it went on to say that Kling was an "otherwise qualified person," capable of meeting the program's requirements and that "possession of a handicap is not a permissible ground for assuming an inability to function in a particular context." Further, the court held that pending the outcome of the suit against the school the young woman should be admitted as the hardship endured by her in being denied admission far outweighed that of the school in admitting her. A considerable time had elapsed since she was denied admission (18 months) and the school had an outstanding reputation which would provide excellent training and increased career opportunities. These factors, coupled with the court's view that she demonstrated a probability of success when the trial was heard, resulted in enjoining the school from denying her admission.

Kling began a nursing program at a community college. When the federal court handed down its decision in favor of the plaintiff in 1980 the college offered to admit her but refused to accept any of the community college credits. The plaintiff declined the offer and sought money damages. In 1985 a federal appeals court held that the plaintiff was entitled to money damages.[42] The court noted that the college physician had failed to evaluate the plaintiff on an individual basis.

Rights of the Handicapped Employee

Another case dealing with discrimination in employment is presented here because of its reliance on Section 504 rather than on other employment discrimination legal principles. The case, *Trageser v. Libbie Rehabilitation Center* is complex in that it had to interpret the intent of Congress when it created amendments to Section 504 in 1978.[43]

Novella Trageser, a registered nurse, had worked at the defendant facility since 1971 and was promoted to director of nurses in 1975.[44] The facility was a private corporation which operated a nursing home which was the recipient of substantial federal monies in the form of Medicare, Medicaid, Veterans Administration, and welfare payments. The fact that Trageser was a "private" employee rather than a government employee appears to be a significant factor in the outcome of the case as the court applied the 1978 regulations which precluded a private employee redress unless it was shown that the primary purpose of the federal financial assistance was to create jobs or where the discrimination in employment necessarily causes discrimination against the primary beneficiaries of the federal aid.

Tragaser had progressive retinitis pigmentosa. In April 1976 the Virginia Department of Health conducted a site inspection. During the visit a state inspector noted that Trageser's eyesight had deteriorated since the last visit and inquired what the home intended to do about it. The administrator brought it to the attention of the board of directors at a June meeting and the board voted to dismiss her. When Trageser was informed of the board's decision she resigned. She subsequently brought suit alleging her Section 504 rights had been violated. She sought reinstatement, back pay, and an injunction against payment of federal financial assistance to the facility unless she was reinstated.

When the case was first heard the court agreed that the termination of her employment constituted a discharge and not a voluntary resignation. However, the court held that it was clear that Congress deliberately meant to limit the legal redress of an employee of a private institution who alleges employment discrimination to those situations in which the primary objective of the federal financial assistance was to provide jobs. Although Trageser's discharge occurred in 1976 and the amendments to the Rehabilitation Act were not enacted until 1978 the court applied them to her case. The case has been the subject of criticism because it so narrowly interpreted congressional intent so as to preclude relief to a private employee, but not to a government employee, who has been discriminated against in employment. The criticism is based on the argument that one of the main purposes of the 1973 Rehabilitation Act was to prevent or redress employment discrimination. However, in 1979 the U.S. Supreme Court refused to review the *Trageser* decision. An interesting aside to the case is that although the discharge was initiated by the action of a state health inspector it is not known whether the state itself would have imposed any sanction if the nursing home had continued to employ the nurse.

Summary

Section 504 of the Rehabilitation Act passed in 1973 had a great impact on education rights, including the right of a handicapped individual to obtain a nursing education. The North Carolina Davis case was the first case applicable to a nursing setting and it is to be narrowly interpreted. The *Kling* case, decided shortly after *Davis*, held that a "controlled" illness could not be used to exclude an individual from a nursing program.

Section 504 also precludes discrimination of the handicapped in the workplace. Both the school and the workplace must make reasonable accommodation to place the individual. However, a school will not be forced to significantly change its curriculum to the detriment of its program objectives and an employer may have a legitimate reason for refusing to hire a handicapped individual. The facts in the Section 504 cases are just as important as in the negligence cases. The act is a vehicle intended to "mainstream" handicapped individuals into both the work force and the educational system.

DISCIPLINARY PROCEEDINGS BEFORE A NURSING BOARD

There is considerable case law in the area of disciplinary proceedings before licensing boards. Every nurse needs to know that a license to practice nursing is a property right that is protected by the U.S. Constitution. No one may be deprived of life, liberty, or property without due process of law. Due process entails notice and an opportunity for a hearing. The law requires due process whenever a nurse's license is suspended. revoked or some other limitation is imposed upon the licensee's scope of practice. In writing about the value of a nursing license to a nurse one writer recently wrote: "The right to practice nursing is a valuable property right and is provided constitutional protection. Even when the amount of money involved is small or the reprimand or penalty minor, considerably more may be at stake for the nurse. The attorney should move with great caution in recommending that the nurse submit to censure without challenge or that the nurse (or the insurer) "pay up." The record of the nurse affects not only current work relationships, but also future employment situations since it may be used to preclude licensing in another state."[45]

As an administrative agency, boards of nursing derive their authority from enabling legislation. This authority includes approval and supervision of nursing educational programs, promulgation of rules and regulations, issuance of rulings or advisory opinions, granting licenses, reviewing petitions, and conducting hearings. Rules and regulations, while not law, have the "force of the law" whereas "rulings" and "advisory opinions" do not have the status of law or its force. Each state is responsible for defining statutory terms. The definitions are found in the statute itself or in companion rules and regulations. Administrative agencies are regarded as the "fourth" branch of the government, the first three being the judicial, legislative, and executive branches.

Disciplinary hearings are conducted according to state laws; they are less formal than a trial but afford some of the protection of a court proceeding. Most states have an "open meeting" law which assures public access, however, there are situations in which the public is excluded by having the hearing conducted in an executive session. The standard for the admissibility of evidence during the hearing are found in the state's administrative procedures law.[46] The informal nature of a board hearing can be illustrated by the holding in a recent Pennsylvania case which stated that, "Agencies shall not be bound by technical rules of evidence at agency hearings, and all relevant evidence of reasonable probative value may be received. Reasonable examination and cross-examination shall be permitted."[47]

Because one of the reasons for the existence of a licensing board is for protection of the public, a board's decision to revoke or suspend a license will generally be upheld unless the nurse can show that the board exceeded its delegated authority; the nurse was deprived of rights; the board's decision was unsupported by the evidence; or, as in the *Tuma* case, the statute or regulations failed to specifically define the behavior in question. Review of the case law involving disciplinary proceedings points toward the allowance of wide discretion in disciplinary actions taken by licensing boards.

No health care professional should go before a hearing board without the counsel of an attorney when notice has been given that the reason for the hearing is in response to a complaint by a consumer, employer, or other professional, or when an allegation of a crime or unauthorized practice is made. License revocation is the most serious action as it prohibits the nurse from practicing. A nurse may petition the board to lift the revocation after the stipulated period. Any decision by a licensing board that results in interference with the right to practice may be appealed. The appeal process differs from state to state, but some type of appeal is always available. When the stakes are high it is unwise for any health care professional to go before a regulatory agency without the benefit of legal counsel as the petitioner may be precluded from asserting an argument or right because it was not brought up at the initial proceedings. Important rights may be waived and statements made which are not in the best interest of the petitioner.

Due Process

The notice requirement of due process includes the right to know the nature of the allegations made against the practitioner. It is not uncommon for a nurse to waive protected rights or admit to wrong-doing before legal counsel has been obtained.

In *Lieb v. Board of Examiners for Nursing*, a Connecticut nurse who alleged that she was unable to defend herself because of improper notice was unsuccessful in appealing her license revocation.[48] The woman, a registered nurse, charted Demerol as having been given to a patient when in fact she took it herself. Shortly thereafter she was interviewed by drug control agents after waiving her constitutional right to remain silent and admitted the transgression. She signed a waiver and voluntarily gave her statement. During the interview she admitted to taking Demerol at another institution almost 20 years previously. She stated that at that time she was beset by severe physical problems and had been subsequently fired. A month after the interview she received a summons to appear before the licensing board to answer charges against her.

The notice of the charges indicated that the prohibited conduct included, "conduct which fails to conform to the accepted standards of the nursing profession including, but is not limited to the following: (1) fraud, (2) incompetence, (3) physical illness or loss of motor skills, (4) emotional disturbance." The notice of the charge also stated that she could be represented by legal counsel and present evidence in her behalf. She was not represented, testified on her own behalf, and introduced an affidavit from a psychiatrist. The following month the board issued its findings and revoked her license.

The nurse alleged that the board went beyond the scope of the notice in taking into account the events of 1957 and that she had not prepared a defense. The court held that her argument had no merit as she freely admitted it in testimony at the hearing, as well as in the voluntary written statement made to the agents. After her admission, the only question that remained was the sanction which would be rendered by the board. The board's review of all the evidence before it was proper. The case illustrates an attempt by an attorney, retained after the fact, to negate the impact of evidence that the nurse was not legally compelled to give.

Even when the board sanction is based on a criminal conviction the nurse must be given notice and have a hearing before it can take any action on the nurse's license.

A recent New York case, *Durante v. Board of Regents of State University*, held that the board sanction against a nurse who had been previously convicted of criminal activity was not unfair.[49] The board determined that the nurse should have his license suspended for 2 years, but ordered that he should be placed on probation for 2 years instead. The nurse appealed the probationary status.

In 1967 he was convicted under federal law for possession of marijuana, in 1969 he was convicted for smuggling marijuana into the country, and in 1975 he was convicted of criminal possession of a gun. The nurse based his appeal on the fact that in 1977, at the time of the board hearing, the laws relevant to marijuana were laxer than at the time of his conviction and there was no evidence at the trial for the possession of a weapon that it was intended for use. The appeals court held that the nurse could not relitigate the convictions in a disciplinary proceeding as his actions had already been litigated in court.

The courts have held that conviction of a federal felony is accepted grounds for revocation even when the crime was committed in another state.[50] Some states have included a provision in the nursing licensing law that a conviction of a crime in any jurisdiction directly related to the practice of nursing or to the ability to practice nursing will be grounds for revocation.[51]

Authority of the Board

There are a number of cases challenging board decisions. An interesting, but factually narrow Tennessee case held that the board of registration in nursing had no authority to revoke the license of a registered nurse for practicing as a lay midwife.[52]

> In *Leggett v. Tennessee Board of Nursing*, a nurse was licensed to practice in the state, but did not have a graduate degree nor was she certified by any national nurse-midwife organization. She testified that graduate study for nurse-midwifery was available to her. She also knew that nurse-midwifery was an "expanded" nursing function and that the board had a rule related to such practice. She had delivered over 50 babies and testimony demonstrated that she had medicated patients with pitocin which was a controlled substance not available to laypersons without prescription. She did not have jointly written protocols with a physician. An important fact in the case was that she never held herself out to the public as a nurse-midwife.
>
> Although the board admitted that a nurse licensed to practice in the state could deliver babies as a lay midwife, it sought to apply a rule promulgated by it which inherently recognized nurse-midwifery as one of the expanded roles in nursing. The board alleged that the nurse willfully violated its rule. The rule stipulated that the Nursing Practice Act did not prohibit licensed nurses from expanding their roles. It prohibited a nurse from performing professional acts for which the nurse was unprepared. It further stipulated that those whose expanded role involved the management of "medical aspects of a patient's care must have written medical protocols, jointly developed by the nurse and the sponsoring physician(s)."
>
> The court held that the nurse did not come within the scope of the rule. The legislature specifically excluded the practice of midwifery from the definition of medicine and the generic definition of professional nursing did

not include midwifery. Thus, the board could not argue that the nurse's conduct was unprofessional in the generic definition context. The board unsuccessfully argued that, even though the legislature did not choose to include lay midwifery practice within its jurisdiction, it had jurisdiction since midwifery is a "health related activity" closely akin to nursing. Disagreeing with the board's position, the court said that under state law a woman could be delivered by a nurse-midwife, a physician, or a lay-midwife. Just because she also happened to be a nurse she should not be precluded from delivering babies any more than a nurse should be precluded from occasionally working as a secretary or receptionist.

Further, the court said that, "There is no showing that performing the services of midwife independently of the profession of nursing in any way adversely affects the skill or ability of a Registered Nurse in the performance of her profession as a Registered Nurse." The court reasoned that the board had no authority to second-guess the legislature when it appears clear that it elected not to regulate the practice of lay-midwifery by statute. Specifically addressing the pitocin issue, the court held that because the nurse was not practicing under title of a nurse the board would not be the authority to discipline or sanction her for an activity unless it could show that her action would affect the quality of nursing care when she practiced as a nurse.

However, in *Leigh v. Board of Registration in Nursing* the Massachusetts Supreme Court when confronted with essentially the same facts reached a different result.[53] The board's decision to suspend a nurse's license for practicing midwifery was upheld. The plaintiff who was a registered nurse assisted in more than 600 home births. The state had no laws regulating the practice of lay midwifery, and lay midwives assisted in normal uncomplicated home births. Regulations governing the practice of nurse midwifery precluded nurses from participating in home deliveries.

The plaintiff graduated from a collegiate nursing program in 1969 and worked in obstetrics in a hospital setting. In 1977 she began to practice as a lay midwife. After 1977 she also did a little hospital private duty nursing. The nurse was aware of the regulations governing the practice of nurse midwifery which came into existence in 1980. The nurse had not completed a formal nurse midwifery program and was not certified. In September 1982 the plaintiff was assisting at a home birth which became complicated because of a prolapsed cord. She called an ambulance to transport the woman to a hospital. A disagreement arose between the nurse and paramedics about the management of the prolapse during the transport to the hospital. The procedures the nurse was recommending for the treatment of the prolapsed cord were correct.[54] This episode resulted in her receiving a "show cause" complaint from the nursing board in May 1983. The show cause complaint put the plaintiff on notice that the board of nursing intended to take action against her nursing license. The board cited the nurse for gross misconduct. Two hearings were held in the fall of 1983. Shortly thereafter the board informed the plaintiff that her license had been suspended for a period of at least 1 year. The nurse invoked her right to have the board's decision reviewed by a single justice of the state supreme court. The justice vacated the board's decision and sent the case back to the board for further consideration because the board failed to adequately state the reasons for its decision as required by the state's administrative procedure act. The board reaffirmed its decision stating that the basis for the decision was the nurse's failure to comply with the state's nursing practice act and the rules and regulations in effect since 1980, which set out the criteria for the practice of nurse midwifery in the "expanded role."[55] Nurses in Massachusetts may not perform activities in the "expanded role" unless they comply with the requirements as set out in the rules and regulations. The regulations define practice in an expanded role as,

> professional nursing activity engaged in by a registered nurse in accordance with these regulations and involving the employment of advanced skills including the evaluation, diagnosis, and treatment of patients with diseases and adverse health conditions. It also means the management of therapeutic regimens for acute and chronic problems associated with such diseases and conditions. It does not mean activity which the Board recognizes constitutes generic professional nursing and permits registered nurses to engage in the Commonwealth.[56]

The regulations require satisfactory completion of a formal educational program designed to prepare nurse midwives. The program must be acceptable to the board. In addition, the nurse midwife must have current certification by a nationally recognized accrediting body approved by the board.

The plaintiff argued that the nursing board had no jurisdiction over her because she was not practicing nursing, but rather, "professional midwifery." In addition, she argued that the regulations violated her state and federal constitutional rights, as well as the due process rights of the pregnant women. The plaintiff further argued that the statute and regulations were an illegal restraint of trade.

The court held that the laws did not violate the nurse's equal protection rights just because they failed to restrict lay midwives, but did prohibit nurse midwives from attending home births. The court found that although the legislature did not enact laws relative to lay midwifery it had a legitimate interest in requiring its preference that births attended by nurse midwives take place in licensed facilities. The legislature had a right to state its preference for hospital births where nurses are going to assist in these births. The fact that the legislature did not choose to regulate lay midwifery did not render the nurse midwifery statute unconstitutional. The legislature elected to limit nurse midwifery activities.

Another argument offered by the nurse was that the pregnant woman's due process rights were being violated by precluding noncertified nurses' attendance at home births. The court said that the statute and regulations did not require the woman to either give birth in hospitals or force them to obtain the services of physicians over lay midwives. The legislature adopted a reasonable approach by stipulating that births attended by nurses should be in the safest place, that is, hospital settings.

Finally, the court held that the statute and regulations were not an illegal restraint of trade because the restraint placed on nurses by the laws was necessary to the successful implementation of the legislative scheme to promote hospital births over home births when nurses were providing nurse midwifery services. When the activities were to further the scheme of the legislature they were exempt from antitrust (illegal trade restraint) liability.[57] The *Leggett* case was not cited in the *Leigh* decision. However, it should be noted that the *Leggett* decision was not decided by the state supreme court but rather by an intermediary court. In addition, one state is not obliged to follow or even take notice of another state's decision.

The issue in another case, *State of Florida v. McTigue,* was whether a regulatory board exceeded its delegated legislative authority in promulgating a rule applicable to lay midwifery.[58] The Florida legislature opted to regulate the practice of lay midwifery and enacted a statute requiring that the applicant show proof of having attended a stated number of deliveries under the supervision of a duly licensed physician. After passage of the statute the agency promulgated a rule that required a written statement from a Florida physician that the applicant had been supervised, and required the applicant to supply the names and addresses of the women. When the plaintiff, who had attended a 2-year physician's assistant program in New York, was denied authority to practice as a midwife he brought suit. All of his experience in lay midwifery occurred in the state of New York.

The court held that the rule constituted an unauthorized exercise of delegated authority. It held that a statement from a licensed physician from any state would meet the statutory requirement. The regulatory agency modified the statute by adding the requirement of a statement from a Florida physician. Such a requirement served to bar an individual who was formally trained, but who had no experience as a midwife in Florida. The court also struck down the requirement that an applicant supply the names and addresses of the women he had delivered in New York. Recognizing the role of the agency to protect the public, the case held that neither rule would serve that purpose.

Narcotics

The concept of rehabilitation is particularly important when the license revocation occurs because of drug dependence or alcohol abuse. Increasingly boards of nursing and medicine are receiving complaints of drug abuse and impaired practitioners. Most frequently the complaint comes to the attention of the board when an employer reports an employee or a consumer files a complaint. Colorado law requires a facility to report both known and suspected drug thefts.[59] The purpose of the Colorado statute is designed to require those who have knowledge of drug theft to report such knowledge to the authorities.

Increasingly, problems with hospital narcotics have been the subject of board disciplinary actions.

In *State of Washington v. Sheldon*, the court ordered a new trial for a nurse who was suspected of taking drugs from a hospital medicine cart.[60] In the suit for possession of a controlled substance the judge's instruction on knowledge of the drugs was ambiguous and confusing. Drugs were found in the nurse's purse persuant to a legal search by a police officer, but the nurse denied knowledge of the drugs.

However, in a recent Mississippi case, *Hogan v. Mississippi Board of Nursing*, the state supreme court held that the board could not revoke a nurse's license for the failure to account for Demerol.[61] The nurse-anesthetist was accused of misappropriating the narcotic when the board found that she did not reasonably account for missing ampules which she checked out of the pharmacy. The chief pharmacist testified that he sometimes did not check to see if individuals signing out narcotics from the pharmacy did it as per hospital policy. Further testimony showed that in the past the pharmacist had been reprimanded by the pharmacy board for this.

The nurse-anesthetist also testified that she was not informed of any specific waste procedure and that she disposed of the unused portion by dropping the syringe in an empty intravenous bottle. She also testified that there were times when she found the narcotic closet and anesthesia cart unlocked. The Supreme Court said the board could find that the nurse was unable to reasonably account for the missing narcotics, but there was no proof that she converted them to her own use. It also held that the inability to account for all the narcotic supply was the inevitable result of a "porous" hospital procedure for such accuracy and securing of the narcotics.

In *Stevens v. Blake* an Alabama court held that one appealing a disciplinary decision of the Board of Nursing was not entitled to a jury trial.[62] The court also said the nurse's due process rights were met even where some Board members were not present at the hearing. In revoking the nurse's license the court found that the evidence supported a finding that she engaged in unprofessional conduct likely to cause injury to the public health when she self-administered a narcotic while on duty.

A board of nursing is not bound by the recommendation of the hearing officer as illustrated by another Alabama case. In *Alabama Board of Nursing v. Herrick*, decided at about the same time, the court held that the board did not abuse its discretionary authority when it revoked a nurse's license because of intoxication while on duty in an emergency room.[63] A hearing officer recommended that the nurse's license be suspended for 3 months, but the board ordered it revoked. There was evidence that there were other occasions of intoxication while on duty.

In cases involving past misuse of narcotics the board of nursing is concerned with the extent of rehabilitation before a decision to lift the sanction is made. Rehabilitation may apply to cases other than the narcotic cases. The concept is important whenever there is an issue of public safety.

An intriguing case which illustrates the factual importance of the rehabilitation concept involved a nurse who had engaged in antiwar activities.[64]

> A registered nurse was convicted of destruction of Selective Service records and was sentenced to 3 years in a federal reformatory. A state statute existed which called for revocation or suspension of the license of a convicted felon, "if the Illinois Department of Registration and Education determines, after investigation, that such person has not been sufficiently rehabilitated to warrant the public trust." Prior to the 3-year conviction the nurse had served 14 months on a similar conviction in another state. On her parole release in 1971 she worked at a health center until her second conviction. The Illinois Board of Nurse Examiners dismissed the complaint for revocation when the nurse's attorney successfully argued that the agency had presented no evidence on the issues of rehabilitation and public trust as required by the statute. The inclusion of the rehabilitation and public trust provision recognizes that not all felonious crimes automatically preclude a right to remain a licensed nurse.

Authority to Discipline for Activities Which Occurred in a Foreign State

It is becoming increasingly common for a state to take action on the license of a health care provider even where the conduct complained of arose in another state.[65] A number of states have provided legal sanction for such discipline by enacting legislation or promulgating rules and regulations. Florida law, for example, stipulates that disciplinary action may be taken for having a license to practice nursing revoked, suspended or otherwise acted against, including the denial of licensure, by the licensing authority of another state, territory, or country.[66]

> A New York licensed pharmacist in *Heller v. Ambach* had his license to practice revoked after he was convicted by a New Jersey court for the indiscriminate sale of controlled drugs at a pharmacy owned by him in New Jersey.[67] The drug was a cough suppressant substance containing codeine. He contended that the crimes he pleaded guilty to in New Jersey would not constitute crimes under New York law and thus could not be relied upon to establish unprofessional conduct. He had raised no objection at the administrative level hearing, nor did he answer the charges orally or in writing. When he sought review of the decision at a later proceeding it was held that he had waived the opportunity. The revocation was upheld as it was not shown that it was excessive punishment and the discipline was justified for protection of the public.

Unprofessional Conduct

In recent years there have been a number of cases involving the interpretation of the term, "unprofessional conduct" as it is used in different statutes and regulations relevant to health care professionals. Some states specifically set out the behavior which constitutes unprofessional conduct whereas, others simply rely on a broad application of the term.[68] Even where the specific conduct is set out in the statute or regulation the law frequently includes a statement that unprofessional behavior is not limited to the identified conduct. Considerable deference is given to a regulatory board whose primary objective is to protect the public.

What constitutes unprofessional conduct is generally established by the testimony of qualified experts. A Minnesota court held that, "Unprofessional conduct is conduct which violates those standards of professional behavior which through professional experience have become established, by the consensus of the expert opinion of the members, as reasonably necessary for the protection of the public interest."[69]

A Nebraska statute empowered the nursing board to deny a nursing license on proof that the applicant was guilty of unprofessional conduct.[70] However, unprofessional conduct was not defined by either statute or regulation.

> The registered nurse in *Scott v. Nebraska Board of Nursing* appealed the board decision against her and the sole issue before the state high court was whether the denial was supported by evidence of unprofessional conduct. In essence, the board had to demonstrate that it was acting within its powers and that it was not acting arbitrary, capricious, or unreasonable.
>
> The nurse, who was licensed to practice in New York and did practice there before going to South Dakota, was denied a permanent license by Nebraska authorities based on complaints issued by the South Dakota Board. At the Nebraska hearing the nurse was represented by counsel and presented evidence in her behalf. The board produced affidavits and expert testimony setting out the unprofessional conduct and noncompliance with nursing standards. Among the findings issued by the board were the following: patient abandonment, refusing to comply with established hospital policy, unwillingness to attend hospital education programs, failure to comply with reasonable employment policies such as dress code and work schedules, failure to seek and accept guidance in work-related activities, and a number of documented deviations from accepted nursing practice. The Supreme Court held that it could not substitute its judgment for that of the board because the legislature delegated this function to it. The court had authority to overturn the board's decision only if it was shown that their decision was contrary to the evidence before it.

A 1979 case, *Leukhardt v. Commonwealth State Board of Nurse Examiners*, dealt with an unusual situation when the actions of a nurse were criticized.[71] The decision of the Pennsylvania Nursing Board to formally reprimand a registered nurse was not upheld when it was appealed. The wife of a confused man who was in the intensive care unit initiated the complaint after she saw the nurse strike him during a linen change. The wife also initiated a civil suit for money damages against the nurse and the hospital, based on the same incident. Pennsylvania law authorizes the board to take disciplinary action when it finds that a licensee has wilfully violated the professional practice statute or regulations promulgated by the board. The board relied on the following regulation: "The registered nurse assesses human responses and plans, implements and evaluates nursing care for individuals and families for whom the nurse is responsible. In carrying out this responsibility, the nurse performs all of the following functions: . . . Carries out nursing care actions which promote, maintain, and restore the well-being of individuals."

After a hearing the board issued a finding that the nurse had slapped the patient in order to induce him to release his tight grasp on her arm, but that other means existed by which she could have induced him to release his grasp. The board concluded that her actions "constituted a violation of nursing care standards and a disregard for the underlying philosophies, duties and obligations of a nurse. . . ." On appeal the court found that the board had not weighed the following evidence. The man was disoriented and had seized the nurse's arm in a viselike grip which prevented her from using it to hold him in position. Three nurses in all were required to change his linen and he was flailing his extremities and was in danger of falling. The nurse testified that she "tapped" the patient on the back to get him to release his grasp as she was supporting the heaviest part of him and needed both arms to do so. The other nurses collaborated her testimony. The nurse had tried to pry his fingers from her arm and requests by all the nurses failed to get the patient to release the arm. Although the board conceded that the blow to the patient's shoulder was solely for the purpose of making him release his hold, it ignored evidence which would make the nurse's action reasonable under the circumstances. The appeals court held that contrary to the board's conclusion the nurse's actions were calculated to promote her patient's well-being, not impair it.

Florida law stipulates that "unprofessional conduct shall include any departure from, or the failure to conform to, the minimal standard of acceptable and prevailing nursing practice." In *Sap v. Florida State Board of Nursing*, the Florida licensing board sought to discipline a licensed practical nurse (LPN) for leaving the door to the medicine closet open and for leaving the medicine cart in patient's rooms and in the hallways unattended.[72] Although the nurse denied these transgressions there was evidence introduced which would support the allegations. The nurse also admitted to a medication overdose and physical abuse of a nursing home patient.

After the hearing the hearing officer who was the "trier of fact" submitted his order which stated that there was inconclusive evidence as to the medicine closet and cart incidents. Additionally, he found that the facility did not have a formal policy requiring that the doors be locked or that the cart should be constantly attended or secured. The board rejected the officer's findings and suspended the nurse's license. When the case was appealed the court remanded it back with instructions that the hearing officer should determine whether, or not, the complaints were supported by the evidence. Following such clarification the board would then be in a position to find that the nurse's conduct did or did not comply with practice standards. The case distinguishes the role of the hearing officer to hear and rule on the evidence from that of the board which was to accept the officer's findings and determine what, if any, discipline is warranted. The case also illustrates the need for all parties involved in an adjudicatory hearing to identify the scope of authority of the respective participants. In this case, the board had to accept the evidentiary findings of the hearing officer.

Each state must adopt and comply with rules promulgated to assure a fair hearing.[73] In the event that a nurse is called to appear before a licensing board it is essential that the rules under which the proceeding is to be conducted be reviewed. Failure to completely understand the rules may preclude a fair hearing or negatively impact on future recourse. If the nurse's legal authority to practice is the subject of the hearing it is well to keep in mind that the hearing is a quasijudicial procedure.

Perhaps the most well-known case dealing with the question of unprofessional conduct is *Tuma v. Board of Nursing*.[74] The legal issue was one of constitutional due process although the factual situation involved counseling of a terminally ill patient. The Idaho nursing practice statute stipulated that action could be taken against a nurse's license to practice for "immoral, unprofessional or dishonorable conduct." The acts that delineated unprofessional conduct included any practice or behavior of a character likely to deceive or defraud the public, obtaining of any fee or compensation by fraud, deceit, or misrepresentation; and advertising by any means whatsoever of the practice of nursing in which untruthful or misleading statements are made. Tuma's actions did not fall within the scope of these published prohibited activities and thus the board was left with an undefined provision.

Tuma supervised nursing students in a hospital clinical setting in conjunction with her position as a nursing instructor at the College of Southern Idaho. Because Tuma was particularly interested in working with dying patients, she assigned a patient who was about to begin a course of chemotherapy in an attempt to reverse malignant myelogenous leukemia. The patient had been diagnosed with cancer 12 years previously and had been informed by her physician that her only hope for survival was chemotherapy which was to begin March 3, 1976.

Tuma and a student nurse met with the patient and discussed the side effects of the treatment, as well as alternative treatment. The patient had already consented to the treatment. Tuma did not offer any advice with respect to whether the patient should withdraw consent or try another form of treatment. The patient requested that Tuma return that evening and meet with her family and give them the same information, including the work being done at a hospital in Salt Lake City using Chaparral and Laetrile. Tuma agreed, although she told the patient the discussions of the alternative treatment "wasn't exactly ethical." The chemotherapy was started but was discontinued at 8 P.M. when the physician was informed of the events by the daughter-in-law. The physician requested the name of the nurse, but did not discuss with the patient her apparent change of attitude.

The discussion with the family that evening included the side effects of chemotherapy, and such alternatives as natural foods, herbs, and Laetrile. Tuma pointed out that the woman might have difficulty in securing the treatment, including transfusions, if she left the hospital. After the discussion the parties concluded that the patient should remain hospitalized and chemotherapy was reinstated at 9:15 that evening. The patient died 2 weeks later.

The physician complained to the hospital and College authorities and Tuma was removed as an instructor. The hospital personnel department complained to the board of registration and alleged that Tuma had interferred with the physician–patient relationship. The nursing board requested documentation of the events from all parties involved in it. Although the hospital personnel department tendered a letter to the family they did not respond or participate in the disciplinary proceedings. In accordance with their authority the board drafted a petition and scheduled a hearing.

The Idaho Code specified that the Board appoint a disinterested person to serve as the hearing officer. The appointment of a disinterested party presumably would assure an impartial decision. The officer was not a nurse. His responsibility was to issue a conclusion based on findings of fact. After certification of the findings the board could impose a penalty, or not, on its own. The officer concluded that Tuma's action constituted "unprofessional conduct" and the board suspended her license for 6 months. She was allowed to practice pending the outcome of the appeal. Tuma's appeal to an intermediary court failed and she ultimately appealed to the state supreme court.

Tuma successfully argued that neither the legislature or the board gave notice of acts that would constitute unprofessional conduct. In the absence of written guidelines as to the conduct which was prohibited Tuma could not know that her discussions, as perceived by her as patient counseling, would be perceived as constituting unprofessional conduct. Additionally, the existence of guidelines would guide a tribunal in deliberations that involved allegations of unprofessional activities. Tumas's argument was strengthened by the fact that the board was on record as endorsing a standard of care requiring a nurse to "promote, and participate in, patient education based on the individual's health needs, and involve the individual and family for a better understanding and implementation of immediate and long term goals." The court was not persuaded by testimony that Tuma admitted "guilt" by stating on three occasions during the day in question that the discussions were not quite ethical or legal. The court viewed these statements as simply an awareness on her part that the discussions of alternative treatment might not be endorsed by the medical profession.

The board objected to the inclusion of Tuma's testimony that she subscribed to the principles of the American Nurses' Association Code. The code, adopted in 1976, serves to inform nurses and their clients of the professions' position regarding ethical matters. Tuma sought to have the Code entered into the proceedings to show a disposition that she subscribed to similar professional tenets.

The court soundly rejected the board's argument that it should determine on a case-by-case basis what constitutes unprofessional practice. Such an approach would be "an intolerable state of affairs" and would violate the due process concept. The court held that fundamental fairness requires that specific behavior be identified in such a manner that a reasonable professional could determine from it what is to be done or what is likely to constitute a prohibited activity. In deciding the case, the Idaho Court looked to a 1935 Connecticut case which held that the words, "immoral, dishonorable, or unprofessional" are general, and standing alone have no possibility of reasonable certainty.[75]

In a case decided after *Tuma*, an Illinois court held that a dentist was on notice of the types of activities which would constitute unprofessional conduct.[76]

> The case, *Chastek v. Anderson*, cites a significant number of cases in which the term "unprofessional conduct" is upheld and distinguishes them from other cases in which the term failed to meet constitutional requirements. In the Illinois case the dental board issued a complaint against a dentist alleging improper treatment of several patients. The dentist had argued that the statute failed to identify what constituted unprofessional practice and thus, had failed the due process requirement of advance notice of unpermitted conduct. The Illinois statute cited 20 separate grounds for which a dentist could have a license revoked, one of which was unprofessional conduct. The statute specifically set out that its purpose was to protect the health, safety, and welfare of the public. The court held that the clear legislative intent combined with the term unprofessional conduct provided adequate notice that substandard care would constitute such conduct.

Contrasting *Tuma* and similar cases in which the courts held that the term standing alone provided inadequate notice, the Illinois court noted that none of them involved facts of alleged acts of negligence. None of the complaints alleged an unfitness to practice.

The courts will uphold a broad, undefined unprofessional conduct standard where it can be shown that the professional duty is prescribed in terms definite enough to serve as a guide to those who must comply with it. The court will analyze the statute in terms of its purpose. A broad definition inherently delegates to a licensing board the function of evaluating on an individual case basis whether the issue raised involves competency or fitness to practice. In the absence of such a finding it is likely that courts will continue to find broad conduct categories inadequate to satisfy constitutional notice requirements.

Summary

A nurse's license is a valuable property right and constitutional rights require due process in a disciplinary hearing. While the court will frequently defer to the discretionary authority of a board of nursing it will not hesitate to set aside a board sanction if the hearing was not conducted fairly or the order was against the weight of the evidence presented at the hearing. Board hearings are not as formal as courtroom trials. No nurse should go into a hearing in which there is the possibility that a sanction may be imposed. Valuable rights may be lost because of the technical nature of the applicable adjudicatory rules.

While there has always been a substantial number of cases involving physicians, it is only recently that the reported cases involve nurses' rights. A number of cases deal with the interpretation of the Nursing Practice Act, especially in the area of "unprofessional practice." During the last decade states have revised their nursing practice acts and many have expanded the section which deals with board discipline, specifically spelling out the prohibited or questionable behavior.

There is also a new approach when dealing with other state board sanctions. A number of states have enacted provisions that regard infractions in other states, especially those of a criminal nature, sufficient grounds to refuse to grant a license or take other disciplinary action. The *Tuma* case did much to heighten awareness of fundamental fairness when disciplining for "unprofessional" conduct. The case was a simple due process case, not a test case to determine whether a nurse could counsel a patient.

ADVANCED NURSING PRACTICE

In late 1980 the Board of Registration for the Healing Arts in Missouri decided to take legal action against several nurse practitioners and physicians who worked at a family planning and abortion clinic in the state.[77]

> In the subsequent suit, *Sermchief v. Gonzales,* the board asked the court to declare that the nurses at that clinic and several other clinics were engaged in the unauthorized practice of medicine and that the five clinic doctors aided and abetted the nurses in the unlawful conduct. The services routinely provided included: the taking of a history; breast and pelvic examinations; laboratory testing of Papanicolaou smears, gonorrhea cultures, and blood serology; the providing of and giving of information about oral contraceptives, condoms, and intrauterine devices; the dispensing of certain designated medications; and counseling services and community education. These services were provided in accordance with standing orders and protocols.
>
> The Missouri Medical Act was not clearly defined, and, in fact, was vague as most medical practice acts are. The Medical Act stated:
>
> > It shall be unlawful for any person not now a registered physician within the meaning of the law to practice medicine or surgery in any of its departments, or to profess to cure and attempt to treat the sick and

others afflicted with bodily or mental infirmities, or engage in the practice of midwifery in this state, except as herein provided.[78]

The board asked the court to "determine and advise" all parties of the definition of the phrase, "nursing diagnosis." In analyzing the case the Supreme Court had to carefully review the "old" Nursing Practice Act and the 1975 amended act. The amended Missouri Nursing Practice Act defines professional nursing as

> the performance for compensation of any act which requires substantial specialized education, judgment, and skill based on knowledge and application of principles derived from the biological, physical, social and nursing sciences, *including, but not limited to* [emphasis added]
> (a) Responsibility for the teaching of health care and the prevention of illness to the patient and his family; or
> (b) Assessment, nursing diagnosis, nursing care, and counsel of persons who are ill, injured or experiencing alterations in normal health processes; or
> (c) The administration of medications and treatments as prescribed by a person licensed in this state to prescribe such medications and treatments; or
> (d) The coordination and assistance in the delivery of a plan of health care with all members of the health team; or
> (e) The teaching and supervision of other persons in the performance of any of the foregoing. . . .[79]

The following statutes were repealed when the 1975 Nursing Practice statute was enacted:

> 2. A person practices professional nursing who for compensation or personal profit performs, under the supervision and direction of a practitioner authorized to sign birth and death certificates, any professional services requiring the application of principles of the biological, physical or social sciences and nursing skills in the care of the sick, in the prevention of disease or in the conservation of health.[80]
>
> Nothing contained in this chapter shall be construed as conferring any authority on any person to practice medicine or osteopathy or to undertake the treatment or cure of disease.[81]

A trial court held that the services that the nurses provided constituted the "unauthorized practice of medicine." On direct appeal, the Missouri Supreme Court turned aside the trial court ruling and declared that the practices were within those authorized under the state Nursing Practice Act. The court found that the nurses referred a patient to one of the clinic physicians if a condition designated in the clinic standing orders and protocols would contraindicate the use of contraceptives. In that case, further examination and evaluation would be done. The standing orders and protocols were directed to specifically named nurses and were not the same for all the nurses in the various clinics. Both parties requested the court to "define the line" separating the practice of medicine from the practice of nursing, but the court responded that it only address the "narrow" question whether the acts of the nurses were permitted under the Nursing Practice Act or were prohibited by the Medical Practice Act.

Applying basic principles, the court interpreted the meaning of the respective statutes. The court must first determine the "intent" of the legislature when it enacted the statutes. In short, it had to look at the legislative purpose and reason for passing the laws in the first place. It is important to note that the nursing act was an amended statute. Thus, one has to look at the sections deleted and the new sections inserted to determine what was intended by the change. The court stated, "An amended statute should be construed on the theory that the Legislature intended to accomplish a substantive change in the law." The Supreme Court looked at what was and was not in the new legislation.

In a footnote, the court noted that such state legislation "was the ongoing expansion of nursing responsibilities." This specifically referred to the broadening of nursing roles in response to "changes in patterns of demand for health services, and the evolution of professional relationships among nurses, physicians, and other health professions."

The court held that the statutory revision, "reveals a manifest legislative desire to expand the scope of authorized nursing practices." In interpreting the phrase, "including, but not limited to," the Court said that such an open-ended definition of professional nursing "evidences an intent to avoid statutory constraints on the evolution of new functions for nurses delivering health services." This was a key ruling in the case.

The court further noted that physician prepared standing orders and protocols for nurses were so well established and accepted at the time the Missouri statute was enacted that the legislature "could not have been unaware of the use of such practices. The court said, "There can be no question that a nurse undertakes only a nursing diagnosis, as opposed to a medical diagnosis, when she or he finds or fails to find symptoms described by physicians in standing orders and protocols for the purpose of administering courses of treatment prescribed by the physician in such orders and protocols." The court found it significant that, although 40 states had modernized and expanded their practice acts during recent years there was no legal challenge to the nurses' authority to act as the Missouri nurses acted.

Sermchief is an important case because it was the first case to test the new wave of nursing practice acts. Although narrowly interpreted, that is, confined to the facts of the case, it provides significant direction for states that contemplate revising their nursing practice acts to reflect the status of nursing in the scheme of the health care delivery system. It was not unexpected that the court was reluctant to definitively define "nursing diagnosis," that is the proper role for the profession to articulate why the concept exists and what impact it has for nursing. The case was decided less on the legal interpretation of nursing diagnosis than on the distinct differences between the old and the new Nursing Practice Act.

The Arkansas Supreme Court, in *Arkansas State Nurses' Association v. Arkansas State Medical Board*, recently ruled that a regulation of the state medical board was not permitted under its authority granted by the legislature.[82] The regulation limited the number of registered nurse-practitioners who might be employed by a physician. Physicians who violated the regulation could be found to be practicing outside their act. The Arkansas State Nurses Association initiated the suit, seeking to have the regulation declared invalid.

The court held that hiring too many nurse-practitioners did not fall within the malpractice statute. The court also noted that a 1977 statute relative to physicians' assistants stipulated that any one physician may employ two assistants, but the limitation was not applicable to medical group practices where there were many physicians. The nurse-practitioner regulation prohibited groups of two or more physicians from hiring more than two practitioners at any one time.

SUMMARY

While most practicing nurses are keenly interested in cases involving liability law, they should also be aware of the impact of the law on other practice issues. When one reviews the dates of most of the cases reported in this chapter, it is plain that "nurses' rights" is a fairly recent concept.

Employment rights affect every practicing nurse, whether under an employment contract or not. The most recent issue in employment rights is the safety of the work environment for both the nurse-worker and co-workers. Sometimes the nurse is the vanguard, protecting others from potential harm.

In recent years, laws have been enacted that provide some protection in both the work setting and in areas of educational opportunity. However, the rights of nurses when called to appear before a nursing board comprise a significant amount of the case law impacting on nurses. Sometimes, a single case sets precedent. For example, precedent was set in *Backus*, *Davis*, and *Sermchief* because these cases examined such issues as the limits on practice, the right of a handicapped individual to pursue a nursing career, and the scope of nursing practice.

REFERENCES AND NOTES

1. For a reference on the Labor Relations Act, see Munger, M. (May 1974). Labor Relations Act: Implications for nurses. *Association of Operating Room Nurses Journal, 19*(5), 1127. However, see Crenshaw v. Bozeman Deaconess Hospital 693 P. 2nd 487 (MT, 1984), where the requirement of good faith on the part of the defendants was necessary when the suit was not based on a wrongful discharge allegation.
2. Dentzer, S. You can't fire me, I'll sue. *Newsweek*, July 12, 1982, p. 63.

3. Summers, C. (Jan.–Feb. 1980). Protecting all employees against unjust dismissal. *Harvard Business Review, 58*(1), 132. See also Letters to the Editor. (May–June 1980). *Harvard Business Review, 58*(3), 204 (readers' response to the Summers article).

4. See Anon. (1980). Note: Protecting at will employees against wrongful discharge: The duty to terminate only in good faith. *Harvard Law Review, 93*, 1816; Blades, L. (1967). Employment at will against individual freedom: On limiting the abusive exercise of employer power. *Columbia Law Review,* 67, 1404; Anon. (1974). Note: Implied contract rights to job security. *Stanford Law Review, 26*, 335; Anon. (1973). Comment: Towards a property right in employment. *Buffalo Law Review, 22*, 1081; Glendon, M., & Lev, E. (1979). Changes in the bonding of the employment relationship: An essay on the new property. *Boston College Law Review, 20*, 457.

5. Summers, C. (Jan.–Feb. 1980). Protecting all employees against unjust dismissal. *Harvard Business Review, 58*(1), 132.

6. Andress v. Augusta Nursing Facilities, Inc., 275 S.E. 2nd 368 (GA, 1980).

7. Hinrichs v. Tranquilaire Hospital, 353 S. 2nd 1130 (AL, 1977).

8. O'Sullivan v. Mallon, 390 A. 2nd 149 (NJ, 1978).

9. Meierer v. E.I. du Pont de Nemours & Co., 792 F. 2nd 1117 (1986). See also Anon. (1985). Judge sets aside monetary damages awarded to nurse. *The American Nurse, 17*(7), 6; Anon. (1987). Newscaps: DuPont surrenders to South Carolina R.N. *American Journal of Nursing, 87*(8), 1096.

10. For other cases in which the discharged nurse prevailed see the following: Duldulao v. St. Mary of Nazareth Hospital, 505 N.E. 2nd 314 (IL, 1987), where the court held that although there was no written employment contract and the duration of the employment was for an indefinite period, the hospital's actions were not protected by law because the defendant failed to follow its own rules as stated in the hospital handbook. The handbook required the hospital to state the nature of the infraction or shortcoming in writing before any disciplinary action could be taken and this was not done. Sides v. Duke Hospital, 328 S.E. 2nd 181 (NC, 1985), where an appellate court held that a claim by a nurse-anesthetist against a hospital for wrongful discharge and wrongful interference with her employment contract should not have been dismissed by the trial court. The nurse had worked at the hospital for 10 years when a family sued for the wrongful death of a patient. The nurse had refused to administer certain anesthetics to immobilize a patient as ordered by the anesthesiologist. She refused because the dose was excessive. The anesthesiologist gave the medication himself. The patient had a cardiac arrest and suffered permanent brain damage. The nurse was told not to testify about all she knew about the case, however she testified truthfully. After a pretrial deposition the physicians in the hospital became hostile toward her and she was told that her job performance was poor in some areas. Shortly thereafter she was fired. She sued the hospital, her nurse supervisor, and two physicians for wrongful discharge. The court dismissed the claim against the supervisor because she did not have an employment contract with her. The court said the plaintiff's claim against the hospital, even if it was an at will contract, was valid because the hospital could not terminate her for unlawful purposes. The court also said the plaintiff had a valid claim against the physicians for wrongful interference with her contract with the hospital.

11. Edgewood Nursing Center, Inc. v. N.L.R.B., 581 F. 2nd 363 (1978). See also Leikvold v. Valley View Community Hospital, 688 P. 2nd 170 (AZ, 1984), where there was a jury question whether the hospital manual provided for a termination hearing.

12. For other cases in which the discharged nurse did not prevail see the following cases, Sullivan v. University of Mississippi Medical Center, 617 F. Supp. 554 (1985), where the nurse sued the university medical center alleging that because of her handicap it fired her 1 month after she was hired. The federal court held that the nurse had no right to sue the state agency because they were immune from suit. Gleason v. Board of County Commissioners of the County of Weld, 620 F. Supp. 632 (1985), where a nurse

was discharged by the county health department. A federal court held that although her hearing was held after the discharge instead of before the discharge her due process rights had been fully complied with. Her termination was affirmed by both a grievance board and the board of county commissioners. Ewing v. Board of Trustees of Pulaski Memorial Hospital, 486 N.E. 2nd 1094 (IN, 1985), Where a nurse-anesthetist was discharged after almost 10 years. Although the nurse argued that she and the defendant hospital had entered into an employment contract because of statements made in letters from the executive director of the hospital the court held that the letters were not intended to serve as a contract of employment. The defendant presented evidence that the nurse was told that the board of trustees was the only one who had authority to enter into contracts with employees.

Mock v. LaGuardia Hospital-Hip Hospital, Inc., 498 N.Y.S. 2nd 446 (NY, 1986), where nurses who were discharged for union organizing activities brought a defamation suit against the hospital alleging they were defamed at a hearing before the National Labor Relations Board when hospital representatives claimed the nurses were disloyal, untrustworthy, deceitful, and lacked good faith. The nurses were supervisory nurses and under federal laws were categorized as management personnel who "owe a duty of loyalty" to their employer and can be lawfully discharged for labor union activity. The court held the statements were not defamatory.

13. Nelson v. Mustian, 502 F. Supp. 698 (1980).
14. Anon. (Oct. 1981). News: Judge upholds NYC health code ban on holding patients for X Ray. *American Journal of Nursing, 81*(10), 1788.
15. State Employees Association v. Department of Mental Health 365 N.W. 2nd 93 (MI, 1984) at pp. 96 and 97.
16. State Employees Association v. Department of Mental Health, 365 N.W. 2nd 93 (MI, 1984). The other two nurses were ordered reinstated with back pay approximately 6 months after the drowning. The appeals court did not hear legal arguments with respect to their cases because the issues were moot.
17. Stoker v. Tarentino, 489 N.Y.S. 2nd 43 (NY, 1985).
18. Swanson v. St. John's Lutheran Hospital, 597 P. 2nd 702 (MT, 1979).
19. Anon. (Feb. 1980). *Modern Healthcare (Legal Briefs), 10*(2), 92.
20. Slayton v. Comm. of Pennsylvania Unemployment Compensation Review Board, 427 A. 2nd 323 (PA, 1981). See also Amador v. Unemployment Ins. Appeals Board, 677 P. 2nd 224 (CA, 1984). In this case no disqualification was found where a worker refused to perform work he reasonably believed would jeopardize the health of others.
21. Davis v. California Unemployment Insurance Appeals Board and St. John's Hospital, 117 *California Reporter, 463* (CA, 1974).
22. Ibid., at p. 405, citing Deering's Annotated California (Unemployment Insurance) Code 1256.
23. Owens v. Williams, 77 N.E. 2nd 318 (MA, 1948).
24. Byars v. Baptist Medical Center, Inc., 361 S. 2nd 350 (AL, 1978). See also Heying v. Simonaitis, 466 N.E. 2nd 1137 (IL, 1984), where the court held that no grounds for the suit against the physicians and nurses existed.
25. Tennessee Coal, Iron and Railway Co., v. Kelly, 50 S. 1008 (TN, 1909).
26. Rookard v. Health and Hospitals, Corporation, 710 F. 2nd 41 (1983).
27. Sullivan, R. Court reinstates lawsuit by nurse on dismissal from a city hospital. *New York Times*, June 12, 1983, p. 58.
28. Sibley Memorial Hospital v. Wilson, 488 F. 2nd 1338 (1973).
29. Fesel v. Masonic Home of Delaware, 447 F. Supp. 1346 (1978); affirmed at 591 F. 2nd 1334 (1979).
30. Backus v. Baptist Medical Center, 510 F. Supp. 1191 (1981).
31. Annas, G. (Dec. 1981). Male nurses in the delivery room. *Hastings Center Report 11*(6), 20.
32. Buckley v. Hospital Corporation of America, 758 F. 2nd 1525 (1985).

33. 29 United States Code sections 621 to 634 (1967). 29 U.S.C. §631 (1984) protects employees between the ages of 40 and 70.

34. United States Code Annotated §784.

35. For a critical analysis of the Davis case see Hull, K. (1979). The Davis case and the progress of handicapped rights. South Bend, Indiana: National Center for Law and the Handicapped.

36. 42 *Federal Register* 22676-22702 (May 4, 1977); 45 Code of Federal Regulations §§84.1 - 84.61 (1979).

37. Southeastern Community College v. Davis, 99 S. Ct. 2361 (1979).

38. Davis v. Southeastern Community College, 424 F. Supp. 1341 (1976).

39. Davis v. Southeastern Community College, 574 F. 2nd 1158 (1978).

40. American Nurses' Association. (1980). *The Nursing Practice Act: Suggested state legislation*, Kansas City, Missouri: American Nurses' Association (G-142 IM 2/80).

41. Kling v. County of Los Angeles, 633 F. 2nd 876 (1980).

42. Kling v. County of Los Angeles, 769 F. 2nd 532 (1985).

43. For a legal discussion of the complexities of *Trageser,* as well as criticism of the holding, see Kurshan, R. (1981). Employment discrimination under Section 504 of the Rehabilitation Act: Trageser v. Libbie Rehabilitation Center. *Boston College Law Review, 21*(5), 1178; and Anon. (Mar.–Apr. 1979). Private Right of action for employment discrimination under Section 504 curtailed by new amendments. *Mental Disability Law Reporter, 3*(2), 99.

44. Trageser v. Libbie Rehabilitation Center, Inc., 590 F. 2nd 87 (1979). For the latest case involving violation of section 504 rights see, School Board of Nassau County, Florida v. Arline, 107 S. Ct. 1123 (1987), where the court held that a school teacher who had a third relapse of tuberculosis in 2 years was a "handicapped individual" within the meaning of "impaired" in the Rehabilitation Act. The court's ruling made it clear that employers who receive federal funds may not fire employees just because they have a contagious disease. The court held that a substantial risk of infecting other people may disqualify an employee from continued employment, but this determination must be "individualized." The American Medical Association filed a friend-of-the-court brief in which it said that employers must apply reasonable medical judgment to determine how the disease is transmitted, how long the disease will remain contagious, what potential harm exists for other persons, and how likely it is that the disease will be transmitted and cause harm.

45. Walker, D. (1980). Nursing 1980: New responsibility, new liability. *Trial, 16*(12), 43.

46. See, for example, Massachusetts General Laws, Chap. 30A.

47. Commonwealth, State Board of Medical Education and Licensure v. Contakos, 346 A. 2nd 850 (PA, 1975).

48. Lieb v. Board of Examiners for Nursing, 411 A. 2nd 42 (CT, 1979).

49. Durante v. Board of Regents of State University, 416 N.Y.S. 2nd 401 (NY, 1979).

50. Bruni v. Department of Registration and Education, 319 N.E. 2nd 37 (IL, 1974).

51. Florida Statutes Annotated (1979), chap. 464.0125 (1) (c).

52. Leggett v. Tennessee Board of Nursing, 612 S.W. 2nd 476 (TN, 1980).

53. Leigh v. Board of Registration in Nursing, 506 N.E. 2nd 91 (1987). See also, the case facts as indicated in Leigh v. Board of Registration in Nursing, 481 N.E. 2nd 1347 (1985).

54. Massachusetts Supreme Judicial Court, No. 84-71, Memorandum of decision of Justice H. Wilkins (September 4, 1984).

55. Massachusetts General Laws, Chap. 112, §80B-D (1975) and 244 Code of Massachusetts Regulations 4.13(1), (1980).

56. 244 Code of Massachusetts Regulations 4.05(8), (1980).

57. In 1984, House Bill no. 5985 dealing with lay midwifery was introduced, but was not enacted by the legislature. In the wake of the 1987 Massachusetts Supreme Court decision in the Leigh case, bills were submitted to the legislature to permit nurse

midwives to attend home births and calling for state licensing of lay midwives. See Anon. Massachusetts midwife curb upheld. *New York Times*, May 24, 1987, p. 35.

58. State of Florida, Department of Health and Rehabilitative Services, v. McTigue, 387 S. 2nd 454 (FL, 1980).
59. Anon. (Jan. 16, 1981). Denver nurses arrested for hospital drug thefts. *American Medical News*, p. 3.
60. State of Washington v. Sheldon, 684 P. 2nd 1350 (WA, 1984).
61. Hogan v. Mississippi Board of Nursing, 457 S. 2nd 931 (MS, 1984).
62. Stevens v. Blake, 456 S. 2nd 795 (AL, 1984).
63. Alabama Board of Nursing v. Herrick, 454 S. 2nd 1041 (AL, 1984). See also Ledo v. University of the State of N.Y., State Education Department, 478 N.Y.S. 2nd 108 (NY, 1984).
64. Anon. (1976). News section: Panel dismisses complaint against Jane Kennedy. *American Journal of Nursing*, 76(1), 10.
65. See, for example, conviction of a federal felony was grounds for discipline against a physician involved in counterfeiting. Bruni v. Department of Registration and Education, 319 N.E. 2nd 37 (IL, 1974); Cert. denied, 95 S. Ct. 1573 (1975). See also Matter of Miles v. Nyquist, 377 N.E. 2nd 483 (NY, 1977).
66. Florida Statutes Annotated, Chap. 464.018 (1-c) (1986).
67. Heller v. Ambach, 433 N.Y.S. 2nd 281 (NY, 1980).
68. Maine Revised Statutes, Title 32, chap. 31, §2105; Utah Code Annotated Title 58 chap. 31, (58-31-14) 1979; Florida Statutes Annotated chap. 464.0125 (1) (f), 1979; Oregon Revised Statutes, chap. 678, (678.111), 1977; New Hampshire Revised Statutes Annotated 316-B:12 (Rules and Regulations), 1976.
69. Reyburn v. Minn. State Board of Optometry, 78 N.W. 2nd 351 (MN, 1956).
70. Scott v. Nebraska Board of Nursing, 244 N.W. 2nd 683 (NE, 1976).
71. Leukhardt v. Commonwealth State Board of Nurse Examiners, 403 A. 2nd 645 (PA, 1979).
72. Sapp v. Florida State Board of Nursing, 384 S. 2nd 254 (FL, 1980).
73. See, for example, 801 Code of Massachusetts Regulations 1.00–1.03, Standard Adjudicatory Rules of Practice and Procedure, Massachusetts, 1979.
74. Tuma v. Board of Nursing, 593 P. 2nd 711 (ID, 1979).
75. Sage-Allen Company v. Wheeler, 179 A. 195 (CT, 1935).
76. Chastek v. Anderson, 416 N.E. 2nd 247 (IL, 1981).
77. Sermchief v. Gonzales, 660 S.W. 2nd 683 (MO, 1983).
78. Missouri Revised Statutes. §334.010 (1939 as amended 1959).
79. Missouri Revised Statutes. §335.016.8 (a)–(e), (1976).
80. Missouri Revised Statutes. §335.010.2, (1969).
81. Missouri Revised Statutes §335.190, (1969).
82. Arkansas State Nurses Association v. Arkansas State Medical Board, 677 S.W. 2nd 293 (AR, 1984).

12

EDUCATIONAL LAW

Increasingly in the last decade the courts have been asked to define the right of an individual's access to education. Affirmative action has substantially expanded the right to be admitted to an educational institution. Once one is admitted to an educational facility the due process and equal protection clause of the Fourteenth Amendment provide considerable protection for both the student and the facility. Faculty and student bylaws should include provisions that delineate the rights and obligations of both the institution and the student when a dispute arises between the parties. The case law on student dismissal is extensive. Although there are not a significant number of legal cases based on the Family Educational Rights and Privacy Act of 1974, it serves as a model for other groups and it is reasonable to expect that the protection provided by the Act might be expanded in the future to include other situations, such as employment records. A number of legal issues have arisen as a result of declaring bankruptcy on student loans, In particular, refusing to forward a student's transcript and the impact of a discharge in bankruptcy when application is made to a licensing authority to take a licensing examination. Although nonacademic suits are infrequently instituted, three cases have been included in the chapter to illustrate the nature of such suits. Of course, suits alleging negligence on the part of the educational facility can be brought by the injured student.

ADMISSION

Under the Civil Rights Act, the federal government prohibits discrimination on grounds of race, color or nationality.[1] In addition to state and federal regulations, an institution may have a corporate charter or by-law setting out criteria to be followed in the admission of students. Most of the cases dealing with the admission process involve the concept of affirmative action. The concept of affirmative action is based on the fact that, historically, minority applicants had not been provided the same educational opportunities as nonminority groups. In recent years the student selection process has included criteria for the acceptance of "disadvantaged" and minority students.

Because public educational facilities receive support from the state or federal government, they are not at liberty to conduct their affairs free from governmental scrutiny. Private colleges, on the other hand, did not have to account to the government for such things as their admission criteria. Thus, the student attending a private facility did not have the protection of the due process and equal protection clause of the U.S. Constitution. However, this has changed to some extent as a result of such factors as the student loan program and other governmental assistance given to private institutions. There still remains a difference in the application of state and federal constitutional laws to public versus private institutions. In general, courts have been hesitant to interfere in the internal affairs of both public and private institutions. They have, nonetheless, struck down admission practices and policies where it is shown that the criteria were unreasonable, arbitrary, or violated the law.

One of the earliest affirmative action suits, *DeFunis v. Odegaard*, involved a challenge to the admission policy of a law school.[2] The policy was challenged because it established a type of screening procedure for minority applicants which was distinct from the admission procedure required of nonminority students. There were 1600 applicants for the 150 positions in the state-operated school. The challenging student claimed that the admission policy was racially discriminatory against him and violated the equal protection clause of the Fourteenth Amendment. Thirty-six of the 37 accepted minority students had averages below the challenging applicant. The Equal Protection Clause of the Fourteenth Amendment provides that no state will deny equal protection of the laws to any person within its jurisdiction, thus, state agencies may not discriminate against individuals because of their race, color, religion, sex, or natural origin. The trial court agreed with the applicant's allegation and ordered his admission. The state's highest court reversed the ruling and held that the minority admission procedure was justified and not unconstitutional. The law student remained in the program pending an appeal before the U.S. Supreme Court. When the case came before the Supreme Court, the student was in his last quarter of the law school program and the justices voted not to render a decision on the merits of the case. Disagreeing with the majority justices' decision not to review the case on its merits, Justice Douglas said that there was no constitutional right for any race to be preferred and the challenging applicant had a constitutional right to have his application considered on its individual merits in a racially neutral manner. He stated that, "the Equal Protection Clause commands the elimination of racial barriers, not their creation in order to satisfy our theory as to how society ought to be organized."

Two years later in *Alevy v. Downstate Medical Center*, a state court held that, although a college practiced reverse or benign discrimination, in proper circumstances, such practice was constitutional.[3] The complainant achieved an undergraduate grade point average of 3.47 and was a magna cum laude graduate. On the Medical College Application Test (MCAT) he scored in the 99th percentile in science and 90th percentile in verbal skills. His MCAT test average of 680 was higher than every one of the accepted minority students. The medical school received 6300 applications for the 216 class slots. After an interview at the publicly funded medical school the complainant was placed number 84th on a second waiting list and his chances of acceptance were remote. One of the interviewing faculty members conceded that the applicant's screening code was higher than any of the accepted minority candidates, and that he probably would have been admitted if he were a member of a minority. The applicant instituted a suit, alleging that his qualifications for admission were superior to those minorities admitted and that the medical school had granted preferential treatment in violation of the law by using a different screening code for minorities. The medical school responded to the suit by stating that its admission policies were responsive to the medical needs of the community's large minority population. The *Alevy* case set out two criteria for recognizing reverse discrimination. First, it must be shown that a substantial state interest underlies the preferential treatment policy. Such a scheme must promote some legitimate, governmental purpose, such as the education of minority medical students who will then provide much needed medical services to groups, traditionally underserved. The second criteria held that less objectionable alternatives, which serve the same purpose, should be considered.

Although the state court dealt with the legal issues raised by reverse discrimination it did not order the admission of the plaintiff because there were 114 applicants ahead of him on the waiting list and he could not show any legal harm as a result of the selection process. The case is important because it established guidelines. These were later expanded in the precedent-setting *Bakke* decision.

The concept of reverse discrimination can be traced back to the 1960s when sociological studies showed a relationship between riots and a lack of journalistic coverage, thus, the courts allowed short-term reverse discrimination to educate minority journalists who would report the events in a more comprehensive manner. The court in *Alevy* suggested that a less objectionable alternative, while still advancing the objectives of the educational program, might include decreasing the size of the preference or placing a limit on the time span in which the practice would operate.

In 1978, in *Regents of University of California v. Allan Bakke*, the U.S. Supreme Court, ruling on the merits of reverse discrimination, agreed in principle in the concept of affirmative action.[4] However, it held that the university's special admission procedure for minority applicants was invalid. Previously, the trial and California Supreme Court had ruled that the quota system set out in the medical school admission procedure was invalid. The U.S. Supreme Court applying the Equal Protection Clause held that preference for members of any one group for no reason other than race or ethnic origin is discriminatory for its own sake and forbidden by the Constitution. The highest court said, "The guarantee of the Equal Protection Clause can not mean one thing when applied to one individual and something else when applied to a person of another color; if both are not accorded the same practice, then it is not equal".

Bakke brought suit, challenging the legality of the university's special admission program under which 16 of the 100 positions in the class were reserved for "disadvantaged" minority students. The university had two admissions programs, a regular and special admissions program. The disadvantaged applicants could be considered under both the regular and special admission program, but the nonminority applicants could only be reviewed according to the regular admission program. In the regular admission procedure, there was outright rejection if the applicant's overall undergraduate grade point average fell below 2.5. However, such was not the case for the special admission program applicants. They were not ranked against the regular admission applicants. During a 4-year period, 63 minority students were admitted to the university under the special program, and 44 under the general program. No disadvantaged whites were admitted under the special program, although many applied.

In 1973, Bakke was rejected under the general admission criteria. He had applied late, at which time no general applicants with scores less than 470 were being accepted and his score was 468. At that time, four special slots were still unfilled. He wrote to the chairman of the admissions committee, protesting that the special program operated as a racial quota. The next year, he filed early and although he attained a total screening score of 549 out of a possible 600, he was again rejected. He was not placed on the discretionary waiting list in either year. Bakke brought suit challenging the legality of the special admission program. In his suit, he sought to compel his admission, alleging that the special program operated to exclude him on the basis of his race in violation of the federal equal protection clause, state constitutional provisions, and the Civil Rights Act. The trial court decided not to compel his admission as Bakke did not prove that he would have been admitted "but for" the special program. On appeal, the state supreme court ordered his admission when the university could not demonstrate that he would not have been admitted if the special program did not exist.

In invalidating the special admission program, the U.S. Supreme Court said that a system which operates on a racial or ethnic classification premise calls for the most exacting scrutinization by the courts. The court agreed that there was a compelling interest to justify the consideration of race in the admissions procedure, but race is only one of a number of factors which should be controlling. The court relied on the admissions program as implemented by several of the country's colleges to illustrate how ethnic diversity is promoted to achieve a more heterogeneous student body. For example, each year, Harvard University receives far more applicants to its freshman program than it can admit and most of the applicants are intellectually suited to its educational demands. While for the past three decades the University has subscribed to the belief that diversity is an essential component of the total educational process, it never established a racial quota. The university's "diversity" policy provided for recognition of the contributions which an applicant from a Kansas farming region or a city ghetto could make to the educational process. Recognizing that race or ethnic factors may be among many to be considered, the admissions committee, in examining the applicant's file, may be persuaded to accept a racial minority student over a similarly desirable applicant because of a unique contribution the student may make in the total scheme of the education process. When looking at a qualified candidate, "race may tip the balance" in favor of the minority applicant over a nonminority applicant. That balance may tip in the applicant's favor in examining his ability to overcome a factor such as economic adversity. The critical criteria are often individual qualities or experiences which are not dependent upon the race factor, but sometimes associated with it.

While not establishing target quotas, Harvard's admissions committee is aware of the impact of numbers. Acceptance of a small number of minority students tends to prevent "mainstreaming"; that is, keeping the numbers of any ethnic group so insignificant that the students will naturally seek support from each other, rather than interact with the college community as a whole. Additionally, "clustering" of any group will set up roadblocks to their achieving their potential.

The U.S. Supreme Court held that the special admission program was invalid because it violated the Equal Protection Clause of the Federal Constitution. The court stated:

> A classification which aids persons who are perceived as members of relatively victimized groups at the expense of other innocent individuals is permissible only when there are judicial, legislative, or administrative findings of constitutional or statutory violation. The purpose of helping certain groups whom faculty of state medical schools perceived as being victims of societal discrimination did not justify a

classification, for admissions purposes, which imposed disadvantages upon white applicants who bore no responsibility for whatever harm the beneficiaries of the special admission program were thought to have suffered.

The court identified as the principle defect of the special program, the fact that it denied to the nonminority applicant the right to individual consideration without regard to his race. The fatal flaw of the preferential procedure was its disregard of individual rights. No matter how strong Bakke's qualifications, including his own potential for contribution to educational diversity, he was never given the chance to compete with the preferred applicants for the special admission seats.

Denial Based on Gender

In a 1982 5-to-4 decision the U.S. Supreme Court held that a state statute which excluded male nurses from enrolling in a state-supported college nursing program violated the Equal Protection clause of the Fourteenth Amendment.[5]

In *Mississippi University For Women v. Hogan*, an all-women's state college was created by the Mississippi legislature in 1884 and since its inception limited its enrollment to women. In 1974 the college began a baccalaureate nursing program. In 1979 the plaintiff, a nondegree nurse who worked as a nursing supervisor in a city where the college was located, applied to the program. The college denied him admission although he was otherwise qualified. The denial was based solely on his gender. The college told him he could only audit the courses.

Finding for the male nurse, the Supreme Court held that the exclusionary policy, based solely on sex, denied the plaintiff equal protection of the laws. Although prior decisions have upheld laws that apply a gender test the party, seeking to uphold the sole gender law carries the burden of showing an "exceedingly persuasive justification" for such a classification. Such a burden is met by showing that the classification serves "important governmental objectives and that the discriminatory means employed are substantially related to the achievement of those objectives." It is possible that the objective itself may be illegitimate, such as, exclusion of a presumed innately inferior group. Assuming the objective is legitimate and important, the court next determines whether the means to achieve the objective is valid.

The college argued that the legislature intended to recognize "educational affirmative action" because historically women were discriminated against when seeking educational opportunities. However, the court held that the denial, rather than compensating women for past injustices, tended to perpetuate a stereotyped view that nursing was exclusively woman's work. In sum, the court held that such gender based limitations could be constitutional, but two burdens must be shown. First, the sex-classification must be justified as necessary to achieve certain objectives. Second, the discriminatory means must substantially relate to the achievement of the objectives.

School Catalog

One court has ruled on the legal significance of a school catalog in the admission process.

> In *Steinberg v. Chicago Medical School,* an applicant to a medical school who had been rejected filed suit against the school, claiming that it had failed to evaluate his application according to the academic criteria set out in the school catalog.[6] The university had accepted the required $15.00 application fee. The words in the catalog stated:
>
>> Students are selected on the basis of scholarship, character, and motivation without regard to race, creed, or sex. The student's potential for the study and practice of medicine will be evaluated on the basis of academic achievement, MCAT results, personal appraisals by an advisory committee, and the personal interview, if requested, by the Committee on Admissions.
>
> The applicant alleged that the defendant used nonacademic criteria, that is, the ability of applicants or their family to pledge or make payment of large sums of money to the medical school. The court held that the wording in the catalog constituted an offer to contract (enter into dealings with each other) and the conduct of the parties sufficiently established the existence of an agreement. The court held that a contract between a private educational institute and the student confers duties on both parties which cannot be arbitrarily disregarded and the agreement to the contract will be legally enforced.

Summary

The laws that protect a student with respect to admission to a school are based on either the Civil Rights Act of 1964, state law, or agreements published by the school. Traditionally public schools have provided greater constitutional protection than private schools, but this distinction is less firm than previously because of government ties to the private school through such programs as the student loan program.

Most of the admission suits deal with constitutional challenges to a school's affirmative action program because the program creates a different admission procedure for minority applicants. However, affirmative action programs have been held constitutional. A New York court in the *Alevy* case addressed the issue of reverse discrimination and set out criteria for overcoming reverse discrimination. First, it must be shown that a significant state interest, such as education of minority students, must underly the preferential treatment policy. Second, the school must consider the least objectionable means to accomplish its objective.

In 1978 the U.S. Supreme Court in the *Bakke* case, although recognizing the concept of affirmative action, held that the University of California's special admission procedure for minority applicants was invalid. The flaw in the University's special admission procedure for minority students was that it outright precluded nonminority applicants from consideration under its preferential admission procedure.

The next significant admission case, *Mississippi University for Women*, was decided in 1982 by the U.S. Supreme Court when it held that denying admission based solely on gender violated the Equal Protection Clause of the Fourteenth Amendment. In order for such a practice to overcome constitutional challenge, the objective must meet a "persuasive justification" test, and the means to achieve the objective must be valid.

Although most of the school catalog cases are instituted in dismissals, one case held that the wording in a catalog constituted a contractual offer and the school was duty bound to comply with its own terms.

DISMISSAL

The cases on dismissals illustrate a wide range of legal issues including the significance of a school catalog, honor code violations or other issues of integrity, academic and clinical failure and under what circumstances the courts will review these decisions, failure to grant a degree, and grade determination. Inherent in most of the cases is the application of the constitutional protection of the due process and equal protection clause of the Fourteenth Amendment. The Fourteenth Amendment protects "liberty" and "property" rights and is increasingly invoked in suits brought against educational institutions. A nursing education and the right to practice nursing are examples of constitutionally protected rights.

Early legal decisions afforded greater constitutional protection to public facilities than private institutions, and while this distinction is still recognized, it is not as compelling as previously.

Federal due process rights may not be applicable where the institution is private although factors such as participation in the federal student loan program are sufficient to show the necessary "state action" allowing application of federal law. In instances where the federal due process law does not apply, a state constitutional due process provision may offer similar protection for the student.

Due process rights are classified as either substantive or procedural and the dismissal cases involve both categories. *Procedural* rights may be violated as a result of failure on the part of the institution to provide an opportunity for a hearing prior to dismissal for disciplinary reasons. *Substantive* rights are violated where the student can demonstrate that the faculty acted with "bad faith" or in an arbitrary manner in citing specific grounds for dismissal.

The courts have refrained from becoming involved in matters of school dismissals for academic failure, unless the faculty acted in bad faith. In the matter of due process rights, the courts have made a distinction between dismissal or suspension for academic reasons as opposed to dismissals for disciplinary reasons. Due process rights attach to dismissals for non-academic reasons, such as discipline. However, case law holds that the application of due process rights are limited when the dismissal is based solely upon academic deficiency. Due process rights are limited to notice of impending failure, but do not include a right to a hearing after the fact of failing. In the absence of any contradicting school policy the courts view clinical experience determinations as part of the academic grade. Although there are few cases alleging bad faith in arriving at a clinical grade determination, the area may be vulnerable under the right factual situation.

In *Prendergast v. Rush-Presbyterian-St. Luke's Medical Center,* a master's degree student brought a suit against a college for unfairly denying her the right to continue her nursing education.[7] The criteria for graduation required that the student successfully complete three specific courses. She received a grade of "A" and "F" on two different term papers and was given a failing course grade. The college would not allow her to enroll in the next sequential required course and she instituted legal proceedings. She sought a court order to prevent the college from interfering with her continued studies, pending a review of her failing grade by the faculty. The grade review determined that "C" was a proper course grade and the court entered the following order: that the permanent grade be recorded as "C"; the plaintiff be reinstated as a student in the nursing program to fulfill the requirements for graduation; and that during the remaining course of studies, the plaintiff be treated in the same manner and graded according to the same standards and requirements as those imposed on other nursing graduate students. Accordingly, the plaintiff voluntarily dismissed the legal complaint against the university. She enrolled in the next nursing course, and received a "D" as a final grade. All other students received grades of "A" or "B." Thus, she filed an amended complaint, alleging that the university had induced her to dismiss her original suit by fraudulent misrepresentation, and had violated the court order. The defendant university was unsuccessful in arguing that the plaintiff's original complaint could not be reinstated because she had not been granted that right when the court issued their order. The student's original legal action was revived because the court determined that the terms for the dismissal of the original complaint was agreed on by the parties and the college was bound to comply with the specific conditions of the agreement.

School Catalog

A New York court, in *Atkin v. Traetta,* interpreting the specific language of a school catalog, held that a nursing school faculty had a responsibility to the public to create academic standards because the nursing courses involved clinical practice.[8] The students did not prevail in their suit. A group of nursing students at a community college, sought to enjoin the college from applying a grade change to them.

The nursing faculty of the associate degree program became concerned about the large number of students who lost matriculation or failed to graduate from the nursing program because of low grades in nursing courses. School policy then existing allowed a student to progress from one nursing course to another, even if they received a grade of "D-minus." A faculty group within the nursing department studied the grading policy and proposed a change which was accepted by the appropriate committees. The policy change required a grade of "C minus" before a student could progress to more advanced nursing courses. The policy, which was adopted in November 1972 and was to become effective in the fall of 1973, was communicated to the students via the school catalog, as well as by other school network means. Six students who received "D" grades and were prevented from enrolling in advanced nursing courses, sought to stop the college from applying the policy to them. Their argument was that they enrolled in the program prior to the change and the new policy was a "change in the curriculum under the terms of the catalog." A paragraph in the catalog stated that where the college has adopted a change in curriculum requirements, students who entered prior to the curriculum change have the option of conforming to either the new or old curriculum requirements.

The court addressed several issues including the right of the faculty to protect the public and the legal significance of a curriculum change when it alters the terms of a school catalog. A high court held that the faculty had acted in a reasonable manner in making the change and it did not arbitrarily effect the students because an extended period of time elapsed before it became effective. The students were put on notice of the change well in advance of its implementation. That court held that, "Under the terms of the catalog, the change didn't constitute a curriculum change. Even if it did, it appeared that the faculty was merely establishing minimum standards of academic competency in the public interest". A lower court had held that no harm would be done by maintaining the old grading standard because the state licensing examination would ultimately determine a nurses' fitness to practice. However, the higher court said that because the nursing program involved direct patient care and the licensing exam only assures minimum criteria, the faculty had a responsibility to establish minimum standards of academic competency to protect the public.

An important fact in the case was that there were two separate committees, one to study the curriculum and another to evaluate a student's academic standing. It was the Committee on Course and Standing, not the

Committee on Curriculum, which proposed the policy change. The college argued that grades were not germane to the "curriculum changes." The case involved a legal interpretation of specific wording in a school catalog and the court accepted the college's arguments in rejecting a practical construction on the meaning of the word "curriculum."

Lyons v. Salve Regina College dealt with the interpretation of the word "recommendation" which appeared in the college catalog and other school directives.[9] A senior nursing student, who had received "mostly A's and B's" in her studies, missed several days of a required nursing course which had a clinical component. The absence was not due to illness. The student alleged that she continued in the course after receiving assurance from an instructor that she would receive an "incomplete," and not an "F" grade at the end of the course. The instructor subsequently denied having given such assurance. When the student received the failing grade, she appealed to a three-member faculty committee, as stipulated in the college catalog, registration materials, and other academic information sources. The wording in the catalog which was relied on by the student read, "After the case is presented to the three-member grade appeals committee, the recommendation of the committee is made to the dean." A memorandum from the dean to the student stated that she could register conditionally but it would be revoked if the decision of the grade appeals committee went against her. Two members of the committee recommended that the student be given an "incomplete" with an opportunity to make up the missed course requirements, while the third member recommended that the failing grade stand and the student could apply for reinstatement. After receiving the committee's majority recommendation the dean dismissed the student from the nursing program. The student transferred to another program in the college and graduated with a degree in psychology.

Both parties to the legal action agreed that the rules of the college constituted a contract. The legal issue was whether the dean breached the contract by failing to follow the recommendation of the grade appeals committee. Ruling against the former nursing student, the court said that the term "recommendation" should not be converted from an expression of the committee's opinion into a mandatory order whereby the dean could not render the ultimate decision. In discussing whether the words in the catalog constituted language of a contractual nature the court said, "Principles of commercial contract law were not to be rigidly applied to construe provisions of the student catalog nor to define a contractual relationship between student and college."

In interpreting the language in school catalogs, the cases have generally held that the law of contracts need not be rigidly applied in all its aspects, even though some elements of the commercial contract doctrine may be used in identifying the student-university relationship. The relationship is unique and it must necessarily be different at different schools and not bound by strict commercial principles. However, there may be a more persuasive argument for applying strict contract principles when the student–university relationship involves private schools.[10]

In *Mahavogsanan v. Hall* a graduate student from Thailand was successful in a suit to compel the granting of a degree.[11] The court agreed that the student's argument that the language found in the university's catalogue constituted a contract that was binding on the university. At the time of her enrollment the requirements for graduation were set out in the general school catalog. The university required completion of 60 hours of a prescribed course of studies with a grade of at least "B." When the student began her studies, a provision in the catalog stated: "Academic regulations, other than degree requirements, are subject to change at the end of any quarter. A student will normally satisfy the degree requirements of the catalog in effect at the time of entrance." The university, applying a new policy, withheld her degree, pending a satisfactory completion of a comprehensive examination of her course work. The university maintained that the examination was not a degree requirement, but simply a standard of performance to evaluate her ability to master the subject matter. The university argued that it reserved the right to change or add standards of performance at any time.

The student was told of the additional requirement 2 weeks before the first comprehensive examination date and only 6 weeks prior to completion of the last of her course work. The court found that the change was not a modification of an academic regulation, but was, in fact, a change in the requirements for a degree. In view of the student's language problem, the court found that the short notice of the examination requirement did not allow the student sufficient time to prepare for them. The comprehensive examinations tested abilities and materials which she may not have necessarily received during her course work. The court did not find fault with the increased requirement applied prospectively, but only to their retroactive application to the plaintiff whose language problem accentuated the hardship caused by the lack of notice. The lack of timely notice constituted a lack of due process.

In *University of Texas Health Science Center v. Babb*, a Texas court ordered the university to apply the academic standards as set forth in the 1978–1979 school catalog which was the year the plaintiff student entered its nursing program.[12] At the time the student entered the nursing program classes were conducted under the semester system and the catalog provided that if a student's grade-point average for the total number of hours falls below 2.0 the student will be placed on scholastic probation. It further provided that a student could obtain a degree by complying with the requirements in the catalog in effect when the program was begun or the catalog governing any subsequent year, provided that the student completes the work for the degree within six years of the date of the applicable catalog. A subsequent revision in the 1979–1981 catalog contained a restriction that was not in the earlier catalog. The new restriction read, "A student with more than two D's in the quarter will be required to withdraw."

Just before the end of the 1979 fall term the student was told she was failing one of her courses. She was advised to withdraw and seek readmission. She did so and reentered under the school's newly organized quarter program. However, she received a "withdraw failing" grade for her fall, 1979 semester grades. She then successfully completed a total of six 3-hour courses under the new quarter system in order to make up the withdraw failing grade.

During the course of study under the quarter system the student received two "D's" and she was dismissed from the program. She was not permitted to discuss her dismissal with the dean. In her subsequent suit the student argued that the 1979–1981 catalog, with its "no more than two D's" requirement, should not apply to her as she originally entered under the 1978–1979 catalog criteria. The student did not argue that the university standards were unreasonable or that the University could not change its promotional standards. Her argument was that she should not have been judged by the 1979–1981 criteria.

The Texas court held that the university's catalog constituted a written contract and the student had a right to rely on the 1978–1979 retention and promotional terms created by the university. The 1978–1979 catalog did not permit the university to dismiss a student based on the number of bad grades; it only required a student to maintain a 2.0 grade-point average.

The school catalog may set out rules and regulations dealing with other than academic standards, and violation of the rules may be grounds for dismissal. A Massachusetts court held that violation of a reasonable college rule was sufficient grounds to dismiss a student in the last semester of his senior year.[13] In *Coveney v. President and Trustees of Holy Cross College,* the school had a rule, published in the student handbook, which prohibited students from interfering with the rights of other students. In the case the violation occurred when the plaintiff went into a female student's dormitory room without permission and later refused the rightful occupants from entering the room. The rightful occupant of the room had become intoxicated at a dormitory party and had been taken to her room by friends. The plaintiff, a male student, and two other male students went to her room and prevented other students, including a rightful occupant, from entering the girl's room by holding the door closed. The plaintiff never gave an explanation of his presence in the room.

The student dean informed the plaintiff that he could voluntarily withdraw from the school or face expulsion. Before the student was expelled he requested a hearing before the college judicial board which was refused. He then filed suit and obtained a temporary restraining order from the court which permitted the student to temporarily attend classes. The student was then granted a hearing before the president of the college. The college asked the student to dismiss the court suit in consideration for the hearing, and sign a release holding the college harmless from any liability for future disciplinary actions. The student signed the release. After the hearing the college president upheld the expulsion. Of the other two male students involved in the incident, one voluntarily withdrew and the other received his degree, but at a later date.

In reviewing the case, the state high court held that the college did not violate any of the plaintiff's due process rights and the release was valid. Upholding the recognized legal rule that a college, even a private one, may not arbitrarily or capriciously dismiss a student, the court held the college regulation was a recognized ground for dismissal. The court held that a college must have broad discretion in determining the appropriate range of sanctions for a policy violation. Addressing the plaintiff's argument that permitting one of the students to graduate was arbitrary as to the plaintiff, the court held that differences in discipline may reasonably exist. The student who was permitted to graduate did not bar entry into the room.

Courts have regarded terms set forth in school catalogs as binding contracts. A few, however, have held that the language in the catalog should not be rigidly applied in all its aspects. Sometimes the courts will go beyond the language in the catalog as it did in the *Atkin v. Traetta* case and permit a college to change its promotional standards and make them retroactive where the nursing courses involved a clinical practice component. This was done in the *Atkin* case because the college owed a "responsibility to the public." The threshold question must always be whether the rule or change in rule was reasonable and whether implementation of the rule is done with fundamental fairness.

Scholastic Achievement and Clinical Performance

The courts have been uniform in refusing to review the manner of grading a student or the setting of degree requirements. In matters of scholarship, the school authorities are uniquely qualified by training and experience to judge a students performance. However, the courts will offer relief in instances where the student can show that the college acted in bad faith. Review will be granted by the courts where the decision, supposedly for academic deficiency, was in fact made arbitrarily, capriciously, and in bad faith. The first reported case was brought by a medical student against a Vermont college in 1965.

In *Connelly v. University of Vermont and State Agricultural College*, a third-year medical student, dismissed from school, alleged that the dismissal was based on reasons other than the quality of his class and clinical work.[14] He had received grades of 82 and 87 in a pediatrics-obstetrics course prior to an illness which caused him to lose a month of course work. He made up the work, but was advised on completion that he had failed and could not proceed to the fourth year. His petition to the college's committee on advancement for permission to repeat his third year's work was denied. The student argued that his teacher determined, in advance of the make-up work, that he would not give plaintiff a passing grade regardless of the quality of his prior work or make-up tests. The student alleged that his work in the course was comparable to and in many instances superior to the work of other students who received a passing grade. The court, in ruling that there appeared to be genuinely disputed issues of fact, held that the student had a right to have the issue of bad faith on the part of the College tried in court. In this precedent-setting case, the court said that, generally, it would not review cases where the student was delinquent in his studies or was unfit for the practice of medicine because it viewed such matters to be wholly within the jurisdiction of the school authorities as the college, and not the courts, is in the best position to evaluate the proper standard of scholarship and a student's ability. However, the court ruled that where the school authorities are motivated by malice or bad faith in dismissing the student, or where the dismissal was arbitrary or capricious, the issue is one that is subject to judicial review.

In 1971, a foreign student studying veterinary medicine brought a legal suit to compel a university to give him a degree.

The court in *Balogun v. Cornell University* refused to substitute its judgment for the college's academic committee where the facts showed that the student be ranked last in his class and had had difficulty throughout the entire program, especially with clinical requirements.[15] After reviewing his academic performance the faculty voted 39 to 1 not to graduate the student. They also voted not to allow him to register for any more courses in the program. The University had published in the school catalog that it reserved the right to review student progress. The catalog included a statement which said that the college has a responsibility to maintain a standard of excellence as determined by the faculty and, although a weighted average of 70 percent is passing, a determination that a student has done satisfactory or unsatisfactory work is based on an appraisal of the student's record and potential. The record showed that the standard procedures of review of academic achievement and professional potential were equally applied to all members of the plaintiff's class. The faculty showed that their actions were a rightful exercise of honest discretion in the review of his performance. The student was unable to show gross error on the part of the faculty.

In *Greenhill v. Bailey*, a former medical student alleged that he had been deprived of his due process rights when he was not allowed to appear before hearings for promotion into his final year of study.[16] The plaintiff, who was admitted as an advanced student, had not been originally accepted into the school because he ranked below its required grade average. He was, however, accepted in the College of Osteopathic Medicine and Surgery and he ranked near the bottom of his class for the 2 years he was there. After his transfer to the medical program his academic record was weak. He passed a pediatric course with the lowest grade, twice failed an obstetric and gynecology course, and failed a clerkship in internal medicine. The plaintiff alleged that his dismissal, without a hearing, was improper. He alleged that the fact that he passed Part II of the National Boards demonstrated that the faculty acted arbitrarily and in bad faith. Ruling in favor of the college, the court said faculty judgments were not based on any single test and that many factors are involved in the determination that a person has or does not have the ability to function successfully as a physician. The court found that faculty judgment was based on close personal contact with the student and observation of conduct on patient rounds, handling of their cases, responses to actual medical problems, and other pertinent matters. The court stated: "The plaintiff's difficulties were foreseeable. In view of his academic history, the student's admission was an error which should not be compounded by requiring the medical school to keep and graduate a student who in the collective judgment of proper authorities is not qualified." In responding to the student's allegation that he had no prior notice of failing the clerkship, the court held the decision was not made until he completed the clerkship. The fact that he had daily discussions, conferences, and suggestions made should have alerted the plaintiff to his impending problems.

In the past, nursing faculty have been somewhat concerned about failing a student in the clinical component of a course because, unlike a written test evaluation, a significant portion of the evaluation process is based upon subjective data. It is not uncommon for a student to achieve good grades in the classroom, but be unable to apply essential health care knowledge to a patient care situation. This is frequently identified by faculty as a failure to demonstrate sufficient clinical aptitude for professional practice.[17] Even though an evaluation is more subjective than objective, the courts will lean toward academic freedom and independence of educational management. The burden of proof that a school had a bad motive in the dismissal is on the student who is alleging that fact.

In *Gaspar v. Bruton*, a student in a practical nursing program sought a permanent restraining order to prevent the school from dismissing her because of clinical inaptitude.[18] Two weeks after being informed of her dismissal she brought suit, alleging deprivation of due process, and that her dismissal was unreasonable, and capricious. The student was placed on probation at the completion of two-thirds of the program and was dismissed 2 months later. When she was placed on probation she was advised that she had to correct a number of identified deficiencies or she would be dismissed. On the day of her dismissal, she met with the superintendent and three of her instructors who informed her of the fact. Subsequently she was given a detailed justification for the action by the superintendent and informed that she could question the instructors who were then available, but she declined.

The school was successful in obtaining a judgment in its favor by showing that, although the student was a "B" student in the classroom, she could not achieve a number of course and school objectives. The school maintained that the student's performance in the clinical area was unsatisfactory and submitted the written evaluations of at least five instructors who wrote that, in their opinion, she could not properly function as a practical nurse. The areas of unsatisfactory performance included inability to prioritize assignments, failure to adequately observe postoperative patients and monitor their care, inability to carry out proper aseptic technique when caring for newborns and patients with infections, and a continuing inability to accurately record patient findings. Course and level objectives identified clinical practice areas which the student would need to master to remain in good standing. In a hearing before the Board of Education, at the request of the student's attorney, the student did not call any witnesses on her behalf and generally denied the alleged clinical deficiencies attributed to her. In addressing the due process issue, the court said that such a right vested with the student by virtue of the fact that a contractual relationship existed between the student and the school, as well as the fact that the school was a public facility. However, in a legal sense, the student was provided much more due process than is necessary in cases involving academic termination or suspension. "All that is required is that the student be made aware prior to termination of his failure or impending failure to meet those standards. The faculty were required to examine the students to determine whether they performed to the conditions entitling them to a diploma. Their decisions are conclusive, providing that their action has been in good faith."

When a school issues a diploma or degree to its students it, in effect, certifies to society that the student possesses the knowledge and skills necessarily required to practice a given discipline.

In *McIntosh v. Manhattan Community College*, the court held that it would not substitute its opinion for the college's policy that no student should receive a nursing degree unless the student passes a required nursing course.[19] The student received a failing grade of 69.713 and the passing grade was 70.00. The student who had taken the course twice petitioned the court to either rule on whether two of her "incorrect" answers were correct or to "round-off" her grade to a passing grade. The court held that the refusal to round-off the grade was not arbitrary or capricious. Responding to the plaintiff's argument that an examination question that required her to choose between two possible correct answers as a means of testing the student's judgment was not arbitrary. In addition, the plaintiff failed to offer any evidence that would demonstrate that her two answers were as correct or more correct than the designated answers.

In spite of detailed promotional policies, some students reach the end of their educational program before they are dismissed. It is not uncommon for faculty to promote students who are marginal in hope that they will attain increased proficiency as they progress in the program. The courts recognize that, particularly in the health care professions, public interest requires that the school graduate students who have attained identified educational goals. However, there are limitations on the right of a university to withhold a degree.

In *Jansen v. Emory University*, a former dental student, who had been conditionally promoted to his final year of study, brought suit against a private university, alleging violation of his due process rights when he was dismissed at the end of the last quarter.[20] He ranked 103 out of 106 students and had repeated his junior year. At that time he was informed that his progress would be evaluated quarterly and he would be dismissed if acceptable progress was not shown. During his senior year he was advised that his "standards, conscientiousness and professional integrity" were in question as a result of several documented patient care situations. He received a "D" in the fall and winter clinical courses. Just prior to the faculty vote to dismiss him the dean of the dental school had signed papers certifying that he was expected to graduate and thus be eligible to take the dental licensing exam. The university catalog included the statement, "Attendance at Emory is a privilege and not a right, however, no student will be dismissed without Due Process." The student argued that the due process he received was deficient. The court, ruling in favor of the university, held that the wording in the catalog was not meant to include expansive due process rights in view of the fact that the university was private. The court said that the university did not waive its right to dismiss a student by promoting him. In view of his academic history, the student knew his progress would be evaluated and he could not complain when the judgment of the faculty ultimately was unfavorable to him.

Illinois state law stipulated that the granting of a degree by a state-run university was discretionary and not mandatory. However, where the student could show that the university acted maliciously and in bad faith by arbitrarily refusing to award a degree, the court will provide the student with a legal remedy. The plaintiff in *Tanner v. Board of Trustees of University of Illinois* was a Ph.D. candidate and had completed the required course work, including the submission of a written doctoral dissertation.[21] A thesis committee was formed to evaluate the student's dissertation and to conduct comprehensive oral and written examinations. After completing his oral examination, he completed the written examinations which had been submitted by three members of the five member evaluation committee. The student was then informed that he would have to be reevaluated in a single, written examination. When he agreed to this requirement, he was informed that the examination would contain an oral, as well as a written component. A short time later, he was told that he would have to begin the entire evaluation process because his initial thesis examinations and dissertation were unacceptable because the thesis committee was never formally recognized by the graduate college. Although state law precluded the awarding of money damages because the college was a state-run facility the court held that the student was entitled to legal redress.

In 1978, the U.S. Supreme Court in *Board of Curators of University of Missouri v. Horowitz* held that no hearing was required to dismiss a medical student at a publicly supported university for an academic deficiency.[22] The Supreme Court has not determined what process is due a student attending a professional school who suffers a disciplinary dismissal. However, the Supreme Court has held that high school students, facing a 10-day suspension for misconduct, were entitled to "some kind of notice" as well as "some kind of hearing."[23] The court said that procedural due process would be satisfied by an informal meeting held shortly after the misconduct. The due process requirements may be satisfied, even if held minutes after the misconduct, if the student is informed of the alleged misbehavior and allowed to present his version of the situation.[24] Where the dismissal on disciplinary grounds involves an extended period of time, the due process safeguards must necessarily be more extensive. This is particularly true, when the disciplinary measures will preclude the student from progressing to the next successive course or delay graduation.

Honor Codes

Most schools include in their published materials statements on academic honesty, as well as the disciplinary measures for violation of the honor code. An honor code is particularly important when the educational program is one which prepares a person in one of the health care disciplines because of the public trust placed in health care providers. Dismissal for nonacademic reasons, such as an honor code violation, requires broader application of due process rights. Mere notice that a student is being dismissed for an honor code violation will not suffice. The student has a right to a formal appeal procedure including the right to question witnesses and have witnesses testify in his behalf.

In *Slaughter v. Brigham Young University*, a student attending a private university was dismissed for a violation of the school's rules of conduct.[25] The honor code stipulated that students should observe "high principles of honor, integrity and morality" and be honest in all behavior. The university, a religious affiliation, identified honest behavior as, "not cheating, plagiarizing or knowingly giving false information." The student, a doctoral candidate, used his professor's name as co-author of articles the student had written. In fact, he had done all the work on which the articles were based before coming to the university and the professor did not participate in either the preparation or review of the articles. The student had previously been unsuccessful in getting the articles published using his own name. The court found that the regulations were reasonable, clear and definite, and the due process requirements for a hearing were met.

An Ohio case, *Bleiker v. Board of Trustees of Ohio State University* upheld the dismissal of a student after a finding that she had received adequate notice and a hearing prior to her discharge.[26] The student, who was a veterinary student in her last year of study at a tax-supported university, had been accused of violating the university's honor code. The student was dismissed for two semesters and her readmission was contingent upon certification of normal health status. She was receiving psychiatric counseling. The honor code provision forbid the "misrepresenting of one's work or fraudulently or unfairly advancing one's academic status." An instructor reported that changes in the student's examination answer sheet violated the honor code. At one stage of the hearing, a psychiatrist, employed by the university and who had seen the student, expressed an opinion that, rather than an attempt to deceive, the student was manifesting a typical stress response. The student was notified of the hearing 3 days in advance and had a witness testify in her behalf. At the hearing she was allowed to examine the examination sheet in question and had the opportunity to question the instructor who filed the code violation complaint.

The court agreed that extended or permanent dismissals require formal procedures. The issue confronting the court was "just how much more formality is guaranteed by the Fourteenth Amendment." The court translated that question into the following test: "Were the procedures used sufficient to protect the student from an erroneous deprivation of her property interest to continue her education without interruption?" The court found that, under the facts of the case, the student was afforded procedural protections which would keep at a minimum, the risk of erroneous deprivation of her interests. However, the court stated that the University would be well advised to adopt, as a matter of routine, the additional procedures the plaintiff sought to invoke. Such formal procedures, the court said, may contribute significantly to protecting important private interests. The procedural safeguards which the plaintiff's counsel alleged should have been provided include a written statement of the allegation; a written record of the hearing with a detailed written statement of the findings; inspection of physical evidence, such as her examination sheet, prior to the hearing; representation by her own legal counsel; and notice of the hearing well in advance of the scheduled date.

Physical Incapacity

The trend has been that the courts will more closely review cases where the dismissal is for a cause unrelated to academic performance. The courts recognize the importance of higher education to professional advancement and employment opportunities and it will scrutinize the actions of educational institutions in nonacademic dismissals.

The court in *Tedeschi v. Wagner College* held that a student should have been afforded the opportunity of a formal hearing where the dismissal from a private college was for disciplinary reasons.[27] The student had been dismissed because of her irrational and disruptive conduct in classes. The court did not invoke any constitutional right, but rather relied on the published rules of the college. The guidelines provided that in the event a student is suspended or expelled for any cause other than academic failure, he will have the right to be heard by a student–faculty hearing board. The guidelines further stipulated that the board would then present its findings to the college president for a final determination. Although the college had met informally with the student, it did not comply with its own procedural rules. Ordinarily, a hearing serves the purpose of allowing both parties in a dispute to air their conflicting versions of the events so that a balanced judgment can be formed. The student should have had the opportunity to justify her behavior, and the informal meetings, although held with administrative faculty, were not considered an acceptable substitute for the hearing board. The court held that the published guidelines would be reduced to a meaningless exercise if the administrative officials could avoid its own rules by substituting a procedure which provided less protection than the guidelines.

An earlier case, *Grimard v. Carlston*, held that informal meetings with the school authorities were sufficient, where the forced withdrawal resulted from a temporary physical impairment which interfered with the clinical component of the nursing program.[28] The plaintiff was enrolled in a four-semester nursing program at a state community college. The school's policy required the immediate withdrawal of any student who became unacceptable to the program for health reasons. The student fractured his ankle 2 months into the second semester and had to use first, crutches and then a cane. The clinical instructor said that it was impossible for the student to do the necessary patient care activities in a safe manner. The school authorities held several informal discussions with both the student and his attorney, but they maintained the position that the course would have to be completed after the student recovered from his accident. The student's suit sought to enjoin the forced withdrawal and, in addition, sought to compel the school to provide him with remedial help to catch up with missed coursework. The court held that the student's continued enrollment constituted a property interest, but that interest was not violated, even though the hearing was informal. The court found that the school's strong interest in protecting patients from potential harm resulting from the student's physical incapacity warranted the forced withdrawal. Further, the school's decision not to allow him to do clinical assignments was appropriate to protect patients even in advance of a hearing. A more formal hearing would not have contributed to the school's determination of the student's ability to perform the patient care activities.

In a recent case involving the dismissal of a nursing student from a private Rhode Island college a federal district court held that the young woman's suit should not be dismissed.[29] The defendants in *Russell v. Salve Regina College* had argued that they were entitled to have the suit dismissed without a trial on the merits. The nurse sued the college and seven faculty members including the dean and a clinical coordinator. She sought to recover damages for loss of income and for intentional infliction of emotional distress. She relied on both federal and Rhode Island law in her claim.

The woman was admitted to the private college by early decision and began her studies in September 1982. At her admissions interview she told the school that she planned to matriculate in the nursing program. The curriculum of the college was designed so that the student would initially concentrate in liberal arts studies and the nursing curriculum would begin at the beginning of the second year. According to health records in the college's health services unit the plaintiff was 5 feet 6 inches in height and weighed slightly over 300 pounds. She maintained "respectable" grades throughout the program.

When the student began the formal nursing program in the fall of 1983 (her sophomore year), the college alleged her weight became a problem which interfered with her clinical responsibilities. There was a problem getting uniforms and scrub gowns. The faculty made use of the student to demonstrate nursing procedures incident to the care of obese patients. During this period the faculty had discussions with the student and lectured her about the desirability of weight loss. The student categorized these frequent and prolonged discussions as "torment" and "humiliation," whereas the faculty described the activities as "expressions of concern" or "forthright statements of school policy."

At the beginning of her junior year in the fall of 1984 the student entered into a contract that stipulated that her continuation in the nursing program was contingent on her losing 2 pounds a week. Under the terms of the contract the student was to meet with the clinical coordinator weekly with "evidence of progress in the weight loss program." However, her weight never fell appreciably below 300 pounds. An escalating level of tension developed between the plaintiff and some of the defendants. In August 1985 the student received a letter from the coordinator advising her that she was being dismissed from the nursing program. The student resumed her nursing studies at another school and completed the program without incident.

The federal court held that the woman's claims based on violation of her due process rights and an unconstitutional interference with her protected liberty and property rights could not prevail nor could her claim of discrimination of a handicapped person prevail. This was because the college which was private was not a "state actor." In order for the private institution to come within the constitutional mandates or federal law the plaintiff would have had to show their activities constituted "state action." Although the college was the recipient of a library grant and its nursing program was subject to approval by a state agency, these were deemed insufficient to constitute a state action. The "requirement of 'state action' demands more than some (modest) interplay between the public and private sectors." In striking down the handicapped discrimination claim, the court said that a college which received federal funding only indirectly, for example, through tuition subsidies to students. would only be subject to suit for violation of its financial aid program indiscretions. The plaintiff did not allege that the college discriminated against her in matters affecting scholarship assistance or other financial aid. In fact, the college received an "insignificant" amount of money to administer its Pell Grants (student loan program) which the court found too little to constitute a "funding of the school's nursing program" as required under the federal discrimination law. Thus, the court held that the student had no rights under either the federal constitution or federal law.

Further, the court held that the woman's claim that the college in dismissing her lacked "good faith and fair dealing" in its relationship with her must fail because the state does not recognize wrongful dismissals based on this theory of recovery. However, the court held that the woman's claim of *intentional* infliction of emotional harm was recognized given her claim that she suffered nightmares, sleeplessness, nausea, vomiting, diarrhea, gastric upset, and hypoglycemic attacks in the wake of the defendant's conduct. In alleging intentional infliction of emotional harm the plaintiff must show that the defendant's actions were "outrageous in character" and so extreme in degree that they go beyond all possible bounds of decency. The test the courts frequently apply is that "recitation of the facts to an average member of the community would arouse his resentment against the actor, and lead him to exclaim, 'outrageous!'."[30] However, a claim for *negligent* infliction of emotional distress would not prevail because the state did not recognize the legal theory in either state law or case law.

The court also held that the relationship between the plaintiff and the college was such that the plaintiff could reasonably have expected to be allowed a considerable degree of privacy, at least to intimate and personal matters. In addition, the state has a privacy act in effect since 1980.[31] The privacy law states that the invasion must be of "something that is entitled to be private or would be expected to be private." The court stated that the fact of the woman's obesity was obvious, but the college's "continual" inquiry into her progress with the diet, scrutiny of her personal weight loss records, exaggerated interest in her diet, and preoccupation with her perceived lack of self-discipline were grounds for a jury to find invasion of privacy.

In her claim against the college itself the court found that the relationship between the student and the university is contractual in nature and this came into existence when the student began her matriculation. The plaintiff alleged nonperformance of an agreement to educate. The court looked to whether the "implied" agreement between the college and the student was sufficient to support this claim. The college argued unsuccessfully that the woman failed to comply with the requirements in the college handbook which required each student to inform the clinical coordinator of any health problems. In fact, before a clinical placement, each student was to sign a form prepared by the college that vouchsafes full disclosure of any medical abnormalities. In accordance with the handbook, the coordinator has discretion to determine whether a student's participation in the clinical area is contraindicated because of health reasons. The form signed by all students states "I will accept the decision of the Clinical Agency Coordinator and Department Chairman as final as to whether or not I can function in the Clinical Area."

The court found that the college has an obvious interest in ensuring that no student poses a health risk to herself or others, however, the court said that the only possible bases for prohibiting the woman from her clinical experience were either "(a) that her obesity would impede satisfactory performance of her duties, or (b) that her appearance would be a poor example for patients." The court said that it was for a jury to determine whether the decision to expel the woman, at least as it relates to the handbook language, was the product of reason or caprice. In short, it was a factual issue for the triers of fact whether the school's claim that the woman's obesity reduced her proficiency to such an extent so as to justify her dismissal. The college argued that the student failed a required clinical course "directly related" to her obesity. There was an allegation that her weight hindered her ability to perform such tasks as the administration of CPR.[32] The woman introduced evidence that the day before the dismissal a letter was sent to the school in which a supervisor at a Connecticut hospital where the woman had been working wrote that she "looked and acted in a very professional manner. Her attendance was excellent and her performance very good. I would be most pleased to hire her as a professional nurse. In fact, I expect to be able to offer her a position for June of 1986."

Addressing the document signed by the woman in which she agreed to lose 2 pounds each week the court said the contract is "at best a useful piece of evidence to assist in constructing the jigsaw of contractual terms, and at worst a piece of paper which is meaningless except as proof of the defendant's malevolence." The validity of the execution of the contract may be weakened by such factors as the student's allegation of duress and coercion and her state of mind at the time she signed it.

In sum, the court held that the woman had no rights based on due process or discrimination rights as federal laws were not applicable. However, she did have rights as guaranteed by the state's privacy act, as well as rights grounded in intentional infliction of emotional harm and nonperformance of an agreement to educate. Thus, the court held that her suit should proceed to be heard at a trial on its merits.

Summary

The number of legal theories available to a student challenging a dismissal from a school are more extensive than those available for an admission criteria challenge. In addition, the law makes a distinction between a private school (one not receiving tax monies) and a public facility. A tax supported school must comply with the federal constitution guarantee of due process rights. Of course, where a private school has provided for due process protection the courts will enforce such provisions. In addition, a number of courts have held that basic due process rights apply, even to private schools.[33] The courts may also require due process rights of a private school where the school receives public monies, thus making the school a "state actor" for the purpose of applying constitutional protection for the student. The courts have also held that they will not become involved in academic dismissals unless the plaintiff can show that the school acted in bad faith.[34] Due process rights also apply to academic dismissals as well as disciplinary dismissals. The reason the courts are reluctant to interfere in academic dismissals is because they believe that the school and its faculty is in the best position to set its own academic standards.

Case law has held that a school may change its academic or degree requirements during a student's course of study, but notification to the student must be timely. Academic changes, especially in programs where the safety of the public is involved, will be upheld. Where a university changes its published academic criteria the courts will review the wording in both the old and new catalog. The wording contained in the school catalog and other academic information sources will be closely scrutinized by the courts in the academic dismissal cases. In addition, courts will look at the facts of the case to determine whether the school fairly implemented the new policy. Where, however, a catalog contains language permitting a student already enrolled to comply with either the old or new criteria the student will not be required to meet the new criteria.

Some nursing and medical students have challenged their dismissal because of a clinical failure. The courts will not find for the plaintiff unless it is shown that the student was unaware of his failing status. Also, the courts will not fault a school for promoting a marginal student and subsequently finding that the student has not demonstrated academic or clinical growth. A school is permitted to review a student's collective progress and finding deficiencies the subsequent dismissal will be upheld.

NONACADEMIC SUITS AGAINST SCHOOLS

A law student in *Wilson v. Continental Insurance Company* brought a negligence suit against a university, alleging that a program in mind control caused him to have serious mental problems.[35] The university offered the course to minority law students to assist them in establishing study habits and other behavior discipline deemed necessary for success in the program. Before the course was arranged, the school asked the university counseling center to determine whether they wanted to recommend the course. The center gave the program an "adverse recommendation," but did not cite reasons for its lack of endorsement. The university went ahead with the program. The student, who had no history of any mental problems, suffered serious psychologic problems 3 weeks after beginning the course. He had to undergo 6 months of psychiatric treatment. On return to the law school, he suffered similar psychiatric problems and had to withdraw again. He alleged, among other things, that the university was negligent in not doing any prepsychologic evaluation tests prior to the course. The court, ruling in favor of the university, said that no legal duty existed on the part of the school to protect the student from a harm that was not foreseeable. To require the University to conduct base-line psychological tests on its students would place an unreasonable burden on the educational system. The court noted that mental disturbances can be caused by a myriad of reasons, particularly with the rigors of law school.

In suits challenging school policy, the courts have held that the policy must be reasonable to be valid.

In *Sellman v. Baruch College of City University of N.Y.*, a student enrolled in a city college instituted a legal action to have the student bylaws invalidated.[36] The student government constitution required candidates for elective office to be registered for a minimum of 12 credits and maintain a 2.5 grade average. The plaintiff had a 2.1 average and was a part-time student enrolled for 6 credit hours. He alleged that the bylaws infringed upon his constitutional rights. In ruling in favor of the college, the court held that the fundamental purpose of the institution was to educate students and the bylaws further promoted the legitimate interests of the college. There existed a legitimate interest in limiting the elective position to those students whose ties to the School demonstrated a sufficient degree of commitment to and participation in school affairs. Full-time students comprised 90 percent of the student body and it was not unreasonable to take the position that a student taking less than 12 hours would be unable to adequately understand or represent the interests of the full-time students. The court said that participation in student government activities is a demanding and time-consuming endeavor. It is reasonable to conclude that involvement in such time-consuming activities may be detrimental to the academic progress of those students whose grades are only barely above the passing grade. The purpose of the bylaw was not to penalize, but to direct the students energies towards academic studies and to insure that those who govern are not forced into early resignation by academic failure.

In another suit, *Swidryk v. Saint Michael's Medical Center,* a first year resident in obstetrics and gynecology sued the medical education director at the hospital where the resident was serving his residency in obstetrics for education malpractice.[37] The resident was sued for malpractice in the delivery of a baby and blamed the director for alleged inadequacies in the program. In initiating suit against the director the resident alleged that he was negligent in failing to properly supervise the resident program and that he breached a contractual duty to provide a suitable environment for the obstetric educational experience. The court held that the resident failed to state a cause of action in either contract or tort law which is recognized. In addition, the court stated that it would be against public policy to review the day-to-day management of graduate medical programs and the system in place to assure quality medical education was sufficient. State laws existed which provided for review and implementation of medical education.

Summary

Nonacademic suits are far less prevalent than those instituted for alleged admission or dismissal wrongs. Of course, a suit in negligence for a physical injury sustained by the student can always be brought.

STUDENT LOANS

There are a number of issues associated with student loans which are of concern to nursing schools. All of these revolve around the collection of the loans or the appropriateness of measures taken by schools to compel students to repay their loans. In recent years the government has begun to crack down on both schools and debtors because of the misuse of education loans and the failure on the part of the students to repay the loans.

Student loans are administered by the Education Department and the Veterans Administration. Schools have been faulted for retaining students whose grade-point average is less than 2.0 and for otherwise not enforcing their own academic standards.[38] Recently governmental officials have begun to file civil suits against debtors who have defaulted on student loans or failed to pay other educational benefits.[39] In 1981 the U.S. Senate asked the General Accounting Office (GAO) to do an indepth study of the loan collection problems in the Health Professions and Nursing Student Loan Programs.[40] The GAO's study faulted the schools for placing too little emphasis on collecting the loans. In response to the GAO study, the Department of Health and Human Service's published policy was that after March 1983 schools exceeding a 5 percent collection delinquency rate would receive no new program funds and would be unable to issue new loans.

Because most of the student loan cases arise from the bankruptcy courts it is helpful to understand a few basic concepts for enacting the Federal Bankruptcy Code. The code was enacted to make it easier for businesses and individuals to obtain relief from overwhelming debts. Because the Bankruptcy Code is a federal law its legislative purpose (to provide relief) cannot be circumvented. The law established a right to declare bankruptcy and precludes penalizing one who has had a debt discharged by a bankruptcy proceeding. The objective of the code is to give debtors a "new opportunity in life and a clear field for future effort, unhampered by the pressure and discouragement of pre-existing debts."[41]

Not all debts are automatically discharged when an individual files bankruptcy. Student educational loans are not discharged unless the debtor can prove that payment of the loan will impose an undue hardship on him or his dependents. In many of the cases the ex-student has invoked a constitutional protection.

> In *Lee v. Board of Higher Education in the City of New York* a student challenged the constitutionality of a city college's policy of denying transcripts to those students who, rather than repaying an education loan, had obtained a discharge of the loan obligation in bankruptcy court.[42] The court held that the policy deprived the student of the protection guaranteed by the equal protection clause of the U.S. Constitution. The case also held that the Bankruptcy Act, as a federal law, was supreme to the public college's administrative rules.

> In another case, *Matter of Bruce*, a university sought to get a court order preventing a student from discharging a loan in bankruptcy.[43] The university sought to have the loan categorized as the kind which was not covered by the federal Act. The bankruptcy court held that the student loan which was made directly by the university and was not insured or guaranteed by any federal agency was the type loan which could be discharged under the Bankruptcy Act.

Discharge of the student loan may have implication for the licensing or certification procedure.

> In *Application of Gahan*, an unmarried law school graduate, who had obtained a series of student loans under a federally funded guaranty program, was denied admission to the bar on grounds of insufficient moral character, after he had been permitted to discharge $14,000 in bankruptcy.[44] Or-

dinarily student loans are paid off or amortized over a 10-year period with 7 percent interest and in this case the student had agreed and expected to repay the loan after graduation. The student's payments were $175 monthly and he had no other debts.

Upon graduation from law school he was admitted to the practice of law in California and obtained a position which paid $14,000 for a period of 9 months after which he was out of work for a period of 2 months. During the time of employment he made some payments, but subsequently defaulted on the debt. He secured a loan from a bank which he paid off because he intended to borrow from the bank again in the future. During the 2-month layoff period he mortgaged a 1959 Jaguar automobile to a friend for a loan of $2500 and he deposited the sum in two credit-exempt savings accounts. He then filed for bankruptcy and the student loan was discharged.

After the discharge he secured another law position which paid $18,000. He subsequently applied for admission to the Minnesota bar and was denied admission. One of the criteria for admission stated that "no person shall be admitted to practice law who has not established to the satisfaction of the Board of Examiners that he is a person of good moral character." At issue in the case was whether the filing of the bankruptcy petition demonstrated a lack in moral character.

The court held that the *fact* of his bankruptcy may not be considered in judging his moral character and the bankruptcy proceeding itself should not be a basis for denying his admission. However, his actions, apart from the bankruptcy proceeding, demonstrated a disregard for the rights of others. He didn't pay debts even when he was reasonably able to do so. Applicants to the bar, said the court, who flagrantly disregard the rights of others and default on serious financial obligations, such as student loans, are lacking in good moral character if the default is neglectful, irresponsible and can not be excused by a compelling hardship that is reasonably beyond the control of the applicant. The court held that his failure to assume his obligations, when he was economically capable of doing so, reflected adversely on his ability to perform the duties of an attorney. The court noted that a student loan is entrusted to a person and repayment provides stability to the student-loan program and guarantees the continuance of the program for future student needs. A flagrant disregard is indicative of a lack of moral commitment to the rights of other students, as well as creditors. Such flagrant financial irresponsibility reflects adversely on the applicant's ability to manage financial matters, and subsequently a fitness to practice law. The court found that it was appropriate for the board to prevent problems from such irresponsibility by denying admissions, rather than seek to remedy the problem after it occurs and victimizes a client.

The *Gahan* case is contrasted with *Florida Board of Bar Examiners re: Groot* in which a discharge in bankruptcy did not prevent admission to the practice of law where it was shown that the applicant suffered a compelling hardship.[45] The applicant, who was recently divorced with two young children, had to support two households and had to borrow from his family when his own personal resources became exhausted. The court held that the circumstances surrounding the default justified the bankruptcy petition as the intent of the bankruptcy law was to allow him to use his money to meet present responsibilities and not past obligations.

There are a number of suits dealing with loan or scholarship repayment where the recipient failed to perform a "pay-back" service obligation.

In *U.S. v. Haithco* the government brought an action against a Michigan registered nurse because she failed to live up to the requirements of a National Health Services Corps (NHSC) scholarship requirement.[46] In 1978 while a student at the Michigan State University School of Nursing, the defendant applied for one of the NHSC scholarships. The scholarship program was established by Congress to promote health services in rural and urban underserved populations. The NHSC scholarship contract was signed by the defendant which obligated her to serve a 2-year period in an area designated by NHSC. She received $7432.00 for the academic year 1978 and $7610.40 for 1979. The defendant received materials specifically informing her of the pay-back obligation. Sixty days before her graduation, notice was sent to her reminding her of the obligation. According to the Corps she was to serve in the Indian Health Service (IHS) which meant that she would be providing services to American Indians or Alaskan Natives. According to federal laws and the contract language itself breach of the scholarship contract would result in the defendant paying three times the scholarship funds, plus interest. There was an waiver clause for extreme hardship or where compliance would be "unconscionable" or "impossible."

The NHSC notified the defendant that an IHS position facility was to open in Red Lake Hospital (Minnesota) in September, 1980, and asked the defendant to confirm her interest in this facility. The defendant completed her nursing program in June 1980. Attempts to negotiate with the nurse were unsuccessful and she was advised of the default clause in the NHSC contract. The nurse, then filed for waiver of the contract, citing hardship. However, she failed to supply the necessary documentation to support her waiver request. In March 1981 she was notified that she owed $45,127.20 (triple the $15,042.40 scholarship plus the accrued interest). Ultimately, the debt was referred to a collection agency. In October 1983 she was advised that if she committed herself to serve at an IHS site the obligation would be fulfilled, however the defendant failed to respond to this offer. Thus, a suit was instituted for the amount of $75,941.34.

The court held that the damage provision in the scholarship contract did not operate as an unenforceable penalty. It said that the nurse voluntarily and knowingly made a commitment in exchange for the funds and she reneged on that commitment. Noting that she had a right to seek a waiver she never followed through on sending the required information for processing of the waiver. The court said that it was irrelevant that she wanted a more convenient placement in terms of her family, her marriage, or her desire to further pursue her education. The scholarship program is ultimately designed to serve needs larger than the personal needs of the recipient. The court found that the defendant had earned between $21,000 and $25,000 yearly since 1983 and had incurred essentially no individual debt.

In a similar case against a physician, a federal court held that the failure of the government to accept pay-back service at a New York hospital, not in a medically underserved area, was not arbitrary and capricious.[47] The physician in *Mattis v. U.S.* received $40,000 in scholarship monies and had his pay-back obligation deferred while he completed a residency in emergency medicine. The court said that while the defendant would have preferred placement in New York or at one of the hospitals he identified as providing emergency care and at which he preferred to serve, he was contractually obligated to practice where the government assigned him.

In summary, the government, in order to continue a viable student loan program, has recently held both the schools and the debtor accountable. The schools have been cautioned to enforce their academic standards so that the monies will be applied to deserving applicants and further, to be more viligant in the collection of loans. The courts have closely scrutinized the motivation and circumstances in discharging a student loan debt. However, they have not permitted the use of bankruptcy in justified cases to serve to withhold transcripts or prevent licensure. There is also case law dealing with the validity of the penalty clause and the obligation clause of government scholarship loans. The government takes the position that the recipient receives a benefit from the government when the scholarship is given, and barring grounds for waiver the obligation to serve in a medically underserved area is firm. The case law is clear that while the NHSC may negotiate placement to some extent the recipient is obliged to serve where the government assigns the individual.

In 1987 the Department of Education notified recipients of student loans who are in default that they would be billed for the costs of collecting the obligation if legal proceedings are instituted.[48] The new policy applies to loans administered through the schools, not those from individual banks. This latest effort is made to collect on student loans, on Federally Insured Student Loans, and on the National Direct Student Loans program. Loans from financial institutions do not come within the new policy. In addition, in an attempt to more aggressively collect on student loans the government has confiscated the tax refunds of those in default and deducts payments from the paychecks of federal employees in default. Individuals who are 6 months behind in loan payments are considered in default. The default amounts were estimated to be $5.9 billion by mid-1987.

PRIVACY OF RECORDS

In 1974, Congress enacted the Family Educational Rights and Privacy Act, which is more commonly referred to as the Buckley Amendment.[49] The act specifically provides protection in two broad areas: individual access to educational records and release of educational records to third parties. Prior to this legislation neither students or their parents had access to the student's educational and school records. Before the federal law, a few states had enacted legislation which provided essentially the same protections as the 1974 law and a few provided greater protection than the federal law. However, most states did not provide any protection. If the federal law does not apply, an individual may be protected by existing state law. The federal law regulates only federally supported colleges and public school systems. Federal support may be in the form of student loans to the facility or monies in the form of federal grants. If the institution takes federal monies, the Buckley Amendment applies. A state law may provide more protection than the federal law, but it may not provide less. The federal law applies to students currently or previously enrolled in the institution.

The legislation denies federal funds to an educational institution that prevents parents or students over the age of 18 the right to review their records. The access provision only applies to materials provided after January 1975. Federal funds are also barred where the institution has a rule or practice of releasing certain information about the student without the written consent of the student or parent. If the parent claims the student as a tax deduction or assumes the financial responsibility of the education, then the parent has a right of access to the record, even in the absence of the student's consent. If the student is over 18, the records may be released to the parents, if the student consents. Students do not have a right to review the financial statement submitted by the parents, unless the parents have consented.

Access to academic and educational records includes the entire record, including health and counseling records. Interoffice memorandums are not considered part of the student record unless they are placed in the record. An applicant to a school does not have a right of access. The right to review the record does not vest until the student is accepted into the program. An applicant seeking to review any of his references would not be able to under the provisions of the federal law. Many schools discard information obtained during the admission process in the event the application is not accepted. A former student is also allowed access. Therefore, unless the right of access has been waived, the student has a right to review any references the facility receives or sends to third parties after the student has graduated from the school. Some educational facilities notify persons who have written letters of reference for inclusion in a former student's college placement file, that the individual has reserved the right of access.

The original legislation did not have a waiver of rights provision. Shortly after the legislation was enacted it was amended to allow students to waive their right of access to letters of reference. The amendment was included after educational groups expressed their concern about the value of letters of reference if the student had access to them once they were accepted into the school's program. Many school officials believed that letters of reference should be kept confidential between the university and the individual who wrote the letter. Universities frequently include the waiver forms in the materials sent to students applying for admission. However, the applicant need not sign the waiver. The waiver of the right of access to letters of reference cannot be made a condition for acceptance.

There are exceptions to the student or parent consent requirement when releasing educational records information to third parties. They include release to other school officials within the facility and having an educational interest in the record, state and federal regulatory agencies, officials of other schools in which the student intends to enroll, organizations that are reviewing the records for potential financial aid, educational researchers, and in compliance with a court order. There are two threshold requirements attached to these exceptions. First, the student's record must include the names of those requesting the specific information and their legitimate interest in acquiring the information, and second, the information is given only if the recipients promise not to disclose the information beyond the stated reason. This second requirement must be communicated in writing to the party requesting the information. A record of the names of those requesting information and their reasons must be kept within the student's files.

When a student makes a request to review the record the school must grant the request within 45 days and the school authorities may not destroy the records during this time. Where the requested document contains information on another student, the school authorities have the right to eliminate that information from the record before it is released. The right to inspect confers the right to take notes or have photocopies made. A school would be well advised to establish the protocol to be followed during the actual review process, and reasonable policies relevant to photocopy costs.

The act allows the student to have a record that contains inaccurate information amended. If the school refuses to correct the record, the student has a right to a formal hearing. The formal appeal process should be established by the school officials and communicated to the student in the school manual. Results of the formal hearing should be recorded and formalized in writing and copies given to the disputing parties. If the student disputes the results of the hearing, direct appeal can be made to the federal agency that administers the act.

Some information is not automatically considered confidential. Information which is public directory in nature may be released to third parties without the consent of the student. However, the nature of information that qualifies as "directory information" must be communicated to the student in order to provide the student sufficient opportunity to object to the release of specific directory information. Ordinarily, directory information, includes general information, such as, name, address, area of study, and participation in school activities, such as sports, clubs, and awards.

Summary

Prior to enactment of the Family Educational Rights and Privacy Act, only a few states had passed laws establishing similar rights and privacy provisions. The significance of a privacy law which existed prior to the 1974 federal act is that it may provide broader protection than the federal law and, so long as the state provisions do not conflict with the federal law, the state law must be complied with. The thrust of the federal act is that access to the student's record or family financial statements is regulated and there are limitations on release of such information to third parties. The penalty for noncompliance with the Federal Act is the denial of federal funds.

SUMMARY

The majority of the cases involving students and professionals schools deal with admission and dismissal procedures. Most of the admission cases are based upon the concept of affirmative action, and raise constitutional issues. Preferential treatment policies will survive constitutional scrutiny if the school can show that a substantial state interest justifies the policy. For example, the objective to provide needed medical services to a historically underserved group is an example of a compelling state interest. Also, the criteria for selection must consider the least objectionable alternatives in formulating the admission policy. In the *Alevy* case the court suggested that a less objectionable alternative may include placing a time limit on the special admission policy.

In 1978 the United States Supreme Court upheld the concept of affirmative action, but held that the special admission policy quota system adopted by the University of California was invalid. In another important admission case the U.S. Supreme Court in 1982 held that the failure of a school to permit men to obtain a nursing degree violated the equal protection clause of the Fourteenth Amendment. However, the court held that gender-based admissions may be constitutional where such policy is necessary to achieve a justifiable school objective, and the discriminatory means directly relate to the objective.

The case law on school dismissals is more extensive than the admission cases. The courts have shown a reluctance to second-guess dismissal decisions by the faculty because of the belief that schools have the right to establish their own policy for retention and setting academic achievement. In most of the cases that set aside the dismissal decision the students were able to show that their due process procedural rights were not met. A violation of substantive rights on the part of the faculty is more difficult to show. There is a need to show bad faith on the part of the faculty in order for a student to prevail in a substantive dismissal case. The school catalog may be used in both the admission and dismissal cases. The school catalog dismissal cases involve both academic and nonacademic standards.

Collection of student loans has generated a significant amount of case law and much of it deals with whether a student can dismiss an educational loan in a bankruptcy proceeding. As in all cases the courts will look to the facts of the case in determining whether a student loan may be discharged. Increasingly, where government loans are involved the process of collection has been intensified and the government has stipulated that the collection procedure by the schools must be carried out with more diligence.

The privacy of educational records was highlighted in 1974 when Congress enacted the Family Education Rights and Privacy Act. The act provides protection against unauthorized access and release of information to third parties. When an issue of privacy is raised, both federal and state privacy laws should be reviewed in order to determine the extent of the law.

REFERENCES AND NOTES

1. Title VII of Civil Rights Act of 1964, 42 U.S.C. §2000d et seq.
2. DeFunis v. Odegaard, 416 U.S. 321 (1974).
3. Alevy v. Downstate Medical Center, 384 N.Y.S. 2nd 82 (NY, 1976).
4. Regents of University of California v. Allan Bakke, 98 S.Ct. 2733 (1978).
5. Mississippi University for Women v. Hogan, 102 S. Ct. 3331 (1982).
6. Steinberg v. Chicago Medical School, 371 N.E. 2nd 634 (IL, 1977).
7. Prendergast v. Rush-Presbyterian-St. Luke's Medical Center, Rush University et al., 397 N.E. 2nd 432 (IL, 1979).
8. Atkin v. Traetta et al., 359 NY 2nd 120 (NY, 1972). Ritz, A., & McMahon, R. (Sept./Oct. 1976). Commitment to standards ends in the courts. *Nurse Educator,* 22–24.
9. Lyons v. Salve Regina College et al. 565 F. 2nd 200 (1978).
10. Slaughter v. Brigham Young University, 514 F. 2nd 622 (1975).
11. Mahavogsanan v. Hall, 401 F. Supp. 381 (1975).
12. University of Texas Health Science Center v. Babb, 646 S.W. 2nd 502 (TX, 1982).
13. Coveney v. President and Trustees of Holy Cross College, 445 N.E. 2nd 136 (MA, 1983).
14. Connelly v. University of Vermont and State Agricultural College, 244 F. Supp. 156 (1965).
15. Balogun v. Cornell University, 33 N.Y.S. 2nd 838 (NY, 1971). See also Stoller v. College of Medicine, 562 F. Supp. 403 (1983).
16. Greenhill v. Bailey, 378 F. Supp. 632 (1974).
17. Sofair v. State University of N.Y. College of Medicine, 377 N.E. 2nd 730 (1978).
18. Gaspar v. Bruton, 513 F. 2nd 843 (OK, 1975).

19. McIntosh v. Manhattan Community College, 433 N.E. 2nd 1274 (NY, 1982). See also In the Matter of Patti Ann H. v. N.Y. Medical College, 453 N.Y.S. 2nd 196 (NY, 1982). See also, Johnson v. Cuyahoga County Community College, 489 N.E. 2nd 1088 (OH, 1985), where the court held that a nursing school did not act in an arbitrary and capricious manner in refusing to raise the student's 73.7 percent grade average to a passing grade thus giving her the opportunity to take the July 1983 state board examinations. See also, Essigmann v. Western New England College, 419 N.E. 2nd 1047 (MA, 1981), where the court held that a law student's due process rights were not violated in the method of grade computation used by the faculty. The school's policy was to compute course grades by including failing course grades, even if the student elected to repeat the course and obtained a passing grade on the second attempt. The court stated, "As a matter of common sense, a student who passes a course only after failing and repeating it is not academically equal to the student who takes the course but once and passes. Thus, it is neither arbitrary nor unfair to adopt a grading system which reflects this difference."

20. Jansen v. Emory University, 440 F. Supp. 1060 (1977).

21. Tanner v. Board of Trustees of University of Illinois, 363 N.E. 2nd 108 (1977).

22. Board of Curators of University of Missouri v. Horowitz, 435 U.S. 78, 98 S. Ct. 948 (1978). See also Regents of the University of Michigan v. Ewing, 106 S. Ct. 507 (1985), where in a medical school dismissal case the court said the "decision was made conscientiously with clear deliberation, based on an evaluation of his entire academic career at the university." See also Schuler v. University of Minnesota, 788 F. 2nd 510 (1986). Where the court said the *Board of Curators v. Horowitz* standard of notice or warning and "careful and deliberate consideration" was met. In addition, the hearing was conducted in appropriate manner. Although the hearing did not follow the procedure set out in the university's rules such departure was not arbitrary or capricious. It should be noted that in this case the woman received a hearing although *Board of Curators* held that hearings were not required in academic dismissals. See also, Mauriello v. University of Medicine and Dentistry of New Jersey, 781 F. 2nd 46 (1986), where the court held in an academic dismissal that it was not "beyond the pale of reasoned academic decision-making."

23. Goss v. Lopez, 95 S. Ct. 729 (1975).

24. Ibid., p. 741.

25. Slaughter v. Brigham Young University, 514 F. 2nd 622 (1975). Cert. denied, 96 S. Ct. 202 (1975). See also, Patterson v. Hunt, 682 S.W. 2nd 508 (TN, 1984), where a Tennessee Court of Appeals held that the dismissal of three dental students for alleged honor code violations comported with their due process rights. Two of the students admitted at a hearing that they participated in the plan to cheat in an examination and a third student, who did not cheat in the examination, admitted that he violated the honor code by informing one of the dismissed students of the time the correct answers would be posted. One of the students asked another student to obtain the answers to the examination and give them to him while he was taking the examination. The second student did so after finding out from the third student when the answers would be posted. The third student, who did not wish to see a copy of the answer key, only informed the second student where the answer key was posted. It was posted after the examination had begun. Each student signed the following honor code document before entering the school:

I, the undersigned, signify that I have read the Honor Code and By-Laws of the Honor Council and hereby pledge my support of them. I understand what is expected of me as a student of the University of Tennessee College of Dentistry and realize that a plea of ignorance will not be acceptable by Honor Council. If I have reason to suspect that a breach of the Honor Code has been committed, I will take action in one of the following ways: (1) Issue a personal warning to the suspect with the knowledge of a member of the Honor Council. (2) Issue a personal warning to the suspect through a member of the Honor Council.

26. Bleiker v. Board of Trustees of Ohio State University, College of Veterinary Medicine, 485 F. Supp. 1381 (1980).
27. Tedeschi v. Wagner College, 404 N.E. 2nd 1302 (NY, 1980).
28. Grimard v. Carlston, 567 F. 2nd 1171 (1978).
29. Russell v. Salve Regina College, 649 F. Supp. 391 (1986). See also Harvey v. Palmer College of Chiropractic, 363 N.W. 2nd 443 (IA, 1984), where a court ordered that a dismissed student's trial for alleged breach of contract, fraud, and intentional infliction of emotional distress be set aside and a new trial ordered. The school's judiciary council imposed a suspension for unprofessional conduct and the administration increased the punishment to dismissal. There was evidence at the trial that council and school had not complied with the procedures in the student handbook and that one of the council members demonstrated bias in arriving at his decision. The higher court found that there were sufficient irregularities in the way the case was initiated and in the appointment and composition of the council.
30. Anon. (1965) Restatement (Second) of Torts, §46. American Law Institute, Washington, DC.
31. Rhode Island General Laws §9-1-28.1(a),(b). (1980 and as amended 1985).
32. Fee, G. Ousted student sues for $2 million. *Boston Herald American*, October 21, 1985, p. 5.
33. See, Carmody, D. College erred in suspensions, a court rules. *New York Times*, August 2, 1987, p. 49, where a federal appeals court held that a private college in New York was required to provide students, who conducted a 3-day sit-in at the college, a hearing before suspending them. In that case the college's disciplinary rules had been rewritten to comply with a 1969 state education law which required colleges to file their disciplinary rules with the state. The submitted rules were mandated to include the possibility of suspension for breaches of order. The students remained at their sit-in even after the college secured a court order ordering them to leave. The students were told that if they did not leave they would be suspended.
34. Irby, D., Fantel, J., Milam, S., and Schwarz, M. (Jan. 15, 1981). Legal guidelines for evaluating and dismissing medical students. *New England Journal of Medicine, 304*(3), 180.
35. Wilson V. Continental Insurance Company et al., 274 N.W. 2nd 679 (1980). See also Central Security Mutual Insurance Company v. De Pinto, 681 P 2nd 15 (KA, 1984).
36. Sellman v. Baruch College of City University of N.Y., 482 F. Supp. 475 (1979).
37. Swidryk v. Saint Michael's Medical Center, 493 A. 2nd 641 (NJ, 1985).
38. Anon. Report criticizes education loan. *New York Times*, Dec. 27, 1981, p. 30.
39. Anon. 173 Carolinians sued for student aid debts. *New York Times*, May 9, 1982, p. 24.
40. Anon. (Jan. 1983). GAO faults universities, HHS for delinquent student loans. *Hospital Medical Staff, 12*(1) 21.
41. Perez v. Campbell, 402 U.S. 637 (1971).
42. Lee v. Board of Higher Education in City of New York, *Bankruptcy Reporter, 781* (1979).
43. Matter of Bruce, 3 *Bankruptcy Reporter, 77* (1980). See also, In re Lee, 71 *Bankruptcy Reporter, 833* (1987).
44. Application of Gahan, 279 N.W. 2nd 816 (MN,1979).
45. Florida Board of Bar Examiners re: Groot, 365 So. 2nd 164 (FL, 1978).
46. U.S. v. Haithco, 644 F. Supp. 63 (1986).
47. Mattis v. U.S., 648 F. Supp. 137 (1986).
48. Anon. A higher penalty on student loans. *New York Times*, July 19, 1987, p. 26.
49. Family Educational Rights and Privacy Act, 20 U.S.C. 1232g, 45 C.F.R. 99 (1974).

APPENDICES

NURSING GUIDELINES FOR USE OF RESTRAINTS IN NONPSYCHIATRIC SETTINGS
Massachusetts Nurses Association*

The professional nurse as a health team member who monitors the patient's condition twenty-four hours a day is in a central position to assess the patient's potential for injury and evaluate the need for restraint. Restraint should be considered only as a temporary means of intervention, and evaluation of need is continuous. The nurse is responsible for knowing policies pertaining to the use of restraint in the clinical setting in which she practices.

Restraint is defined as the use of a chemical substance, mechanical device, and/or physical restriction by one or more persons which limits the activity of another.

A. Assessment of Risk Factors
  1. Physiological Data
     a. Neurologic deficits
     b. Alteration in senses
     c. Distortion of ability to interpret the environment
     d. Debilitation
     e. Medications, including interaction of multiple drugs
  2. Behavioral Data
     a. History of falls
     b. History of confusion; cognitive changes
     c. Hallucinations
     d. Abusive behavior (past or present)
     e. Agitation
     f. Drug or alcohol abuse
     g. Combativeness or aggressive tendencies
B. Determination of Nursing Diagnosis
  1. Potential for injury
     a. Harm to self
  2. Potential for violence
     b. Harm to others
C. Development and Implementation of Plan of Care
  1. Emergency use of minimum physical restraint to ensure safety
  2. Consideration of alternatives to use of restraint
     a. Companionship—staff, family, friends, volunteers

---

* Reprinted with permission of the Massachusetts Nurses Association, a constituent of the American Nurses' Association.

       b. Manipulation of the environment—change in room, improved lighting, accessible means of communication (call light or other)

       c. Diversion—television, radio, music

       d. Transfer home or to familiar surroundings

   3. Plan of nursing care is developed for period of restraint and is based on needs which result from the type of restraint applied

       a. Patient preparation and teaching regarding the use of restraint

       b. Family preparation and teaching regarding rationale and use of restraint

       c. Collaboration with the physician as indicated

       d. Appropriate choice and application of least restrictive restraint

       e. Assessment of skin, cardiovascular, respiratory, neurologic, and musculoskeletal integrity as determined by type of restraint

       f. Assessment of physiologic response to chemical restraint (medications) including therapeutic responses and side effects

       g. Assessment of emotional response to restraint

       h. Interventions appropriate to maintain physiologic integrity, i.e.:

         (1) Periodic release of restraint

         (2) Range of motion

         (3) Protective padding

         (4) Maintenance of hygiene

D. Evaluation

   1. Evaluation of outcomes of care is continuous and is reflected through documentation in the following areas:

       a. Appropriateness and effectiveness of restraint methodology

       b. Appropriateness and effectiveness of nursing intervention

       c. Mental status and behavioral response

       d. Physical response to restraints, i.e., skin, cardiovascular status, respiratory status, response to medication, etc.

       e. Patient and family response to use of restraint

       f. Continuation of need for restraint or alteration in method

       g. Achievement of desired outcome

Bibliography

DiFabio, S. (May 1981). Nurses' reaction to restraining patients. *American Journal of Nursing, 81*(5), 973–975.

Feist, R. (Dec. 1978). A survey of accidental falls in a small home for the aged. *Journal of Gerontological Nursing*, 15–17.

Restraint and seclusion regulations. 104 CMR 3.12 (Dept. Mental Health), (MA).

Tadsen, J. & Brandt, R. (Mar. 1973). Rules for restraints. Hygiene and humanity. *Modern Nursing Home*, 57–58.

Wolanin, M. D., & Phillips, L. (1981). *Confusion, Prevention and care* (pp. 106–107, 541). St Louis: C. V. Mosby.

GUIDELINES FOR COLLABORATION OF PHARMACISTS AND NURSES IN INSTITUTIONAL CARE SETTINGS
American Society of Hospital Pharmacists
and American Nurses' Association*

This document describes the benefits and responsibilities of pharmacy and nursing collaboration within the institutional setting. The value of this collaborative effort is reflected in the quality of patient care. The responsibilities of the nurse and the pharmacist are to their respective professions; their accountability is to their patients. As members of the health care team, nurses and pharmacists collaborate with other professionals and members of other disciplines. The complexity of drug therapy requires consultation between nurses and pharmacists on a regular basis.

Pharmacists are well acquainted with the complex problems associated with drug therapy and possess knowledge concerning medications that is useful to nurses in providing patient care. Pharmacists' intensive basic and continuing education in drug therapy, practical application of this knowledge, and presence in institutions make them the appropriate health professional to supply drug information. Since nurses are responsible for direct patient care and are in close contact with the patient, they can provide valuable information regarding beneficial and adverse responses to drug therapy.

In order to promote the exchange of information between nurses and pharmacists, the following guidelines are proposed:

1. Orientation for nurses and student nurses to the institution should include introduction to the pharmacy so that the available services can be discussed and demonstrated.
2. Orientation for pharmacists and pharmacy students should include introduction to a patient care unit so that its services can be discussed and demonstrated.
3. Collaboration between the nurse and the pharmacist should occur on a regular basis whenever either professional is developing a program to which the other can contribute. Interprofessional collaboration should also occur whenever the perceived roles of the professionals overlap, e.g., in patient education, monitoring adverse drug reactions, cardiopulmonary resuscitation, nurse–pharmacist rounds in critical care areas. and nursing care plans.

Nurses equipped with adequate drug information and knowledge of the patient are able to administer drugs properly and detect the occurrence of desirable or undesirable drug effects.

It is important for the pharmacist to work in collaboration with the nurse when medications are administered. The following are examples of information that should be provided to the nurse by the pharmacist:

---

* Reprinted with permission of *American Journal of Hospital Pharmacy*, 37 (Feb. 1980). Copyright © 1980, American Society of Hospital Pharmacists, Inc. All rights reserved.

Information on new drugs

Information on investigational drugs used in the institution

Drug side effects and therapeutic risks

Contraindications to particular drug therapy

Compatibility and stability of drugs, including intravenous admixtures

Drug computations

Drug metabolism, excretion, and blood level data (and likelihood of a cumulative effect)

Drug interactions (including drug/drug, drug/food, and laboratory test modifications)

Effect of patient age and pathophysiology on drug action

Drug information services should include the following:

1. A pharmacist should be available on site or on call 24 hours a day to provide drug information when needed. It is important that nurses have sufficient information to instruct patients in the use of their medications. Telephone communications should be used only if personal contact in the patient-care area cannot take place.
2. The pharmacist should consult with the nurse, preferably by personal contact, in regard to drugs prescribed for specific patients. The information exchange is best provided in the patient-care area, where the pharmacists can obtain patient data from other professionals, the patient, and the patient's records, as well as from the nurse. The pharmacist should record information that is important to the patient's medication regimen in the patient's record. Specific allergies to drugs should be highlighted on the patient's record.
3. Drug information bulletins and newsletters compiled by pharmacists should be distributed to the nursing staff.
4. Each nursing unit should be provided with reference material on drugs, e.g., *American Hospital Formulary Service*, and the staff should be instructed on the efficient use of these resources. A current formulary, accessible in the patient-care area, should be provided and should contain information about drugs used in the institution.
5. Pharmacists should participate with nurses and physicians in review of patients' medications in relation to patient need therapeutic duplications and possible drug interactions. This can be done either by making rounds or jointly reviewing records, including the drug history. The pharmacist should maintain a drug profile which can be useful in this review.
6. A program of continuing education on drug therapy should be provided by pharmacists in the institution. New information on drugs and informaton on new drugs should also be provided.

Pharmacists and nurses can both be involved in providing patient education. A collaborative team effort should be made in the development of programs for patient education. Counseling, teaching, and informing patients on their drug therapy should be a part of the patient education program in all institutions.

Communication among health professionals should begin during their educational years. Pharmacy and nursing organizations should offer periodic joint continuing education programs that provide drug information and program-ming on patient education and other areas where these two professions can share information. As fellow professionals, nurses and pharmacists should strive toward the common goal of quality patient care.

Approved by the ASHP Board of Directors on April 21, 1979 and by the ANA Congress for Nursing Practice on July 12, 1979; developed by the Joint Commit-tee of the American Nurses' Association and the American Society of Hospital Pharmacists.

References

1. Anon. (July 1968). ASHP statement on the hospital pharmacists and drug information services, *American Journal of Hospital Pharmacists, 25,* 381–382.
2. Anon. (1972). *Drug information: Literature review of needs, resources, and services,* DHEW pub. no. (HSW) 72-3013. Washington, DC.

Appendix C

LIFE SUPPORT GUIDELINES
Los Angeles County Bar Association
and Los Angeles County Medical Association*

Pulling the plug. Physicians caring for gravely ill or injured persons faced with that step have found little guidance from either code or case law, according to Les Rothenberg, co chair of the joint ad hoc Committee on Biomedical Ethics of the Los Angeles County Medical and Bar Associations.

To assist physicians and hospitals in setting policies in this area, the committee developed guidelines for the discontinuance of cardiopulmonary life-support systems under specified circumstances. The council of the medical association adopted the guidelines unanimously on March 2, and the county bar association Board of Trustees approved them on March 11, 1981.

The guidelines set forth five general principles which should govern decision making in this area and three sets of circumstances in which decisions to discontinue the use of cardiopulmonary life-support systems can be made without prior approval by the courts.

The five general principles are:

1. It is the right of a person capable of giving informed consent to make his or her own decision regarding medical care after having been fully informed about the benefits, risks and consequences of available treatment, even when such a decision might foreseeably result in shortening the individual's life.

2. Persons who are unable to give informed consent have the same rights as do persons who can give such consent. Decisions made on behalf of persons who cannot give their own informed consent should, to the extent possible, be the decisions which those persons would have made for themselves had they been able to do so. Parents (or the guardian) of a minor child, or the conservator of an adult patient, must consent to the decision. Family members of adult patients should always be consulted, although they have no legal standing under present California law to make such decisions on behalf of the patient.

3. A physician may discontinue use of a cardiopulmonary life-support system (i.e., mechanical respirator or ventilator) and is not required to continue its use indefinitely solely because such support was initiated at an earlier time.

4. The dignity of the individual must be preserved, and necessary measures to assure comfort be maintained at all times.

5. It is the right of individual physicians to decline to participate in the withdrawal of life-support systems. In exercising this right, however, the physician must take appropriate steps to transfer the care of the patient to another qualified physician.

The three specific sets of circumstances outlined in the guidelines are:

---

* From Anon. (April 1981). Agreement reached on life support guidelines. *County Bar Update, 1*(4). Reprinted with permission of the Los Angeles County Bar Association. Guidelines were developed by the Joint Committee on Biomedical Ethics of the Los Angeles County Bar Association and the Los Angeles County Medical Association and were approved by the governing bodies of both organizations.

1. Brain Death

Section 7180 of the California Health and Safety Code states: "A person shall be pronounced dead if it is determined by a physician that the person has suffered a total and irreversible cessation of brain function." This statute also requires that a second physician independently confirm the death and that neither physician be involved in decisions regarding transplantation of organs.

a. The physicians should document in the medical record the basis for the diagnosis of brain death.

b. The patient should be pronounced brain dead before disconnecting the respirator or ventilator.

c. It is desirable to explain the brain death law to family members and other interested persons before this procedure is implemented.

2. California Natural Death Act

Sections 7185 through 7195 of the California Health and Safety Code (the California Natural Death Act) provide that cardiopulmonary life-support systems must be withdrawn from patients who have signed a "valid and binding" Directive to Physicians. For further information, physicians should consult the Guidelines on the California Natural Death Act adopted by the California Medical Association and the California Hospital Association (CHA). These guidelines are reproduced in the CHA Consent Manual.

3. Irreversible Coma*

Cardiopulmonary life-support systems may be discontinued if all of the following conditions are present:

a. The medical record contains a written diagnosis of irreversible coma, confirmed by a physician who by training or experience is qualified to assist in making such decisions. The medical record must include adequate medical evidence to support the diagnosis;

b. The medical record indicates that there has been no expressed intention on the part of the patient that life-support systems be initiated or maintained in such circumstances; and

c. The medical record indicates that the patient's family, or guardian or conservator, concurs in the decision to discontinue such support.

The comfort and dignity of the patient shall be maintained if death does not occur on discontinuation of cardiopulmonary life-support systems.

---

* While paragraphs (1) and (2), dealing with brain death and the California Natural Death Act, are based on provisions of the California Health and Safety Code, this paragraph, dealing with irreversible coma, is not based on any California statute or court decision, but rather reflects our view of good medical practice and the current standard of medical care in Los Angeles County.

GUIDELINES FOR HOSPITALS AND PHYSICIANS ON *DO NOT RESUSCITATE* ORDERS
*Medical Society of the State of New York**†

The following are intended *only* to be guidelines for physicians and hospitals. Hospital medical staffs and governing bodies are encouraged to develop policies consistent with their respective by-laws and rules and regulations.

Definition

DNR (Do Not Resuscitate) means that, in the event of a cardiac or respiratory arrest, cardiopulmonary resuscitative measures will not be initiated or carried out.

Background

1. An appropriate knowledge of the serious nature of the patient's medical condition is necessary.
2. The attending physician should determine the appropriateness of a DNR order for any given patient.
3. DNR orders are compatible with maximal therapeutic care. A patient may receive vigorous support in all other therapeutic modalities and yet a DNR order may be justified.
4. When a patient is capable of making his own judgments, the DNR decision should be reached consensually by the patient and physician. When the patient is not capable of making his own decision, the decision should be reached after consultation between the appropriate family member(s) and the physician. If a patient disagrees, or, in the case of a patient incapable of making an appropriate decision, the family member(s) disagree, a DNR order should not be written.

Implementation

1. Once the DNR decision has been made, this directive shall be written as a formal order by the attending physician. A verbal or telephone order for DNR cannot be justified as a sound medical or legal practice.
2. It is the responsibility of the attending physician to insure that this order and its meaning are discussed with appropriate members of the hospital staff.
3. The facts and considerations relevant to this decision shall be recorded by the attending physician in the progress notes.
4. The DNR order shall be subject to review at any time by all concerned parties on a regular basis and may be rescinded at any time.

---

* Approved by the Medical Society of the State of New York on September 9, 1982.
† Reprinted with permission of the Medical Society of the State of New York.

DO NOT RESUSCITATE GUIDELINES
Minnesota Medical Association*†

These guidelines have been drafted by the Ad Hoc Committee on Death of the Minnesota Medical Association. It is widely recognized that in some clinical situations the initiation of potentially life-prolonging treatment is inappropriate. While there may be a variety of situations in which it is justifiable to withhold or withdraw medical treatment, the guidelines presented here cover only one specific aspect of the dilemmas created by modern medical technology, issues surrounding the question of whether or not to initiate cardiopulmonary resuscitation (CPR) when the patient experiences an acute cardiac or respiratory arrest.

Definition

DNR (do not resuscitate)—in the event of an acute cardiac or respiratory arrest, no cardiopulmonary resuscitative measures will be initiated.

Considerations

1. An appropriate knowledge of the patient's medical condition is necessary before consideration of a DNR order.
2. The attending physician should determine the appropriateness of the DNR order for any given medical condition.
3. DNR orders are compatible with maximal therapeutic care. The patient may be receiving vigorous support in all other therapeutic modalities and yet justifiably be considered a proper subject for the DNR order.
4. When the patient is competent, the DNR decision will be reached consensually by the patient and physician. When the patient is judged to be incompetent, this decision will be reached consensually by the appropriate family member(s) and physician. If a competent patient disagrees, or, in cases of incompetency, the family member(s) disagrees, a DNR order will not be written.

Implementation

1. Once the DNR decision has been made, this directive shall be written as a formal order by the attending physician. It is the responsibility of the attending physician to insure that this order and its meaning are discussed with appropriate members of the hospital staff.
2. The facts and considerations relevant to this decision shall be recorded by the attending physician in the progress notes.
3. The DNR order shall be subject to review on a regular basis and may be rescinded at any time.

---

* Approved by the Minnesota Medical Association Board of Trustees on January 24, 1981.
† Reprinted with permission of the Minnesota Medical Association.

DO NOT RESUSCITATE GUIDELINES
*Medical Association of the State of Alabama**

It is widely recognized that in some clinical situations the initiation of potentially life-prolonging treatment is inappropriate. While there may be a variety of situations in which it is justifiable to withhold or withdraw medical treatment, the guidelines presented here cover only one specific aspect of the dilemmas created by modern medical technology, issues surrounding the question of whether or not to initiate cardiopulmonary resuscitation (CPR) when the patient experiences an acute cardiac or respiratory arrest.

Definition

DNR (do not resuscitate)—In the event of an acute cardiac or respiratory arrest, no cardiopulmonary resuscitative measures will be initiated.

Considerations

1. An appropriate knowledge of the patient's medical condition is necessary before consideration of a DNR order.
2. The attending physician should determine the appropriateness of the DNR order for any given medical condition.
3. DNR orders are compatible with maximal therapeutic care. The patient may be receiving vigourous support in all other therapeutic modalities and yet justifiably be considered a proper subject for the DNR order.
4. When the patient is competent, the DNR decision will be reached consensually by the patient and physician. When the patient is judged to be incompetent, this decision will be reached consensually by the appropriate family member(s) and physician. If a competent patient disagrees, or, in cases of incompetency, the family member(s) disagrees, a DNR order will not be written.

Implementation

1. Once the DNR decision has been made, this directive shall be written as a formal order by the attending physician. It is the responsibility of the attending physician to insure that this order and its meaning are discussed with appropriate members of the hospital staff.
2. The facts and considerations relevant to this decision shall be recorded by the attending physician in the progress notes.
3. The DNR order shall be subject to review on a regular basis and may be rescinded at any time.

---

* Reprinted with permission of the Medical Association of the State of Alabama.

WRITTEN ORDERS DESCRIBING CARE FOR CRITICALLY ILL AND/OR TERMINALLY ILL PATIENTS
*Texas Medical Association**

At sessions of the Texas Medical Association House of Delegates in May 1981, the following resolution was approved concerning written orders describing care for critically ill or terminally ill patients:

WHEREAS, There are substantial ethical and legal responsibilities involved with decisions to prescribe care for critically ill and/or terminally ill patients; and

WHEREAS, It is important to have a consensus and sharing of feelings with all those involved in the decision (patient, family, hospital staff and physicians); and

WHEREAS, A physician's decision in these matters will be based primarily upon medical information; and

WHEREAS, It is unlikely that firm and rigid guidelines for "no CPR" decisions can be formulated; therefore be it

RESOLVED, That the Texas Medical Association encourage medical staffs to develop general guidelines; and be it further

RESOLVED, That these guidelines may include:

1. Resuscitation of many terminally ill patients is not medically indicated.

2. The need for clear documentation of the reasons for this medical decision is of primary importance. This is the physician's responsibility.

3. To the extent possible, guidance from the patient, family and the hospital staff should be sought.

---

* Reprinted with permission from the Texas Medical Association.

Appendix H

WITHOLDING OR WITHDRAWING LIFE PROLONGING MEDICAL TREATMENT
American Medical Association Council on Ethical and Judicial Affairs*†

The social commitment of the physician is to sustain life and relieve suffering. Where the performance of one duty conflicts with the other, the choice of the patient, or his family or legal representative if the patient is incompetent to act in his own behalf, should prevail. In the absence of the patient's choice or an authorized proxy, the physician must act in the best interest of the patient.

For humane reasons, with informed consent, a physician may do what is medically necessary to alleviate severe pain, or cease or omit treatment to permit a terminally ill patient whose death is imminent to die. However, he should not intentionally cause death. In deciding whether the administration of potentially life-prolonging medical treatment is in the best interest of the patient who is incompetent to act in his own behalf, the physician should determine what the possibility is for extending life under humane and comfortable conditions and what are the prior expressed wishes of the patient and attitudes of the family or those who have responsibility for the custody of the patient.

Even if death is not imminent but a patient's coma is beyond doubt irreversible and there are adequate safeguards to confirm the accuracy of the diagnosis and with the concurrence of those who have responsibility for the care of the patient, it is not unethical to discontinue all means of life-prolonging medical treatment.

Life-prolonging medical treatment includes medication and artificially or technologically supplied respiration, nutrition or hydration. In treating a terminally ill or irreversibly comatose patient, the physician should determine whether the benefits of treatment outweigh its burdens. At all times, the dignity of the patient should be maintained.

Issued March 15, 1986

---

* Opinion statement issued by the Council on Ethical and Judicial Affairs on March 15, 1986.
† Reprinted with permission of the American Medical Association Council on Ethical and Judicial Affairs.

AUTONOMY RIGHTS OF PATIENTS
*Massachusetts Medical Society**†*

The Massachusetts Medical Society recognizes the autonomy rights of terminally ill and/or vegetative individuals who have previously expressed their wishes to refuse treatment and intravenous fluids and gastrointestinal feeding by tube, and that implementation of these wishes by a physician does not in itself constitute unethical medical behavior provided that appropriate medical and family consultation is obtained.

Issued July 17, 1985

---

* Resolution passed July 17, 1985.
† Reprinted with permission of the Massachusetts Medical Society.

GLOSSARY

Affidavit. A written statement which is confirmed under oath. For example, see the sworn statement of the physician in the Quackenbush case, p. 317.

Agency. The fiduciary relation which results from the manifestation of consent by one person to another that the other shall act on his behalf and subject to his control. An example is the relationship of an employee and employer.

Appeal. A resort by a party for the purpose of obtaining a review and retrial of the legal issues. For example, in the Atkin case, p. 462, the lower court held for the six students and the higher state court reversed the lower court and ruled in favor of the faculty.

Appellant. The party who appeals the decision of a lower court to a court of higher jurisdiction. An example is when a losing party appeals a trial court decision to the next court level.

Appellee. The party against whom an appeal to a higher court is taken.

Assault. An intentional act designed to make the victim fearful and which produces reasonable apprehension of harm.

Battery. The touching of one person by another without permission (e.g., doing a D & C when permission is granted only for a pelvic exam).

Best interest test. One of the evidentiary standards or test criteria which courts apply in medical treatment cases. See the Chad Green case, p. 391, where the court applied this test. See also the O'Connor case, p. 234, where this test was abolished as a standard for involuntary commitment.

Borrowed servant. Holds the person who temporarily borrowed the nurse from her employer liable for the nurse's negligence where the nurse specifically carried out the borrower's directions. This doctrine frees the "master" from liability and is an exception to the "master and servant" rule whereby the master/employer is liable for the servant's negligent acts. See the Minogue case, p. 83.

Burden of proof. The legal requirement charging the plaintiff or the defendant with the responsibility of meeting the burden of persuasion. See the Florida civil statute which sets out the burden placed upon the plaintiff to show a deviation from professional standards, pp. 42 and 43. See also the cases involving the Res Ipsa Loquitur theory.

Captain of the ship doctrine. A legal doctrine which was first articulated in 1949 and which holds a surgeon responsible for the actions of all those who assist him in the surgery. The doctrine has been weakened in recent years because the courts have recognized the individual roles of those present in the operating room.

Case law. The body of judicial cases concerning a particular legal subject which have evolved from the courts.

Charitable immunity. A legal doctrine which protects a charitable organization from a negligence suit in part or in toto. The principle behind this doctrine is that a charitable hospital should not have to use its limited financial resources in defending itself. In recent years this doctrine has been weakened. Sovereign immunity applies to public facilities and charitable gives private, nonprofit hospitals immunity from tort liability. See p. 163.

Civil law. Part of American law which does not deal with crimes.

Civil suit. A legal cause of action brought to establish a right or to seek legal redress for harm in the form of money damages.

Clear and convincing evidence. An evidentiary standard or test applied to weigh the value or credibility of evidence. See the Eichner case, p. 338.

Common law. The body of law which is comprised of both judicial decisions and the body of principles and rules which derive their authority solely from usages and customs of immemorial antiquity. Distinguished from legislative laws. That which is derived from all the statutory and case law background of England and the American colonies. See the common law definition of brain death, p. 322.

Comparative negligence. A defense theory in negligence cases in which the degree of negligence of the plaintiff is measured against that of the defendant. An example is when the plaintiff was 60 percent negligent and The defendant 40 percent. Over 38 states have adopted the comparative negligence doctrine by either statute or case law. In most cases where the plaintiff contributed 50 percent or more to his injury he will not recover anything against the defendant. The jury apportions the percent. See p. 115.

Complaint. The plaintiff's petition filed with the court which starts the legal cause of action or suit.

Consent. Voluntary agreement by a person deemed competent to make an intelligent choice to allow someone else to do something. In certain circumstances, a guardian may be in a legal position to consent for another.

Consent degree. A legally sanctioned agreement between all the parties to a dispute. See the Wyatt (p. 229) and Pennhurst (p. 231) cases.

Contract. An agreement between two or more persons which creates an obligation or promise to do or not to do a particular thing. A contract embodies a mutuality of agreement, and mutuality of obligation. The written contract contains the agreement of the parties, with any terms and conditions, and serves as a proof of the obligation. See the Steinberg case, p. 459.

Contributory negligence. A defense theory in negligence cases in which the injured person is responsible to some extent for the injury he suffered because both he and the defendant were negligent. To a large extent this theory has been replaced by the doctrine of comparative negligence because it was considered too harsh in that any percent of contributory negligence barred the plaintiff from recovering any money damages. See the Chamberlain case, p. 140.

Corporate negligence. Liability of an institution for its failure to exercise reasonable care in conducting its business, such as monitoring implementation of its bylaws, providing a safe environment and proper equipment, and evaluating the quality of its professional staff. Distinguished from vicarious liability. See the Bellaire General Hospital case, p. 146.

Crime. Unlawful act committed against society as a whole in violation of a criminal law. Crimes are prosecuted by and in the name of the state.

Cross examination. The oral examination of a witness by the attorney opposed to the party who called the witness and done after the calling party has elicited his testimony. Ordinarily, the opposing attorney's examination is limited to the matters which were elicited on direct testimony examination of the witness.

Custom and usage. Custom is a course of action which has attained the "force of the law" and has gained acceptance because it is done with regularity. Usage is following a uniform course of conduct which is reasonable. The two terms are generally used together. See the preamble statement of the California nursing practice act, p. 55.

Damages. A pecuniary award or compensation awarded by the court or jury for the loss or harm the plaintiff has suffered. In a negligence case it will include pain and suffering and economic factors. See the University Community Hospital case, p. 147.

Defamation. The injury to a person's reputation/character by willful and malicious statements made to a third person. Inclusive of both **libel** (written word/cartoons) and **slander** (spoken word).

Defendant. The individual against whom legal recovery is sought in a civil or criminal case.

Deposition. A pretrial stenographic record of testimony elicited from either a plaintiff, defendant, or other nonparty to a suit which is taken under oath and which may be used as testimony at a trial.

Dicta. In a legal case the language which goes beyond that necessary to the decision in the case. It is judicial comment or opinion which is not considered germane to the legal holding of a case.

Discovery. Pretrial activities done to gain knowledge of the facts of a case. These include written and oral answers to questions and review of documents. See p. 10.

Discretionary judgment. Authorized or delegated judgments. Sometimes referred to as "independent" judgments. See pp. 72 and 80.

Dissenting opinion. Taken by an appellate justice a formal position which disagrees with the majority court holding. For example, the dissenting opinion in Maslonka I became the majority opinion when it was appealed, p. 97.

Due process. A legal concept requiring that legal proceedings or quasi-legal proceedings will be conducted in accordance with legal rules and principles which protect the individual's rights. The 14th Amendment of the U.S. Constitution is the "due process clause." See p. 431 and the Donaldson case, p. 228.

Elements of negligence. The legal concepts which must be proven in a negligence suit are the following:

Duty. An obligation imposed by law requiring one person to conform to a certain standard of conduct for the protection of another against an unreasonable risk. In addition, the plaintiff must establish that a legal relationship exists between the plaintiff and the defendant.

Breach. A derilection of the duty owed. A failure to perform up to the established standard of care.

Causation. The careless act must be the direct or immediate (proximate) cause of the injury. See the DeFalco case, p. 75.

Foreseeable. The injury which resulted from the negligent act must be the natural and probable result of the negligent act and one which an ordinary prudent person ought to have foreseen as likely to occur as a result of the negligence. See the Hartman case, p. 134.

Harm or damages. Injury to another, including medical expenses, pain and suffering, loss of income and/or decreased earning capacity, mental suffering, and wrongful death.

Elopement. When a patient leaves a facility without the knowledge of those responsible for his care. For example, when a resident wanders away from a nursing home. See the Young case, p. 49.

Ethics. The principles of right and wrong conduct as they apply to professional problems.

Evidence. Testimony, writings, material objects, or other things presented to the senses that are offered to prove or disprove a fact in a legal proceeding.

Expert witness. One who is skilled in some art, science, trade, profession, or other human activity and possesses peculiar knowledge concerning it. Possessed of knowledge not generally known by ordinary persons. See p. 27.

Fact(s). Actual and absolute reality, as distinguished from mere supposition or opinion. The reality of events or things the actual occurrence or existence of which is to be determined by the evidence. Many facts in a trial are in dispute. A jury is the "trier of facts." For example, see the Darling case, pp. 56 and 57 where the plaintiff testified that the nurses did not monitor his leg, and the nurses testified that they did, but did not record the monitoring process.

Federal courts. The courts of the United States as opposed to the state court system. Federal cases will be cited in either the *Federal Supplement* or the *Federal Reporter* according to the level of appeal. See the Slaughter case, p. 471.

"Force of the law." Lacking the legal status of a law, but having the weight of a law. For example, rules and regulations are not legal statutes, but they are specifically mandated to implement the law. See p. 432.

Foreseeable. That which is reasonably to be expected if certain actions are done or not done. For example, it is foreseeable that patients without identification bracelets will be mixed-up in the operating room and will have the wrong operation. It is not essential that the *exact* harm be foreseen.

Good faith. A legal concept which encompasses, among other things, an honest belief, the absence of malice, and the absence of design to defraud or to seek an unconscionable advantage over another. See the Farrell case, p. 346.

Guardian ad litem. A special guardian appointed by the court to represent the interests of an infant or incompetent in any litigation. See the Saikewicz case, p. 334.

Incorporation by reference. When the writer makes reference within the records to a document, not normally a part of the records, and it becomes an integral part of the records. See p. 216.

Independent duty. An obligation or duty which must be met by a particular individual although another has the same or overlapping obligation or duty. See Long, p. 110, and Pettis, p. 196.

Independent recollection. Where there is no documentation of an event, but some extraordinary factor triggers the memory of the individual to recall the event. For example. when triplets are born on New Year's Eve. See also the Wagner case, p. 203.

Injunction. A legal procedure whereby one party petitions the court to stop another from doing a particular act. For example, in 1983 a federal court enjoined HHS from implementing proposed regulations requiring clinics to notify the parents of minors if the clinic had prescribed any birth control devices. See p. 292.

In loco parentis. The legal doctrine which provides that under certain circumstances the courts may assign a person to stand in the place of parents and possess their legal rights, duties, and responsibilities towards a child.

Interrogatories. A discovery device consisting of written questions about the case submitted by one party to the other party and which are to be answered under oath. They may be used as evidence at a trial.

Intervening cause. An independent cause or factor which intervenes between the original wrongful act or omission and the injury; a defense theory. It turns aside the natural sequence of events, and produces a result which would not otherwise have followed and which could not have been reasonably anticipated. See Kaiser, p. 136, and Norton, p. 86.

Jury instructions. A direction given by the judge to the jury concerning the rules or principles of law applicable to the case and given at the close of the evidence. It is also referred to as "the charge" to the jury. It is common for one party or another to contest the particular phrasing of the instruction and base their appeal on the instruction.

Latent defect. A hidden defect; one which could not be discovered by reasonable and customary inspection. For example, an IV pole which lacks the metal strength to support three glass IV bottles. See also p. 145.

Liability. A legally recognized responsibility one is bound in law or justice to perform. In negligence law it is an obligation one assumes for the loss to another through either a failure to act or acting inappropriately. Thus, the term liable is more appropriate to civil cases, whereas guilt is more germane to criminal cases.

Liability insurance. A contract to have someone else pay for any liability or loss thereby in return for the payment of premiums. Such insurance may be obtained on an occurrence basis or a claims made basis. An **occurrence basis policy** means that the nurse is covered so long as the incident occurred when the premiums were being paid. For example, if the incident occurred in January 1987 and the nurse was paying the premiums at that time she would be covered if suit was brought in January 1988 and she was no longer paying the premiums. A **claims made basis policy** means that the coverage is not retroactive to the time of the incident and coverage is contingent upon premiums being paid. For example, in order for the nurse to be covered for an incident which occurred in January 1987 she must be making premium payments at the time the suit was filed in court 1 year later.

Litigation. A trial in court for the purpose of contesting or establishing legal rights and duties between the parties to a suit at law.

Malpractice. Professional misconduct or an unreasonable lack of skill in discharging professional duties which results in injury or harm to another. The failure to meet the standard of care of a reasonable professional.

Mature minor rule. Legal recognition that an individual who is a minor, below the age of majority, is capable of fully understanding the implications of consent or lack of consent. The rule was first recognized in 1956. See Lacey v. Laird, 139 N.E. 2nd 25 (OH, 1956). See also p. 284.

Mental incapacity or mental incompetency. When it is determined that a person has an essential privation of reasoning faculties, or when a person is incapable of understanding and acting with discretion in the ordinary affairs of life. See p. 315. Incapacity means the lack of physical or intellectual ability, such as in the situation of minors. See line of medical treatment cases. See Chapters 9 and 10. Adjudicated incompetency means that the court has declared the individual mentally incompetent.

Negligence. The failure to use such care as a reasonably prudent and careful person would use under similar circumstances. The standard of care in a negligence case is the "reasonable man standard," that is, that degree of care which a person of ordinary prudence would exercise in the same or similar circumstances. See p. 27.

Noncompliance. Failure of the patient to follow instructions. For example, when a patient willfully fails to follow instructions concerning a prescribed medication schedule it will be argued that the patient was noncompliant and contributed to subsequent injury. See p. 104.

Parens patriae doctrine. The role of the state as sovereign and guardian of persons under legal disability. See the In re the Mental Health of K.K.B. case, p. 254.

Patent defect. In a consumer context, a defect which is plainly visible or which can be discovered by such an inspection as would be made in the exercise of ordinary care and prudence; for example, a wheelchair with wheels which turn unevenly. See also p. 145.

Physical evidence. Tangible objects, such as equipment, pictures, demonstrative charts, and "day in the life" videotapes which are offered in evidence to prove or disprove a fact.

Plaintiff. The person who initiates suit against the defendant seeking legal redress in the form of money damages or other legal relief.

Power of attorney. The creation of an agent, chosen by the patient while mentally competent, who has authority to make medical decisions in the event the person granting the power to another becomes unable to make decisions. The authority is formalized in a written instrument.

Preponderance of evidence. Evidence which is of greater weight or more convincing than the evidence which is offered in opposition to it; that amount of evidence necessary for a plaintiff to win in a civil case—means that the damage injury was more than likely the defendant's fault. See Thompson v. U.S., 368 F. Supp. 466. See also p. 239.

Prima facie evidence. Evidence, which at face value, is sufficient to establish a given fact. It is subject to contradiction, but, if not contradicted, will suffice for the proof of a particular fact. See pp. 239 and 59.

Privilege. A particular advantage which releases one from the performance of a duty or obligation or exempts one from a liability which would otherwise be incurred. See Owens case, p. 417.

Probable cause. Reasonable cause, that is, having more evidence for than against; a reasonable ground for belief in the existence of facts warranting the complaint. See p. 239.

Procedural due process. Fourteenth Amendment safeguards which afford an individual the right of reasonable notice and the opportunity to be heard when the individual's constitutional rights are to be affected. See pp. 445 and 446.

Proximate cause. The primary or moving cause in an injury; the last negligent act contributory to an injury without which such injury would not have resulted; act or omission immediately causing or failing to prevent the injury. To constitute proximate cause the event cannot be broken by any other intervening cause. See the Norton case, pp. 85–87.

Res ipsa loquitur. A legal doctrine which permits the issue of negligence to go to the jury without expert witness testimony. To successfully argue the application of this doctrine, (a) the accident or occurrence producing the injury must be of a kind which ordinarily does not happen in the absence of someone's negligence; (b) the injuries must be caused by an agency or instrumentality within the exclusive control of the defendant(s); and (c) the injury-causing accident or occurrence is not due to any voluntary action or contribution on the part of the plaintiff, i.e., where surgery was done on one part of the body and the patient was burned on another part of the body. See Carranza v. Tucson Medical Center, 662 P. 2nd 455 (AZ, 1983). See also the Southwest Texas Methodist Hospital case, p. 164.

Respondeat superior doctrine. Translates as "let the master answer." Means that the master (employer) is liable for the wrongful acts of his servant (employee) where the employee was acting in the course of his employment. For example, the employer is liable even where the nurse administers a medication by a route which is outside of the hospital protocols sheet.

Risk management. Initially, a business concept which identified and evaluated the probability of financial loss in order that such loss could be prevented. In health care the concept is used to identify and evaluate liability exposure to prevent financial loss. See the American Hospital Association definition, p. 213.

Safety statute. A law enacted to protect a specified class of persons from a particular type of harm. For example, a law permitting school nurses to administer adrenalin to school children who are allergic to bee stings. See the Leahy case, p. 59.

Standard of care. In negligence law, that degree of care which a reasonably prudent person should exercise under the same or similar circumstances. Where a person's conduct falls below that standard, he may be liable for the injury resulting from his conduct. In professional malpractice cases, the standard of care is applied to measure the competence of the professional. The traditional standard for nurses is that she exercise an average degree of skill, care, and diligence exercised by members of the same discipline, practicing in the same or similar locality in light of the present state of nursing knowledge and practice skills.

Standard of proof. The evidentiary standard required in a particular type of case. For example, in Massachusetts the level of proof for civil commitment is high; that of beyond a reasonable doubt. This standard is the same as for criminal cases. See p. 233. In civil cases, such as malpractice cases, the standard of proof which must be met by the plaintiff is a "preponderance of the evidence" which means that the damage was more likely caused by the defendant's fault than not.

State court. Those courts which make up the state judicial system in contrast to the federal courts. State court cases decisions will be cited in the respective state reporting system. See the Booty case, p. 120.

Statute. An act of the legislature declaring, commanding, or prohibiting something. A legislative declaration differs from judicial law (court decisions) and executive declarations (Presidential orders). For example, the "good samaritan law" in Massachusetts is found in the Massachusetts General Laws, Chapter 112, § 12B.

Statute of limitations. The statutory or regulatory time limit that a plaintiff has to bring a legal suit. The doctrine permits an extention where the wrong could not be reasonably "discovered" within the time frame. In addition, the majority of states allow a longer time frame when the plaintiff is a minor. See p. 5.

Subpoena. A command by the court to appear at a certain time and place to give testimony upon a certain matter. Thus, a subpoena is the vehicle to command a witness to a court or give testimony in court or at a deposition. In addition, a subpoena duces tecum commands that a witness produce documents in his possession. See p. 12.

Substantive due process. Fourteenth Amendment safeguards which protect an individual from arbitrary and capricious decisions which affect life, liberty, or property. See Tanner case, p. 470.

Substituted judgment doctrine. In medical treatment cases a subjective test applied to determine the supposed wish of the incompetent patient. See p. 253. See also the Saikewicz case, p. 334, and the Jobes case, p. 385.

Summons. The legal document used to commence a civil action and which is served on the party by a sheriff.

Trier of fact. The role of a jury in a trial is to make findings of fact, that is, to decide whether to believe the patient's testimony or the nurse's testimony. The jury's role as trier of fact contrasts with the judge's role which is to make rulings of law, for example, a judge decides, as a matter of law, whether a physician may testify as to the standard of care in a nursing malpractice case. In a trial without a jury, the judge serves as the trier of fact and rules on the law.

Vicarious liability. Liability of a corporation or facility for the negligence of its employees. Based on the concept that the employer has the legal right (duty) to exert some control over the employee's work. The concept encourages an employer to monitor and supervise the acts of its employees.

SUBJECT AND CASE INDEX